Manual of Austere and Prehospital Ultrasound

Benjamin D. Nicholson
Michael J. Vitto • Harinder S. Dhindsa
Editors

Manual of Austere and Prehospital Ultrasound

Springer

Editors
Benjamin D. Nicholson
Department of Emergency Medicine
Virginia Commonwealth University
School of Medicine
Richmond, VA
USA

Michael J. Vitto
Department of Emergency Medicine
Virginia Commonwealth University
School of Medicine
Richmond, VA
USA

Harinder S. Dhindsa
Department of Emergency Medicine
Virginia Commonwealth University
School of Medicine
Richmond, VA
USA

ISBN 978-3-030-64286-0 ISBN 978-3-030-64287-7 (eBook)
https://doi.org/10.1007/978-3-030-64287-7

This Springer imprint is published by the registered company Springer Nature Switzerland AG
The registered company address is: Gewerbestrasse 11, 6330 Cham, Switzerland

Introduction to Manual

Introduction

To begin, we must say thank you. The *Manual of Austere and Prehospital Ultrasound* is first and foremost written to improve your ability to care for the most critically ill and injured patients you encounter. We believe that ultrasound application represents the highest level of patient care and your willingness to embrace this exciting technology is admirable. In the next few pages, we will outline the goals of this text, where we see ultrasound fitting into clinical practice, and our vision for the future of ultrasound in the out-of-hospital environment.

In the austere and prehospital environment, the addition of new equipment or technology must match an increase in knowledge. The most efficient systems match improvements in either and follow a line of efficiency, indicated in blue in Fig. 1 above. A second means of ensuring efficiency in out-of-hospital care is to ensure that this equipment/knowledge efficiency mirrors changes to patient care. These two concepts are the foundation for this text. It aims to provide the knowledge necessary to fully utilize the new generation of portable, relatively inexpensive ultrasound devices while focusing on diagnostic studies, procedures, and monitoring that will impact patient care.

The text is structured around the concept that any ultrasound study must fall into one of three broad categories. It must help a provider better diagnose a condition,

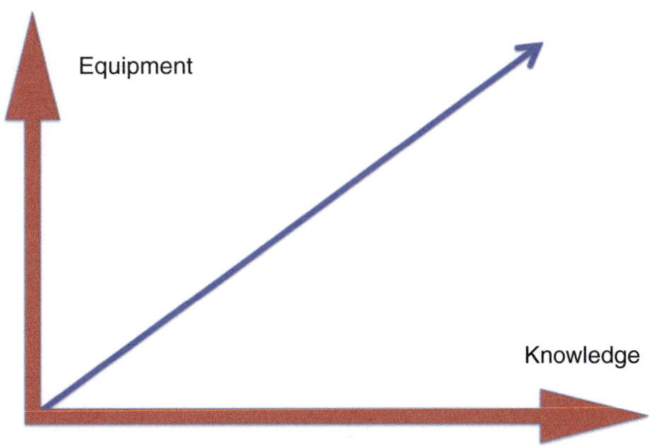

Fig. 1 Relationship between equipment and knowledge expansion with the proposed line of efficiency

perform safer procedures, or better monitor a patient. Wherever possible, patient complaints are used to categorize the diagnostic studies. Given the span of prehospital and austere care, some sections will include material that is more applicable to remote settings and providers caring for patients for prolonged periods. These sections are highlighted as "Advanced Topics." Finally, we have put together information on building an ultrasound program from the ground up, including initial training, credentialing expectations, developing a quality improvement and assurance program, and caring for equipment.

For all topics in this book, discussion with your medical team and obtaining hands-on training is best practice, prior to implementing.

Happy scanning.

Richmond, VA, USA Benjamin D. Nicholson
Richmond, VA, USA Michael J. Vitto
Richmond, VA, USA Harinder S. Dhindsa

Contents

Contributors

Christopher F. Allison Department of Emergency Medicine, Maine Medical Center, Portland, ME, USA

Jay B. Baker Special Operations Command Europe, APO, AE, USA

Sean Burns Emergency Department, Boston Medical Center, Boston, MA, USA

Andrew Cathers Department of Emergency Medicine, UW Madison, Madison, WI, USA

Sarah C. Crockett Department of Emergency Medicine, Dartmouth Hitchcock Medical Center, Lebanon, NH, USA

Harinder S. Dhindsa Department of Emergency Medicine, Virginia Commonwealth University School of Medicine, Richmond, VA, USA

Hubert R. Draper Department of Defense, Army, Fort Bragg, NC, USA

James Caleb A. Ersando Department of Defense, Army, Fort Bragg, NC, USA

David Evans Department of Emergency Medicine, Virginia Commonwealth University, Richmond, VA, USA

Brandon M. Fetterolf 1st Special Forces Command, US Army, Fort Bragg, NC, USA

Douglas C. George Division of Emergency Medicine, University of Vermont Medical Center, Burlington, VT, USA

Catalina Gonzalez-Marques Brigham and Women's Department of Emergency Medicine, Boston, MA, USA

Fredrik Granholm Department of Emergency and Ambulance, Sundsvall County Hospital, Sundsvall, Sweden

Justin Grisham Department of Emergency Medicine, Madigan Army Medical Center, Tacoma, WA, USA

Matthew Jensen VCU Health Critical Care Transport Network, Richmond, VA, USA

Michael Joyce Department of Emergency Medicine, Virginia Commonwealth University, Richmond, VA, USA

Konrad Karasek Department of Emergency Medicine, Boston Medical Center, Boston, MA, USA

John G. Knight Jr Department of Emergency Medicine, San Antonio, TX, USA

Alex Kranc Emergency Department, Lexington Medical Center, West Columbia, SC, USA

Randy M. Kring Department of Emergency Medicine, Maine Medical Center, Portland, ME, USA

Ricky C. Kue Massachusetts Urban Search and Rescue Task Force-1 (MA-TF1), Beverly, MA, USA

Megan Leo Department of Emergency Medicine, Boston Medical Center, Boston, MA, USA

Amir Louka Department of Emergency Medicine, VCU Medical Center/VCU Health, Richmond, VA, USA

Stephanie K. Louka VCU Health, Richmond, VA, USA

David C. Mackenzie Department of Emergency Medicine, Maine Medical Center, Portland, ME, USA

Kelly Mayo Department of Emergency Medicine, Boston University School of Medicine, Boston Medical Center, Boston, MA, USA

Amanda Medoro Department of Emergency Medicine, University of New Mexico, Albuquerque, NM, USA

K. Meera Muruganandan Emergency Department, Boston Medical Center, Boston, MA, USA

Matthew Neth Department of Emergency Medicine, OHSU, Portland, OR, USA

Benjamin D. Nicholson Department of Emergency Medicine, Virginia Commonwealth University School of Medicine, Richmond, VA, USA

Laurel O'Connor Department of Emergency Medicine, University of Massachusetts Medical School, Worcester, MA, USA

Joseph R. Pare Department of Emergency Medicine, Boston University School of Medicine, Boston Medical Center, Boston, MA, USA

Michael D. Perreault Department of Emergency Medicine, Madigan Army Medical Center, Tacoma, WA, USA

Katherine Rodman Department of Emergency Aviation, VCU Health, Richmond, VA, USA

Nikolai Schnittke Department of Emergency Medicine, Oregon Health and Sciences University, Portland, OR, USA

Kendall Shaw Department of Emergency Medicine, Virginia Commonwealth University Health System, Richmond, VA, USA

Zachary P. Soucy Department of Emergency Medicine, Dartmouth Hitchcock Medical Center, Lebanon, NH, USA

Robert Stenberg Emergency Department, Cleveland Clinic Akron General, Akron, OH, USA

Lori Stolz Department of Emergency Medicine, University of Cincinnati, Cincinnati, OH, USA

Lindsay Anne Taylor Department of Emergency Medicine, Virginia Commonwealth University Health System, Richmond, VA, USA

Jordan Tozer Department of Emergency Medicine, Virginia Commonwealth University Health System, Richmond, VA, USA

Michael J. Vitto Department of Emergency Medicine, Virginia Commonwealth University School of Medicine, Richmond, VA, USA

Jacob Wayman Department of Emergency Medicine, Virginia Commonwealth University, Richmond, VA, USA

Nicholas E. Weinberg Department of Emergency Medicine, Dartmouth Hitchcock Medical Center, Lebanon, NH, USA

Luke Welle Department of Emergency Medicine, University of New Mexico, Albuquerque, NM, USA

Jenna M. B. White Department of Emergency Medicine, University of New Mexico, Albuquerque, NM, USA

Part I

Introduction and Background

Physics and Knobs

Michael Joyce and Robert Stenberg

Introduction

Understanding the physics behind how an ultrasound machine obtains images may seem like an unnecessary endeavor, but having a solid understanding of what is behind the image can help make interpretations easy and quick. In fact, most of what we use to diagnose pathology is based on an object changing the way the sound behaves, and thus distorting our image.

Ultrasound is mechanical waves at frequencies beyond what the human ear can detect. Our ears top out at around 20,000 hertz (Hz). Diagnostic imaging starts around 1 million Hz, or 1 megahertz (MHz) and usually goes up to around 15–20 MHz deepening on application. All of the probes in use for point of care ultrasound are variable frequency probes; meaning you can adjust the frequency of them to improve your image. Having a solid foundation in the relationship between frequency, resolution and depth will help you obtain top quality images.

Principles

Sound applications are all over our world, including such things as police radar guns, sonar on large navy ships and echolocation in animals. All of these applications, including diagnostic medical ultrasound rely on the principal that sound velocity through a medium is a constant, and thus you can calculate how long it should take for sound to travel to an object and back. Simple applications, such as

M. Joyce (✉)
Department of Emergency Medicine, Virginia Commonwealth University, Richmond, VA, USA
e-mail: john.joyce@vcuhealth.org

R. Stenberg
Emergency Department, Cleveland Clinic Akron General, Akron, OH, USA

B. D. Nicholson et al. (eds.), *Manual of Austere and Prehospital Ultrasound*,
https://doi.org/10.1007/978-3-030-64287-7_1

sonar on a boat, do not require any further modification by a computer. Just time the sound, listen for it to come back, and you get a distance. The sound is always travelling through the same medium (water) and thus always behaves the same. Unfortunately, for diagnostic ultrasound, the sound must travel through multiple different mediums making for lots of changes in how the sound propagates, but fortunately, we can use these differences to help us interpret what we are seeing inside the body.

In point of care ultrasound, the sound image is usually created by a piezoelectric crystal that can both create the sound by converting electricity into a mechanical sound wave and re-absorb the sound and change it back to an electrical signal, therefore acting as an all in one device. Newer machines are starting to use silicone chips to accomplish the same feat, which has brought down the price and size of machines.

Ultrasound does this sound production/collection in two main fashions: continuous wave, and pulse wave echo.

Continuous wave is what is used in "doppler machines" to check for fetal heart tones and pulses, but also with more complex flow measurements such as vascular studies on diagnostic ultrasound. For continues wave, there is constantly sound being sent out and also being read. This allows for us to determine changes in frequency only (the Doppler effect), but not distance (if you are always sending sound, there is no way to decipher when a wave has returned that you sent out). The familiar example of Doppler effect is the ambulance approaching us and then going away. As the ambulance approaches, the frequency increases and the sound frequency (pitch) becomes higher and higher. After it passes, the frequency slowly decreases and the sound pitch gets lower and lower. Diagnostic ultrasound uses this principle to determine both the direction and the speed of the moving object – in our case the blood. If the frequency is increasing, the blood is coming towards you and if the frequency is decreasing, it is moving away from you. The machine can also determine how rapidly the frequency is changing and determine the speed as well!

This type of ultrasound was all we had at first, and is very similar to the simplistic sonar machines in boats. With the advent of rapidly improving computers however, pulse wave echo was invented. Instead of always sending and always listening, now the machine will send out a pulse of sound waves, and then wait for them to come back. Now – it can calculate just how far away that image is by timing how long it takes to return. Then, it does this again, and again, and again, until it has a map of all the things in its line of sight. If you speed this process up sending thousands of pulses per second, you can get a live image of all the objects in front of you. Now we have diagnostic ultrasound!

The next step then is to get that sound into the body at different depths. As we have discussed, the sound must travel through different tissues to get to our target organ or object. The further the sound has to go, the harder it is for the sound to get there. If it has to travel through skin, adipose, muscle, a kidney, more adipose and then to the aorta, a lot of the sound is going to bounce off and not make it, or will run out of energy. This happens by a multitude of different reasons, such as absorption, refraction, reflection and scatter. A higher frequency sound succumbs to these problems much easier than a lower frequency sound. A good example is to think of treble and bass notes in music. A singer who is singing a very high pitch (high frequency) note will be heard very clearly by people right in front of them, but those off at a distance may not even hear it as it disperses. A bass note from a large subwoofer however, can be heard blocks away – but does not carry the same clarity. The same thing happens in diagnostic ultrasound. If we use really high frequency sounds, it does not go far, but gives us very good resolution. If however, we need to get way down deep, we can use a low frequency sound to travel further, but in trade give up some of our resolution.

Thus, on the machine, the depth button is really just the frequency button! If you turn the dial to increase your depth, you are decreasing the frequency, and vice versa. To obtain an ideal image, you should use only the lowest frequency needed. So if your target image is at the very top of your screen, decrease the depth until you only see the object of interest on the screen, and your resolution will dramatically improve!

The final principal that is essential to understand so you can obtain great images is gain. Gain is not contrast! When you increase the contrast on your TV for example, you are increasing the ability to differentiate two different pixels by changing each pixels level of brightness. In ultrasound, we cannot just change our pixels like a TV can because we are relying on the sound that returns to make our image. If not much sound returns (due to absorption, refraction, scatter, etc) then our image will look very dark. What we can do then, is turn up the gain, which increases the perceived intensity of the signal that is interpreted. So if the signal at first registered to the machine as 5/10 intensity, turning the gain up can make it look like a 7/10 intensity. This is great, but it also increases the signal from all the objects coming back because it cannot decipher which pixel we want to see better like a TV. Thus, there is a sweet spot with gain, and if you add too much, all you will see is 10/10 intensity everywhere, or a white screen! If your gain is too low though, you will see all 1/10 intensities and a black or very dark screen. Thus, you should find a gain that allows you to see the most objects without making them all white.

Image Optimization

Now that we understand how the image is created, before you interpret the image you must optimize it. This is an often-overlooked step by new sonographers. When you place the probe on the patient and see the image you were hoping for, you can get excited and start trying to make the diagnosis immediately. However, you are placing yourself at a great handicap. Optimizing all of the following things will make for images that can be interpreted with much higher accuracy!

Probe Selection

Selecting a probe to match your application is essential. There are innumerable probes on the market, but all have certain things in common that you need to decide on. The first is the frequency. As we discussed, a higher frequency will only travel a short distance, but provide a very high quality image. These probes are good for imaging near the surface, such as skin, muscle, nerves, extremity vessels and eyes. Lower frequency probes are used for deeper imaging, such as in the abdominal cavity and the thoracic cavity. The second major characteristic is the footprint. This is just how big the sound transmitting area is. A smaller footprint, can get into smaller places, but only give a very narrow image width. A larger probe can give a large viewing area, but can be difficult to get all the crystals touching the skin and thus the sound into the body.

Ideally, you would have one probe that can do low frequency and one probe that can do high frequency, but this is not always an option. In austere environments, if you had to pick one probe to bring with you, a lower frequency probe is likely best as it can still see superficial structures, just with less resolution. As mentioned however, new silicone chips are coming on the market, and these chips are able to span a much wider frequency range (such as 1–15 MHz!).

In short, select the probe that can provide the highest frequency image for your application if you have multiple to choose from. If imaging between structures, such as the ribs to see the heart, you will also need a smaller footprint.

Depth

Once you have selected your probe and found your image, you need to adjust the depth. As we already discussed, changing the depth is just changing the frequency. To optimize your depth, place the target object so it takes up most of the screen. Any depth beyond the structure you are looking at means your frequency is lower than it needs to be, and thus sacrificing resolution. An example is looking at the heart. If you have the heart taking up the top half of the screen, but the bottom half of the screen is all structures deep to the heart, your depth is too deep and your image could be better. Alternatively, if you are cutting off the bottom part of your heart and can only see half, you do not have enough depth to see all the potential pathology and may miss something important!

Gain

Now that you have the image at the right depth, you should change the gain so that you can see as many structures as possible without making the whole screen white. Frequently, you will find yourself increasing the gain until you see what you were looking for. Again, using the heart as an example, if you cannot tell the difference between the walls and the chambers, your gain is too low. If however, the inside of the chambers look white just like the walls, then your gain is too high!

Focal Zone

The focal zone is the area of the screen where the computer dedicates the most processing power and listening skills to make the image clearer. Most point of care machines do not give you the ability to adjust the focal zone (in an attempt to keep costs low), and the focal zone is therefore right in the center of your screen. If you do not have a focal zone adjustment, place the object of interest exactly in the center of the screen and you will be using the best computing power available for image creation.

Artifacts

Now that we have an optimized image, we must consider artifacts that are being created. Even though we have toted how amazingly smart ultrasound imaging is, in reality it is still very basic and makes a lot of mistakes. The majority of artifacts are produced secondary to assumptions the machine is making while receiving the sound. The machine assumes that any sound that comes back has travelled on a straight line into the tissue and then back. But we know, sound can bounce around and come back from different locations. Or – sound can hit a wall and none of the sound can get past. Or the sound can hit some fluid and not bounce back at all and instead travel right through it before bouncing back. The machine does not know this, but you do and can use these artifacts to interpret what is going on. If sound hits a poor transmitter (bone), all the sound bounces back and is displayed as very bright hyperechoic (*hyper*-lots *echoic*-sound). If all the sound transmits really well say through a fluid filled structure, then no sound bounces back and you get a dark hypoechoic (*hypo*-few *echoic*-sound) signal. Lets look at some of the artifacts this creates.

Shadowing

Shadowing, or acoustic shadowing is when there are no images seen beyond a structure. The common example is bone, such as ribs. The ultrasound waves are highly absorbed or reflected, and no ultrasound is propagated past them. Shadowing can be differentiated further into clean and dirty. Clean shadowing is traditionally seen where there is no signal seen past the region, such as bones or renal/biliary calculi. Dirty shadowing, is typically secondary to gas, and some sound still gets through but much less than would be expected.

Reverberation

When sound bounces between two highly reflective structures, the machine repeats the image downward. This is commonly seen with highly reflective foreign bodies such as metal or glass. In normal lung, A-lines can also be seen, which is reverberation of the parietal pleural line.

Mirror Artifact

Mirror artifact literally produces a mirror type image of something seen nearer to the probe. Clinically, this is often seen above the diaphragm, and is normal. If there is absence of mirror artifact superior to the diaphragm, and replaced by a hypoechoic area, there is suspicion or a pleural effusion. Similar to reverberation, where the ultrasound beam strikes a highly reflective surface. The beam then bounces back and forth between structures causing a delayed return to the transducer, and the transducer then thinking it is deeper than it actually is.

Edge Artifact

Also known as edge shadowing or lateral edge shadowing, occurs from refraction as a beam obliquely hits a tissue boundary. This is classically seen in circular structures as the gallbladder, where the lateral edges of the hyperechoic wall produce shadowing beneath it. If not recognized properly, this can be mistaken as a stone due to the shadowing posterior to it.

Posterior Enhancement

Enhancement is seen in large fluid-filled structures. It can often be seen in a full bladder. It happens as the fluid transduces the sound faster and attenuates less than the machine expects, and increases the signal that it thinks it sees.

Aliasing

This is an error seen in doppler imaging, and in many other scenarios outside of ultrasound. It is a problem of under sampling, when something is moving faster than what is trying to observe it. Real world examples include when wheels are spinning so fast, to the human eye, they look like they are going backwards. In ultrasound and film, the frame rate is too slow to interpret which way it is going.

Image Acquisition/Probe Movements

Finally, when obtaining your image, you must be able to manipulate the probe to find and improve your image or to visualize entire structures. Since your plane of sound is only in two dimensions, to view an entire three-dimensional image you must scan through the structure. You would never only look at a single slice of a CT image, and thus you must create all the different slices and put them together in your head with ultrasound. This is arguably the hardest skill in ultrasound, and can only be perfected by lots and lots of hands on practice.

There are a few principles to know here, and to have common language across sonographers. To start, the probe marker should be towards the patient's right if scanning transversely, and towards the patient's head when scanning in the sagittal or coronal plane. To search for a structure of interest, it is best to start by ***scanning,*** which is essentially moving the probe left, right, up or down without changing the angle or rotation of the probe. This will help you visualize an entire area in the body and find the structure you are looking for. Once you have found the image, you can then **fan** through the organ to create your slices. This is accomplished by anchoring the probe to the skin, and then changing the angle of the sound to the left, right, up or down. This will keep the organ of interest in the center of the screen, while creating different planes through it.

If performing a procedure with the ultrasound, it is best to keep the probe and probe marker on the screen to the left to prevent disorientation.

Before you start scanning, you should become familiar with the knobs on your machine. Since each machine is different, it would be impossible to explain them all in this text. However, with your knowledge of how the machine works now, you can find all the important ones very quickly. Locate the depth and gain buttons, determine the probe you are using, the mode you want to use (Doppler vs pulse echo), where the freeze image buttons and save video clip buttons are, and you will be ready to start scanning!

Part II

Introduction to Considerations for Specific Environments

The following section is aimed at introducing a variety of unique out-of-hospital environments and the challenges providers face working in these settings.

Ground Emergency Medical Services (EMS) includes systems across the spectrum of out-of-hospital care including prehospital systems as well as interfacility transfers.

Helicopter EMS focuses on the challenges flight crews face providing critical care transport of severely injured and critically ill patients.

Military special operations continue to work in the far forward environment. As major large scale combat operations shift to smaller operational footprints across a wider area, special operations medical providers find themselves caring for critical patients for longer periods of time and needing to care for illness and injuries not related to combat wounds. The concept of prolonged field care has been introduced to describe the challenges of this new type of operational environment.

Urban search and rescue teams respond to a range of natural and manmade disasters that impact both the local population as well as the health infrastructure.

The environment is paramount to determining the applicability of any new technology. As various out-of-hospital providers consider adding ultrasound to their practice, it is important that the benefits of ultrasound be fully consider alongside the challenges this technology may create. Ultrasound remains a powerful imaging technology that benefits patients in the hands of appropriately trained providers.

Ground Emergency Medical Services

Benjamin D. Nicholson, Harinder S. Dhindsa, and Michael J. Vitto

Introduction

Ground EMS in high income settings includes a wide range of types of programs, response characteristics, patient complaints, and transport times. Ultrasound may provide a benefit to certain patients in certain situations, but implementation likely comes at a cost that may not be reasonable for certain situations.

In this chapter we will introduce certain situations that are unique to the ground EMS environment and should be considered before implementing ultrasound in ground EMS systems. Topics to be considered include: cost of acquiring equipment; training related costs; challenges of both career and volunteer EMS agencies; providing oversight including quality assurance and quality improvement programs; protocol development.

Cost

Implementing ultrasound in the ground EMS environment involves costs that include both training and equipment. EMS departments will also need to include budgets for updating equipment as new technology becomes available, ensuring that there is appropriate storage of images and the associated costs. Training costs will include initial training and recurrence. Training will also need to be provide if additional scans are added to protocols such as a department moving from eFAST to

B. D. Nicholson (✉) · H. S. Dhindsa · M. J. Vitto
Department of Emergency Medicine, Virginia Commonwealth University School of Medicine, Richmond, VA, USA
e-mail: Benjamin.nicholson@vcuhealth.org

B. D. Nicholson et al. (eds.), *Manual of Austere and Prehospital Ultrasound*,
https://doi.org/10.1007/978-3-030-64287-7_2

echocardiogram to ultrasound guided IVs. As with implementing anything new, these costs come at the expense of decreased opportunity to train in other areas and update other equipment.

Volunteer and Career Considerations

In the United States, many EMS agencies still rely heavily on volunteers and the unique challenges of this work force must be considered before implementing ultrasound. Challenges include the ability of all providers to make initial training, buy in of volunteer providers to adding a new skill, ability to maintain competency in this skill if they are only working a limited number of hours per week, month, or year. Each of these challenges must be considered prior to implementing an ultrasound programs. While it is easier to mandate training of career providers, this comes at the cost of overtime, potentially increasing burn out, and taking away from their personal time. Mixed departments may find this particularly challenging as they have different standards for what they can require of each provider. If the new skill were technology is rolled out to career only, volunteer providers may feel slighted.

Medical Director Oversight

Medical directors must provide sufficient oversight of the providers and his commute challenging in large department. This includes a sufficient quality assurance in quality improvement program and initially likely 100% quality assurance review of all ultrasound scans and decisions made by providers based on the scans. Medical directors must have appropriate training themselves and ultrasound skills in order to review, educate, and improve provider use of ultrasound. Protocol development is key to any ultrasound program and must take into account which scans will be performed, how they will be interpreted, and the safe limits to which ultrasound will be applied.

Conclusion

Each department must consider the significant costs associated with implementing new technology and balance this against the size of the potential patient population who would benefit from a specific ultrasound guided study or procedure. For many departments, this evaluation would be in favor of not implementing an ultrasound program. An engaged medical director is also necessary to ensure appropriate oversight and quality improvement processes are in place. There is a paucity of high quality literature evaluating ultrasound in the prehospital environment and immense opportunity for interested researchers.

Helicopter Emergency Medical Services

Katherine Rodman and Matthew Jensen

Approximately 85 million Americans live more than 1 hour away from a level one or level two trauma center [1]. In order to serve these disparate and geographically isolated communities, the use of helicopter emergency medical services (HEMS) has become ubiquitous in the United States. Whilst the proliferation of HEMS has become controversial in recent years, the utilization of rapid transportation to definitive care can, and has been, lifesaving for innumerable patients. Broadly speaking, civilian HEMS is used for two reasons. Firstly, the speed at which the patient can be moved from either the scene of an accident or critical access hospital to a regional specialty or trauma center. Secondly, the ability of the critical care providers on the helicopters to bring hospital-level care to the patient, thus accelerating the patient's care timeline [2].

It is estimated that there are 400,000 rotary wing medical transports each year in the United States, utilizing a wide range of different single-engine and multi-engine airframes [3]. The most commonly employed airframes for HEMS in the US include single-engine Bell 206/407, and Airbus's AS-350 and EC-130, and multi-engine platforms Bell 222/230/412/429, Airbus BO-105/BK-117/EC-135/EC-145/AS-365, and the Agusta A-109/139 [3]. The decision to choose one airframe over another is born out of geographical, topographical, mission profile, and financial considerations.

The program the authors work for utilizes an Airbus EC 135 and EC145 to carry out approximately 1300 scene and interfacility flights per year. These aircraft are staffed with a single pilot, critical care registered nurse, and paramedic and carry a single patient in a combination of visual and instrument flight rules missions. The

K. Rodman (✉)
Department of Emergency Aviation, VCU Health, Richmond, VA, USA
e-mail: Katherine.Rodman@vcuhealth.org

M. Jensen
VCU Health Critical Care Transport Network, Richmond, VA, USA
e-mail: Matthew.Jensen@vcuhealth.org

B. D. Nicholson et al. (eds.), *Manual of Austere and Prehospital Ultrasound*,
https://doi.org/10.1007/978-3-030-64287-7_3

interior of these two aircraft features two-rear facing seats with an optional configuration of a third aft forward-facing seat on the patient's left. The onboard inverter provides direct current power for medical equipment, including a mounted Hamilton T1 ventilator, Zoll Propaq MD cardiac monitor, and multiple Braun BodyGuard infusion pumps. The advanced critical care equipment on board also includes a cooler containing an Abbott iSTAT device with point of care laboratory testing supplies, and a TIC cooler containing packed red blood cells. These pieces of equipment, whilst important for delivering tailored patient care, all consume valuable space within the cabin.

There are several significant potential or perceived benefits to the use of point of care ultrasound (POCUS) in HEMS. Most intuitively is the ability for flight crews to utilize the technology to identify the presence of traumatic injuries or medical and surgical pathology that may require intervention and treatment urgently to preserve life or reduce the likelihood of morbidity and mortality. Clear examples of this would be the presence of blood in Morrison's Pouch following blunt trauma necessitating transfusion of blood products, the absence of lung slide in a patient about to be converted to positive pressure ventilation and so requiring pneumothorax decompression to prevent tensioning, or a developing pericardial tamponade requiring ultrasound-guided pericardiocentesis to stave off cardiac arrest. The use of ultrasound has been validated as being highly sensitive and specific for internal hemorrhage when used by trained providers [4, 5].

Similarly, the use of ultrasound in the flight environment can provide clinical information that allows for the earlier diagnosis of critical pathology. Historically, the ability to see inside a patient and visualize causative pathology has been the purview of hospitals alone, but the migration of small, portable, and affordable ultrasound devices outside their four walls has made it possible to make diagnoses much earlier. The acceleration of an informed diagnostic process to the prehospital environment may bring about more nuanced and tailored patient care. This is exemplified by the hypothetical hypotensive and tachycardiac patient. It may reasonably be assumed that the patient is hypotensive secondary to volume loss, either severe dehydration or internal bleeding, and that the heart rate is compensatory and beneficial. By performing a *Rapid Ultrasound in Shock and Hypotension* exam or similar, it may be revealed that the patient is actually suffering from a profound aortic dissection and that the key to them surviving transport to hospital is decreasing the percussive impact of systole against the dissecting lumen through the use of beta blockade. In this example, the use of ultrasound in the HEMS environment would transform the treatment decision made by the flight crew and directly impact patient care.

Unlike interfacility transfers where HEMS are facilitating the transport of a patient between sending and receiving physicians and hospital units, scene requests require flight crews to attend an oftentimes undifferentiated patient and then choose the appropriate facility to deliver them to for definitive care. This decision can be challenging as closer, non-specialty facilities may not be appropriate for certain conditions, to include stroke, myocardial infarction, and trauma. The role of HEMS is to provide advanced critical care to patients whilst rapidly transporting them to the most appropriate facility, and as such this may require overflying closer hospitals. Ultrasound can play a role in assisting this decision making, as the patient with a grossly positive eFAST following a motor vehicle accident may potentially be better serviced by a longer flight time that terminates at an American College of Surgeons accredited level one trauma center, rather than a closer level two or three trauma center.

The introduction of POCUS into the HEMS environment can add another layer of procedural assistance during transport. Whilst the gold standard for confirming placement of endotracheal tubes (ET) has been established with the use of end tidal CO_2, the utilization of ultrasound as an adjunct to $EtCO_2$ for ensuring correct ET placement has been demonstrated to be a valid confirmation tool by flight crews, and may have additional benefit in low cardiac output states, hypothermia, or large pulmonary embolism [6–8]. Additionally, ultrasound has been shown to aid providers in establishing vascular access in vasculopathic patients [9, 10]. As the population ages, and their comorbidities increase, the ability to quickly and easily achieve intravascular access in an ill patient may decrease. For the difficult vascular access patient in a life-threatening situation the use of intraosseous access has increased in prevalence, though this procedure may not always be appropriate or indicated. In these situations, using the linear probe on the ultrasound may enable providers to access vasculature that is deeper within tissues and administer intravenous therapy without the trauma and potential sequalae of intraosseous access.

When consideration is given to implementing any new device, equipment, or technology, the balance of possible advantages must be weighed against the possible disadvantages the introduction may bring. Whilst the potential gains ultrasound can bring to HEMS are myriad, the corresponding potential losses stack up in equal number. The most immediately obvious is the space within the patient-care cabin that the device occupies. The Commission on Accreditation of Medical Transport Systems requires that all equipment be secured within the cabin to reduce likelihood of it striking and causing injury to- or death of- crew and patient in the event of a hard landing or crash [11]. The amount of L-Track (also known as *brown line*, or just *track*) available for strapping within air medical aircraft is limited, and priority must be given to equipment and supplies essential for carrying out the mission profile. Additionally, the ultrasound would be best secured and stored within the aircraft adjacent to a power supply to mitigate the limited battery life of the device. The combination of both available space for secure storage and 110 V power outlet may not be readily accessible in many airframes and configurations.

The aeromedical transport environment is a remarkably complex and expensive beast at baseline with estimates of the annual cost of keeping a base open in the region of $3,000,000 [3]. As medical technology advances and additive devices enter the critical care transport world, the overheads will only continue to rise with no real prospective of relative insurance and Medicare reimbursements [12]. The cost of adding ultrasound to an already expensive HEMS program can be prohibitive, even for hospital-based programs such as the authors' [4]. Historically, the price tag of introducing ultrasound to a multi-aircraft network has been so high as to require inclusion within hospital Capital Budget rather than discretionary spending. This necessity of requiring hospital executive suite approval for the addition of POCUS onto helicopters decreases the likelihood of expenditure approval and so has restricted the introduction of ultrasound to HEMS. As the cost of ultrasound has decreased over recent years, budgeting for the devices has become easier to manage at a program level. Additionally, in acknowledgement of the prohibitive cost of ultrasound the developers and retailers of POCUS machines have offered non-traditional renting options for hospitals and programs which has increased the availability of prehospital ultrasound. As such, ultrasound has the potential to become exponentially more accessible within the aeromedical environment and its use more ubiquitous.

As with any new skill, procedure, or use of technology there is an initial and recurrent training requirement for providers. It has been demonstrated that with just several hours of didactic and practical instruction, paramedics were proficient at obtaining and interpreting images useful for cardiac standstill, pneumothoraces, and pericardial effusion [13]. Similarly, with an initial six-hour training session, emergency medical services providers were shown to develop the ability to perform and interpret FAST and abdominal aortic exams with 100% agreement between the crew and physician reviewers [14]. The totality of pertinent ultrasound knowledge and skill set requires more than 6 hours of FAST and AA instruction, however, and like any competency requires ongoing and refresher training to ensure adequacy of image acquisition and interpretation. The addition of even abbreviated initial training for the cadre of flight crew, however, and the provision of frequent skill checks and refresher training sessions may prove to generate too large a financial burden for a service to bear.

In order to develop a high yield and functional prehospital ultrasound program, the establishment of quality assurance and quality improvement systems with physician involvement is paramount. The initial training and education must include an emphasis on both image acquisition and interpretation, and the trainees' scans and analysis must be vetted and determined to be adequate by a physician with a background of accredited ultrasound training. Each scan then performed by the HEMS crews on a patient must be saved securely and uploaded into a HIPPA-compliant dedicated system for timely physician-based QI/QA. The authors' Network utilizes the popular radiologic program QPath (Telexy, Blaine, WA USA) for this purpose. This ongoing quality assurance ensures contemporaneous review of the images and interpretation flight crew utilize to inform their diagnoses, therapies, and decision making, allowing for early identification of deficiencies or areas for improvement. As the intent of the HEMS ultrasound utilization is to inform patient-centered decision making, the introduction of such a QI/QA program must be established prior to the roll out of the POCUS into the HEMS environment to make certain that no opportunity for sub-optimal image acquisition and interpretation exists. This need for a, or several, qualified and appropriately trained physicians to be so intimately involved in the QA/QI process places additional demands on program medical directors and may necessitate the onboarding of additional physician staff. The time, resource, and financial burdens of this requirement must be considered when a program decides to introduce POCUS into their critical care transport system.

The old dichotomy of "stay and play or load and go" has largely been discarded as the ability to provide meaningful care en route has developed over recent years, though the notion that prehospital critical care is a time sensitive affair remains true. For every test, procedure, or therapy performed by flight crews there is an opportunity cost and so clinical decisions regarding pretest probability must form part of the ultrasound use matrix. Given the time sensitivity associated with HEMS operations, the introduction of ultrasound should not increase scene times or delay transport and treatment. Studies have shown that in less than 180 seconds most focused ultrasound exams can be completed and do not delay leaving the scene [4]. This ability to perform a significant number of diagnostic and therapeutic exams with the POCUS must not distract the prehospital provider, however, and discipline is required to carry out only the exams that have a high pretest probability and may lead to patient-oriented decision making.

Finally, the POCUS device chosen must be suitable for the environment it's being deployed into. There are several factors that the HEMS program must ruminate on before a device purchase or rental agreement is pursued. Table 1 delineates some of the more important features pertinent to the flight world. Patient transport duration, acuity of patients, and overall flight volume will determine your scan-to-charge time ratio and may impact device selection. A busy service that flies many consecutive short legs with sick, undifferentiated patients will require a device that can perform more scans on a single charge than a program that flies relatively fewer patients over more time. The availability of inverter powered 110 V outlets within the cabin, however, can mitigate battery life limitations. The scans intended to be

Table 1 Comparison of the three most popular POCUS devices [15–18]

Device	Battery life	Available probes	Available modes	Available scans	Weight
Sonosite iViz	60 minutes scanning, 8-hour standby	Linear array Phased array	2D with color Doppler M mode	Abdominal Cardiac FAST Lung OB/GYN Vascular Musculoskeletal	520 grams
Philips Lumify	Utilizes host device battery; ranges from 2 hours 30 minutes (Samsung Galaxy S2 tablet) to 5 hours 30 minutes (Samsung Galaxy S4 tablet)	Sector array Curved array Linear array	2D with color Doppler M mode	Abdominal Cardiac FAST Lung OB/GYN Vascular Musculoskeletal	Host device Dependent
Butterfly iQ	120 minutes scanning, 5 hours to charge	Single probe with capacitive micro-machined ultrasound transducers	M mode B mode Color Doppler	Abdominal Cardiac FAST Lung OB/GYN Vascular	313 grams
				Musculoskeletal	

performed and the environment in which the images will be acquired will be a determinant on the required image quality. Simple eFAST exams may be achievable with a lower image quality or resolution than detailed cardiac exams, and easier to acquire in an AW109 with its relatively smaller patient cabin windows and less ambient light than the Bell 407 with its large forward canopy, lack of partition between forward and aft cabins, and large windows. Similarly, the available probes and modes will determine the exams able to be performed and so the machine must fit the mission profile of the program. As with the introduction of any medical device into an aeromedical aircraft, such as mechanical ventilator or fluid warmer, the programs maintenance department will need to perform run up checks with the device in the aircraft and turned on to ensure compatibility with avionics. The current generation of POCUS utilize commercially available Android and Apple devices and so can be protected with external rubber cases, increasing their robustness and durability.

Whilst the potential exists for prehospital point of care ultrasound to impact helicopter emergency medical services operations in several key ways, namely the ability to improve diagnostic accuracy, guide therapy, and inform decision making, the hurdles, challenges, and limitations associated with its introduction and use must be weighed and considered. A HEMS program planning its way forward with an ultrasound program should ensure they have the space within the patient care cabin for the device, that they have the training and educational resources available for both initial and refresher training, the financial backing of their organization for the purchase or rent of the machine, and physician involvement for robust quality assurance and improvement processes. It is only with all these factors considered and accounted for that a helicopter emergency medical service can set up its ultrasound program for success.

References

1. Association of Air Medical Services. H.R. 3378 / S. 2121: ensuring access to Air Ambulance Services Act. 2017. Retrieved from https://aams.org/h-r-3378-ensuring-access-air-ambulance-services-act-2017/.
2. American College of Emergency Physicians. Policy statement: appropriate and safe utilization of helicopter emergency medical services. Dallas: American College of Emergency Physicians; 2018.
3. Association of Air Medical Services. Fact sheets and FAQs. 2015. Retrieved from https://aams.org/member-services/fact-sheet-faqs/.
4. El Sayed MJ, Zaghrini E. Prehospital emergency ultrasound: a review of current clinical applications, challenges, and future implications. Emergency Medical International. 2013. Retrieved from https://doi.org/10.1155/2013/531674.
5. El Zahran T, El Sayed MJ. Prehospital ultrasound in trauma: a review of current and potential future clinical applications. J Emerg Trauma Shock. 2018;11(1):4–9.
6. Nicholson B, Vitto M, Louka A, Dhindsa H, Rodman K, Lovelady J, Baker K. Feasibility of obtaining in-flight evaluation of endotracheal tube placement with ultrasound during helicopter transport. Air Med J. 2018;37(4):238. https://doi.org/10.1016/j.amj.2018.04.011.
7. Grmec S. Comparison of three different methods to confirm tracheal tube placement in emergency intubation. Intensive Care Med. 2002;28(6):701–4.

8. Brun PM, Bessereau J, Cazes N, Querellou E, Chenaltia H. Lung ultrasound associated to capnography to verify correct endotracheal tube positioning in prehospital *(sic)*. Am J Emerg Med. 2012;30(9):2080. https://doi.org/10.1016/j.ajem.2011.10.023.
9. Weiner MM, Geldard P, Mittnacht AJC. Ultrasound-guided vascular access: a comprehensive review. J Cardiothorac Vasc Anesth. 2012;27(2):345–60.
10. Lamperti M, Bodenham AR, Pittiruti M, Blavias M, Augoustides JG, Elbarbary M, Pirotte T, Karakitsos D, LeDonne J, Doniger S, Scoppettuolo G, Feller-Kopman D, Schummer W, Biffi R, Desruennes E, Melniker LA, Verghese ST. International evidence-based recommenations on ultrasound-guided vascular access. Intensive Care Med. 2012;38(7):1105–17. https://doi.org/10.1007/s00134-012-2597-x.
11. Commission on Accreditation of Medical Transport Systems. Eleventh edition accreditation standards of the Commission on Accreditation of Medical Transport Systems. 2018. Retrieved from https://www.camts.org/wp-content/uploads/2017/05/CAMTS-11th-Standards-DIGITAL-FREE.pdf.
12. Bergen A. Air medical services cost study report. Palm Harbor: Xcendra; 2017.
13. Chin EJ, Chan CH, Mortazavi R, Anderson CL, Kahn CA, Summers S, Fox JC. A pilot study examining the viability of a Prehospital Assessment with UltraSound for Emergencies (PAUSE) protocol. J Emerg Med. 2013;44(1):142–9. https://doi.org/10.1016/j.jemermed.2021.02.032.
14. Heegaard W, Hildebrant D, Spear D, Chason K, Nelson B, Ho J. Prehospital ultrasound by paramedics: results of field trial. Acad Emerg Med. 2010;17(6):624–30. https://doi.org/10.1111/j.1553-2712.2010.00755.x.
15. FUJI FILM, SonoSite Inc. SonoSite iViz spec sheet. June 2016. Retrieved from https://www.sonosite.com/sites/default/files/2181_US_iViz_Spec_Sheet_v52.pdf.
16. Philips. Lumify v1.8 device compatibility list. July 2019. Retrieved from http://incenter.medical.philips.com/doclib/enc/11387700/Lumify_Tablet_Compatibility.pdf%3Ffunc%3Ddoc.Fetch%26nodeid%3D11387700.
17. Philips. Philips Lumify overview. 2019. Retrieved from https://www.usa.philips.com/healthcare/product/HC795005/lumify/overview.
18. Butterfly Network Inc. Butterfly iQ specs. 2019. Retrieved from https://www.butterflynetwork.com/specs.

Military Special Operations and Prolonged Field Care

James Caleb A. Ersando, Brandon M. Fetterolf, Hubert R. Draper, John G. Knight Jr, and Jay B. Baker

Chapter Content

The special operations environment presents challenging circumstances for its assigned medical providers. The areas of operation (AO) span various terrain encompassing air, maritime, and ground operations; each with their own unique challenges. Special operations forces (SOF) are tasked to accomplish a great breadth of capabilities often with less available equipment, limited resupply capability, personnel, and time. Their operations span multiple continents with varying hostile forces and often in denied or austere areas. Ultrasound has arguably become one of the most important capabilities for the SOF medical provider given the growing recognition of its expanding uses combined with the complexity of the SOF mission. Furthermore, it may act as one of the only advanced triage tools that can help provide important decision-making dispositions for providers and commanders.

A variety of non-Physician personnel receive training in ultrasound use across the SOF medical community. This expands ultrasound capability down to the point-of-injury (POI) provider who is likely not operating under direct physician guidance. These point-of-injury providers include a variety of special operations medics

J. C. A. Ersando (✉) · H. R. Draper
Department of Defense, Army, Fort Bragg, NC, USA

B. M. Fetterolf
1st Special Forces Command, US Army, Fort Bragg, NC, USA
e-mail: fettero1@msu.edu

J. G. Knight Jr
Department of Emergency Medicine, San Antonio, TX, USA

J. B. Baker
Special Operations Command Europe, APO, AE, USA

B. D. Nicholson et al. (eds.), *Manual of Austere and Prehospital Ultrasound*,
https://doi.org/10.1007/978-3-030-64287-7_4

and in rare cases physician assistants or nurses who are cross-trained in these procedures. These providers are presented with unique challenges and considerations when conducting combat operations.

Due to the nature of SOF operations, medical treatment and evacuation is a contingency in mission planning and execution. SOF should be prepared to effectively care for their casualties but this is not the mission's primary focus. Consequently, the ability to carry every ideal medical device and supply to tackle any potential medical scenario is unrealistic. Although SOF medical teams do exist, they may be far removed from the ground forces and require medical evacuation to their location. In many theaters, access to these levels of care may not occur for hours, perhaps even days. In austere environments where weight and space are at a premium – and oftentimes the provider is limited to the equipment they can bring in on their back – an ultrasound is one of the most valuable tools at their disposal. Considerations must be made for the size, weight, and even the method of carrying the ultrasound; video quality and battery life may be sacrificed for portability. Ideally an ultrasound should be able to fit in a pouch of an aid bag or even within the medical providers' apparel.

To maintain the element of surprise, prototypical SOF missions are conducted during hours of darkness. This environment supports the need to maintain low visibility and signature as they proceed through operations. Comparatively, the utilization of an ultrasound in the civilian environment would likely occur much sooner in a patient evaluation than their SOF counterparts due to tactical considerations. Poor timing could lead to devastating results for personnel on the ground. Other low-light considerations occur during flight operations when pilots need minimal light interference from equipment during periods of darkness.

Durability of the equipment is another chief concern while operating in the resource limited environments. When the availability of replacement equipment ranges from weeks to months, ruggedized ultrasounds are key. Similar to laptops that are being deployed in the hands of SOF elements, compact ultrasound machines and probes are becoming more sturdy and able to withstand rougher treatment.

Another key consideration in resource limited environments is the access to power to operate medical equipment. An obstacle encountered by one SOF medical team was the inability of local infrastructure to support the power requirements of a portable x-ray machine. When their x-ray was plugged into the available outlet the first attempted image resulted in loss of power for the entire building structure. This scenario yielded great opportunity for use of ultrasound to achieve similar diagnostic results which in this case involved the evaluation of a potential long bone fracture.

Optimal evaluation with ultrasound requires a barrier medium between the ultrasound probe and structure being examined. Military medical logistics are underdeveloped in many locations SOF providers are deployed. Creativity and unconventional medium uses can be employed when supplies are limited. Examples include water-based lubricants, plain water, petroleum jelly, hand sanitizer, Flarp ®, bag filled with water based medium, and even gelatinous foods from a meal, ready-to-eat (MRE).

As ultrasound becomes utilized more remotely by independent providers, consultation through telemedicine – for example the ADVISSOR program – has proved an advantageous resource. There are several programs in place throughout the Department of Defense (DoD) that allow military medical providers in the field to communicate through text, e-mail, voice, video or a combination of these modalities. These medical personnel can share ultrasound cases in real-time to receive expert consultation. This allows providers to expand their ultrasound techniques to best care for their patient, especially in cases of more complex pathology.

Anecdotes from SOF providers capture these challenges and substantiate validity to upcoming applications of the ultrasound. In one case, medics working as members of a far-forward special operations resuscitation team in support of counter-ISIS operations in the Middle East validated the use of a small, portable ultrasound as a valuable tool in the austere setting to assess thoracoabdominal trauma. This team frequently resuscitated casualties in mud-brick buildings or in the back of vehicles and, in one instance, performed eFAST exams on two casualties with intra-abdominal hemorrhage from a dismounted IED blast. The casualties were subsequently evacuated to a higher level of care and underwent successful laparotomies following REBOA (Resuscitative Endovascular Balloon Occlusion of the Aorta) placement. Ultrasound is recommended to rule out hemopericardium prior to REBOA placement, in addition to its use as an adjunct for endovascular catheter insertion to successfully implement the procedure [1]. The diverse applications of ultrasound in this environment enabled numerous patients to be sufficiently resuscitated and sent to the next appropriate echelons of medical care.

In the significantly different setting of a small austere clinic in Africa with prolonged transfer times, one SOF medic was successful in using ultrasound to assess a foreign object impaled in the wrist of a young local woman. Ultrasound aided in the problem solving of potential damage to nearby vital anatomical structures and any possible remaining material upon removal. Although the current literature is mixed on the utility of ultrasound and detecting foreign bodies in soft tissue, with foreign body composition playing a significant factor, there is promising research supporting its use in these situations [2–5]. Ultrasound may be utilized for detection and removal depending on depth, size, and composition of the foreign body. Ultrasound has proven and will remain as an essential tool for assessing common injury patterns in austere settings.

Additional applications of the ultrasound in austere environments include ocular and thoracic scanning. Ocular ultrasound can be useful in foreign body evaluation, retinal detachment, assessment of optic nerve sheath all which are highly possible injuries in the special operations environment. SOF medics in Central America utilized these exams to aide treatment of patients in a resource-limited hospital. More literature supports the measurement of the optic nerve sheath diameter as an accurate surrogate for intracranial pressure [6, 7]. Blast injuries provide another unique application for ultrasound. Although many different intrathoracic pathologic processes may manifest from blasts, ultrasound may also be useful in the management scheme of pulmonary edema in the absence of radiography. With the rapidly evolving advancements in ultrasound techniques, it can be anticipated that use of ultrasound will become increasingly invaluable to special operations medical personnel and will continue to have a large impact on patient management in these far forward and austere environments.

All in all, the ultrasound machine continues to gain significant momentum in the prehospital and SOF operational environments. It can aid in disposition, severity of injury or illness, and can help drive treatment. The forward strides in technology combined with ever-improving quality, durability, and smaller size makes this a valuable tool in any SOF medic's backpack.

References

1. Baston C, West TE. Lung ultrasound in acute respiratory distress syndrome and beyond. J Thorac Dis. 2016;8(12):E1763–6. Available from: https://www.sciencedirect.com/science/article/pii/S0422763814200719.
2. Geria R. Ultrasound guided procedures – V. foreign body localization. Ultrasound guide for emergency physicians. 2008 [cited 2019 Mar 17]. Available from: https://www.acep.org/sonoguide/foreign_bodies.html.
3. Hill R. Ultrasound for the detection of foreign bodies in human tissue. Ann Emerg Med. 1997;29(3):353–6. https://doi.org/10.1016/S0196-0644(97)70347-0.
4. Kaylor DW. The utility of bedside ultrasound for the detection of soft tissue foreign bodies in the Emergency Department. Ann Emerg Med. 2005;46(3):79. https://doi.org/10.1016/j.annemergmed.2005.06.293.
5. Schlager D. Ultrasound for the detection of foreign bodies. Ann Emerg Med. 1991;20(2):189–91. https://doi.org/10.1016/S0196-0644(05)81220-X.
6. Lenaghan P. 84 Point-of-care ocular sonography to detect optic disc swelling. Ann Emerg Med. 2011;58(4):S205–6. https://doi.org/10.1016/j.annemergmed.2011.06.110.
7. Lashutka MK. The relationship of intraocular pressure to intracranial pressure. Ann Emerg Med. 2004;43(5):585–91. Available from: https://www.annemergmed.com/article/S0196-0644(03)01314-3/pdf.

Considerations for Ultrasound in the Urban Search and Rescue (USAR) Environment

Ricky C. Kue

Introduction

The field of urban search and rescue (USAR) was formally developed in the 1990's as a response to the growing concerns over organized response to building collapses and victim entrapment as a result of natural disasters such as earthquakes. In that time, the system developed in the United States under the Federal Emergency Management Agency (FEMA) is comprised of a national network of 28 Task Forces positioned throughout the country in nearly 19 states (Fig. 1). This program is known as the National Urban Search and Rescue Response System, which looked at regions at highest risk for earthquakes and building collapses within the United States and develop strategically located assets to best respond. These teams can be called upon into service in response to support heavy search and rescue capabilities at the request of local jurisdictions. Teams are able to deploy within 6 hours of notice and be self-sustained for 72 hours of operations. A typical USAR task force type-1 team is made up of 80 personnel (Fig. 2) specialized in a variety of disciplines providing technical search, rescue, hazmat management, structural engineering, communications, logistics, canine search/recovery as well as emergency medical capabilities [1]. In essence, USAR can be best described as the science of locating, reaching, medically treating, and safely extricating deeply entombed survivors of collapsed structures [2].

The USAR Medical Team

The medical team within a USAR task force is comprised of emergency physicians (referred to as medical team managers) and paramedics (referred to as medical specialists) who have undergone specialized training focused on medical care in a

R. C. Kue (✉)
Massachusetts Urban Search and Rescue Task Force-1 (MA-TF1), Beverly, MA, USA

B. D. Nicholson et al. (eds.), *Manual of Austere and Prehospital Ultrasound*,
https://doi.org/10.1007/978-3-030-64287-7_5

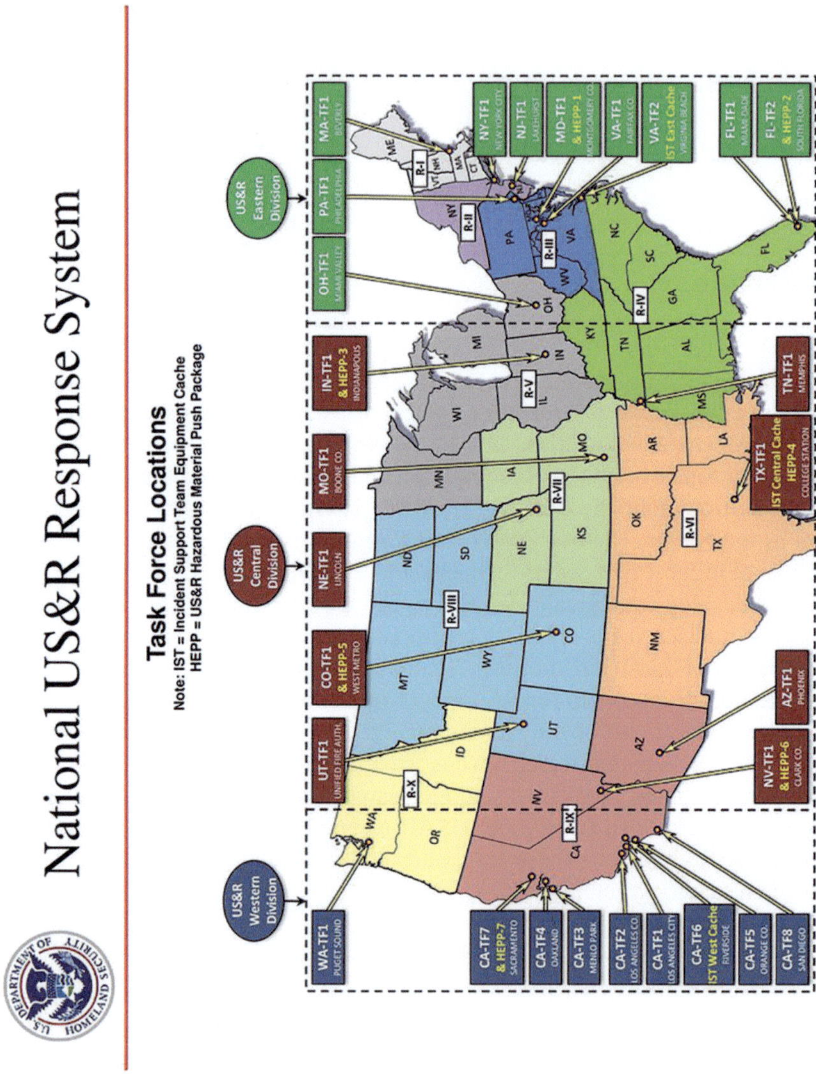

Fig. 1 Locations of FEMA US&R Teams in the United States. (https://www.fema.gov/task-force-locations)

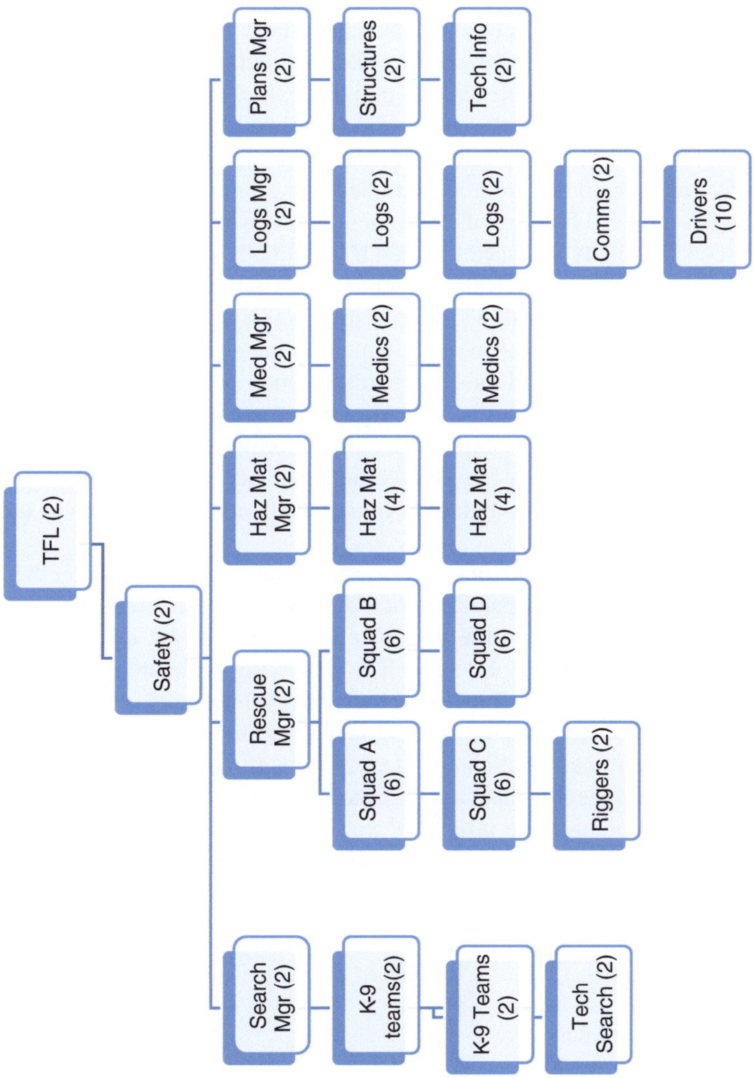

Fig. 2 Typical organizational chart for a FEMS US&R Type 1 team (80 person). TFL Task Force Leader, Med Mgr Medical Manager (Physician)

confined space and management of clinical conditions typically seen as a result of building or structural collapse. While numerous "rescue" incidents can occur on a routine basis in the prehospital environment and readily handled by conventional emergency medical services (EMS) assets, these incidents typically are a result of mechanisms such as a fall, motor vehicle crash or rollover, or entrapment from industrial machinery. Medical care delivered within the USAR environment typically refers to patient care on injuries as a result of "heavy" building collapse which lead to significant entrapment from rubble piles and building materials, prolonged entrapment for up to days and the anticipation that extrication to definitive care will be technically complex and take lengthy periods of time [2, 3]. The technical rescue and extrication process itself can accelerate the pathophysiologic insults to the victim and may cause rapid deterioration and death in an otherwise stable appearing patient who has survived for days of entrapment [2]. Most victims that survive to the point of rescue will likely not have suffered traumatically catastrophic injuries that would likely have required surgical intervention within the "golden hour." Instead, these victims will have clinically significant injures that are survivable if managed but easily aggravated due to the prolonged time they have gone without care, effects of the environment as well as the technical rescue and release from entrapment. In the end, the mechanism of injury due to heavy structural collapse and extended time needed to locate victims and perform extrication all prolong the scene time of these victims resulting in a predictable prolonged field care scenario that requires calculated critical care medicine to stabilize physiologically complex victims as the rescue process is on-going (Fig. 3).

While the victim entrapped from a heavy structural collapse has been the basis for developing the medical capabilities of a USAR task force, recent years have shown an increased change in the typical mission profile for teams. Increased response to hurricanes and floods as well as executing wide-area searches have become commonplace for USAR team deployments. While many of these incidents do not involve significant collapse, medical teams are finding themselves involved with providing urgent care medicine to deployed team members as well as emergency medical care to victims that cannot get to definitive care. In these settings, the medical care has become more typical of that seen in an emergency department, however with less resources. These mission profiles have resulted in teams looking

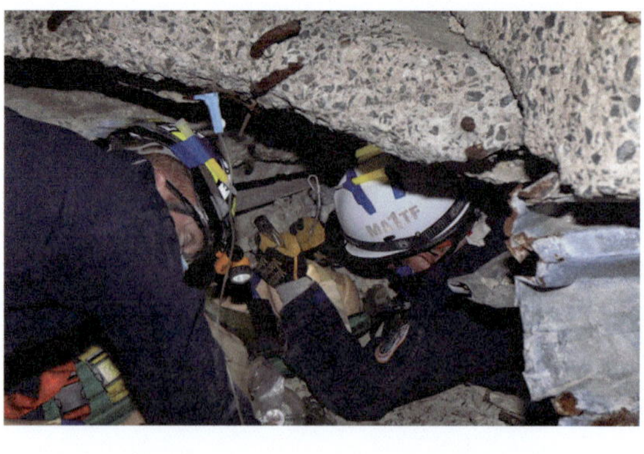

Fig. 3 An example of the typical USAR patient care environment. Two USAR Medical Specialists are working to secure the airway of a victim still entrapped within the confined space of a rubble pile during a training exercise

for resources and capabilities normally found in an emergency department including bedside ultrasound.

Ultrasound in the USAR Environment

In the past, application of point-of-care ultrasound (POCUS) in the USAR environment has been limited by the technology. Delivery of medical care in the USAR environment typically occurs in confined space settings, greatly limiting the ability to bring everything to the patient. As technology has improved recently, the availability of handheld sized POCUS devices that can offer high resolution images comparable to full size machines found in most hospital have made POCUS in the confined space/USAR environment a reality. Recently, the improvement of ultrasound technology with respect to size, portability and durability, the use of ultrasound in the austere setting for specific indications has steadily increased and described in thee literature [4–6]. Despite the rapid advancement of POCUS technology, the current scope of practice for FEMA USAR medical teams do not include ultrasound training nor is the technology required on the FEMA equipment cache list. At the time of this chapter's publication, most teams that have integrated POCUS into their capabilities have done so on their own and with physicians who have the training and competence of using POCUS as part of their daily clinical practice.

Due to reasons described in previous sections of this chapter, the typical USAR confined space patient will inherently have delays which prolong scene time as well as time to definitive care. POCUS for emergency medical providers have been helpful in making rapid decisions based on specific findings on specific types of exams. However, given the USAR working environment constraints, the value of POCUS may not be in a rapid transition to definitive care after recognition of occult hemorrhage. Rather, the value of POCUS in the USAR prolonged field care environment is the ability to perform higher sensitivity serial exams to look for clinical change over time. Studies have looked at the value of integrating ultrasound into mass casualty triage processes in order to help identify those patients who may benefit from higher triage category after identification of hemoperitoneum during prehospital FAST examinations. Most have shown limited change in clinical management based on positive FAST exams [7–11]. Walcher et al. noted a change in clinical management for 30% of patients based on a positive prehospital FAST exam with high sensitivity and specificity for hemoperitoneum [7]. Chart analysis from another study described how approximately 10% of patients triaged as "yellow" using the START algorithm had positive FAST findings with very few having any change to their clinical course of action with at a level I trauma center [10].

For the USAR medical team, positive trauma ultrasound findings provide additional data to help guide management of the confined space victim. Negative findings can help rule out presumptive diagnoses on the differential and allow the medical team to avoid unnecessary interventions while addressing other clinical possibilities not yet ruled out. Positive ultrasound findings may help the USAR medical team better triage patient treatment priorities if multiple victims are encountered. With environmental limitations in the confined space setting such as low lighting, high noise due to active heavy rescue operations and limited access to patient anatomy, the use of ultrasound offers additional clinical data that can be obtained without the use of traditional diagnostic tools such as stethoscopes. It also offers clinical information comparable to other traditional diagnostic tools such as chest radiography in a smaller, compact unit that can be brought to the entrapped patient's bedside.

Clinical Indications: Undifferentiated Shock

It can be expected that after a major building collapse, the usual patient that USAR medical teams will encounter may have suffered significant traumatic forces. While the usual mechanism of injury will consist of crushing or blunt force trauma, other injuries as a direct result from blast overpressure if any explosions were involved as well as penetrating trauma as a result of blast injuries can be expected. The challenge with these patients is that the situational predicament tends to result in entrapment and prolonged extrication. It also results in limited access and assessment of victims. Due to expected delays in reaching still live victims as well as expected prolonged extrication times, many of these patients will be volume deplete even before any hemorrhage has occurred. If exsanguinating hemorrhage has occurred, it is unlikely these victims will survive. Rather, many victims encountered by USAR medical teams have not suffered life-threatening hemorrhage. Instead, the hemorrhage process has been tamponaded by some compressive force or the blood loss in insidious. Being able to apply eFAST protocols will help the medical team differentiate the type of volume loss a victim is experiencing. Use of ultrasound in abdominal trauma can help guide management and improve outcomes [7, 8]. The information of knowing whether a victim's shock is due to intra-abdominal blood loss versus overall low volume due to a decompressed inferior vena cava (IVC) during patient care in a confined space would be added value to the decision-making process on patient acuity, immediate volume needs and whether other anatomical locations of blood loss need to be considered.

Clinical Indications: Renal Perfusion and Crush Syndrome

The clinical condition of most concern to USAR medical teams as a result of massive compressive forces to large amounts is the crush syndrome. Described in detail at the outset of the London Bombings in 1941, it was becoming apparent to rescuers and medical providers that casualties buried under rubble for days would suddenly be freed only to succumb to death from their injuries immediately upon release or later on in the hospital as a result of acute renal failure (ARF). This "crush syndrome" is the direct result muscle tissue compression and necrosis. Compressive times required to develop crush syndrome are typically hours with as little as 2 hours of compression. Crush syndrome results in a characteristic syndrome of rhabdomyolysis, inducing myoglobinuric ARF, also known as traumatic rhabdomyolysis [12]. Crush kills in a few ways. Immediately upon release from compressive forces, there is massive shifting of remaining blood volume into previously tamponaded third spaces. If the victim is not adequately volume resuscitated prior to entrapment release, their blood pressure will be sure to bottom out the moment these forces are released. Crush syndrome also kills during the release of entrapment when otherwise damaged muscle cells are re-perfused, resulting in return circulation of cardiotoxic potassium and calcium shifts. The destruction of muscle tissue and the influx of myoglobin, potassium, and phosphorus into the circulation results in the classic picture of traumatic rhabdomyolysis/crush syndrome. The syndrome is characterized by hypovolemic shock and hyperkalemia [12]. Finally, crush syndrome can ultimately kill a victim later in their clinical course in a predictable manner if myoglobin is not adequately cleared from the plasma and ARF ensues.

The mainstay of treatment for crush syndrome patients has focused on early intravenous fluid resuscitation prior to entrapment release to minimize the effects of hypovolemic shock due to excessive volume shifts, administration of intravenous alkalinizing agents such as sodium bicarbonate to improve the excretion of myoglobin from the body and management of life-threatening arrhythmias due to the effects of potassium, calcium and phosphorus [12]. Use of ultrasound imaging for the evaluation of renal injury as well as its perfusion has been described in the literature [13, 14]. The utility of these applications while more beneficial in the hospital setting, may have limited use in the confined space austere environment. It is unclear whether surrogate ultrasound measures of renal perfusion have any value added to the management of these patients in the acute phase of care. Clinical markers currently used, such as level of mentation, hemodynamic markers, urine output continue to offer valuable clinical data in the absence of reliable renal ultrasound techniques in the austere environment. Additionally, use of ultrasound in major earthquake events described in the literature focused more on the utility of FAST examinations as part of a larger triage methodology to identify patients a t higher risk for surgical intervention rather than in applications related specifically to crush syndrome pathology or renal function [14–16].

Clinical Indications: Undifferentiated Dyspnea

The differential diagnosis for dyspnea in patients within the confined space environment is broad and can range from minor to life threatening. By far, one of the most common causes of dyspnea in the confined space patient is dust impaction. Confined space case reviews have described the dyspnea described by patients due to the suspension of dust particles and debris within the atmosphere of the environment [3]. This is due to the particles released during both the initial collapse and destruction of building materials as well as during the rescue phase in which rescuers utilize machinery to gain patient access through the same pile of debris. These particles pose a health and occupational hazard to both victim and rescuer. They also serve as triggers for any underlying pulmonary disease such as asthma or other reactive airway diseases. The usual treatment is supportive, with mechanical cleansing of the oral and nasal passages of dust, respiratory protective equipment and supplemental oxygen. Where ultrasound comes into use is the ability to differentiate other life-threatening diseases entities as a result of collapse such as development of blast lung due to blast over-pressure exposure or primary pulmonary trauma such as tension pneumothorax or hemothorax. Use of ultrasound during eFAST for identification of tension pneumothorax as evidenced by absence of lung sliding "comet" tail artifacts is easily recognized by the POCUS operation and can also be used as a serial exam during re-assessment of decompensating patients. Looking for other ultrasound findings to identify pulmonary edema in the dyspneic patient may be helpful as the delayed onset of primary blast lung injuries in exposed patients begin to develop. Ultrasound has been shown to offer utility in differentiating specific findings in the pulmonary windows to help differentiate these clinical entities and may have benefit as an adjunct to more traditional physical examination methods of assessing the lung given auscultation may not always be accurate or possible in the confined space environment [17–19].

Conclusions

Prehospital application of POCUS in the USAR environment is promising. While not currently a standard part of medical team training or capabilities, the major advances of POCUS technology have allowed USAR physicians to consider the use of this technology given its ability to identify specific conditions as it relates to trauma. With the sensory and physical constraints of a confined space environment, use of ultrasound gives the USAR medical team a rapid and reliable answer to ruling out life-threatening conditions such as abdominal trauma, pulmonary edema due to blast injury, tension pneumothorax as well as general volume status. While the ultimate determining factor of scene time for confined space patients is based on length of extrication time, useful information in eFAST and other POCUS protocols can give the medical team managers more information that can assist the rescue team managers and task force leaders with accurate and timely information on patient clinical conditions which could then determine further technical rescue decisions. Ultrasound thus becomes an extension of the medical team's diagnostic capabilities in patient assessment and determination of clinical status rather than a simple point-of-care test used to make "yes/no" decisions about disposition. Ultrasound is integrated as part of the patient re-assessments during prolong field care and used similar to other diagnostic tools to help identify and monitor life-threatening conditions, as well as guide therapy and interventions in the absence of more sensitive diagnostic tools found in the hospital setting. Additionally, as USAR teams find themselves engaged in other types of search and rescue missions unrelated to building collapse, most medical teams can integrate POCUS into their sick call/urgent care operations similar to how POCUS is currently used in many emergency departments. This has included missions such as wide area searches, hurricane response, swift water and surface water rescues. In missions where local medical resources become limited, the USAR medical teams will provide day-to-day urgent care services to team members and first responders. US applications commonly used in the emergency department such as procedural applications, soft tissue and musculoskeletal applications including fracture or foreign body identification can be utilized in the field. As the ultrasound technology makes bringing it into the field more feasible, so will the increase of its use in the USAR environment.

References

1. Bea K. Urban search and rescue task forces: facts and issues. CRS Report for Congress. Updated 24 Apr 2006.
2. Barbera JA, Macintyre A. Urban search and rescue. Emerg Med Clin North Am. 1996;14:399–412.
3. Petinaux B, Macintyre A, Barbera J. Confined space medicine and the medical management of complex rescues: a case series. Disaster Med Public Health 190-197. Preparedness. 2014;8:20–9.
4. Nelson B, Melnick E, Li J. Portable ultrasound for remote environments, part 1: feasibility of field deployment. J Emerg Med. 2011;40:190–7. https://doi.org/10.1016/j.jemermed.2009.09.006.
5. Nelson B, Melnick E, Li J. Portable ultrasound for remote environments, part 2: clinical indications. J Emerg Med. 2011;40:313–21. https://doi.org/10.1016/j.jemermed.2009.11.028.
6. Zahran T, El-Sayed M. Prehospital ultrasound in trauma: a review of current and potential future clinical applications. J Emerg Trauma Shock. 2018;11:4–9. https://doi.org/10.4103/JETS.JETS_117_17:10.4103/JETS.JETS_117_17.
7. Walcher F, Weinlich M, Conrad G, et al. Prehospital ultrasound imaging improves management of abdominal trauma. Br J Surg. 2006;93:238–42.
8. Jørgensen H, Jensen C, Dirks J. Does prehospital ultrasound improve treatment of the trauma patient? A systematic review. Eur J Emerg Med. 2010;17:249–53.
9. Stawicki S, Howard J, Pryor J, et al. Portable ultrasonography in mass casualty incidents: the CAVEAT examination. World J Orthop. 2010;1:10–9.
10. Sztajnkrycer M, Baez A, Luke A. FAST ultrasound as an adjunct to triage using the START mass casualty triage system: a preliminary descriptive study. Prehosp Emerg Care. 2006;10:96–102.
11. Ma O, Norvell J, Subramanian S. Ultrasound applications in mass casualties and extreme environments. Crit Care Med. 2007;35:S275–9.
12. Gonzalez D. Crush syndrome. Crit Care Med. 2005;33:s34–41.
13. Keven K, Ates K, Yagmurlu B, et al. Renal doppler ultrasonographic findings in earthquake victims with crush injury. J Ultrasound Med. 2001;20:675–9.
14. Sarkisian A, Khondrkarian R, Amirbekian N, et al. Sonographic screening of mass casualties for abdominal trauma and renal injuries following the 1988 Armenian earthquake. J Trauma. 1991;31:247–50.
15. Dan D, Mingson L, Jie T, et al. Ultrasonographic applications after mass casualty incident caused by Wenchuan earthquake. J Trauma. 2010;68:1417–20.
16. Mulvey JM, Awan SU, Qadri AA, Maqsood MA. Profile of injuries arising from the 2005 Kashmir earthquake: the first 72 hours. Injury, Int J Care Injured. 2008;39:554–60.
17. Noble VE, Lamhaut L, Capp R, et al. Evaluation of a thoracic ultrasound training module for the detection of pneumothorax and pulmonary edema by prehospital physician care providers. BMC Med Ed. 2009;9:3.
18. Zechner P, Aichinger G, Rigaud M, et al. Prehospital lung ultrasound in the distinction between pulmonary edema and exacerbation of chronic obstructive pulmonary disease. Am J Emerg Med. 2010;389:e1–2.
19. Brun P, Bessereau J, Levy D, et al. Prehospital ultrasound thoracic examination to improve decision making, triage, and care in blunt trauma. Am J Emerg Med. 2014;32:817e1–2.

Part III

Introduction to Diagnostic Studies

The diagnostic section focuses on studies that can identify pathology and aid in diagnostic dilemmas. These studies were selected to focus on diagnosing pathology that will alter timing of transport or evacuation, destination selection, or the provision of care in the out-of-hospital environment. Sections that are titled as advanced topics for austere providers focus on studies that are more applicable to prolonged patient care outside of a typical developed healthcare setting including disaster response, wilderness medicine, and the military. Ultrasound is a tremendously powerful tool and there are many additional studies that advanced providers may find useful; however, these studies were considered beyond the scope of this text.

Shortness of Breath

Michael J. Vitto, Benjamin D. Nicholson, and Harinder S. Dhindsa

Introduction

Shortness of breath is a common patient presentation for pre-hospital providers. Treatment pathways require the providers to determine a suspected diagnosis and treatment given physical exam findings and patient histories. Given patients with multiple co-morbidities, unknown or unfamiliar histories, and difficulty using lung auscultation in noisy environments, ultrasound has emerged as a potential tool to assist in diagnosis. Thoracic and lung ultrasound can rapidly determine potential diagnosis. When used in conditions such as asthma and congestive heart failure, there are specific ultrasound findings that can help with treatment plans. Pneumonia, pneumothorax, pleural effusions, and pulmonary edema all can be visualized and differentiated using ultrasound.

Lung ultrasound is a quick and relatively straightforward exam with high lifesaving potential. Lung ultrasound allows for rapid determination of patients with respiratory distress. Given ease of access to a patient's upper chest wall for other pre-hospital interventions such as the twelve lead EKG, needle decompression, and cardiac monitors. Patients with rapid transport times or longer transports times can all benefit from lung ultrasound and serial lung ultrasound while evaluating for diuresis effects, endotracheal tube migrations, and possible enlarging pneumothorax. This chapter will introduce lung ultrasound and the views that can be used on patients in the pre-hospital and austere setting.

M. J. Vitto (✉) · H. S. Dhindsa · B. D. Nicholson
Department of Emergency Medicine, Virginia Commonwealth University School of Medicine, Richmond, VA, USA
e-mail: michael.vitto@vcuhealth.org

B. D. Nicholson et al. (eds.), *Manual of Austere and Prehospital Ultrasound*,
https://doi.org/10.1007/978-3-030-64287-7_6

Anatomy

The normal chest wall consists of the twelve bilateral ribs enclosing the two lungs. There are seven true ribs, three false ribs, and two floating ribs on each side. The right lung consists of three lobes (upper, middle, and lower) and the left lung consists of two lobes (upper and lower). The left lung also has a lingula segment. The lungs are enclosed by the parietal and visceral pleural which makes up the pleural sac. The pleural cavity is the potential space between these pleurae and can contain a small amount of fluid.

Image Acquisition and Interpretation

Terminology

A-Lines

A-line are reverberation artifacts due to reflection of the ultrasound waves. The A-lines are created by reflections off of the pleura. They are seen as echogenic horizontal lines, which are separated by an equal distance between each line. The A-lines can be seen throughout normal lungs (Fig. 1).

B-Lines

B-lines are comet-tail vertical lines that extend from the lung pleural line to the bottom of the ultrasound monitor screen. These lines move with sliding lung. Normally up to three B-lines will be seen per field of view. More that three B-lines per rib space can be seen in patients with pulmonary edema (Fig. 2).

Transducer Selection

The linear, curvilinear, and phased array transducers can all be used for lung ultrasound. Given the superficial structures in the chest wall, the high-frequency linear

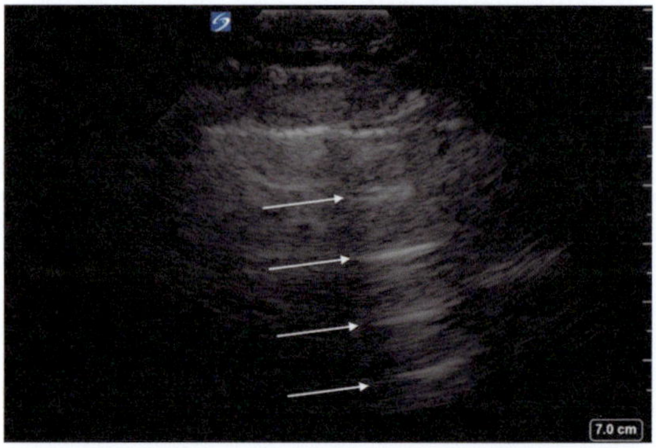

Fig. 1 A-lines: Normal lung findings include horizontal A-lines (arrows) throughout the lung caused by reverberation artifact from the pleural line. (From Creditt, *Clinical ultrasound: a pocket manual*)

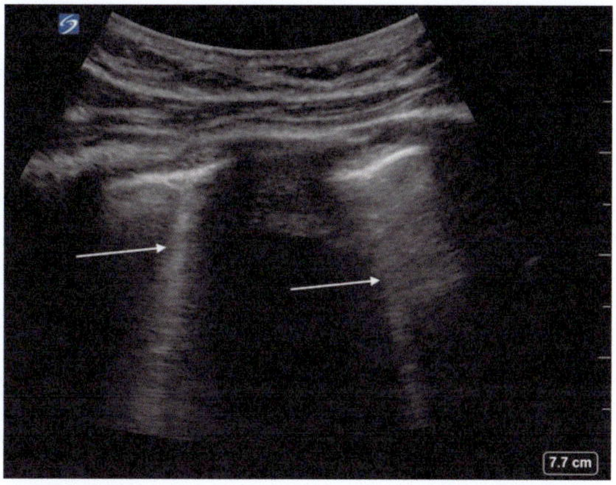

Fig. 2 B-lines: B-lines extend from the pleural line down to the bottom of the screen without fading. Up to three B-lines per lung field is considered normal. (From Creditt, *Clinical ultrasound: a pocket manual*)

transducer gives good visualization of the pleura and lung fields. The low frequency curvilinear transducer has a larger footprint and can visualize multiple rib spaces and deeper fields. The low frequency phased array transducer has a smaller footprint to image between tight rib spaces and also allows for deeper field views.

The marker dot for all of these transducers should be pointed at the patient's head during evaluation of the bilateral lungs. This dot will correspond to the marker dot on the left side of the ultrasound monitor screen. In this configuration, the left side of the screen will be imaging toward the direction of the patients head (cephalic), the right side of the screen will be imaging towards the direction of patients feet (caudal). The top of the screen will show anterior or superficial structures, and the bottom of the screen will show posterior or deep structures.

Positioning and Anatomic Considerations

Patients can be imaged while siting upright or laying flat. Imaging should include anterior, lateral, and posterior chest positions for full lung evaluation. Gravity considerations should be made if looking for air (such as pneumothorax) or fluid (such as pleural effusion). Air will rise to the top. In the upright patient a pneumothorax will be best visualized near the lung apex and pleural effusions near the lung bases. In the supine patient, air and pneumothorax will be seen in an anterior view, while pleural effusions will be located in a posterior view given that fluid will be affected by gravity and travel to the lowest point.

Standard Lung Ultrasound Views

A complete lung exam should include four zones on each side, eight total zones. The anterior lung, lateral lung, posterior lung, and costophrenic angles should be evaluated on both the left and right side (Fig. 3).

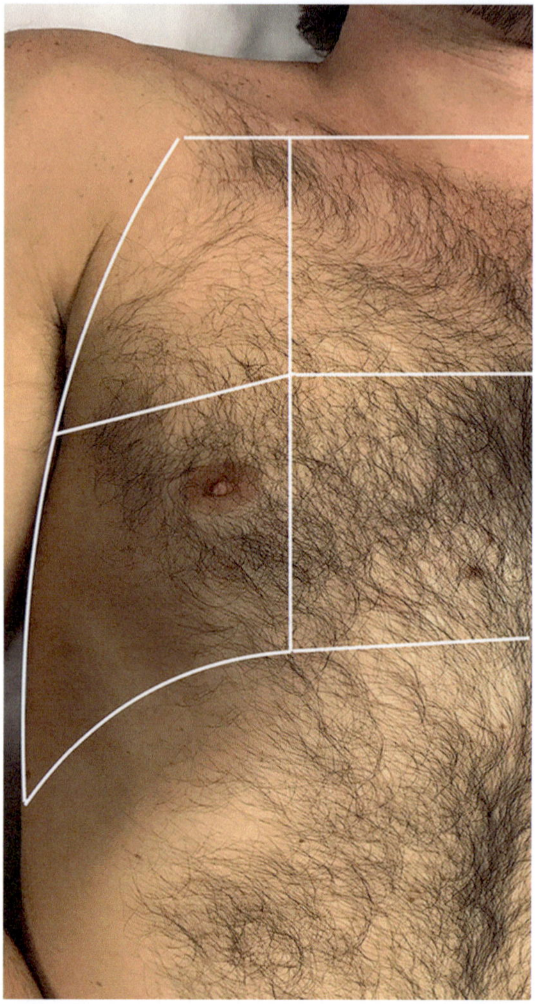

Fig. 3 Lung zones: Anterior and lateral lung zones are outlined here. When imaging the lung, it is important to evaluate multiple zones for completeness. (From Creditt, *Clinical ultrasound: a pocket manual*)

The transducer should be held vertically with the marker dot pointed towards the patient's head (cephalic). Lung sliding will occur as the visceral pleural slides against the parietal pleura. This occurs during normal respirations. The depth should be adjusted so that the objects of interest, in this case the lung plural line is visualized in the middle of the screen. Ribs will be present and can be identified by a hyperechoic rim and posterior shadow. The hyperechoic horizontal line connecting between the two ribs will be the plural line. The lung will slide back and forth horizontally. The ultrasound gain can be decreased to better visualize the bright pleura. The user should shift and slide the transducer caudal down the chest wall to visualize multiple rib spaces while keeping the ultrasound transducer vertical with the marker dot towards the patient's head. This can be continued down the lateral chest wall and the posterior chest wall to obtain a full lung exam (Fig. 4).

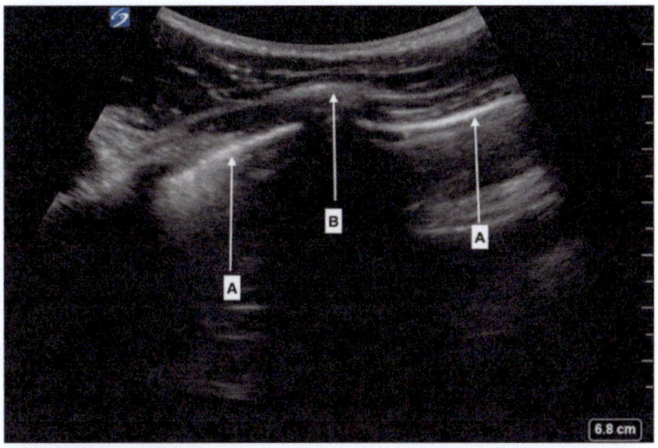

Fig. 4 Normal pleural line: Normal pleural line is hyperechoic and linear (**a**) located between rib shadows (**b**). (From Creditt, *Clinical ultrasound: a pocket manual*)

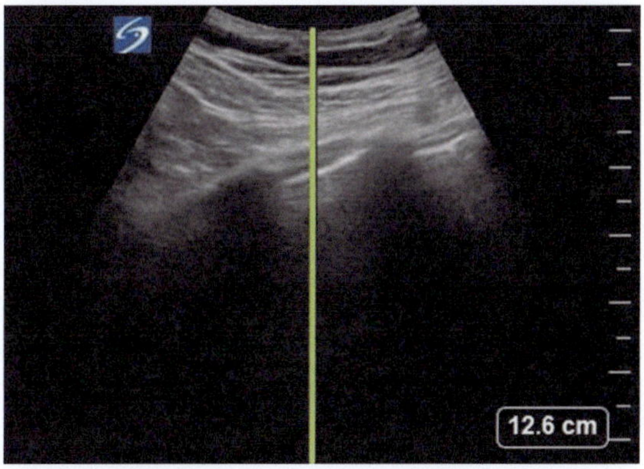

Fig. 5 M-mode with correct spike position: The M-mode spike should be placed between the two rib shadows overlying the hyperechoic pleural line. (From Creditt, *Clinical ultrasound: a pocket manual*)

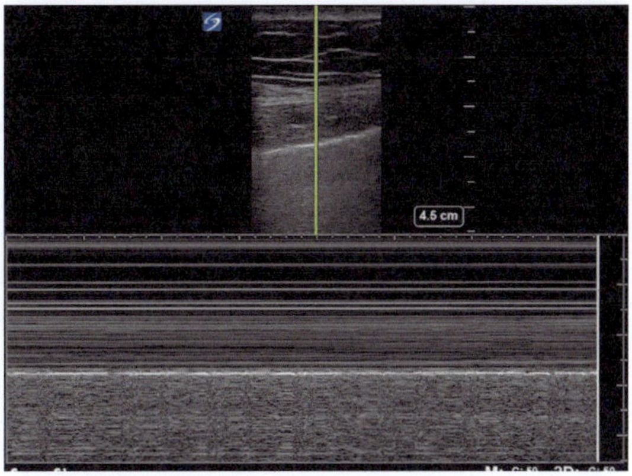

Fig. 6 Normal sliding lung M-mode "seashore sign": M-mode ultrasonography of a normal lung demonstrates the static chest wall in the top half of image and movement of the lungs in the bottom half consistent with normal respiration. Sometimes referred to as "seashore" sign. (From Creditt, *Clinical ultrasound: a pocket manual*)

To assist in identification of sliding lung, motion mode or "M-mode" can be used on the ultrasound machine to show a time motion display of the movement. The M-mode spike should be dropped between two ribs on the screen so that it perpendicularly crosses the pleural line. Once started, M-mode horizontal lines represent the non-moving chest wall and granular patterns shows movement of the lung deep to the pleural line (Figs. 5 and 6).

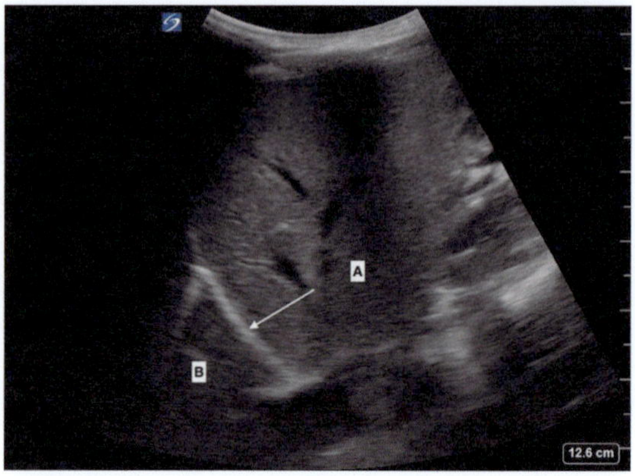

Fig. 7 Right costophrenic angle: The hyperechoic diaphragm (arrow) is seen separating the liver (**a**) and lung tissue (**b**) at the costophrenic angle. (From Creditt, *Clinical ultrasound: a pocket manual*)

To identify the costophrenic angles, place the transducer to the inferior and posterior lateral area of the patient. The transducer marker dot will be pointing towards the patient's head. The images will show where the diaphragm meets at the lung base with the liver on the right side of the patient and spleen on the left side of the patient. The diaphragm will be a hyperechoic linear structure superior to the liver and spleen. The base of the lung parenchyma will be seen superior to the diaphragm (Fig. 7).

Pathology

Pneumothorax

A pneumothorax is the separation of the lung pleura away from the chest wall, and results in a collapsed lung. A pneumothorax can be caused by a spontaneous process, a traumatic injury, or an iatrogenic process. Under ultrasound evaluation, there will be no lung sliding visualized due to the separation of the visceral and parietal pleural linings. Depending on the size of the pneumothorax, it is possible to move the transducer superior or inferior to locate an area of sliding lung. The size of a pneumothorax can be estimated by how far down the chest wall sliding lung is not present. A 100% pneumothorax will have no sliding lung on that side. A fifty percent pneumothorax will have no sliding lung and then sliding lung will return approximately half way down the chest wall. At the point where lung slide returns, this is call lung point sign. Lung point sign is the transition point between normal sliding lung and absence of sliding lung and shows where the pneumothorax is located. The lung point sign is 100% specific for a pneumothorax, but lung point sign will not always be present especially if there is a very large pneumothorax and when the lung is totally collapsed.

M-mode is useful to confirm the presence or absence of sliding lung. When the M-mode spike is placed over an area of no sliding lung, there will be no movement throughout the image since there is no lung sliding. The image will have an appearance of the anterior chest wall throughout. There will be horizontal lines through the entire images. This is referred to as barcode sign due to the horizontal lines (Fig. 8).

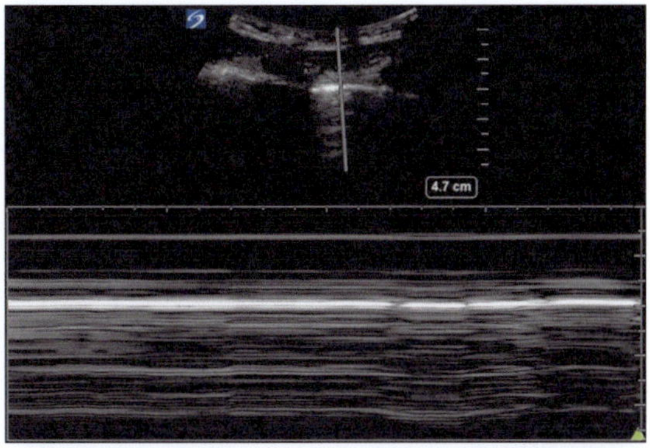

Fig. 8 Barcode sign: M-mode through the pleural line demonstrates no movement as evidenced by the horizontal lines in the bottom half of the image. This is sometimes referred to as "barcode sign" given the similar appearance to retail barcodes. (From Creditt, *Clinical ultrasound: a pocket manual*)

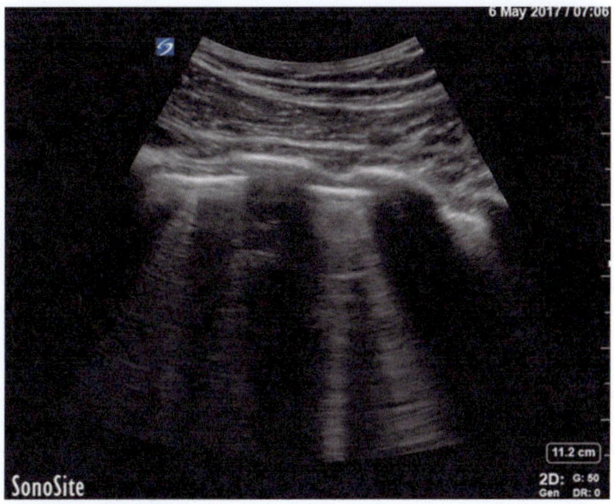

Fig. 9 Pulmonary edema: Diffuse B-lines taking up the entire lung field suggest pulmonary edema in the right clinical setting. (From Creditt, *Clinical ultrasound: a pocket manual*)

Pulmonary Contusions

Pulmonary contusions are caused by trauma to the lung and are an evolving presentation. Trauma can cause interstitial edema to the lung tissue. This will be visualized by ultrasound as B-lines in various rib spaces. This should correspond to sites of traumatic injuries.

Pulmonary Edema

Pulmonary edema is fluid that collects in alveoli of the lung. Pulmonary edema has many causes including patients with congestive heart failure, kidney failure, liver failure, fluid overload, and acute respiratory distress syndrome. In these patients with respiratory distress, lung ultrasound is useful to look for fluid within the lungs. Pulmonary edema is defined by the presence of three or more B-lines that are present in two or more lung fields bilaterally. The more diffuse B-lines in more lung fields correspond to worsening pulmonary edema. Serial lung ultrasounds in patients undergoing diuresis or hemodialysis will show less B-lines over time as the fluid is removed (Fig. 9).

Pleural Effusions

Pleural effusions are fluid collections within the pleural cavity. These fluid collections are gravitationally dependent. Fluid will be seen posteriorly in the supine patient and superior to the diaphragm in the upright or sitting patient. Effusions can be loculated and complex. The pleural effusion on ultrasound evaluation will be anechoic or hypoechoic areas. Consolidated lung may be present floating in the fluid. It can be difficult to distinguish hemorrhagic verses transudative or exudative fluid collections, but given patient history and possible increased internal ultrasound signals in hemorrhagic and exudative collections slight differences can be seen (Figs. 10 and 11).

Pneumonia

Pneumonia is an infection of the lung tissue. Pneumonia can be identified by ultrasound as a consolidation of lung tissue. This appears as a hypoechoic heterogeneous ultrasound signal, which can have a similar appearance to that of the liver. This is referred to as lung hepatization. The lung tissue in a patient with pneumonia can have blurred, irregular margins. Patients with pneumonia on ultrasound may have

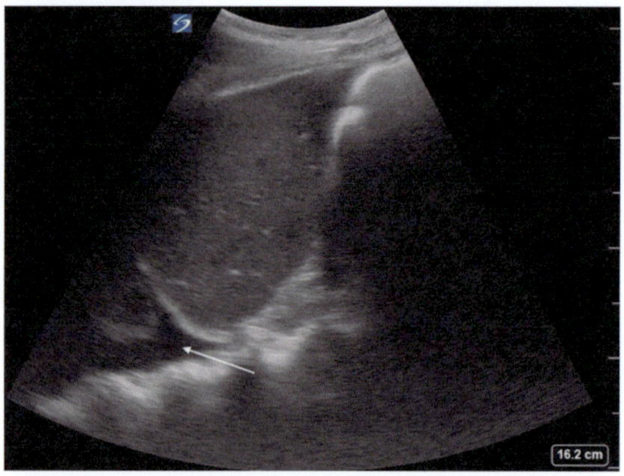

Fig. 10 Pleural effusion: A small pleural effusion (arrow) is noted above the diaphragm. (From Creditt, *Clinical ultrasound: a pocket manual*)

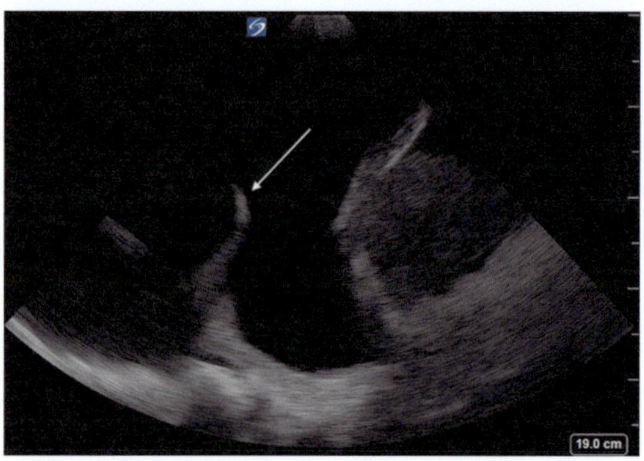

Fig. 11 Floating lung: With large pleural effusions, the lung will appear to be floating in the fluid, creating what looks like a flag flapping in the wind (flag sign). (From Creditt, *Clinical ultrasound: a pocket manual*)

unilateral and focal B-lines. Air bronchograms and fluid bronchograms may be seen. The air bronchograms can be identified as an echogenic tubular structure within the consolidated tissues. The fluid bronchograms are identified as anechoic tubular structures within the consolidated tissues.

Future Opportunities for Research

Opportunities for expanding ultrasound use include work being done in pediatric patients to diagnosis lung conditions such as pneumonia. In addition, the use of serial lung ultrasound in endotracheal intubated patients to evaluated conditions such as endotracheal tube dislodgement or tube migration could be very helpful.

Chest Pain

Jordan Tozer and Kendall Shaw

Introduction

The use of ultrasonography to diagnosis and manage emergent conditions in the hospital setting has been firmly established. In fact, within that setting its use is becoming more widespread, with a focus on the diagnosis of acute cardiac conditions because of the high associated morbidity and mortality. Because of the proven benefits of cardiac ultrasound, termed echocardiography, it is now being implemented in other areas including the prehospital and austere settings. The potential for early diagnosis, early intervention, and change in management through the use of echocardiography is clear.

Cardiac ultrasound is a very broad and technical field. It can take years to master the depth of knowledge within this extensive subject. However, echocardiography can be performed accurately by a novice sonographer with training focused on basic anatomy, basic cardiac function and image acquisition. Patients in any setting can benefit from point-of-care echocardiography to diagnose, guide management, and direct further care for their condition. This chapter will introduce the basic skills needed for obtaining standard echocardiographic views that can be used in the pre-hospital and austere settings. It will present diagnostic pathways and management considerations for common, critical diagnoses that can be made with echocardiography.

J. Tozer (✉) · K. Shaw
Department of Emergency Medicine, Virginia Commonwealth University Health System, Richmond, VA, USA
e-mail: jordan.tozer@vcuhealth.org

B. D. Nicholson et al. (eds.), *Manual of Austere and Prehospital Ultrasound*,
https://doi.org/10.1007/978-3-030-64287-7_7

Anatomy

The heart is a hollow muscular organ that serves as a circulatory pump for the body's blood. The heart works in close conjunction with the lungs to deliver oxygenated blood into systemic circulation. The heart is broadly divided into two sides, the right and the left, each containing one atrium and one ventricle. The right side of the heart receives deoxygenated blood from the systemic venous circulation and pumps it into the pulmonary circulation. The left side of the heart receives oxygenated blood from the pulmonary circulation, and distributes the blood into the high pressure systemic arterial system. The right side of the heart is a much lower pressure system than the left side under normal physiologic conditions, and the heart is structured to accommodate this. As such, the left ventricle (LV) is more muscular than the right and has a larger cavity size.

The pattern of blood flow during the process of central circulation is critical to understanding basic echocardiography. Blood enters the heart from the body through the inferior vena cava (IVC) and superior vena cava (SVC) and drains directly into the right atrium (RA). It then passes through the tricuspid valve and enters the right ventricle (RV). During systole, the ventricular contraction phase, blood is ejected from the right ventricle through the pulmonary valve and into the pulmonary arteries. Blood returns from the pulmonary circulation through the four pulmonary veins and drains directly into the left atrium (LA). During diastole, the ventricular filling phase, blood then flows through the mitral valve and enters the left ventricle. During systole, blood is ejected from the left ventricle through the aortic valve and into the proximal aorta. The aorta ascends posteriorly and then curves inferiorly, making the aortic arch, then descends through the thorax and abdomen. The portion of the aorta from the aortic valve through the branching of the left subclavian artery is known as the ascending aorta and aortic arch; anything distal to the left subclavian artery is known as the descending aorta.

Structurally, the heart is composed of three layers; from outer to inner: the epicardium, the muscular myocardium, and the endocardium. The heart is surrounded by a sac-like structure called the pericardium. The outer layer is the fibrous pericardium which is actually attached to various portions of the thorax by weak ligaments. The inner portion is the serous pericardium, and is further divided into parietal and visceral layers. The visceral layer is synonymous with the epicardium. There is a small amount of serous fluid between the visceral and parietal layers that serves as a lubricant for the heart as it moves through the cardiac cycle.

The heart's position in the thorax creates two important anatomic concepts to understand: its surfaces and its axes. Because of the heart's unique shape it has three surfaces: the inferior/diaphragmatic surface, the posterior surface/base, and the anterior/sternocostal surface. The diaphragmatic surface is formed mostly by the right and left ventricles, with a smaller portion of the right atrium. The posterior surface, also known as the base, is formed primarily by the left atrium. The anterior surface is formed mostly by the right ventricle and to a lesser degree the right atrium.

The long axis of the heart lies from its base to its apex. The terms base and apex are derived from the cone shape of the heart. It is important to note that the heart does not rest on its base, but rather on its diaphragmatic surface. The base of the heart is close to the midline, and the apex of the heart represents the ending point of the left ventricle, usually four centimeters inferolateral to the left nipple near the point of maximum impulse. This orientation of this long axis of the heart can change slightly depending on both anatomic and pathologic features of the patient in question. The short axis lies at a perpendicular angle to the long axis of the heart [1].

Image Acquisition and Interpretation

Probe Selection

For standard echocardiography the phased array probe should be used. This probe has several unique properties that make it ideal for imaging the heart. Primarily, the phased array probe has small face or "footprint", which is ideal for imaging the heart in between the limited space afforded by the ribs. Furthermore, it uses electronic beam steering to "widen out" the beam from the flat probe face, making the field of view larger so that more of the cardiac structure can be imaged. Lastly, the phased array probe uses a high pulsed repetition frequency (PRF), meaning more pulsed sound waves per second. This imaging parameter creates a higher temporal resolution, which is ideal for imaging the dynamic, ever-pumping heart [2].

By convention, when imaging most of the body, the marker dot on the probe is positioned towards the patient's right or towards the head, to correspond to the marker dot which is on the left side of the imaging screen. Because of the unique structure of the heart, and the various imaging axes as mentioned early, the convention is changed for echocardiography. When the ultrasound machine is changed to cardiac mode the marker dot moves to the right of the screen. And when imaging the patient, the marker dot on the phased array probe is moved through a series of positions that correspond to the axes of the heart rather than simply "towards the right" or "towards the head." These positions and the corresponding cardiac images that are obtained will be detailed further in this chapter.

Positioning and Anatomic Considerations

Most providers prefer to scan from the patient's left side, but this is purely operator-dependent. This may be impossible to achieve if working in a small transport vehicle, helicopter or other small working space. Positioning and anatomic considerations vary depending on the view you are attempting to obtain, but several broad parameters apply. The axis of the heart can vary depending on both a patient's overall phenotype and presence of chronic cardiac disease. Tall and thin people tend to have a more vertical long axis, whereas short and obese people tend to have a more horizontal long axis. Additionally, it is worth mentioning that some of the more common chronic cardiac diseases cause a more horizontal axis, such as those with left ventricular hypertrophy due to chronic hypertension. Feeling for the PMI can guide the practitioner in determining apex location and overall axis.

Various positioning methods can be used to increase the viewing window and bring the heart closer to the probe thereby improving image quality. Having a patient put their left arm over their head will broaden the rib spaces, and thus increase the size of several desired scanning windows. Placing the patient in the left lateral decubitus position will allow the heart to be in a more dependent position, which is closer to the chest wall and thus the probe. This can improve all of the cardiac views, but is best for the apical view in particular. Lastly, having a patient inhale or exhale while scanning can facilitate viewing. For instance, inhaling while attempting a subxiphoid view may allow for better alignment of the liver in front of the probe, thus allowing a clearer acoustic window through which to view the heart. In contrast, parasternal and apical views are often improved with exhalation. This can become more important in patients with certain pulmonary pathologies, such as COPD, where exhaling significantly decreases the amount of interference caused by air. These and more view-specific image optimization techniques will be reviewed within each section.

Standard Echocardiographic Views

Parasternal Views

In the two parasternal views, a rib space directly next to the patient's left sternal border is used as a window between bones to view the heart from its anterior surface. There is usually no lung parenchyma between the transducer and heart to cause interference or scattering in this area.

The patient can be supine or in left lateral decubitus position. It may be helpful to have the patient put their left arm behind their head in order to expand rib space and thus widen the window. In these views, respiratory variation will have minimal effect.

Long Axis

The parasternal long axis (PSLA) view is the workhorse for cardiac imaging. It is often the easiest view to obtain and is the view that offers the most diagnostic information. It is very good for evaluating global left ventricular contractility and estimating ejection fraction. It gives information on right ventricular size. This view is also good for obtaining measurements of the left atrium and aortic root. The left atrium may be enlarged in heart failure, mitral regurgitation, and other pathologies. The aortic root can become enlarged in aortic root aneurysm and in some aortic dissections. Evaluating presence of pericardial effusion can also be done in this view, with the presence of posterior fluid being much more sensitive for a true effusion.

To obtain the parasternal long axis view, the probe marker should be oriented towards the patient's right shoulder. The transducer should initially be placed in the

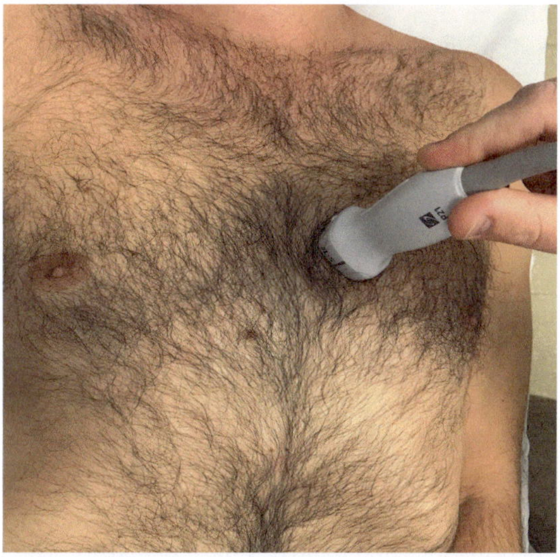

Fig. 1 Parasternal long transducer placement. The transducer is placed on the anterior chest wall at the second or third intercostal space, to the left of the sternum, with the transducer marker towards the patient's right shoulder

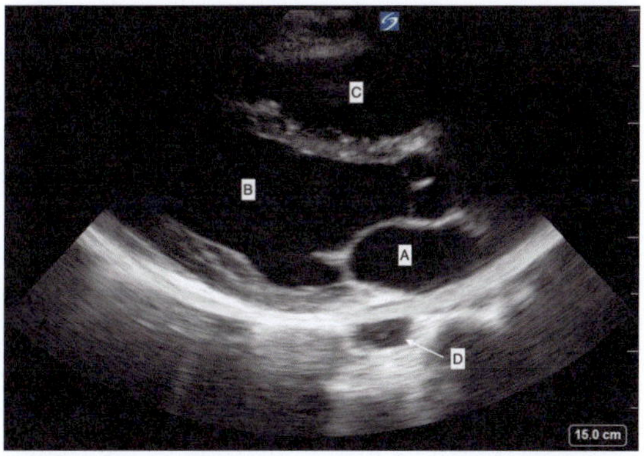

Fig. 2 Parasternal long view. Parasternal long cardiac view in between cardiac cycles with both mitral and aortic valves closed. Blood flows from the left atrium (**a**) through the mitral valve, into the left ventricle (**b**), and out to the body through the aortic valve. The right ventricle is can be see at the top of the screen (**c**). The descending thoracic aorta is posterior to the heart (**d**)

third or fourth intercostal space (Fig. 1). Depending on the patient, moving superiorly or inferiorly by 1–2 rib spaces will be necessary to find the optimal view. As its name suggests, this view is truly parasternal, as the probe should be a maximum of 2 cm from the left sternal border. The probe may need to be fanned or rocked in order to align the probe most closely with the long axis of the heart.

On the imaging display, the apex of the heart will be oriented towards the left side of the screen, and the base of the heart to the right (Fig. 2). The right ventricle will located at the top of the screen. Beneath it, and towards the left side of the screen will be the left ventricle. In a properly oriented image, the left ventricular outflow tract (LVOT), aortic valve, and aortic root should be visible. The left atrium will be beneath the aortic root and to the right of the left ventricle. The anterior and posterior leaflets of the mitral valve should be visible. The proper depth is achieved when a cross-sectional view of the descending aorta is visible posterior to the pericardium.

Once the parasternal long view is appropriately obtained, there are several pieces of information that can be quickly gathered to produce highly useful information about the functional status of the heart: global ventricular function or ejection fraction estimate, which includes mitral valve assessment; the presence of pericardial effusion; and the relative sizes of the RV, LVOT and LA as they relate to each other. When oriented appropriately the RV, ascending aorta, and LA should be approximately the same size in the PSLA. Any violation of this rule usually indicates a pathologic process, such as RV enlargement, aortic root aneurysm, or heart failure.

Short Axis

The parasternal short axis (PSSA) is particularly good at detecting localized wall abnormalities and relative ventricular sizes. The window used for the PSSA will be the same intercostal space location as PSLA, just lateral to left sternal border. The same patient positioning will apply for both parasternal views (supine or left lateral decubitus). In the short axis view, however, the probe marker points towards the patient's left shoulder (Fig. 3). This is most often obtained just after the PSLA, so rotating the transducer 90 degrees clockwise from right shoulder to left shoulder provides the starting point for obtaining this image.

Three distinct planes of the short axis are commonly used in cardiac ultrasound, each achieved by a different degree of fanning along the heart's long axis. In all views, the right side of the heart is at the top left of the screen and the left ventricle is more centrally located, and should appear circular in an appropriately oriented image. The views are discussed in order from base to apex. When fanned towards the base, a view at the level of the aortic valve can be achieved. In this view the aortic valve will be just to the right of the right atrium, centrally located. A normal tri-leaflet aortic valve will look like a "Mercedes Benz sign." At the deepest part of

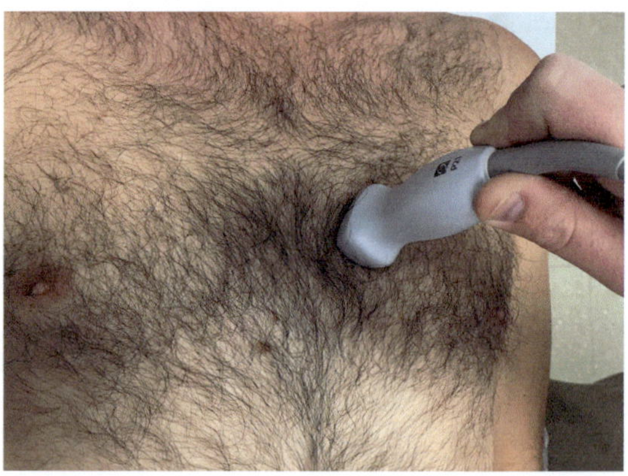

Fig. 3 Parasternal short transducer placement. From the long axis position, the transducer is rotated approximately 90 degrees clockwise so the marker points towards the patient's left shoulder

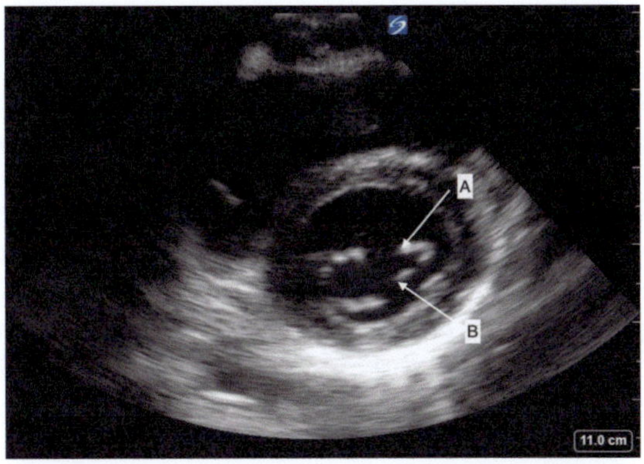

Fig. 4 Mitral valve "fish mouth" in parasternal short view. Mitral valve parasternal short view displaying the "fish mouth" of the mitral valve in short axis. The anterior leaflet (**a**) can be seen above the posterior leaflet (**b**)

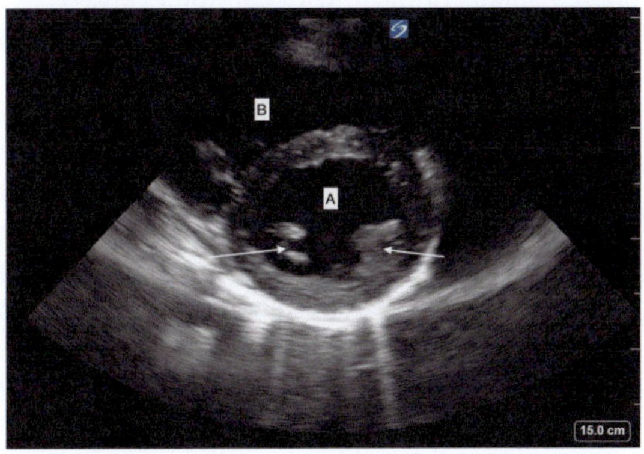

Fig. 5 Parasternal short view. Parasternal short cardiac view at the level of the papillary muscles (arrows). LV cavity (**a**) is circular, not elongated or ovoid. The RV cavity (**b**) can be seen in upper left

the screen, most posteriorly, the left ventricle should be visible. Moving towards the apex, the next view should be at the level of the mitral valve. In this view, the mitral valve is seen in the center of the LV (Fig. 4). The RV is anterior and slightly to the left on the screen. Lastly, when the probe is tilted slightly towards the apex, the LV is viewed in cross-section at the level of the papillary muscles, located at approximately 4 and 8 o'clock on the circular LV (Fig. 5).

The PSSA can be used to evaluate for global ventricular function as well as localized wall motion abnormalities. The LV should move in a concentric fashion during systole. Any gross deviation from that synchronized concentric contraction may represent acute ischemia, old infarct, or electrical rhythm abnormalities such as bundle branch blocks. The relative size of the ventricles is easily approximated in this view as well. The normal ratio of RV to LV is 0.6–1 [3]. When the RV starts to approach or exceed the size of the LV it is indicative of a pathologic process such as acute pulmonary embolism (PE) or chronic pulmonary hypertension (pHTN). If the right sided pressures are high enough, it may cause the septal wall to "bow" outward into the LV, causing the LV to transition from circular appearing to "D-shaped." Additionally, pericardial fluid will be apparent in this view, especially as the heart is fanned through apex to base.

Apical Four Chamber

The apical four chamber view (A4) of the heart images all four chambers of the heart at the same time, as viewed from the apex as its name suggests. It is ideal for directly comparing the right to left sides of the heart, evaluating both LV and RV systolic function, and evaluating for pericardial effusion and tamponade.

The apical four chamber view is the most technically difficult view to obtain, especially for novice providers. While this view can be obtained in a supine patient, the left lateral decubitus position typically will produce superior images as it brings the apex of the heart closer to the chest wall. This view can be obtained in several ways. Often, the probe can be placed in an intercostal space 1–2 cm inferior to the nipple near the PMI, and adjusted accordingly to optimize image (Fig. 6). The optimal position may be more medial in thinner patients, and more laterally located in obese patients or those with cardiomegaly.

This view can also be obtained starting from the PSSA. From the PSSA, the probe can be slid towards the apex, while rotating it slightly in a clockwise position, until the apex is reached. At this point, the probe is fanned to point back towards the base of the heart. This method keeps the heart in view during the transition from PSSA to A4 and may be easier for novice providers. Lastly, palpating for the point of maximal impulse will help guide probe placement, as this typically corresponds with the closest point the left ventricle is to the surface of the skin. In the apical four chamber view, the probe marker will be towards the patient's left side, usually aimed between posterior axilla and elbow.

The ideal apical 4-chamber view will have the apex pointing directly at the transducer, with the septum vertically-oriented, directly in the middle of the screen so that the right side of the heart is on the left side of the screen and vice versa (Fig. 7). The left ventricle will be on the right side of the screen with the left atrium located below it. The right atrium will be located below the right ventricle farther from the probe surface, and the left atrium in a similar position below the left ventricle.

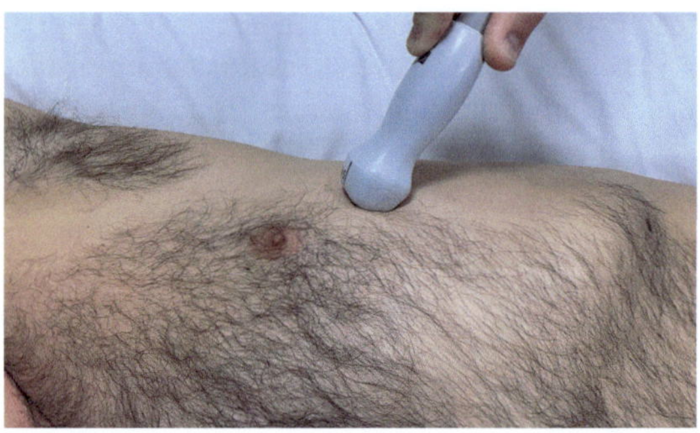

Fig. 6 Apical four chamber transducer placement. The transducer is placed near the point of maximal impulse (PMI) with the marker pointed towards the patient's left elbow

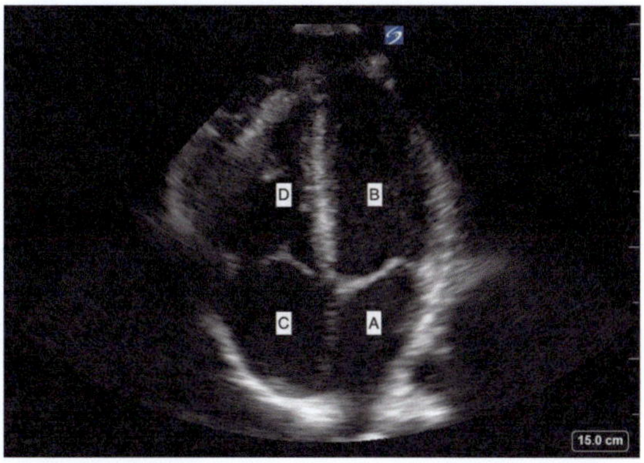

Fig. 7 Apical four chamber view. Apical four chamber view in systole, with apex of the heart located at the top of the screen, base located at the bottom. Ideal orientation is with septal wall (between **d** and **b**) located in vertical orientation, perpendicular to the face of the cardiac transducer. The cardiac chambers are as follows: left atrium (**a**), left ventricle (**b**), right atrium (**c**) and right ventricle (**d**)

Subxiphoid

The subxiphoid view takes a different approach from those previously discussed. In this view, the heart is viewed from the epigastrum, just below the xiphoid process. This approach uses the liver as an acoustic window through which to view the heart from its diaphragmatic surface. By using the liver, a large homogenously echogenic organ, the probe avoids interference from aerated lung and bowel gas. This is typically the view used to evaluated the heart during the eFAST exam. It is helpful in evaluating for pericardial effusion or tamponade and evaluating the inferior vena cava (IVC).

The patient should be supine. Flexing the knees will allow the abdominal musculature to relax and allow for more pressure to be applied with the probe, which may be necessary in more obese patients. Asking the patient to inhale may optimize view by bringing both the liver and the heart more inferior and therefore closer to the transducer.

The cardiac probe marker should be directed to the patient's left and the probe should angled such that it is pointed upward into the chest cavity (Fig. 8). It may be necessary to point the probe slightly towards the patient's left flank, or slide the probe to the patient's right in order to better utilize the liver as an acoustic window.

In this view, the liver will be anterior to the heart, at the top of the screen (Fig. 9). The apex of the heart will be up and to the right of the screen, in contrast to the apical views, in which the apex will be pointed directly at the transducer. The right ventricle will be closest to the transducer after the liver. The left ventricle and left atrium will then be more posterior to the right heart.

To view the IVC from this position, rotate the probe 90-degrees counterclockwise so that the marker dot is oriented cranially (Fig. 10). Then, slide the probe slightly to the right of the patient's midline. A sagittal view of IVC will be posterior to the liver at this angle, and will be seen entering the R atrium on the right side of the screen (Fig. 11). The IVC is usually 1.5–2 cm in anterior-posterior diameter at

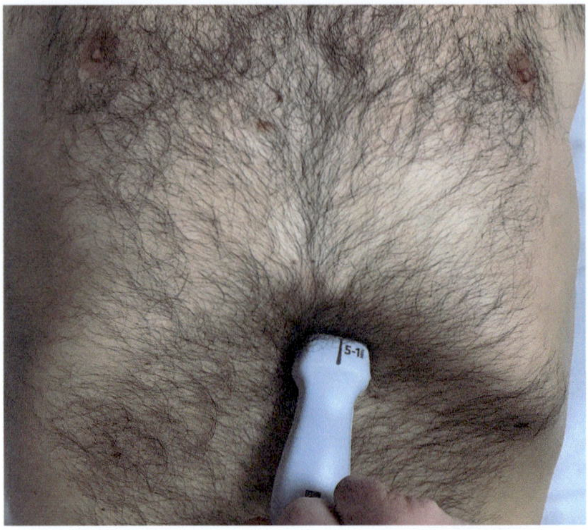

Fig. 8 Subxiphoid transducer placement. The transducer is placed just below the xiphoid process with the marker pointed towards the patient's left

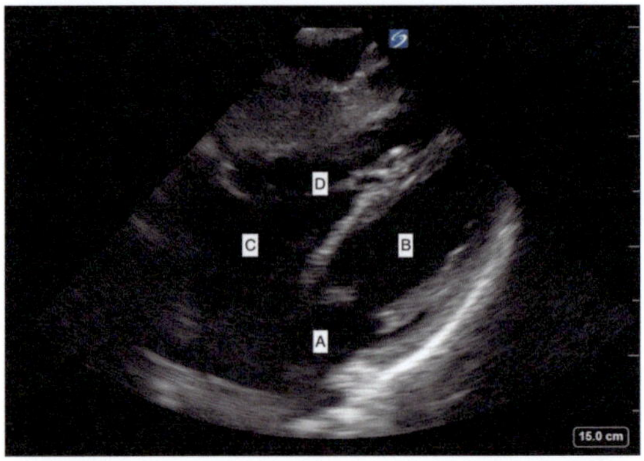

Fig. 9 Subxiphoid view. The subxiphoid cardiac view demonstrates the heart viewed through the acoustic window of the liver. Cardiac chambers are identified as follows: left atrium (**a**), left ventricle (**b**), right atrium (**c**), right ventricle (**d**)

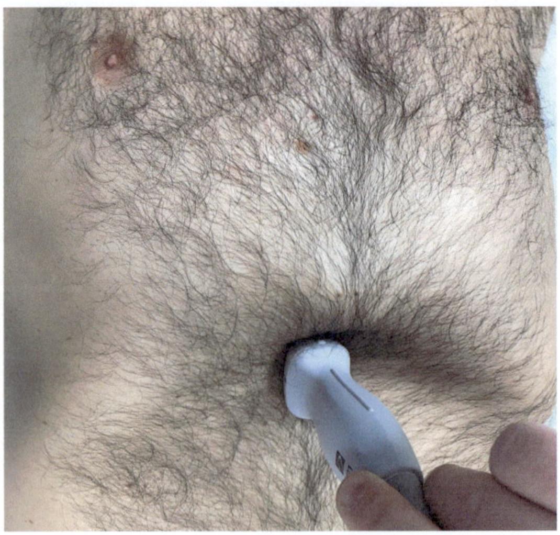

Fig. 10 IVC transducer placement. The transducer is placed just below the xiphoid process, slightly to the right of midline, with the marker pointed towards the patient's head

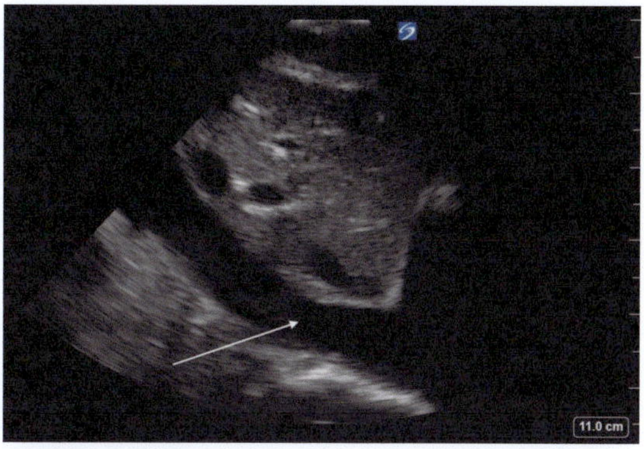

Fig. 11 IVC. The inferior vena cava is demonstrated in long axis passing through the liver and emptying into the right atrium

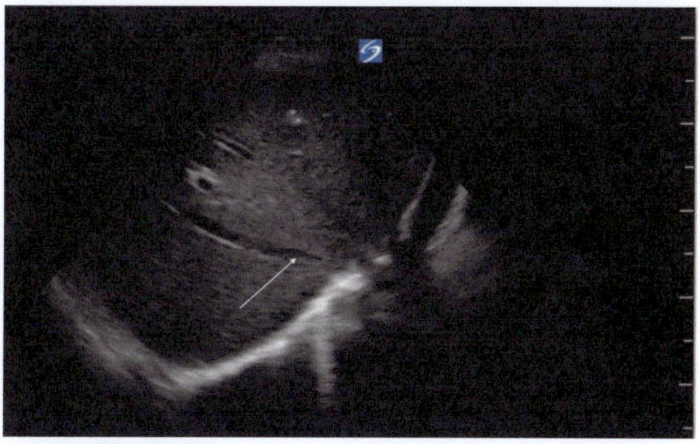

Fig. 12 Collapsed IVC. Collapsed IVC (arrow) passing through the liver on its course to the right atrium. At times, a collapsed IVC can be so small it can be difficult to identify

normal maximum dilation. This is measured 3–4 cm distal from its entrance to the R atrium [3].

The size of the thin-walled IVC usually varies with respirations, collapsing with inspiration and dilating with expiration. A quick visualization of the IVC can provide rapid information into both a patient's cardiac function and volume status. A patient who is hypovolemic may have a small or mostly collapsed IVC (Fig. 12). A patient with an obstructive pathology such as tamponade or pulmonary embolism may have a dilated IVC with minimal respiratory variation (Fig. 13).

Suprasternal

The suprasternal view is a quick and effective way to evaluate for evidence of an aortic dissection. It is fairly specific for this process if it is visualized, but not a sensitive test. Therefore, it should not be considered a "rule-out" examination. In this view, the probe is placed in the suprasternal notch with the probe marker facing towards the left and the probe face pointed downwards into the chest. The probe should be angled as anteriorly as possible. In order to accomplish this, it may be beneficial to tilt the head of the bed to 30 degrees, or even have the patient sit

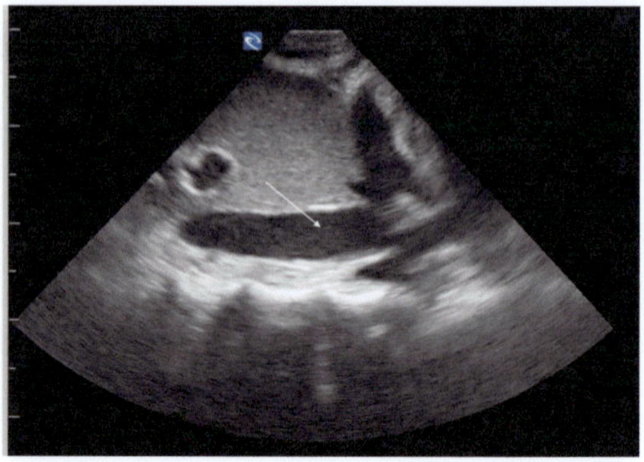

Fig. 13 Dilated IVC. Dilated IVC (arrow) passing through the liver and emptying into the right atrium

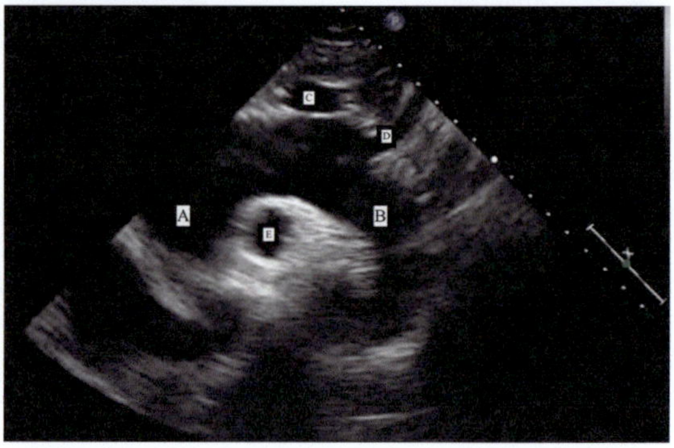

Fig. 14 Suprasternal Notch. The suprasternal notch view shows the ascending (**a**) and descending (**b**) thoracic aorta, with the aortic arch located in between. Also visible here are the brachiocephalic vein (**c**), left carotid artery (**d**), and right pulmonary vein (**e**)

upright and have them extend their neck. The depth of the image will need to be decreased significantly compared to all other cardiac windows.

The aortic arch will be visible with the ascending aorta on the left side of the screen and the descending aorta on the right side of the screen (Fig. 14). From screen left to right, the origins of the brachiocephalic artery, left carotid, and left subclavian arteries will be visible. Beneath the aortic arch, a cross section of the right pulmonary artery will be visible as well.

Pathology

Decreased Left Ventricular Ejection Fraction

Ejection fraction (EF) refers to the percentage of blood volume in the left ventricle that is forced out of the left ventricle into systemic circulation with each systolic contraction. This is the clinical index that is used to evaluate myocardial contractility, and thus offers clinical evidence regarding the overall function of the heart [4]. In general, an EF between 55–65% is considered normal, 45–55% is mildly reduced, 35–45% is moderately reduced, and severely reduced is less than

35%. Heart failure can be classified in several different ways, but the most common way is to dichotomize it into two categories: systolic heart failure or heart failure with reduced ejection fraction (HFrEF) and diastolic heart failure or heart failure with preserved ejection fraction (HFpEF). Systolic heart failure refers to the ability of the LV to contract and squeeze blood out of the heart. Diastolic heart failure refers to the ability for the LV to relax and fill with blood. Systolic heart failure can be related to several causes, including dilated cardiomyopathy (Fig. 15), hypertrophic cardiomyopathy (Fig. 16), severe hypertension and even myocardial infarction. Using ultrasound to evaluate diastolic heart failure is beyond the scope of this text.

The global left ventricular function can be easily assessed by simple visual estimation. In fact, this qualitative assessment has been shown to be as accurate in determining ejection fraction as formal measurements in studies comparing cardiologists to learners with basic training [5]. In order to make this qualitative assessment, three separate estimates should be assimilated. First, during systole the myocardium of the left ventricle should appear to thicken uniformly and the LV chamber size should decrease as blood is pumped out of the heart. If the chamber size appears to reduce by more than 50% then it can be considered normal. If the

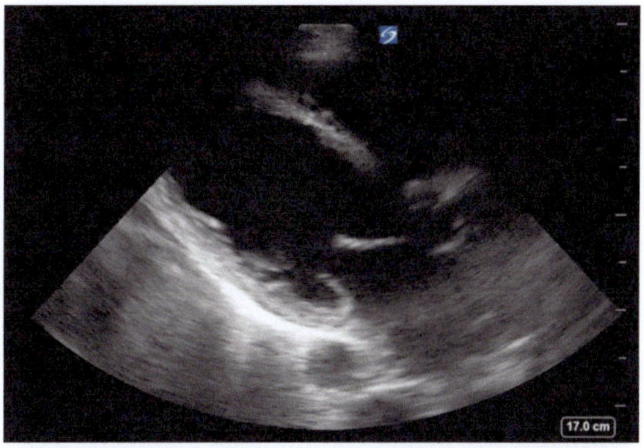

Fig. 15 Dilated cardiomyopathy. Parasternal long axis image demonstrating ballooning of the left ventricle typical of dilated cardiomyopathy

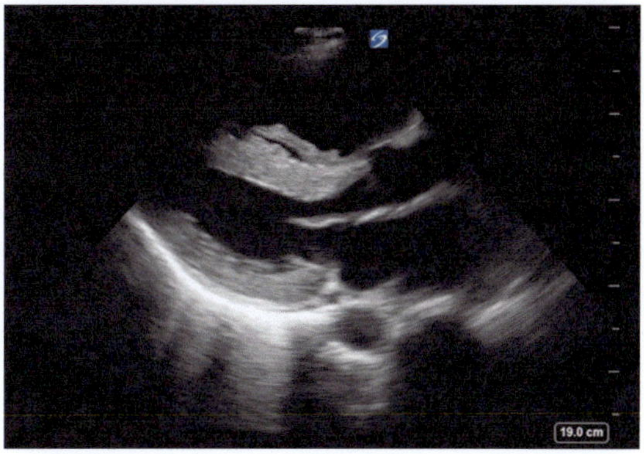

Fig. 16 Hypertrophic cardiomyopathy. Parasternal long axis image demonstrating uniform thickening of the left ventricular walls indicating hypertrophic cardiomyopathy

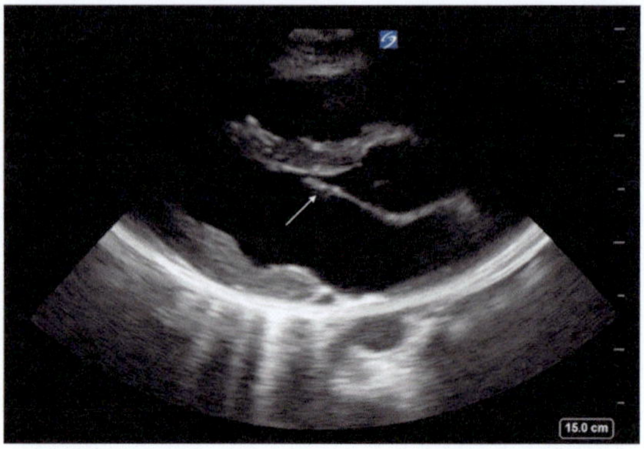

Fig. 17 Mitral valve leaflet touching septum. Parasternal long axis image showing the anterior leaflet of the mitral valve (arrow) touching septum during diastole, which is the common state associated with normal ejection fraction

LV is determined to be squeezing less than 50%, then it is helpful to determine which broad category of systolic heart failure is occurring: mildly reduced, moderately reduced or severely reduced [3]. This is especially critical in patients with no history of heart failure, or in those with severe symptoms who may be experiencing an acute change in heart function, as in a congestive heart failure (CHF) exacerbation. This takes some experience and more focused training, but the same principles apply: visually estimate the percentage change of the left ventricular size.

Next, the contractility and volume status of LV can be estimated by looking at the motion of the anterior mitral valve leaflet. In a healthy individual, the anterior leaflet should closely approach or even touch the septal wall during LV filling (Fig. 17). If there is limited motion of the anterior leaflet, it may indicate that the LV is "congested," i.e., the volume of the ventricle is abnormally high after systole. When this is visually difficult to determine, this motion can be easily mapped in M-mode by placing the scan line over the leaflet tip. Formally, this measurement is termed the end-point septal separation (EPSS). A measurement greater than 7 mm is indicative of moderate to severely reduced ejection fraction [3].

Finally, the mitral annulus at the posterior leaflet should be examined for motion. Normally, the leaflet should have vigorous right to left movement across the screen as the LV contracts during systole and pulls the mitral annulus towards the apex. Little or no movement can indicate poor contractility, and may be a further clue that systolic dysfunction is present.

Using these criteria, the practitioner can develop a qualitative sense of the overall systolic function of the left ventricle. This information is critical to the overall evaluation of the heart. In the setting of an unstable patient, including those with hypotension and/or dyspnea, this evaluation is a crucial first step in determining the root cause. Finding acute heart failure during prehospital evaluation may prompt the provider to escalate care, including the initiation of vasopressors for those with severe hypotension, or positive pressure ventilation for those in severe respiratory distress.

RV Enlargement

Pulmonary embolism causing shock, syncope or vital sign instability is a true emergency with high degree of mortality, yet prompt recognition can sometimes be difficult. The insidious nature of pulmonary embolisms are perhaps their most well-known feature. Dyspnea with normal breath sounds, no clearly defining EKG changes, and no obvious radiographic abnormalities make prompt diagnosis challenging. Only approximately 50% of patients with PE have any complaint of chest pain. In fact, 50% of patients with first time PE will have normal vital signs [6]. However, ultrasonographic detection of acute RV enlargement and strain is highly sensitive for detection of PEs that cause hemodynamic compromise. It is worth noting that chronic pulmonary hypertension can result in right heart strain, but this is typically associated with right ventricular remodeling and hypertrophy, distinguishing it from acute RV dysfunction related to embolism. This section focuses on acute right heart strain due to pulmonary embolism.

Normally, the pressure in the systemic circulatory system is much higher than that in the pulmonary system. Therefore, during systole, the pressure that the LV needs to generate to pump blood against that high systemic pressure is far greater than that in the RV. For example, normal peak systolic measurements of the left and right ventricles are approximately 120 mmHg and 25 mmHg respectively [1]. A similar relationship exists in the atria.

In the case of a pulmonary embolism, the normally low-resistance, high-flow pulmonary vasculature system suddenly becomes obstructed, increasing the RV afterload, or the pressure it has to pump against, significantly. As a result, the systolic and diastolic pressures of the in the right side of heart increase as well. The increased RV afterload can sometimes be so significant as to cause obstructive shock and cardiac arrest. This rise in pressure will manifest itself on echocardiography in several ways.

The relative size of the RV cavity compared to the LV cavity is readily obtained in several views discussed in this text including the parasternal short axis and apical four chamber. A normal ratio is 0.6–1 [3]. The RV can be considered enlarged anytime it starts to exceed this ratio, and certainly if it meets or exceeds the size of the LV. In the PSLA, an enlarged RV may be visible as an elongated RV with flattened interventricular septum (Fig. 18); however, relative ventricular cavity size comparisons are best performed in the PSSA and A4 views [3].

The elevated RV pressures seen in right heart strain can be very prominent during systole, and manifest in ventricular cavity size changes. This can be seen as a flattening of the interventricular septum, resulting in the LV appearing as D-shaped, rather than circular in the PSSA view (Fig. 19). If the relative pressure difference between the two ventricles is even more pronounced, there can even be a "bowing" of the interventricular septum into the LV cavity.

The apical four chamber view is the most accurate in determining the relative sizes of right and left ventricles. Occasionally, off-axis images taken in the other

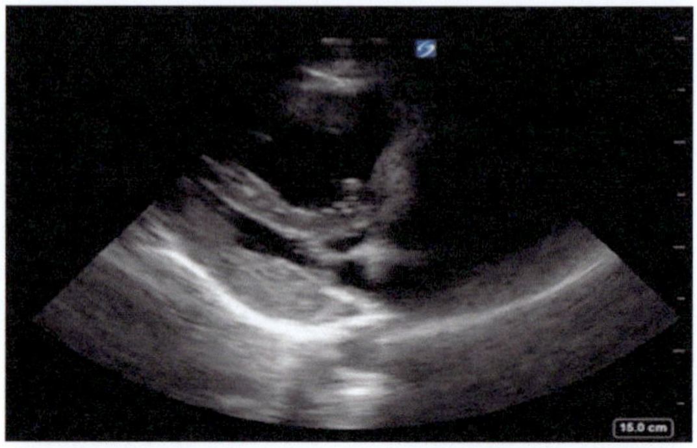

Fig. 18 Parasternal long axis, dilated right ventricle. Parasternal long axis image showing a severely dilated right ventricle with associated left ventricular collapse

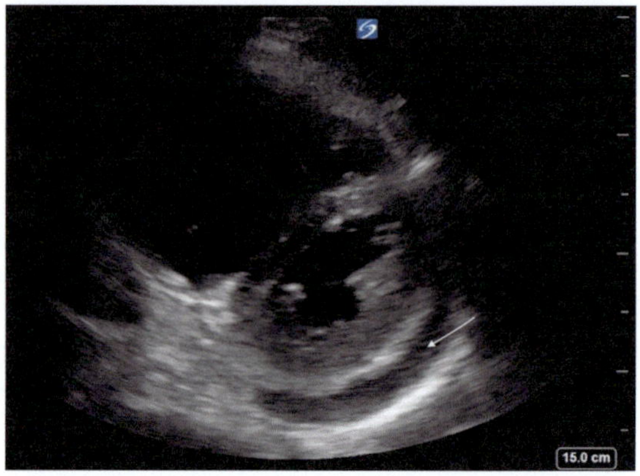

Fig. 19 Parasternal short axis – dilated right ventricle. Parasternal short axis image showing an enlarged right ventricle when compared to the left. This results in septal bowing towards the left ventricle that causes it to appear "D-shaped." Small effusion is denoted by an arrow

cardiac views may give the RV an enlarged appearance, wherein the apical four chamber view removes that potential deception. In this view, the LV should always appear larger than the RV under normal circumstances (Fig. 7). In the case of acute PE, the RV can appear enlarged, which typically indicates a sizable clot burden (Fig. 20). In addition to RV size and septal wall abnormalities, the free wall of the right ventricle may show little to no movement as it struggles to contract against the elevated pressure, best seen in the apical four chamber view. When this occurs the movement of the apex is often spared. This is termed McConnell's sign, and can be used to differentiate acute right heart strain from chronic changes. Chronic right heart strain will result in remodeling of the RV, and the free wall will become hypertrophied and relatively more mobile.

Evaluation of flow across the tricuspid valve is a more advanced mechanism to evaluate for elevated right ventricular systolic pressures (RVSP). When blood flow is obstructed from moving forward in the case of a large PE, not only does the RVSP increase but it causes backwards flow from the ventricle into the atrium, termed tricuspid regurgitation or insufficiency. This can be detected by placing a Doppler color box in the right atrium and looking for flow jets. Qualitatively, a jet flowing from the ventricle into the atrium that reaches the opposite atrial wall is considered severe regurgitation. The quantitative method then requires the continuous wave

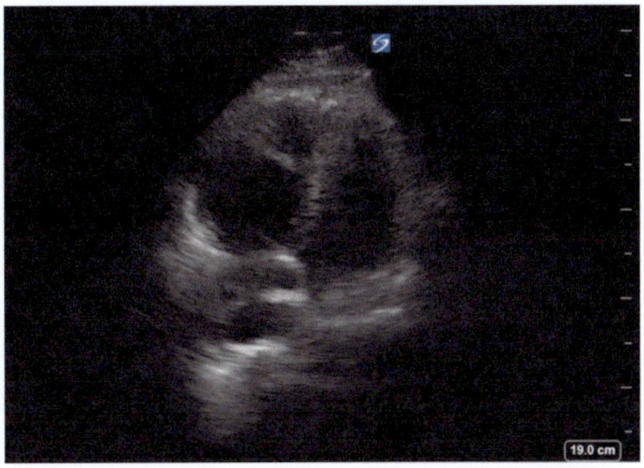

Fig. 20 Apical four chamber – dilated right ventricle. Apical four chamber image showing RV:LV ratio of greater than 1:1, indicating severe RV dilation

Doppler gate be placed in that regurgitant jet to determine actual flow velocities, a more advanced step.

Pericardial Effusion & Cardiac Tamponade

The space between the pericardium and epicardium usually has a very small amount of physiologic fluid that acts to lubricate the heart as it contracts. Normally, that small amount of fluid is less than 50 ml and is undetectable by ultrasound [3]. However, there are many different pathologic conditions that can cause the amount of fluid to build up. When the amount of fluid is significant enough to restrict the physiologic function of the heart, the terminology changes from simple pericardial effusion to cardiac tamponade.

There are many widely varying conditions that can result in a pericardial effusion. The more commonly encountered causes include pericarditis (which itself has many potential causes including infectious and autoimmune), direct injury to the heart in the form of trauma, neoplastic disease, myocardial infarction, many rheumatologic conditions, and renal disease. Depending on the source, pericardial fluid can be hyperechoic, such as in the case of clotted blood or purulence; or it can be hypoechoic, such as most uremic or malignant effusions.

The size of a pericardial effusion is graded by measuring the separation between the epicardium and pericardium. A small effusion is less than 0.5 cm (Fig. 21), a moderate effusion measures between 0.5 and 2 cm (Fig. 22), and a large effusion is greater than 2 cm (Fig. 23) [7, 8]. Two centimeters of separation corresponds to approximately 500 mL of fluid [3].

The heart may have a prominent anterior fat pad located in the anterior precordial space of the right ventricle that is often mistaken for fluid in the PSLA view (Fig. 24). If there is no anechoic substance in the posterior or dependent portion of the pericardial space, or if the anterior anechoic substance appears heterogenous, this is most likely fat [3]. This epicardial fat pad is most common in females, elderly, obese people and diabetics [1].

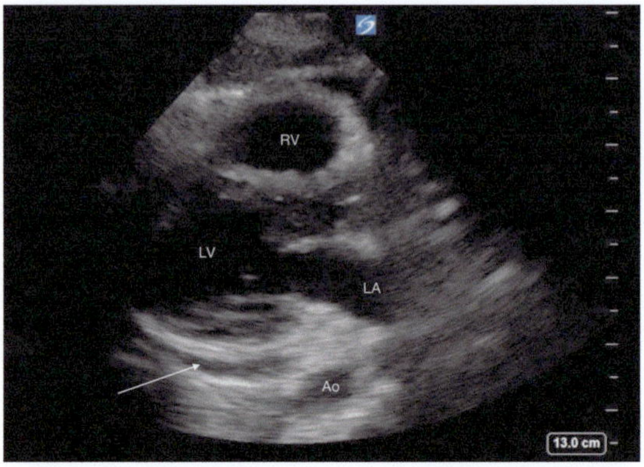

Fig. 21 Small pericardial effusion. Small pericardial effusion (arrow) seen in parasternal long view during diastole. Note the fluid extending anterior to the descending thoracic aorta, differentiating it from pleural effusion. Small effusions typically measure less than 0.5 cm

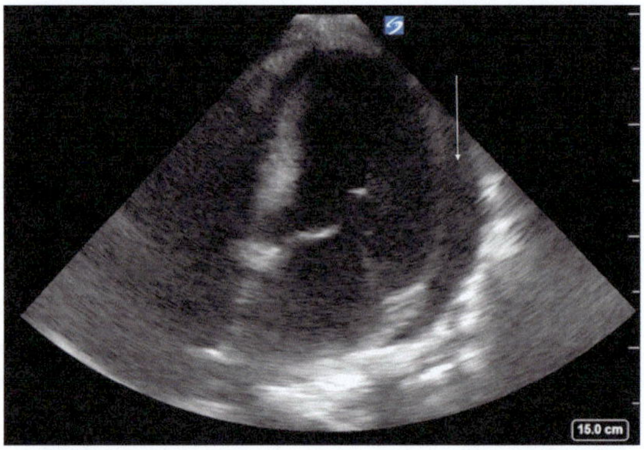

Fig. 22 Moderate pericardial effusion. Moderate sized pericardial effusion (arrow) seen in an apical four chamber view

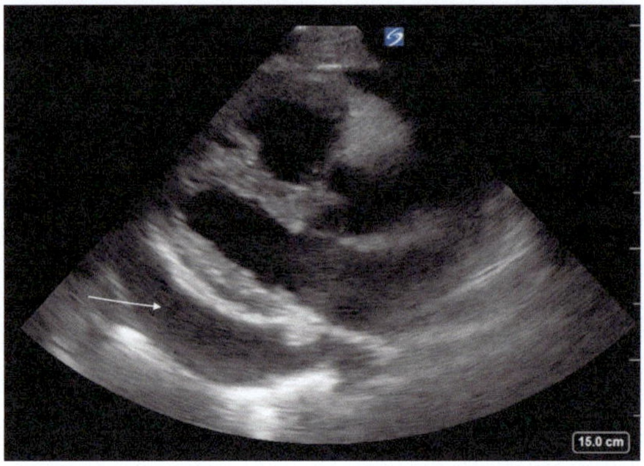

Fig. 23 Large pericardial effusion. A large-sized pericardial effusion is noted here in this parasternal long view. Large pericardial effusions typically measure greater than 2 cm

The pericardium is a semi-flexible sac. It can stretch to accommodate a large amount of fluid if it accumulates at a slow rate, over weeks to months. However, an effusion that accumulates rapidly can cause acute hemodynamic compromise with a much lower fluid burden. Cardiac tamponade occurs when the amount of fluid in the pericardium creates pressure that compromises the ability for the heart to fill with blood. This is a form of obstructive shock.

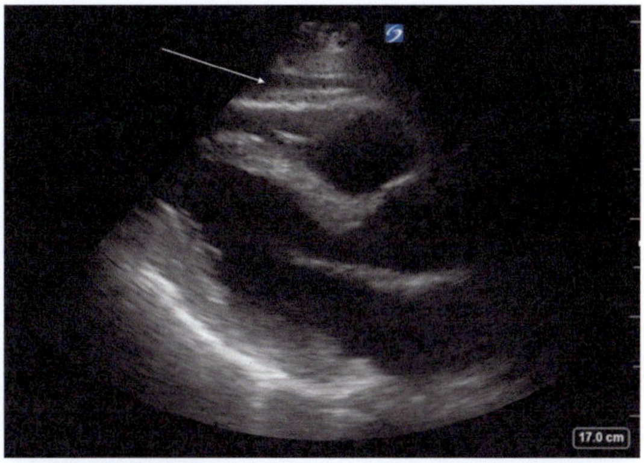

Fig. 24 Epicardial fat pad. An epicardial fat pad may be present anterior to the right ventricle and can be very similar in appearance to a small pericardial effusion in a parasternal long view, often they can be indistinguishable. However, small pericardial effusions will typically be seen posterior to the left ventricle and an epicardial fat pad will be seen anterior to the right ventricle

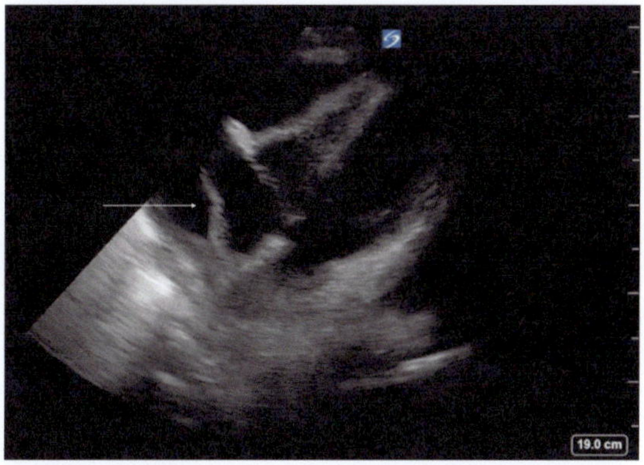

Fig. 25 Right atrial collapse in tamponade. Right atrial collapse (arrow) in pericardial tamponade, demonstrated in the subxiphoid view. This is the most sensitive sign for pericardial tamponade

Because the right side of the heart typically operates under lower pressures, it is susceptible to the inward force of the pericardial fluid before the left side of the heart. Therefore, we use the apical four chamber and subxiphoid views to evaluate for tamponade as they give the best visualization of the right heart. In echocardiography, tamponade is defined as RA collapse during systole and RV collapse during diastole. Right atrial collapse during systole, when it should be filling with blood, is the most sensitive sign for cardiac tamponade as it will usually occur first (Fig. 25) [8]. Diastolic collapse of the RV, its filling phase, is the more specific sign for tamponade and can be easier to detect (Fig. 26).

The IVC should also be evaluated in suspected tamponade. Similar to PE, another common form of obstructive shock, the IVC will be dilated and lack respiratory variation as forward flow of blood is compromised (Fig. 13).

When imaging the heart in PSLA, one common pitfall is to mistake a left-sided pleural effusion for a pericardial effusion. The key distinguishing factor in this view is the relationship of the fluid to the descending thoracic aorta. In both cases, fluid will be posterior to the left ventricle, but a pericardial effusion will track anterior to the descending aorta, whereas a left-sided pleural effusion will stop abruptly at the aorta (Fig. 27).

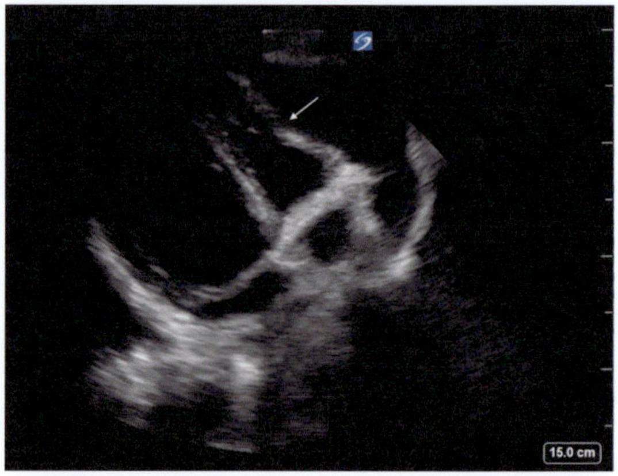

Fig. 26 Right ventricular collapse in tamponade. Right ventricular collapse (arrow) during ventricular filling is seen in this subxiphoid view of pericardial tamponade. This is the most specific sign for pericardial tamponade

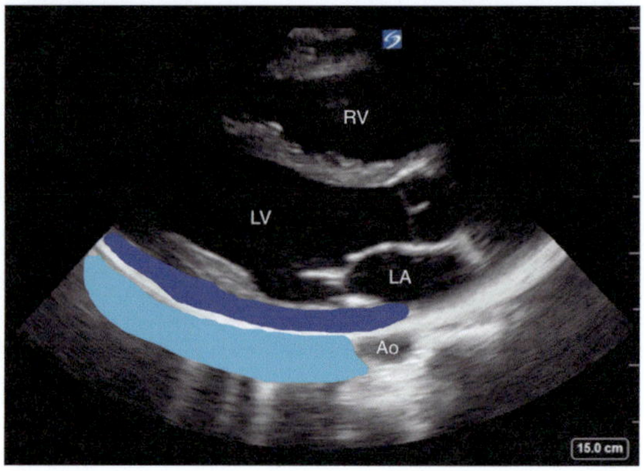

Fig. 27 Pericardial effusion vs. left sided pleural effusion. This parasternal long view demonstrates the distinguishing features of the relative locations where pericardial effusions (dark blue) and pleural effusions (light blue) would appear. Notice the pericardial effusion will travel anterior to the descending aorta, whereas the pleural effusion will not

Pericardiocentesis, draining of the pericardial effusion, should be done emergently in those patients with severe hemodynamic compromise or arrest. Ultrasound can be used to located the largest pocket of fluid to make drainage safer. This may be in the subxiphoid location, as is most commonly taught for this procedure, but an intercostal approach can be considered as well.

Regional Wall Motion Abnormality

Both acute and chronic myocardial ischemia and infarction can cause localized wall motion abnormalities in the region supplied by the affected coronary artery. The area of severely ischemic or infarcted myocardium will not contract, and therefore will appear as asymmetrical or lacking movement during systole. Such asymmetries may be visible in any view, but is most apparent using the PSSA, as this transverse view of the ventricles allows for evaluation of concentric movements almost continuously from base to apex. Areas of chronic ischemia or old infarctions will usually be thinner compared to neighboring regions, due to replacement of myocardium

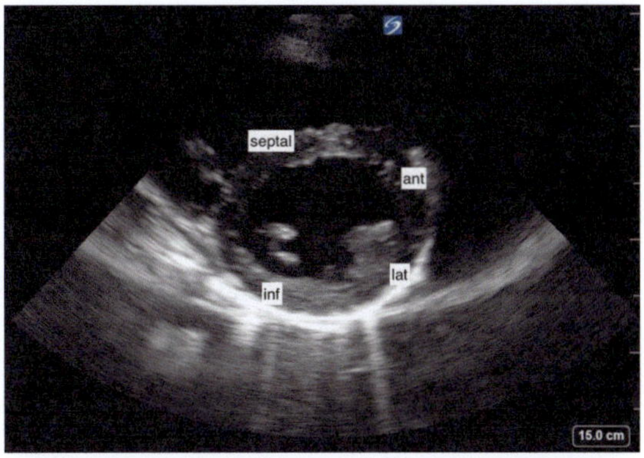

Fig. 28 Walls of LV labeled in parasternal short. Parasternal short cardiac view at the level of the papillary muscles showing the relative wall sections

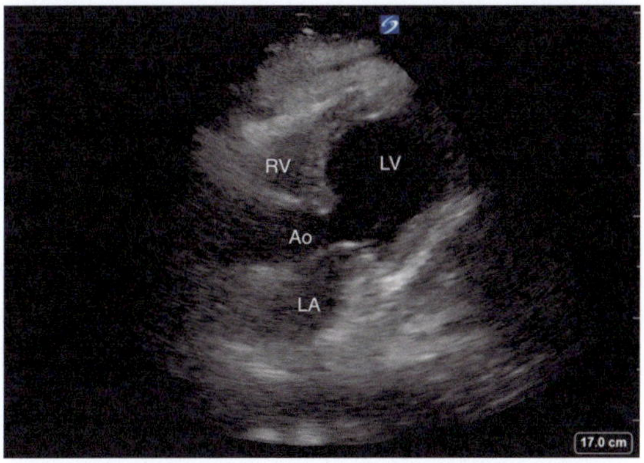

Fig. 29 Takotsubo Cardiomyopathy. Note the isolated apical dilation of the left ventricle (LV) in this subxiphoid view of Takotsubo cardiomyopathy, named after the Japanese word for octopus trap

by fibrotic scar tissue. In contrast, with acute infarctions there will be no difference in thickness of the myocardium at rest, though it will not contract and thicken during systole. EKG is the gold standard for evaluating for myocardial infarction, but in an austere environment in which EKGs or cardiac biomarker testing is not readily available, ultrasound may be the only diagnostic tool. Classically, EKG leads I, aVL, V5, and V6 refer to the lateral wall; leads II, III, and aVF refer to the inferior wall; leads V1-V2 refer to the septal wall; and leads V2-V4 refer to the anterior wall (Fig. 28). In patients in whom EKG findings are difficult to interpret, echocardiography may be useful in confirming suspected infarction. In other environments, ultrasound may be the only diagnostic tool for diagnosing acute myocardial ischemia in those patients with concerning chest pain or similar symptoms.

A rare condition called Takotsubo cardiomyopathy causes acute reversible apical or mid-chamber hypokinesis of the left ventricle. Takotsubo presents with similar symptoms to ACS. EKG findings typically include significant ST elevation of lateral leads, although without reciprocal depression. Otherwise known as stress cardiomyopathy, the ultrasonographic hallmark of this disorder is wall motion abnormalities that do not follow the distribution of any one coronary artery, making the left ventricle appear to balloon out at its apex (Fig. 29). While early recognition is helpful, this condition is treated as a STEMI until proven otherwise by cardiologists.

Aortic Dissection

An aortic dissection occurs when severely elevated blood pressure creates a tear in the arterial wall into which high pressure blood flows, creating a channel between the layers of the arterial wall known as a false lumen. This false passageway can obstruct arterial flow to branches off the aorta, extend into branches off the aorta, obstruct flow to the distal aorta, and even rupture. Aortic dissections are most commonly classified into Stanford Type A and Type B based on the origin of the false lumen. Type A dissections originate in the ascending aorta and involve the aortic arch and its branches. Type B dissections involve the descending aorta distal to the left subclavian. Type A is a true surgical emergency, with a 1–2% increase in mortality with each hour that passes until treatment is achieved [9]. Aortic dissections can have a variety of presentations, but most commonly patient's describe a ripping or tearing sensation in the chest or abdomen that radiates to the back. Other presenting complaints include syncope, new neurological symptoms, and hypotension, and therefore can be difficult to diagnose [9]. Imaging is absolutely crucial to early identification of this potentially fatal pathology, and using ultrasound has been proven to significantly improve time to diagnosis and mortality in suspected aortic dissection [10].

Ultrasonographic evidence of dissection can be difficult to detect. Therefore multiple views should be attempted in order obtain the most information. Evidence includes visualization of the dissection flap, aortic root dilatation, aortic regurgitation and pericardial effusion. A dissection flap will not be visible on ultrasound in the classic fashion that it would be on a CT scan. Often, a flap will be dynamic in position due to differences in blood pressure throughout the cycle. It will appear similar to a valve, moving in and out of the plane of the ultrasound image.

The parasternal long axis and the suprasternal view are best at identifying a type A dissection. The PSLA may show a dilated aortic root that is greater than 3.5 cm, aortic regurgitation using color Doppler, pericardial effusion if the dissection is contiguous with the pericardium, and sometimes a dissection flap. Evidence of acute pericardial effusion should always prompt investigation into the size of the aortic root. The suprasternal view is best at visualizing a type A dissection flap itself. The abdominal aorta should be scanned as well to evaluate for type B dissections. This is a similar scan to aortic aneursym screening, with less emphasis on specific landmarks, and more on scanning through the length of the abdominal aorta. Longitudinal views of the abdominal aorta are more useful for confirming a dissection flap than for screening.

It is important to remember that ultrasound is not a sensitive test for dissection, and should never be used to rule out this condition. However, in the right clinical scenario, visualization of a dissection flap should prompt aggressive blood pressure and heart rate control and evacuation or transport to a center with cardiothoracic surgery capabilities.

Pearls and Pitfalls

Echocardiography is one of the most difficult ultrasound skills to acquire, but perhaps the most critical regarding the management of acutely ill patients. It requires time and practice to master the ultrasonographic anatomy of the heart, the multiple different views, how to adapt these views to different body habitus, and finally to determine pathology. Despite these barriers, it is important to be mindful of that fact that the cardiac views obtained do not have to be perfect to learn useful clinical information. For example, if you wanted to evaluate the source of a patients hypotension, even limited views of the heart can determine if there is a pericardial effusion, enlarged RV, or fulminant heart failure. So, the bottom line is that you do not have to be an echocardiographic master to use ultrasound in the pre-hospital evaluation of a sick patient.

To build on that, the parasternal long axis view of the heart can help you evaluate for most of the pathology that is discussed in this chapter. Typically, it is the easiest to obtain. Remember to use the tips previously discussed to help you obtain this view: move up or down a rib space if the initial attempt is unsuccessful, bring the left arm up, roll the patient toward their left to bring the heart closer to the chest wall, and have the patient expire.

Despite best efforts at optimization, some patients will simply not have diagnostic cardiac views. The types of patients that tend to have very limited cardiac views include those with a history of midline sternotomy, are morbidly obese, have subcutaneous emphysema, have COPD, or are getting positive pressure ventilation. If this type of pathology is encountered, the cardiac exam may be non-diagnostic even under otherwise ideal or optimized conditions.

Finally, the ultrasound machine should be placed in the cardiac mode when imaging the heart. Failure to do so will result in reversed images that may confuse the novice provider. In the apical four chamber view, this will result in the left ventricle appearing where the right ventricle would be in standard imaging, and could result in false diagnosis of enlarged RV or other RV pathology.

Future Opportunities for Research

Cardiac ultrasound in the pre-hospital and austere settings is still an emerging field, with its potential applications yet to be fully realized. Currently, research has focused on examining its current use patterns and feasibility [11–13]. Because ultrasound has the potential to increase diagnostic certainty and allow for therapeutic interventions in the pre-hospital settings, its potential is dramatic. In more austere settings, it may be the only imaging modality available.

Future directions for cardiac ultrasonography in these environments are emerging in several different areas including advanced triage, telemedicine, and early interventions. Regarding advanced triage, especially in the setting of mass casualty events, the use of cardiac ultrasound to identify potentially life threatening conditions that can be intervened upon early can change a victim's status and identify those in whom that early intervention can be life saving [14]. In less acute settings, such as remote villages or other austere settings, cardiac ultrasonography can assist in the decision making to escalate treatment, marshal resources or even transfer a patient to get more advanced care. For example, a patient in whom a large pericardial effusion with evidence of tamponade was identified as the source of hypotension should have a pericardiocentesis performed, but it would not be advisable for the patient to remain in an austere setting if transfer was an option.

Through the use of increasingly advanced ultrasound, wireless technology, and ever-present cell phones, it is easier than ever to transmit ultrasound images in real time. This opens up several different avenues for which ultrasound can be useful in these prehospital or remote settings [15]. First, experts that are physically in a different location from the patient and provider can direct that provider, in real time, in order to assist in obtaining cardiac images, which can be especially useful for less experienced providers. Furthermore, images transmitted in real-time can be used to make early, critical diagnoses that can then direct downstream resource utilization and patient management.

Finally, in a more extreme situation, ultrasound is being used to assist in ECMO cannulization in the prehospital setting in several European countries with promise [16]. This intervention and use of ultrasound requires advanced knowledge and practical expertise, so it is currently limited to only select physician and paramedic teams, but represents another potential for the use of ultrasound in the pre-hospital environment.

Works Cited

1. Mohrman DE, Heller L. The heart pump. In: Mohrman DE, Heller LJ, editors. Cardiovascular physiology. 9th ed. New York: McGraw-Hill; 2018.
2. Penny S, et al. Examination review for ultrasound: sonographic principles and instrumentation. Philadelphia: Wolters Kluwer Health; 2011.
3. Reardon RF, et al. Chapter 6. Cardiac. In: Ma OJ, et al., editors. Ma and Mateer's emergency ultrasound. 3rd ed. New York: McGraw-Hill; 2014.
4. Jaffar A. Anatomical structure of the heart. In: Elmoselhi A, editor. Cardiology: an integrated approach. New York: McGraw-Hill; 2018.
5. Ünlüer EE, et al. Visual estimation of bedside echocardiographic ejection fraction by emergency physicians. West J Emerg Med. 2014;15(2):221–6.
6. Kline JA. Venous thromboembolism. In: Tintinalli JE, et al., editors. Tintinalli's emergency medicine: a comprehensive study guide. 8th ed. New York: McGraw-Hill; 2016.
7. Rasalingam R, Makan M, Perez JE. The Washington manual of echocardiography. Philadelphia: Wolters Kluwer Health/Lippincott Williams & Wilkins; 2013.
8. Otto CM. Textbook of clinical echocardiography. 5th ed. Philadelphia: Elsevier Saunders; 2013.

9. Lo, Bruce. An evidence-based approach to acute aortic syndromes. EB medicine: emergency medicine practice. 2013. Retrieved from www.ebmedicine.net. Aug 2018.
10. Pare, et al. Emergency physician focused cardiac ultrasound improves diagnosis of ascending aortic dissection. Am J Emerg Med. 2016;34:486–92.
11. Rooney KP, et al. Pre-hospital assessment with ultrasound in emergencies: implementation in the field. World J Emerg Med. 2016;7(2):117–23.
12. Hoyer HX, Vogl S, Schiemann U, et al. Prehospital ultrasound in emergency medicine: incidence, feasibility, indications and diagnoses. Eur J Emerg Med. 2010;17(5):254–9.
13. Chin EJ, Chan CH, Mortazavi R, et al. A pilot study examining the viability of a prehospital assessment with ultrasound for emergencies (PAUSE) protocol. J Emerg Med. 2013;44(1):142–9.
14. Wydo SM, et al. Portable ultrasound in disaster triage: a focused review. Eur J Trauma Emerg Surg. 2016;42(2):151–9.
15. Nelson BP, Sanghvi A. Out of hospital point of care ultrasound: current use models and future directions. Eur J Trauma Emerg Surg. 2016;42(2):139–50.
16. Lamhaut L, Jouffroy R, Soldan M, et al. Safety and feasibility of prehospital extra corporeal life support implementation by non-surgeons for out-of-hospital refractory cardiac arrest. Resuscitation. 2013;84(11):1525–9.

Key Literature

Creditt A, et al. Cardiac ultrasound. In: Creditt A, et al., editors. Clinical ultrasound: a pocket manual. New York: Springer; 2018.
Heegaard WG, et al. Ultrasound in prehospital and austere environments. In: John Ma O, et al., editors. Ma and Mateer's emergency ultrasound. 3rd ed. New York: McGraw-Hill; 2014.
Reardon RF, et al. Cardiac. In: Ma OJ, et al., editors. Ma and Mateer's emergency ultrasound. 3rd ed. New York: McGraw-Hill; 2014.

Trauma

Lindsay Anne Taylor

Introduction

Trauma is the leading cause of death in the United States in people younger than 45 years old [1]. Point-of-care ultrasound has been executed by emergency providers in the acute assessment of patients who suffer from blunt and penetrating trauma for many years.

Extended Focused Assessment with Sonography in Trauma (EFAST) is the most accepted algorithm to follow when assessing a hypotensive trauma patient. In the United States the EFAST exam is the imaging test of choice and apart of the Advanced Trauma Life Support protocol developed by the American College of Surgeons. The EFAST assesses potential spaces where blood or air can accumulate around the pericardium, the peritoneum and in the thorax.

In the austere or prehospital setting, the provider relies heavily on their clinical acumen to properly assess and initiate the management of patients. Conditions that a prehospital provider endures can grossly limit the physical examination [2]. Auscultation for breath sounds can be impossible in the noisy environment of an ambulance driving with lights and sirens or in the back of a turbulent helicopter [2].

Prehospital ultrasound (PHUS) is becoming more commonplace and it has been discovered that PHUS of the abdomen and/or thorax has changed the management of many patients. This has been demonstrated to by changing the prehospital diagnosis and treatment, the choice of receiving hospital, or the receiving hospital's response [2]. It has also shown to lower unnecessary procedures and has allowed for more controlled rescues.

L. A. Taylor (✉)
Department of Emergency Medicine, Virginia Commonwealth University Health System, Richmond, VA, USA
e-mail: Lindsay.Taylor@vcuhealth.org

B. D. Nicholson et al. (eds.), *Manual of Austere and Prehospital Ultrasound*,
https://doi.org/10.1007/978-3-030-64287-7_8

In the prehospital setting ultrasound can also be used as an advanced form of triage during mass casualty events in critical multi-trauma patients [3].

The focus of this chapter is to discuss the use of ultrasound for victims of trauma to identify significant internal bleeding or free fluid within the peritoneum, pericardial, or pleural spaces. In addition to the EFAST examination, this chapter will guide you to evaluate other potential sources of lethal hemorrhage including long bone fractures and open book pelvis fractures.

This chapter focuses on using ultrasound to identify injuries on patients suffering from blunt and penetrating trauma. Individual topics covered in this chapter will include the EFAST exam, long bone fractures and open book pelvis fractures.

The EFAST examination covers six acoustic windows for assessing the potential spaces where blood or air can accumulate. These six windows evaluate the pericardium, the peritoneum and/or the pleural space. In an unstable patient identifying these conditions can change management and help expedite the patient's disposition.

Addition injuries that can cause lethal hemorrhage include long bone fractures and open book pelvis injuries. Open book pelvis fractures can be indicative of a retroperitoneal bleed that would not be picked up by a standard EFAST exam [4].

Image Acquisition

When performing an EFAST exam select a low frequency transducer either the curvilinear or the phased array. After the transducer has been selected change the setting on the ultrasound to the abdominal mode.

Pericardium

Start the EFAST exam with evaluation of the pericardium. The pericardium has two layers (the visceral and parietal layer) that normally contain a minimum of 10 mL of physiologic fluid [5]. This is often evaluated using the subxiphoid window but can also be evaluated in the parasternal long axis window on the patient's chest. Starting with the subxiphoid approach place the transducer inferior to the xiphoid process with the indicator marker oriented to match the indicator on the screen. Using moderate pressure angle the transducer superior and fan towards the left shoulder. Once you visualize the heart adjust the depth to visualize the entire heart and the entire pericardium can be seen. Asking the patient to take a deep breath may help. In the subxiphoid window the liver will be in the near field of the screen above the heart. Immediately below the liver is the right ventricle and the right atrium. The most posterior structures will be the left ventricle and the left atrium. The pericardium is hyperechoic (bright white) and a potential space where blood or fluid can accumulate [6] (Figs. 1 and 2).

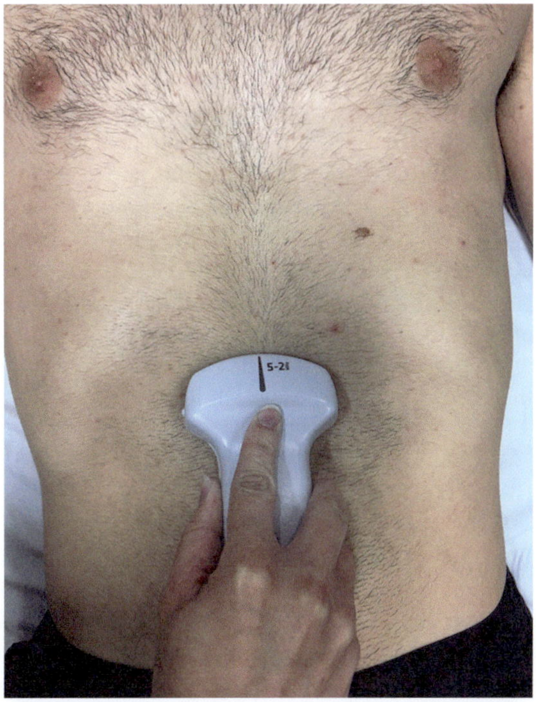

Fig. 1 Subxiphoid EFAST transducer placement: Place the transducer inferior to the xiphoid process with the marker oriented toward the patient's right. Place operator's hand on top of the transducer, use a moderate amount of force to press the transducer into the patient's abdomen, and angle the transducer superior and leftward toward the left shoulder. (From Creditt et al. [6])

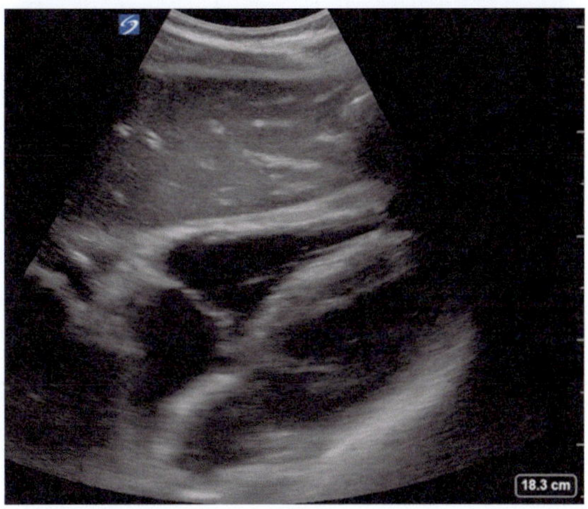

Fig. 2 Subxiphoid EFAST view: Normal EFAST demonstrating a subxiphoid view of the heart. The liver is used as the acoustic window to view cardiac structures and pericardium. The right heart sits closest to the liver. (From Creditt et al. [6])

Lung

Select any transducer to evaluate for lung sliding, however, it is more efficient to continue to use the transducer you started the EFAST examination with. The lungs sit within the thoracic cage made up of ribs and a muscular chest wall. Place the transducer on the anterior chest wall with the marker pointed towards the patient's head near the apex of the lung. Adjust the depth to visualize the ribs shadowing and the pleural line between two ribs. Each lung is surrounded by a visceral and a parietal pleura with a potential space between them. The pleura is a hyperechoic horizontal line between two ribs. Lung sliding occurs when the visceral pleura slides against the parietal pleura during respiration. In normal inflated lungs, sliding appear as small comet tail artifacts showering from the pleural line when the lung inflates and deflates during the respiratory cycle [6].

If you are unable to determine the presence of lung sliding use "M mode" for confirmation. Place the vertical M-mode line through the horizontal pleura between two ribs and press start. The "seashore sign" will occur in normal lung sliding. It appears as horizontal lines in the near field, a hyperechoic pleural line in the middle and a granular pattern in the far field. The granular pattern represents movement of the normal lung during breathing [7].

Right Upper Quadrant

Place the transducer over the patient's right flank between mid-axillary and anterior axillary line with the transducer marker directed towards the patient's head. Visualize the liver and kidney. The kidney with have a hyperechoic lining immediately abutting with the liver. There is a potential space between the liver and kidney called the heptaorenal recess. The hepatorenal recess is usually best imaged between ribs 8 and 11. The diaphragm is seen at the superior edge of the liver (left side of the screen) as a hyperechoic curved stripe that oscillates with breathing. The right lower lung base will be located just above the diaphragm [8].

When scanning through the liver and renal interface, be sure to visualize the tip of the left side of the liver. Free fluid and/or blood most commonly accumulates at the tip of the liver in a supine patient [8] (Fig. 3).

Slide the transducer cephalad to visualize the inferior right hemithorax located above the diaphragm. The diaphragm intersects with the spine in the far field of the screen and the spine should not be seen above the diaphragm (Figs. 4, 5 and 6).

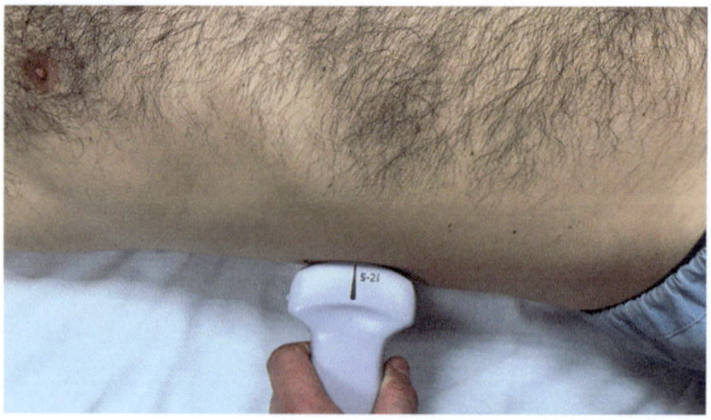

Fig. 3 Transducer placement RUQ: Place the transducer over the patient's right flank between the mid-axillary and anterior axillary line with the transducer marker directed toward the patient's head. (From Creditt et al. [6])

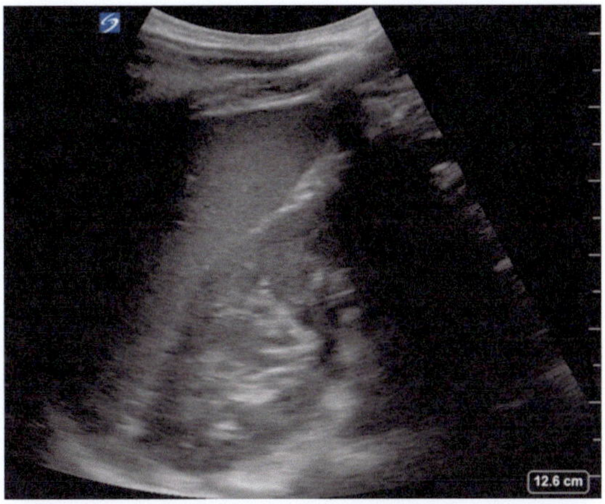

Fig. 4 RUQ normal EFAST: Normal RUQ EFAST showing no free fluid. Imaging should include the tip of the liver, area between the liver and right kidney, and the diaphragm above the liver. (From Creditt et al. [6])

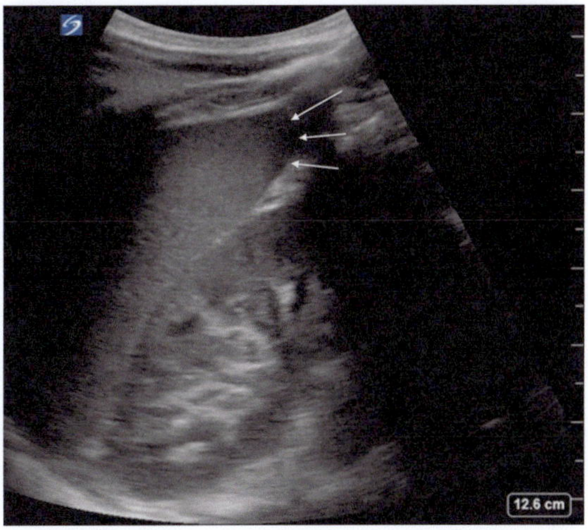

Fig. 5 EFAST liver tip: RUQ view demonstrating the liver tip above the right kidney. Hemoperitoneum can be detected first around the liver tip; therefore, it is important to image this specific area of the RUQ. (From Creditt et al. [6])

Left Upper Quadrant

Place the transducer over the patient's left flank between the mid-axillary and posterior axillary line near the tenth rib space with the marker pointed towards the patient's head. Rotate the transducer clockwise to capture a window between two ribs to reduce the posterior shadowing artifact from the ribs. Visualize the spleen and left kidney. The kidney with have a hyperechoic lining immediately abutting with the spleen. There is a potential space between the spleen and kidney called the splenorenal recess. The diaphragm is seen at the superior edge of the liver (left side of the screen) as a hyperechoic curved stripe that oscillates with breathing. The right lower lung base will be located just above the diaphragm [6, 8] (Fig. 7).

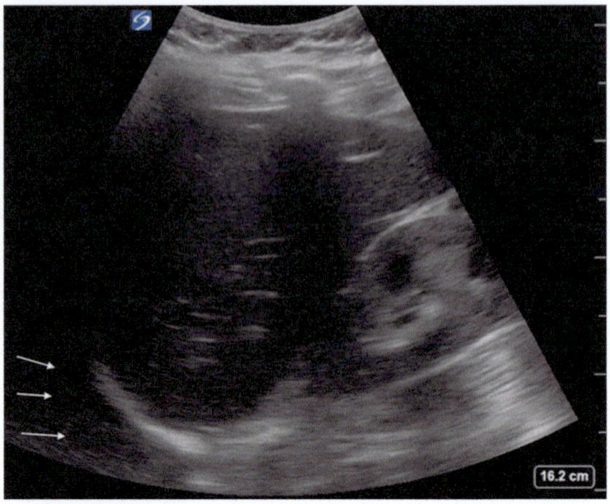

Fig. 6 RUQ EFAST view with hemithorax: Evaluation of the RUQ should include the right hemithorax, visualized above the liver and hyperechoic diaphragm. (From Creditt et al. [6])

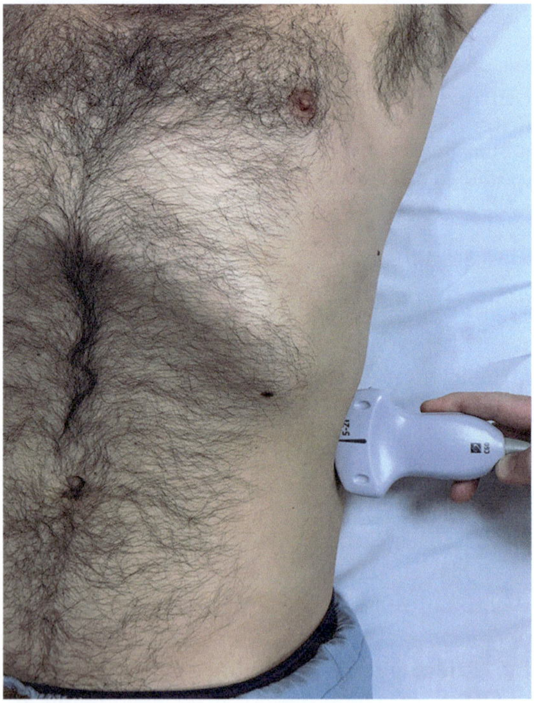

Fig. 7 Transducer placement LUQ: Place the transducer over the patient's left flank between the mid-axillary and posterior axillary line near the tenth rib space with the marker pointed toward the patient's head. (From Creditt et al. [6])

Fluid can also accumulate above the spleen under the diaphragm. This can be a difficult place to assess because of the ribs, but it is an important space as it can be the first place for fluid to accumulate (Fig. 8).

Slide the transducer cephalad to visualize the inferior left hemithorax located above the diaphragm. The diaphragm intersects with the spine in the far field of the screen and the spine should not be seen above the diaphragm [6, 8] (Figs. 9 and 10).

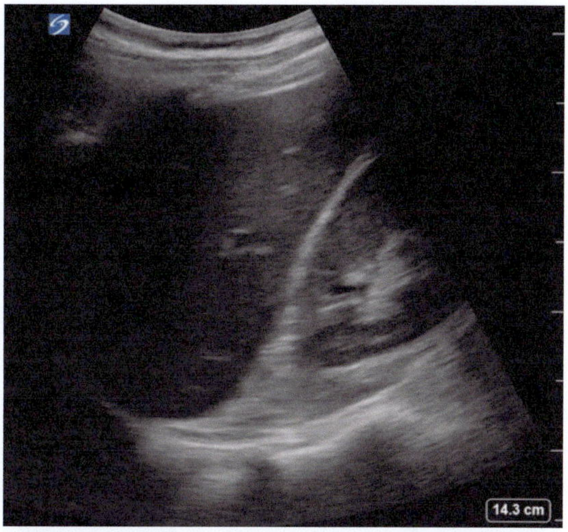

Fig. 8 LUQ standard view: LUQ EFAST view showing no free fluid. Imaging should include the spleen, area between the spleen and left kidney, and views of the diaphragm above the spleen. (From Creditt et al. [6])

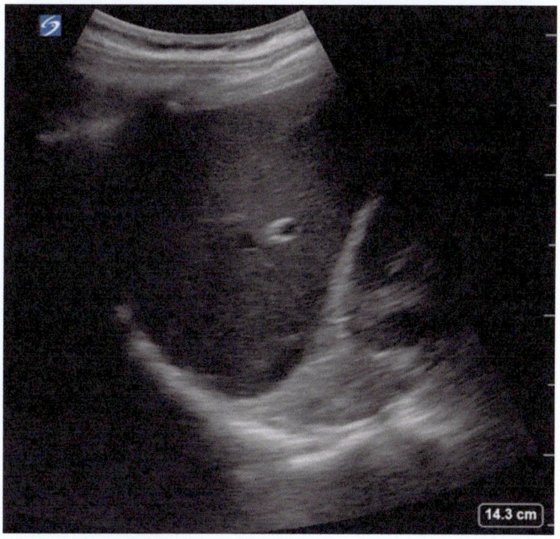

Fig. 9 LUQ EFAST imaging above the spleen: Free fluid will typically accumulate above the spleen first in the LUQ making it important to always image this area. (From Creditt et al. [6])

Suprapubic

In a transverse plane, place the transducer superior to the pubic bone and angle inferiorly with the transducer marker pointed towards the patient's right.

The bladder which will appear as an anechoic (black) collection of fluid contained by an echogenic bladder wall. In the transverse view, the paracolic gutters are located to the right and left of the bladder in the far field, these are two areas of potential space for free fluid to collect [6, 8] (Figs. 11 and 12).

Scan from superior to inferior to visualize the area posterior to the bladder. The uterus or prostate can be also be seen posterior to the bladder in the far field [6, 8].

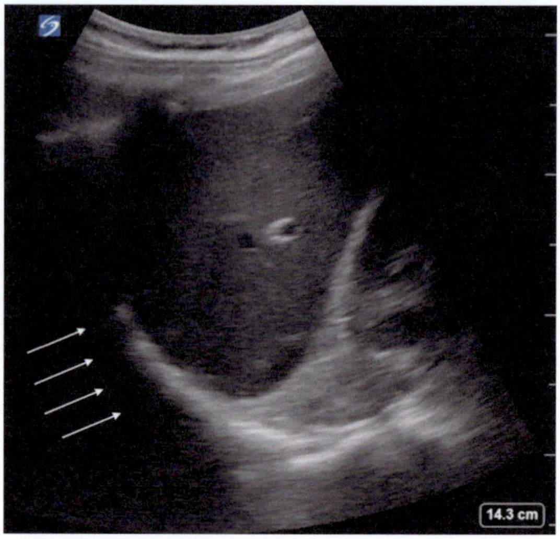

Fig. 10 LUQ EFAST view with left hemithorax: Evaluation of the LUQ should include the left hemithorax, visualized above the spleen and hyperechoic diaphragm. (From Creditt et al. [6])

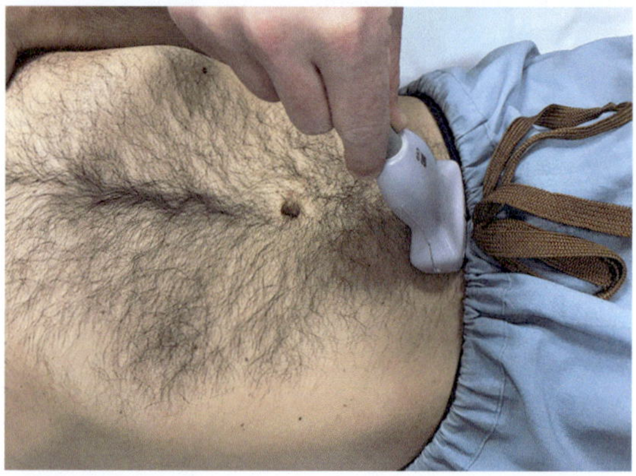

Fig. 11 Transducer placement pelvis, transverse: Place the transducer superior to the pubic bone angled inferiorly with the transducer marker pointed toward the patient's right in the transverse plane. (From Creditt et al. [6])

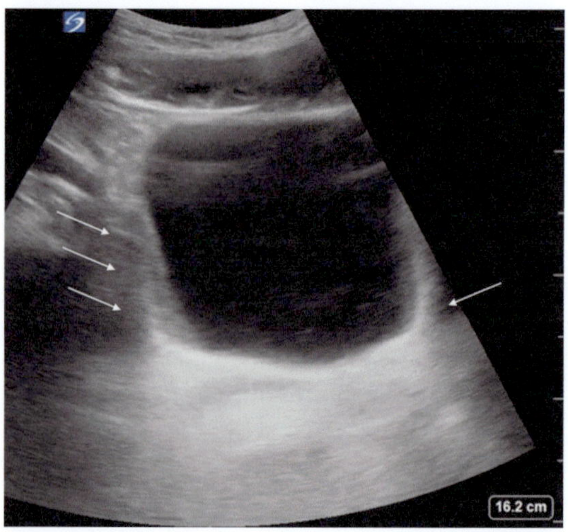

Fig. 12 Paracolic gutters in transverse: Normal pelvis and bladder EFAST view in a transverse plane. Note bilateral paracolic gutters on each side of the bladder. (From Creditt et al. [6])

Rotate the transducer to the sagittal plane with the transducer marker pointed to patient's head. Fan the transducer from right to left evaluating posterior to the bladder for free fluid [6, 8] (Figs. 13 and 14).

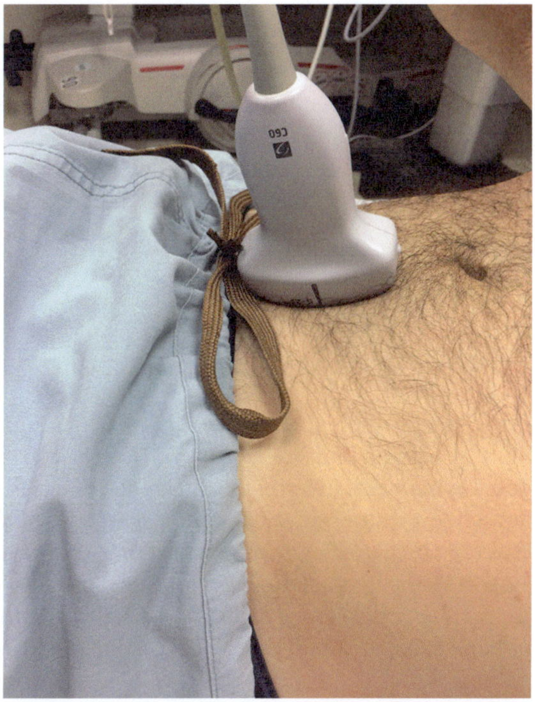

Fig. 13 Transducer placement bladder in sagittal: From a transverse position, rotate the transducer 90° clockwise to image the pelvis in sagittal plane with the transducer marker pointed to patient's head. (From Creditt et al. [6])

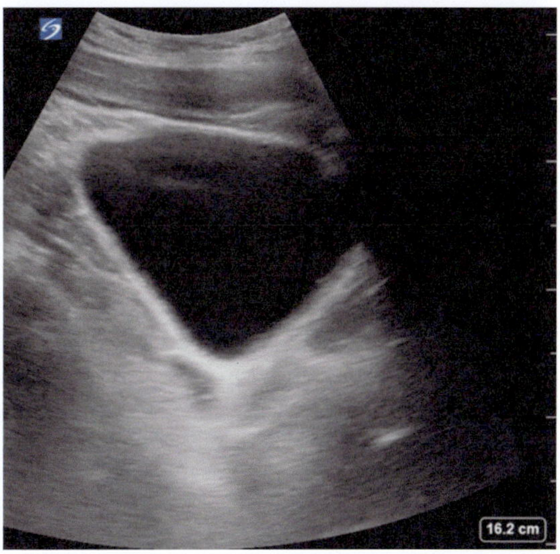

Fig. 14 Sagittal view of bladder: Normal pelvis and bladder EFAST view in a sagittal plane. (From Creditt et al. [6])

Long Bone

When assessing bone with ultrasound select a transducer that will give the appropriate depth. This is usually going to be a linear transducer; however, a curvilinear transducer may be necessary for larger bones such as the femur. Bone will appear in the far field as a hyperechoic structure (the cortex) with posterior acoustic shadowing [9–12]. Scan along the bone of choice beginning in the sagittal plane. Identify the hyperechoic structure deep to the surface of the transducer and slide from proximal to distal keeping the bone in view the entire time looking for continuity of the hyperechoic line. Rotate the transducer to the transverse plane and scan the entire bone again looking for continuity of the hyperechoic structure. A joint will appear as a disruption in the bone; however, the edges will be rounded with a v-shaped divot [9].

Pubic Symphysis

First identify the pubic symphysis by palpating the landmarks of the bony pelvis. Start by using a high frequency 5–10 MHz linear transducer and placing it over the pubic symphysis. Identify the hyperechoic cortex of the right or left hemi-symphysis and slide the transducer toward the opposite hemi-symphysis. There will be an anechoic break in between the two hemi-symphyses [4]. Freeze the frame and measure from bone to bone. A curvilinear transducer may also be used if the patient has excessive subcutaneous adipose tissue and requires a lower frequency transducer to obtain the appropriate depth. The maximum normal width of the pubic symphysis is 25 mm [13–15].

Abnormal Images

Pericardium

There is a potential space between the visceral and parietal pericardium and can accumulate a pathologic effusion. Hemopericardium refers to blood filling this potential space. Other sources of pericardial effusion include infectious, metastatic, uremic, aortic dissection, connective tissue disorders, hypothyroidism, and post-procedural [5]. These effusions may appear as an anechoic or a hypoechoic band between the heart and echogenic pericardium at the inferior border of the heart. A pericardial effusion can be assessed in several windows around the heart, but the two most common views are the subxiphoid window and the parasternal long axis window. In the subxiphoid window the effusion can be visualized between the heart and the liver. In the parasternal long axis window, the fluid can be seen anterior to the RV wall in the near field, but a significant effusion will surround the heart posteriorly and dissects between the posterior wall of the left ventricle and anterior to the descending thoracic aorta [16] (Fig. 15).

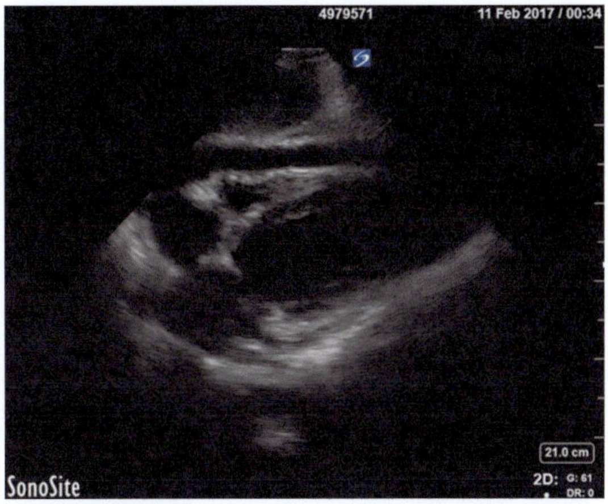

Fig. 15 Pericardial effusion: Anechoic fluid surrounds the right heart indicating a pericardial effusion. (From Creditt et al. [6])

Table 1 Pericardial effusion size categories

Small	<0.5 cm in diameter
Medium	0.5–2.0 cm in diameter
Large	>2.0 cm in diameter

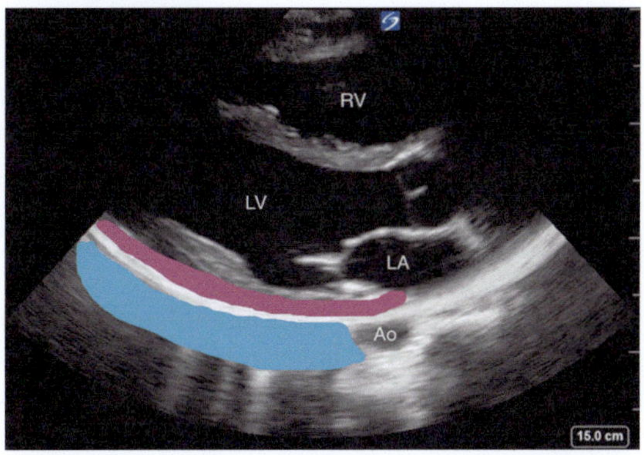

Fig. 16 Comparing pleural fluid and pericardial fluid: In a parasternal long view, pericardial fluid will be present posterior to the left ventricular wall and anterior to the descending aorta. A leftsided pleural effusion will occur posterior to the left ventricular wall and will not be present anterior to the descending aorta. (From Creditt et al. [6])

The size of a pericardial effusion can have an impact on the function of the heart. The size of the effusion should be measured at the end of diastole from the outer wall of the left ventricle to the hyperechoic pericardium [5]. (Table 1).

A left pleural effusion can be confused for a pericardial effusion. A left sided pleural effusion will be in the far field outside the left ventricle, but it will not dissect between the posterior wall of the heart and the descending thoracic aorta [6, 8] (Fig. 16).

In a non-diseased heart, the right atrium and right ventricle function in a low-pressure environment. Cardiac Tamponade occurs when fluid accumulates within the pericardium creating an excessive external pressure that overwhelms the pressure within the cardiac chambers. This type of effusion impairs the ability of the right ventricle to fill during diastole which ultimately causes hypotension and shock

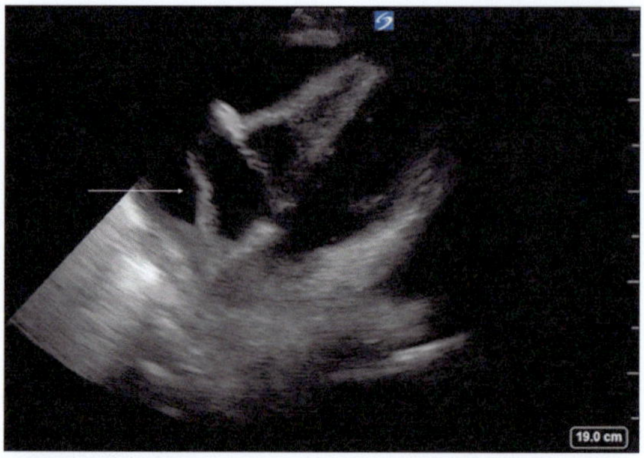

Fig. 17 Right atrial systolic collapse in tamponade: In cardiac tamponade, the pressure within the pericardium exceeds the pressure within the right atrium causing it to collapse during systole. (From Creditt et al. [6])

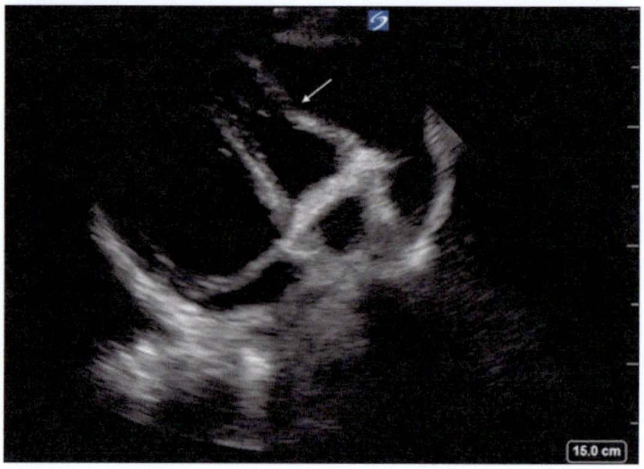

Fig. 18 Right ventricle collapse: In cardiac tamponade, the pressure within the pericardium exceeds the pressure within the right ventricle causing it to collapse during diastole. (From Creditt et al. [6])

[6]. It is often not the amount of effusion surrounding the heart that causes tamponade physiology rather how quickly it accumulates. The most sensitive finding of cardiac tamponade occurs when the free wall of the right atrium collapses during systole. The inversion of the free wall should last greater than one-third of the systolic period [5]. The most specific sign of cardiac tamponade occurs when the right ventricular free wall inverts during diastole [10, 16] (Figs. 17 and 18).

Lung

A pneumothorax can be caused spontaneously or as a result of trauma. Air builds up outside the lung within the thoracic cavity causing the lung to collapse. Air separates the visceral and parietal pleural causing an absence of lung sliding [7].

Slide the transducer down the chest wall until the pleura slides in and out of the intercostal space. The edge of the lung visualized in this intercostal space is called the lung point. The lung point is the transition point at which the partially collapsed lung is visualized during inspiration. The lung point may not be visualized with a large or tension pneumothorax. When the lung point is visualized this has been determined to be 100% specific for pneumothorax [17].

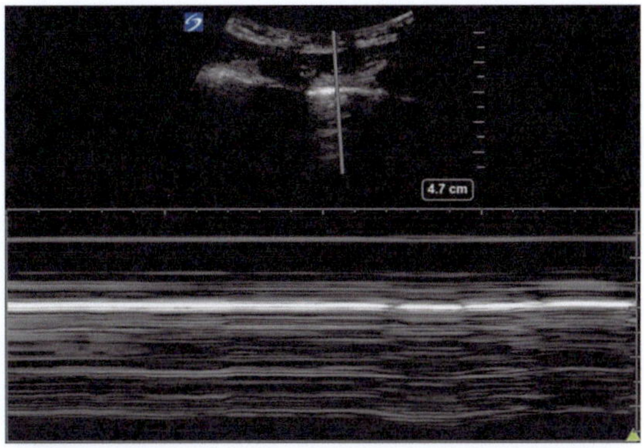

Fig. 19 Barcode sign: M-mode through the pleural line demonstrates no movement as evidenced by the horizontal lines in the bottom half of the image. This is sometimes referred to as "barcode sign" given the similar appearance to retail barcodes. (From Creditt et al. [6])

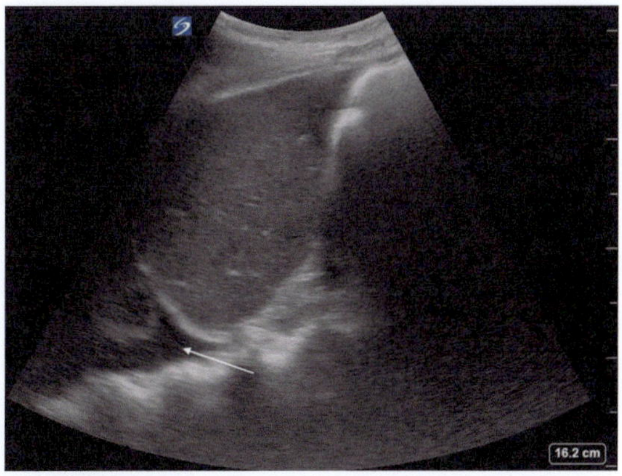

Fig. 20 Positive pleural fluid above the diaphragm: A small pleural effusion (arrow) is noted above the diaphragm. (From Creditt et al. [6])

When trying to confirm a pneumothorax, M-mode can be used as described earlier in the chapter. The intercostal space evaluated will be motionless therefore the chest wall and the lack of lung motion displays as horizontal lines across the screen also known as a "barcode sign" (Fig. 19).

Hemothorax or pleural effusion is the accumulation of blood or free fluid outside of the lung between the visceral and parietal pleura. An effusion appears as an anechoic or hypoechoic collection above the diaphragm within the thoracic cavity. This can be visualized while imaging the right or left upper quadrants during the EFAST exam. When the patient is lying in the supine position the fluid will accumulate posteriorly and inferiorly above the diaphragm. When the patient is sitting upright the fluid will accumulate inferiorly above the diaphragm [6, 8] (Fig. 20).

A large pleural effusion will collapse the lung and cause it to wave back and forth with respiration. This has been coined a "flag" sign [6] (Fig. 21).

Peritoneum

Free intraperitoneal fluid or blood will accumulate in dependent areas of the abdomen first. Blood will be anechoic in an acute setting. These potential spaces include: the hepatorenal recess between the liver and kidney within the RUQ (also known as

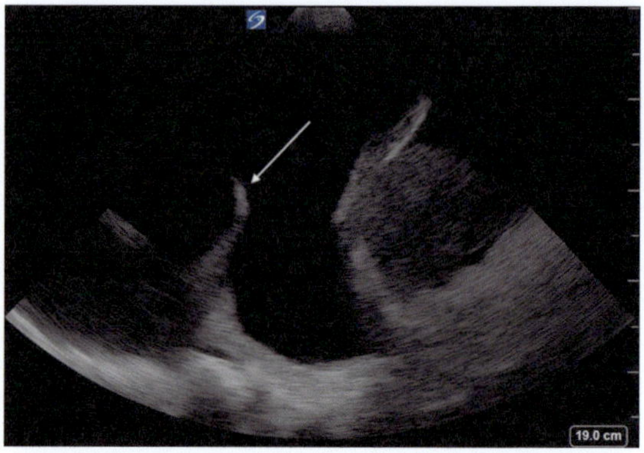

Fig. 21 Large pleura effusion with flag sign: With large pleural effusions, the lung will appear to be floating in the fluid, creating what looks like a flag flapping in the wind (flag sign). (From Creditt et al. [6])

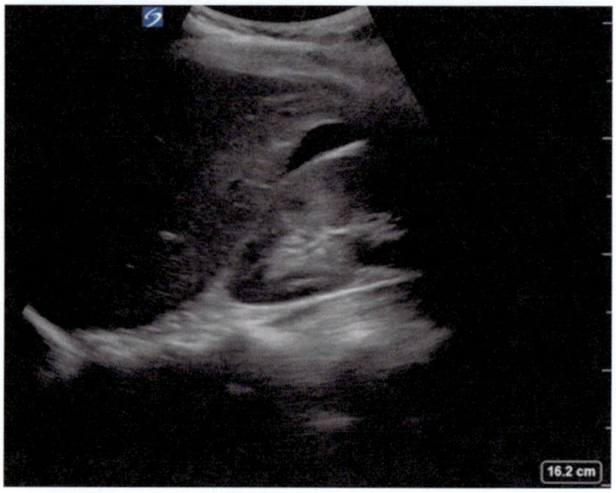

Fig. 22 Positive EFAST Morrison's pouch: Free fluid is located within Morrison's pouch between the liver and right kidney. (From Creditt et al. [6])

Morrison's pouch), the splenorenal recess between the spleen and kidney within the LUQ, the left subphrenic space between the diaphragm and spleen, the pericolic gutters within the pelvis, the rectovesicular pouch (the most dependent area in a supine male), and the rectouterine pouch (also known as the pouch of Douglas and the most dependent area in the supine female) [6, 8] (Figs. 22, 23, 24, 25, 26, and 27).

Long Bone Fracture

Long bone fractures will be identified as a discontinuity to the smooth hyperechoic cortex found in normal bone. This may appear as a subtle disruption without step-off, a subperiosteal hematoma, or an angular deformity [9, 10, 18]. The two main long bones of concern include the humerus and the femur. There may also be a hematoma surrounding the fracture site. This collection of will appear anechoic, hypoechoic or echogenic [9, 10].

Fig. 23 Positive EFAST liver tip: Free fluid is seen here surrounding the liver tip. (From Creditt et al. [6])

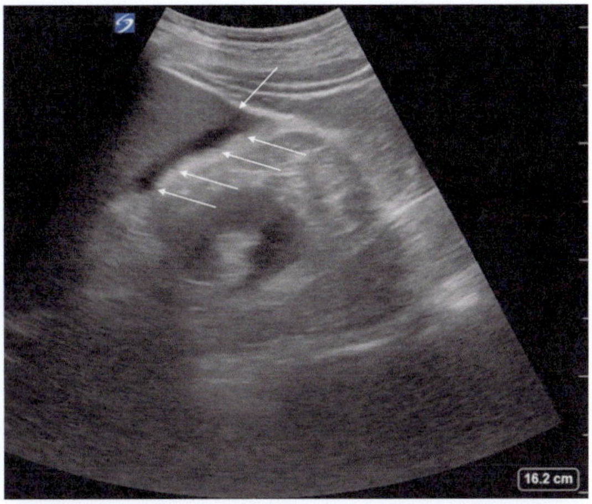

Fig. 24 Positive EFAST LUQ: Free fluid is seen here between the spleen and left kidney. (From Creditt et al. [6])

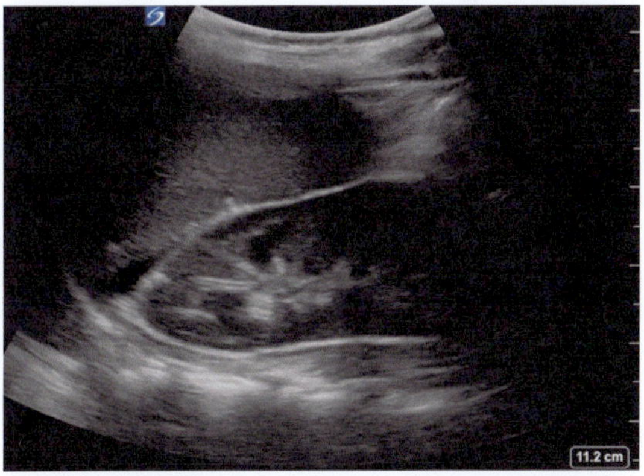

Fig. 25 Positive EFAST LUQ above spleen: Free fluid is located superior to the spleen and inferior to the diaphragm. Fluid will typically accumulate above the spleen first in the LUQ making it important to always image this area. (From Creditt et al. [6])

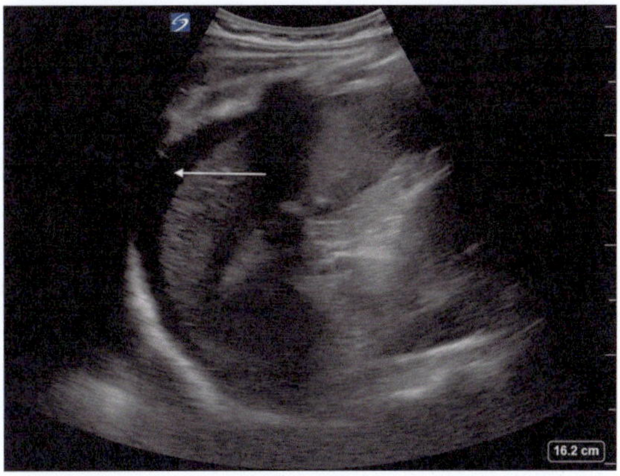

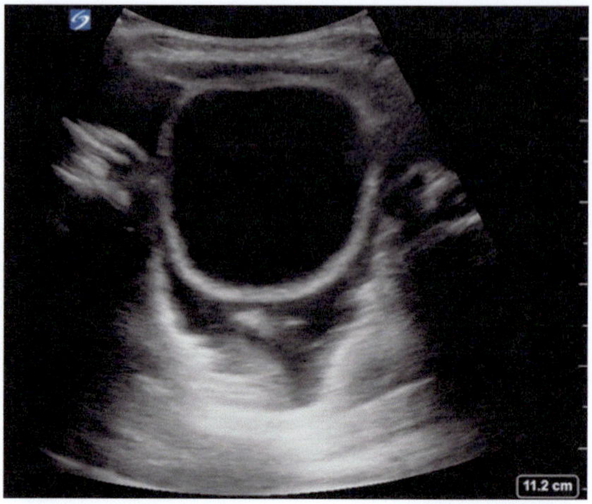

Fig. 26 Positive EFAST bladder transverse: Free fluid is surrounding the bladder in a transverse plane. Note the anechoic fluid posterior to the bladder and in both paracolic gutters. (From Creditt et al. [6])

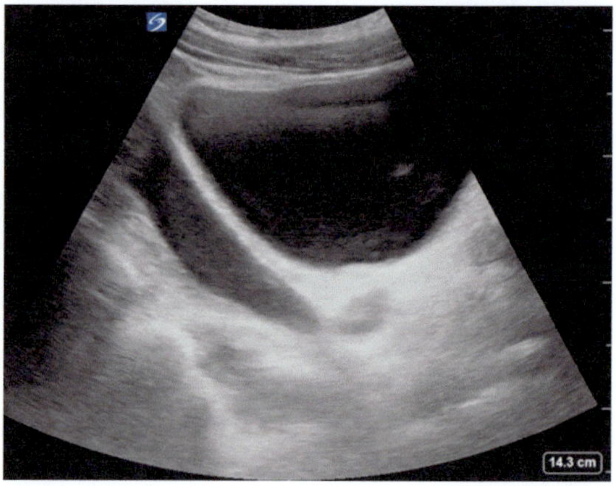

Fig. 27 Positive EFAST bladder sagittal: Free fluid is found around the bladder in the sagittal plane. (From Creditt et al. [6])

Pubic Symphysis (Open Book Pelvis Injury)

Identify the pubic symphysis as described above. Identify the hyperechoic cortex of the right or left hemi-symphysis and slide the transducer toward the opposite hemi-symphysis. Freeze the frame and measure from bone to bone. The maximum normal width of the pubic symphysis is 25 mm [13–15]. If you cannot visualize the opposite hemi-symphysis within the transducer window keep one hemi-symphysis in view and fan the transducer toward the opposite side until visualized [4]. Keep in mind that other pelvic bone injuries may not cause a widening of the pubic symphysis but can still cause lethal hemorrhage, however, ultrasound can identify who will benefit from a pelvic binder in the prehospital and austere setting [4].

Limitations of Current Knowledge and Opportunities for Future Research

Prehospital ultrasound and ultrasound in an austere environment are playing a big role in reducing morbidity and mortality of patients with life-threatening emergencies [19]. By using PHUS first responders can use this diagnostic modality to assist in triage and guide management descisions [2, 3, 19]. Limitations to austere and PHUS include educational didactics, hands-on training and maintenance of skills, cost of equipment, and quality assessment. Furthermore, prehospital and austere ultrasound research is needed to provide evidence on its clinical impact on patient outcomes to make this a standard of care [19]. In addition to didactic and hands-on training for providers, telemedicine/remote guidance can provide an opportunity to guide providers in real time in the austere or prehospital environment [20]. Astronauts have successfully demonstrated implementing remote guidance in ultrasound on the International Space Station [20]. Remote guidance can provide a clinically relevant advancement in the field of austere and prehospital ultrasound.

Key Literature Reviewed

1. Melniker LA, Leibner E, McKenney MG, Lopez P, Briggs WM, Mancuso CA. Randomized controlled clinical trial of point-of-care, limited ultrasonography for trauma in the emergency department: the first sonography outcomes assessment program trial. Ann Emerg Med. 2006;48(3):227–35.
2. O'Dochartaigh D, Douma M. Prehospital ultrasound of the abdomen and thorax changes trauma patient management: a systematic review. Injury. 2015;46(11):2093–102.
3. Lewiss RE, Saul T, Del Rios M. Focus on: EFAST – extended focused assessment with sonography for trauma. https://www.acep.org/Clinical%2D%2D-Practice-Management/Focus-On%2D%2DEFAST%2D%2D-Extended-Focused-Assessment-With-Sonography-for-Trauma/ ACEP News website. Jan 2009. Accessed 20 Apr 2017.
4. Bauman M, Marinaro J, Tawil I, Crandall C, Rosenbaum L, Paul I. Ultrasonographic determination of pubic symphyseal widening in trauma: the FAST-PS study. J Emerg Med. 2011;40(5):528–33.
5. Lewiss RE, et al. Practical guide to critical ultrasound, volume 1. 18 Oct 2018, https://books.apple.com/us/book/practical-guide-to-critical-ultrasound-volume-1/id1439354416.
6. Creditt A, et al. Clinical ultrasound: a pocket manual. Cham: Springer International Publishing; 2018.
7. Husain LF, Hagopian L, Wayman D, Baker WE, Carmody KA. Sonographic diagnosis of pneumothorax. J Emerg Trauma Shock. 2012;5(1):76–81. https://www.ncbi.nlm.nih.gov/pmc/articles/PMC3299161/. Accessed 26 Apr 2017.
8. Ma OJ, Mateer JR, Kirkpatrick AW. Chapter 5: Trauma. In: Ma OJ, Mateer JR, Reardon RF, Joing SA, editors. Emergency ultrasound. 3rd ed. China: McGraw-Hill Education; 2014. p. p61–92.
9. Ma OJ, Mateer JR, Blavais M. Chapter 16: soft tissue. In: Emergency ultrasound. 2nd ed: China: McGraw Hill; 2007.
10. Mallin M, Dawson M. Introduction to bedside ultrasound: volume 2. Lexington: Emergency Ultrasound Solutions; 2013. iBook. https://itun.es/us/ueELM.l
11. Fornage BD. Musculoskeletal sonography. New York: Churchill Livingstone; 1995.

12. Dewitz A. Chapter 18: Musculoskeletal, soft tissue, and miscellaneous applications. In: Ma OJ, Mateer JR, Reardon RF, Joing SA, editors. Emergency ultrasound. 3rd ed. China: McGraw-Hill Education; 2014. p. p503–68.
13. Mirvis SE, Shanmuganatha K. Imaging in trauma and critical care. 2nd ed. Philadelphia: Elsevier Science; 2003.
14. Canale ST. Campbell's operative orthopedics. 10th ed. Philadelphia: Mosby; 2003.
15. Wheeless CR. Wheeless' textbook of orthopedics. Brooklandville: Data Trace Internet Publishing; 2007.
16. Rasalingam R, Makan M, Perez JE. The Washington manual of echocardiography. Philadelphia: Wolters Kluwer Health/Lippincott Williams & Wilkins; 2013.
17. Lichtenstein D, Mezière G, Biderman P, Gepner A. The "lung point": an ultrasound sign specific to pneumothorax. Intensive Care Med. 2014;26(10):1434–40.
18. Griffith JF, Rainer TH, Ching ASC, et al. Sonography compared with radiography in revealing acute rib fracture. AJR. 1999;173:1603–9.
19. El Sayed MJ, Zaghrini E. Prehospital emergency ultrasound: a review of current clinical applications, challenges, and future implications. Emerg Med Int. 2013;2013:1–6.
20. Chiao L, Sharipov S, Sargsyan AE, et al. Ocular examination for trauma; clinical ultrasound aboard the International Space Station. J Trauma. 2005;58(5):885–9.

Undifferentiated Hypotension

Andrew Cathers and Nikolai Schnittke

Introduction

Circulatory shock is hypoperfusion of end-organs due to an underlying illness and is frequently characterized by hypotension. Left untreated, circulatory shock results in rapid multi-organ failure, precipitous drop in blood pressure, and ultimately cardiac arrest. The prevalence of hypotension in nontraumatic, prehospital patients found in one systematic review was only 19.5/1000 EMS contacts, but this population has a disproportionately high mortality rate (33–50%) [12]. The proportion of critically ill patients with circulatory shock is likely to be higher with Advanced Life Support and Critical Care specific prehospital teams, necessitating additional expertise in resuscitation.

Shock is often categorized by its pathophysiologic etiology into distributive, obstructive, cardiogenic, and hypovolemic etiologies. Distributive etiologies reflect a global vasodilatory process in which the intravascular space expands and the residual intravascular fluid is not sufficient to maintain appropriate blood pressure and organ dysfunction. This includes a diverse range of diagnoses including septic shock (most commonly), anaphylaxis, and neurogenic shock. Obstructive shock reflects an increase in afterload (usually abrupt) on the ventricular cardiac output. This includes pulmonary embolism, pericardial tamponade, and tension pneumothorax. Cardiogenic shock refers to inherent failure of the heart to maintain cardiac output. Although this is most commonly due to ischemic heart disease, it can also be due to myriad cardiomyopathies caused by inflammatory, infectious, valvular, stress and trauma-related, or drug-induced etiologies. Finally, hypovolemic shock

A. Cathers (✉)
Department of Emergency Medicine, UW Madison, Madison, WI, USA
e-mail: acathers@medicine.wisc.edu

N. Schnittke
Department of Emergency Medicine, Oregon Health and Sciences University, Portland, OR, USA

B. D. Nicholson et al. (eds.), *Manual of Austere and Prehospital Ultrasound*,
https://doi.org/10.1007/978-3-030-64287-7_9

refers to acute or subacute volume losses in the intravascular space without adequate repletion. Most commonly this refers to hemorrhagic shock, but can also be due to infection, especially gastrointestinal illness.

While the history and physical exam can often point the clinician to the etiology of shock and guide empiric treatment successfully, it is unfortunately often insufficient in the rapid evaluation of shock, especially when the patient is quickly deteriorating. For example, while most trauma patients are presumed to be bleeding until proven otherwise, trauma patients can also suffer from obstructive shock (tamponade, tension pneumothorax) and distributive, neurogenic shock. In the eFAST chapter, we explored the utility and method of utilizing Point-of-Care Ultrasound (POCUS) in evaluating the likely etiology of shock in a trauma patient. In the prehospital setting, POCUS may reduce unnecessary procedures in the field such as tube thoracostomy or needle decompression, which can often pose a risk to both patient and clinician [17, 28]. In emergency department patients with nontraumatic hypotension and shock, POCUS has been shown to substantially decrease the number of possible diagnoses [14] and the time to disposition [10].

The following chapter will build on previous topics to provide an intuitive pathway for using the various ultrasound exams covered previously in order to evaluate causes of shock in both medical and trauma patients. Indeed the first protocols proposed for evaluation of undifferentiated shock drew on the eFAST exam, starting with the Undifferentiated Hypotensive Patient (UHP) protocol in 2001. The concept has been substantially expanded by multiple astute clinicians to include nearly all etiologies of circulatory shock [23]. Here we will start with the sonographic features of the various pathophysiologies of shock, codified in a scanning protocol known as the RUSH (Rapid Ultrasound in SHock) exam. We will then discuss an intervention based approach, which integrates the pathophysiologic findings of the RUSH exam with the guidance of specific interventions, which can be performed in a limited resource environment.

Rapid Ultrasound in SHock (RUSH)

This exam protocol was first developed in 2006 by Weingart et al. [35], and further elaborated by Perrera et al. in 2010 [26]. The protocol is based on the notion that each pathophysiologic etiology of shock (distributive, obstructive, cardiogenic, hypovolemic) will produce physiologic features easily distinguishable by ultrasonography. In order to provide a framework for using ultrasound, the authors use a conceptual "plumbing" model to categorize the sonographic features into three main essential categories: pump, tank, and pipes (Fig. 1):

1. **The Pump:** refers to the function and pathology surrounding the heart. The focused 4-view echocardiographic exam (PLAX, PSAX, A4C, and SX) can rapidly narrow the diagnosis to several etiologies of shock. When assessing the heart, pay particular attention to pericardial effusions, ventricular function, and relative chamber size.

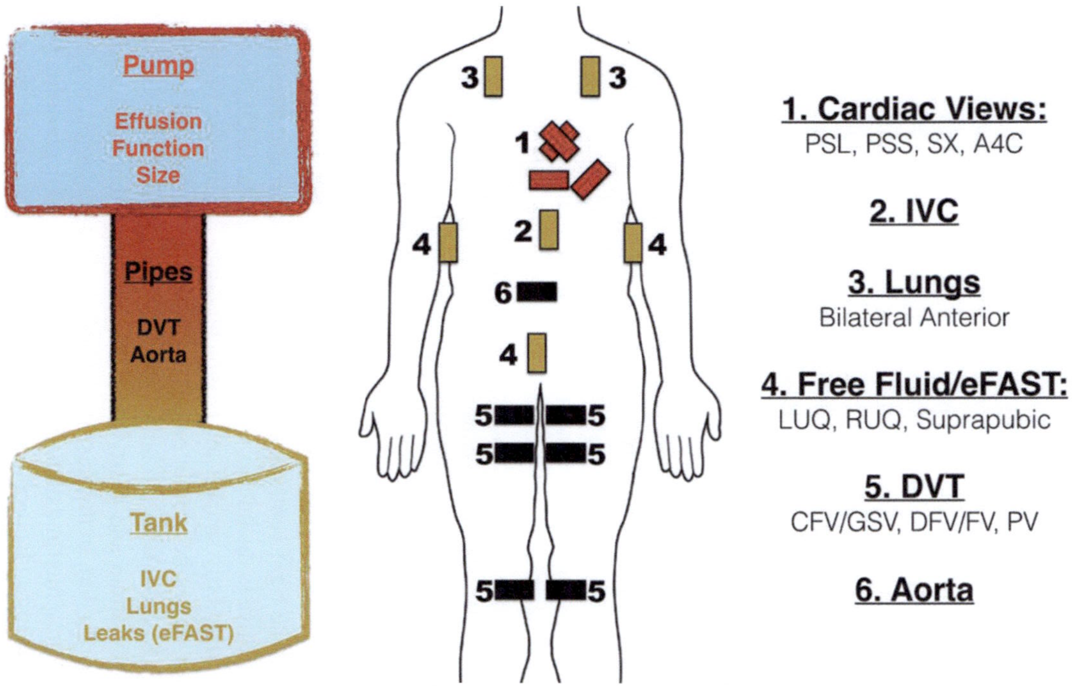

Fig. 1 The RUSH exam. Left: conceptual "plumbing" model of causes of circulatory shock, which can be assessed by ultrasound. Right: Anatomic views to sonographically evaluate the causes of shock as summarized by the RUSH exam

Pericardial effusions can be identified in any of the 4 focused views, however the subxiphoid/subcostal and PLAX views are most frequently utilized because they allow for long axis assessment of the largest amount of pericardium. In the PLAX view, it is helpful to set the depth high enough to visualize the descending aorta. Pericardial effusions can be confirmed as fluid layering anterior to the aorta, whereas pleural effusions will be present posterior to and lateral to the descending aorta. Once an effusion is found, it may be difficult to differentiate tamponade from an asymptomatic effusion in the emergent setting. Due to the relatively low pressures in the right ventricle (RV) compared to the left ventricle (LV), outflow from the RV is preferentially obstructed first. Identification of right heart failure is critical in the detection of this "tamponade" physiology. Collapse of the right ventricle during diastole (when it should normally be filling) is specific for tamponade (75–90% specificity) [2]. By contrast, collapse of the right atrium during late systole (when it should normally be full) may be sensitive to tamponade. Absence of collapse in either chamber carries a 90% sensitivity to rule OUT tamponade physiology in the presence of effusion [22].

For the left ventricle, one ought to focus particularly on systolic function. This is most easily done by observing the movement of the walls of the left ventricle in the PLAX and PSAX views. Cardiogenic shock presents with poor systolic pump function and in this case the walls will appear hypodynamic with poor movement inward during systole. One can also observe the movement of the mitral valve during diastole. In diseases with poor cardiac contractility, the mitral valve will have diminished movement, whereas during normal or hyperactive contractility, the mitral valve will have more pronounced movement, reaching the interventricular septum during end-diastole. In contrast to cardiogenic shock, hypovolemic and distributive shock present the heart with low preload and typically display substantially increased cardiac contractility, referred to as hyperdynamic function [13]. This is seen in the PLAX and PSAX views as near complete obliteration of the ventricular space during systole.

Unlike the left ventricle, the right ventricular wall has much higher compliance so that stress on the right ventricle can be reflected by dramatic alterations in RV morphology. Relative to the thicker walled, concentric, and large LV, the normal RV is thin walled, irregularly shaped and is typically only 2/3 the size of the LV [36]. Acute RV strain, as can be seen in pulmonary embolism will result in acute dilatation of the RV diameter with a relatively thin RV free wall, best seen in the A4C view. Chronic RV strain and heart failure can be seen in chronic lung disease or pulmonary hypertension. In this case the RV also appears enlarged, but the RV free wall will be hypertrophied and thick (>5 mm when measured in diastole). Remember however, that patients with chronic RV failure can also develop acute worsening due to pulmonary embolism or in response to another worsening lung processes, so do not use RV thickness alone to rule out acute pathology and use the clinical picture to risk stratify these patients.

Pearls	Pitfalls
Pericardial effusions are anterior to the descending aorta, while pleural effusions are posterior. Tamponade: assess for right chamber collapse. LV failure: look at wall movement, change in chamber size, and mitral valve movement during diastole. RV failure: look at RV size and wall thickness to assess for acute and chronic RV failure.	Tamponade: It can be difficult to distinguish tamponade from an asymptomatic pericardial effusion. LV failure: when evaluating for systolic function, the mitral valve should remain in view, to ensure you are not led astray by out-of-plane views. RV failure: Remember that chronic RV dysfunction can also have worsening acute decompensation. Use the whole clinical picture to guide interpretation.

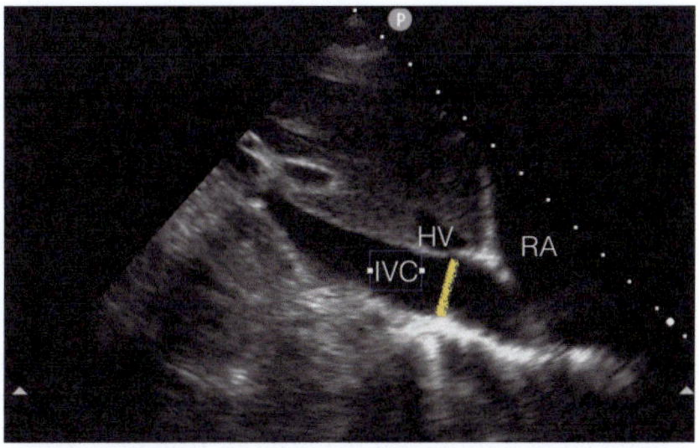

Fig. 2 IVC measurement just proximal to the hepatic vein (HV) before inflow into the right atrium (RA)

2. **The Tank:** refers to the status of the compartments responsible for cardiac preload. For the right ventricle, the tank can be assessed through the inferior vena cava (IVC) and by evaluating for causes of volume loss such as AAA rupture, hemoperitoneum, or hemothorax. For the left ventricle, the tank can be assessed by evaluating lung function and volume status (Fig. 2).

IVC overview The IVC is best evaluated from a modified subxiphoid approach. It is traditionally measured in the sagittal orientation although, if appropriately identified, can also be evaluated in the transverse orientation. The diameter of the IVC varies substantially as it traverses the abdomen, and by convention it is typically measured 1–3 cm distal to the right atrium, just proximal to the confluence of the hepatic vein with the IVC. During evaluation of the IVC, focus on the *size* and *collapsibility* of the IVC.

IVC Size Multiple studies have shown a moderate correlation between IVC size and central venous pressure (CVP) or right atrial pressure (RAP). Traditionally, an IVC maximal diameter < 2.1 cm has been considered small, correlating with a low CVP and an IVC >2.1 cm has been considered large, correlating with a high CVP [29]. However more recent data have emerged suggesting that the normal range may be much wider. These studies suggest that correlation of the IVC with CVP is useful at the extremes. Thus an IVC diameter < 1.5 cm appears to be relatively specific for volume responsiveness, while an IVC diameter > 2.5 cm is specific to lack of volume responsiveness [19].

IVC collapsibility and distensibility In addition to size, the IVC changes diameter during respiration due to changes in venous return. During negative pressure/normal breathing the IVC will collapse during inspiration. During positive pressure/mechanical ventilation the IVC will distend during inspiration. This finding of change in size is generally more pronounced when the RV preload is low (hypovolemic states). A collapsibility or distensibility index can be calculated as a percentage of collapse (IVC_{max}–IVC_{min}/IVC_{min})*100%. Change by >50% is consistent with hypovolemia, while change by <50% will be consistent with hypervolemia [24]. Again, these findings are most reliable at their extremes and care should be used when interpreting these values if they are unclear [7, 27]. In addition, one must make sure that the IVC remains in plane throughout respiration, as it may be difficult to make sure that the change in diameter represents true collapsibility rather than the movement of the IVC out of the sonographic plane. For this, make sure that the patient is breathing normally (do not ask the patient to "take a deep breath") or do the sniff test, by asking the patient to sniff. This will result in less diaphragmatic excursion and out of plane movement.

IVC summary The evaluation of the IVC has been controversial as it is unclear whether IVC appraisal accurately reflects "volume responsiveness" or merely correlates with CVP, which is known to be a suboptimal reflection of actual volume responsiveness [6]. In addition, IVC size can be altered by obstructive shock, and care should be taken to make sure that IVC assessment occurs in concert with cardiac and occasionally DVT evaluation to make sure that the dilated IVC is not a consequence of RV obstruction (tamponade or PE) rather than hypervolemia. Finally, while IVC sonography is helpful at the extremes, intermediate findings may be frustrating. In cases where the IVC does not provide an obvious answer, consider serial dynamic ultrasound during fluid loading to assess for changes in RV preload throughout the resuscitation.

Lungs and the LV "tank" The assessment of the "tank" must also include the compartment containing the LV preload: the lungs. Indeed, the most common way that rapid administration of volume will cause harm is by overloading this compartment, leading to pulmonary edema, hypoxia, and worsening cardiac ischemia in an already critically ill patient. Assessment of the lungs includes evaluation of bilateral B-lines indicating alveolar interstitial syndrome (AIS) and pleural effusions indicating likely preload overload of the LV. It is important to remember that AIS exists on a spectrum: it is often common for ESRD or CHF patients to have some B-lines without any compromise to the LV or oxygenation, however if there are >3 B-lines present in all fields the clinician should be wary of aggressive volume repletion without also addressing the contribution of cardiogenic shock to the overall picture.

While evaluating the lungs, one should also evaluate the pleural line for the presence of sliding and a lung point. Findings suggestive of pneumothorax in a hypotensive patient should raise concern for tension pneumothorax and rapidly change management. In this way evaluation of the "tank" can guide management beyond volume status and aid in the identification of obstructive causes of shock.

Tank losses When there is suspicion for hemorrhagic shock (e.g. trauma, ectopic pregnancy, or other solid organ bleeding) the eFAST exam (including lower lung views to evaluate for hemothorax) can also be a useful adjunct to the assessment of the right ventricular preload tank. In the proper clinical context this may indicate the need for blood product administration rather than crystalloid. On the other hand, in concert with a history of heart failure seen on echocardiogram, this may represent volume overload (ascites, pleural effusion) and may indicated cardiogenic shock. Thus, the evaluation of the tank is closely linked to evaluation of the pump and clinical history and should not be interpreted in isolation.

Pearls	Pitfalls
IVC size and collapsibility are useful in volume assessment at extremes. Consider cut-offs of <1.5 cm with 50% collapsibility and > 2.5 cm with no collapsibility as markers of hypovolemia and hypervolemia respectively. Lungs: Incorporate lung ultrasound for B-lines and pneumothorax into your volume assessment strategy. Tank loss: use the eFAST exam to evaluate for hemorrhagic blood loss in traumatic and atraumatic pathologies.	IVC: do not rely only on the IVC at intermediate values: Do serial exams! IVC: pathology other than volume overload can cause a plethoric IVC. Incorporate cardiac ultrasound to evaluate for obstructive etiology. Lungs: mild B-lines may not represent clinically significant volume overload. Do serial exams! Tank loss: Consider other causes of positive eFAST (ascites, pleural effusion) and interpret using whole clinical picture.

3. **The Pipes:** refers to the evaluation of the distal deep veins and the aorta.

Deep Venous Thrombosis

DVT Background Venous thromboembolism (VTE) is the movement (embolization) of clots to the central venous circulation. This can cause rapid obstructive shock by blocking right ventricular outflow when lodged in the pulmonary arterial vasculature. Clots within the deep venous system (i.e. the proximal veins which run in paired neurovascular bundles with an artery) are most likely to embolize to the pulmonary arteries. The deep veins of the extremities are very amenable to ultrasound evaluation for thrombus.

The clinical scenario is very important to raise the clinician's suspicion for VTE and prompt closer evaluation by ultrasound. Thrombi form in response to disruption of three factors, described by Virchow's triad: immobility/venous stasis (e.g. nursing home patients, prolonged travel, hospitalization/surgery, venous mass effect such as pregnancy), hypercoagulable state (e.g. genetic factors, disease processes such as cancer, hormone medications such as contraceptives) and endothelial cell disruption and activation (trauma, inflammatory disease states such as autoimmune disease, cancer, or infections). Clinically, patients may have leg pain, swelling, skin changes, or a visible/palpable collateral venous "cord".

DVT Ultrasound Anatomy For this exam you will focus on the deep veins of the lower extremity as they pass through the inguinal ligament. Figure 3 shows the anatomy of the deep veins. These veins are paired with an artery throughout their course and can be distinguished from the neighboring artery by compression (veins will compress much more easily than the adjacent artery). As the external iliac exits the inguinal ligament, it becomes the common femoral vein, which runs medial to the common femoral artery (this medial location with respect to the genitalia can be remembered by the mnemonic "venous – penis"). Just distal to this, one will see the greater saphenous vein enter the common femoral vein medially. In this view, the common femoral artery, common femoral vein, and greater saphenous vein will look like a "Mickey Mouse" (Fig. 3). Just distal to the greater saphenous vein, the common femoral vein splits into the deep femoral vein and the femoral vein (sometimes misleadingly called the "superficial femoral vein". Do not be fooled, this vein is very much a deep vein). As these deep veins run behind the thigh they will then form the popliteal vein. The popliteal vein is also a deep vein paired with the popliteal artery, which will sit right under the vein (use the mnemonic "pop – on top" to remember that the vein runs on top of the artery in the popliteal fossa).

DVT Ultrasound Overview In a clinical scenario when VTE is suspected based on exam and history, evaluation of the deep veins of the lower extremity may be helpful in identifying venous thromboembolism as the cause of undifferentiated shock. There are two key principles of the limited DVT exam:

1. *Veins with clot will not be compressible.* To demonstrate compressibility it is important to make sure that the walls of the vein touch, completely obliterating the lumen of the vessel. If you are unable to achieve full compressibility despite significant pressure, this is concerning for a DVT even if you can not see a hyperechoic clot.
2. *DVTs preferentially form in areas just proximal to the confluence of the deep veins.* Based on the anatomy above, there are three regions of confluence: region (1): the common femoral and greater saphenous veins, region (2): the deep and femoral veins, and region (3): the popliteal vein, which originates from the confluence of the deep veins of the calf. While 78% of DVTs are identified in more than one region, 22% can be isolated to one of these regions only and it is important to evaluate all three regions to capture these isolated thrombi [1].

DVT Ultrasound Technique Using a high frequency (linear transducer) start at the inguinal ligament to identify the common femoral vessels and push down focusing on the regions of confluence. Make sure the transducer is held at a 90 degree

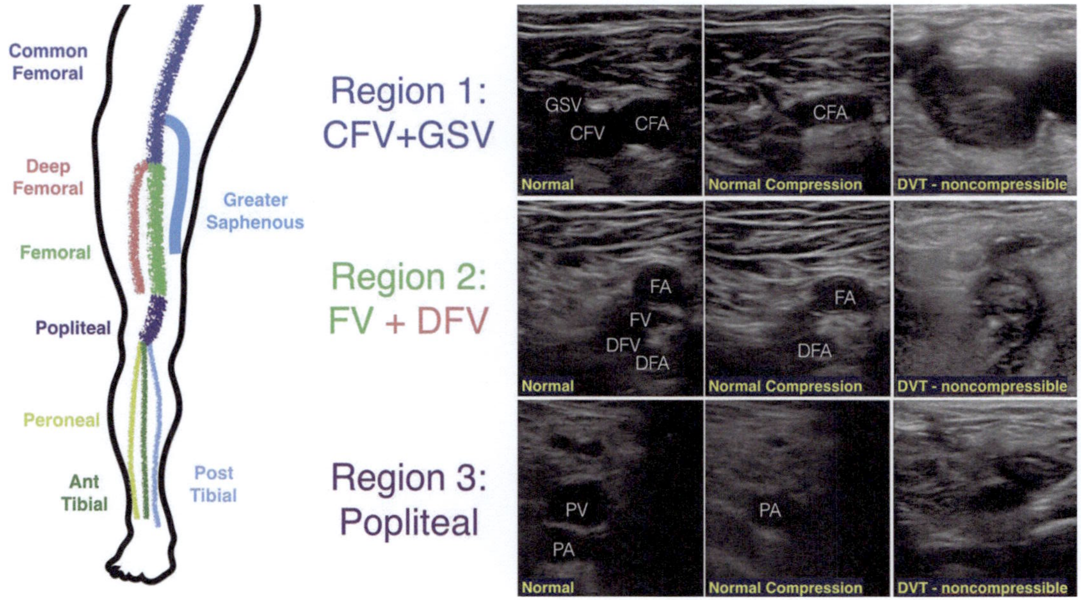

Fig. 3 The DVT exam. Left: Anatomy of the deep veins of the lower extremity. Right: Representative views of the three regions to scan during the focused DVT exam including normal views, normal views with compression, and positive exams with noncompressible, hyperechoic thrombus. CFV/CFA-common femoral vein/artery, GSV-greater saphenous vein, FV/FA-femoral vein, DFV/DFA-deep femoral vein/artery, PV/PA-popliteal vein/artery

angle and that you perform full compression and full release of the veins under direct visualization. Focus on each area of confluence by moving the transducer down about 1 cm at a time to make sure you catch the confluence of the greater saphenous vein and the deep femoral vein. You will then move the transducer behind the knee to find the popliteal vessels and again perform compression through this region to make sure there is no sign of a clot.

Pearls	Pitfalls
Position the patient to maximize venous filling with the extremity in a dependent position, best done through a Trendelenburg position. Externally rotate the hip and flex the knee to open up access to visualise the vessels. Once you see a DVT, stop the exam. Excessive compression may be associated with increased embolization of DVTs to the lungs.	Incomplete compression: most common mistake made by beginners. Make sure the lumen of the vein completely obliterates during compression and reappears with release. Starting with too much pressure: Particularly in the popliteal region, starting with too much pressure may make it difficult to find the vein, since you are compressing it. Assuming that a negative ultrasound means there is no PE. This exam is helpful to rule IN a PE. Unfortunately many emboli can originate from vessels not seen by this exam. In addition, if a large acute clot embolizes to the lungs it may no longer be present in the legs! In up to 50% of patients with pulmonary emboli, no DVT is found with ultrasound [32]. Do not rely on this exam to rule OUT PE as the cause of hypotension.

Aorta

Aorta Background The next structure that is useful to visualize and examine in the undifferentiated shock patient is the aorta. Specifically, the abdominal (rather than thoracic) aorta is most amenable to examination with bedside ultrasound to evaluate for an abdominal aortic aneurysm (AAA). A ruptured AAA can cause profound hemorrhagic shock. As the bleeding is internal and often retroperitoneal, this bleeding and shock can initially be occult and difficult to diagnose.

Dissection of the aorta can also occur, but frequently begins in the thoracic aorta, which is much more difficult to visualize on bedside ultrasound. In addition, many patients with aortic dissections are hypertensive initially, and may not be obvious candidates for the RUSH exam. On ultrasound, aortic dissection may be seen as a hyperechoic linear "flap" in the middle of the vessel lumen, however ultrasound is less sensitive for thoracic aortic dissection than CT scan and there are a number of artifacts that may mimic a dissection flap. While it is important that prehospital and austere environment be familiar with the presentation and pathophysiology of aortic dissection, our discussion in this section will focus on the ruptured abdominal aortic aneurysm (AAA).

The classic patient with a AAA is an older male smoker. However, patients with connective tissue disorders such as Marfan's can also be at higher risk. Other risk factors include positive family history, presence of other vascular aneurysms, atherosclerosis, and advanced age. The incidence of AAA is 4x greater in men than women, but women do seem to have a higher than expected rate of rupture and death [15]. It is believed that AAA-related complications lead to 3 deaths per 100,000, with the general prevalence of AAA in elderly males somewhere between 4–6%. However, many of these aneurysms are small, and at low risk of rupture [8]. Regardless, a high level of suspicion must be maintained for this diagnosis.

AAAs are often asymptomatic until they rupture. As such, many patients are unaware that they have a AAA, even though it has likely been slowly enlarging for years. The majority of aneurysms never rupture, but rupture can lead to profound hemorrhage and cardiovascular collapse. After rupture, mortality rapidly increases every hour, making this a very time-sensitive diagnosis requiring emergent treatment.

Rupture occurs when the weakened vascular wall fails, leading to extravasation of blood. This is often retroperitoneal but can also occur into the peritoneal space. Only 50% of patients with a rupture of their AAA survive long enough to receive medical care – further emphasizing the potential mortality of this disease process. Of those patients that survive to medical care, many of their ruptures are retroperitoneal or partially contained by a hematoma, which can increase the difficulty of diagnosis. Due to the vague symptomatology, up to 30% of all AAAs are initially misdiagnosed, often as renal colic, or musculoskeletal back pain [4]. A high index of suspicion, as well as attention to risk factors, is needed to correctly make the diagnosis.

Due to increased screening in at-risk populations, many patients now may be aware of their AAA even when it is asymptomatic, and so if possible, it can be a pertinent history question to ask the patient or family. Patients often complain of back or abdominal discomfort, along with dizziness, lightheadedness, and other symptoms of early shock. They can also have symptoms of lower extremity vascular compromise or ischemia due to decreased perfusion or intraluminal thrombus embolization.

On physical examination, there may be a palpable, pulsatile abdominal mass located in the midline. A bruit or thrill may possibly be auscultated. In patients with acute ruptures, particularly if it is intraperitoneal, there is often abdominal tenderness and signs of peritonitis, such as rigidity. Retroperitoneal extravasation can lead to classic physical examination findings of retroperitoneal bleeding such as Cullen's sign (periumbilical ecchymosis), Gray-Turner's sign (flank ecchymosis), and Bryant's sign (scrotal ecchymosis). Ruptured AAA should be presumed as the most likely diagnosis in critically ill patients with a presentation consistent with possible ruptured AAA and who are found to have a AAA on US. Occasionally it is possible to visualize clot or asymmetry indicative of a contained AAA rupture, but typically there will be no specific sonographic signs of rupture, so the clinician will need to make the diagnosis clinically by combining the presence of the AAA with the history and exam. In addition, because most AAA's rupture through the posterior wall and therefore retroperitoneally, a FAST exam will often be negative for free intraperitoneal fluid.

Aorta Ultrasound Anatomy This exam will focus on visualization of the abdominal aorta, which can generally be visualized from the epigastrium to the umbilicus.

Although the aorta gradually dilates over time, the generally accepted sizing guidelines remain the same. An aneurysm is defined as a segmental, full-thickness dilation of a blood vessel 50 percent greater than its normal diameter [9]. Most guidelines list the normal diameter of the aorta as under 3 cm [34]. Anything over 3 cm is generally classified as aneurysmal. The larger the size, the greater the risk of rupture. During routine ultrasounds, an aorta of between 3 and 5 cm is closely observed over time, while aortas between 5 and 7 cm are urgent surgical candidates, and aortas greater than 7 cm are emergent surgical candidates. However, it is important to remember that any AAA can rupture, and so the clinical picture must be closely considered with any abnormal finding.

There are several key vessels that can help confirm that the structure being visualized is the aorta. Most proximally, the celiac artery arises anteriorly off the aorta, forming what is called the "seagull sign" in the transverse view. The "wings" are formed by the branching off of the splenic and hepatic arteries. The next key vessel is the superior mesenteric artery (SMA), which appears like a "mantle clock" in the transverse view. Most aortic aneurysms are infrarenal, and so the scan must be done through the iliac bifurcation, which will always be caudal/distal to the previously described vessels.

Aorta Ultrasound Overview Early identification of a ruptured AAA as the etiology of a patient's shock can be extremely helpful. The primary subtype of the patient's shock would therefore be hemorrhagic. The principle of permissive hypotension should be followed, and early administration of blood products is ideal. If blood products are not available, judicious and small boluses of crystalloids should be used, with a goal of maintain perfusion and mentation, but not of attaining a "normal" systolic blood pressure or mean arterial pressure. If possible, the patient should be transferred as quickly as possible to a center with vascular surgery capabilities in order to provide definitive care. Ideally – that center would be pre-alerted by the prior team in order to mobilize the blood bank and surgical teams.

Ultrasonographic visualization of the aorta during the RUSH exam in a patient with undifferentiated shock can be extremely useful. If the aorta is visualized and is not aneurysmal, then ruptured AAA can be effectively excluded from the diagnosis. However, if a AAA is found, then a high index of suspicion must be maintained, and this can be used to guide the patient's resuscitation and disposition.

Aorta Ultrasound Technique Visualizing the aorta is typically best done with the curved abdominal probe. Oftentimes it requires deeper depth than other organs, with up to 15–17 cm of depth required to visualize the most proximal abdominal aorta (as the aorta generally becomes more superficial as it travels distally). A large swath of gel should be applied straight down the midline, from the xiphoid to at least the umbilicus. The probe should be placed just below the xiphoid process with the marker towards the patient's right, in order to achieve a short axis view.

Typically, the easiest structure to identify first is the spinal stripe. This will be a hyperechoic crescent shaped structure very posterior, with a distinct shadow behind it. The aorta typically sits just superior and to the right (patient's left) of the spine. Initially identifying the spinal stripe ensures appropriate depth as well as allowing the aorta itself to be more easily identified. Ideally the celiac artery take-off should be visualized to ensure that the exam is begun appropriately proximally. The probe should be traversed distally to follow the aorta until it bifurcates into the iliac arteries, which typically occurs at the umbilicus. Smooth pressure will maintain steady views as well as encourage bowel gas to move and reduce obscuration. If possible, longitudinal views should also be obtained to provide additional information. This can be particularly helpful as it will allow easy visualization of relative aneurysmal diameter in relation to the rest of the aorta.

A common mistake is to misidentify the inferior vena cava (IVC) as the aorta. Referencing the location of the vessels in relation to the spinal stripe can be helpful to avoid this. Additionally, if viewed longitudinally, the spine should create a "scalloped" appearance under the aorta. Finally, the aorta should vary in a pulsatile manner. However, the IVC can also vary with respiration/ventilation, and so careful attention must be made to differentiate the two.

A final important point is in relation to the measurement of the aorta. Measurements should always be obtained from the outer diameter to the opposite outer diameter. Although this may overestimate AAA size at time, it will prevent mistakenly underestimating size due to contained ruptures or internal thrombus, which can be either acute or chronic.

Pearls	Pitfalls
Use as much depth as needed to identify the spinal stripe, and then find the aorta Apply smooth pressure to maintain visualization and move bowel gas Consider doing a FAST concurrently to evaluate for potential intraperitoneal rupture If the aorta is visualized and is not aneurysmal, then ruptured AAA can effectively be excluded If a AAA is found, then a high index of suspicion must be maintained, and this can be used to guide the patient's resuscitation and disposition.	Inadvertently identifying the IVC as the aorta can lead to misdiagnosis Not measuring the complete aortic diameter can lead to false negatives, particularly in cases of contained ruptures with thrombus – measure from outside to outside Assuming that a patient with a AAA can only be hypotensive from a ruptured AAA and not properly considering other etiologies

Strengths of the RUSH Exam

The RUSH exam provides a conceptually sound approach to identifying the pathophysiology of shock. Each "plumbing" category has features that can lead to the accurate identification of the etiology of shock (distributive, obstructive, cardiogenic, hypovolemic) summarized in the table below. This provides an intuitive mental model for incorporating ultrasound into the management of the hypotensive, critically ill patient. Indeed, use of the RUSH and similar protocols has been shown to facilitate accurate diagnosis [33], change management [30], and reduce time to disposition [10].

	Distributive	Obstructive	Hypovolemic	Cardiogenic
Pump	Hyperdynamic, but can have stress induced heart failure in sepsis	Effusion and tamponade Dilated RV Cardiac thrombus	Hyperdynamic	LV or RV failure
Tank	Flat, collapsible IVC	No lung sliding with lung point Dilated, collapsible IVC	Flat, collapsible IVC Positive eFAST	Dilated, non collapsible IVC Diffuse B-lines, pleural effusions, and ascites
Pipes	No findings	DVT	AAA	No findings

Limitations of the RUSH Exam

Unfortunately the complete RUSH exam includes upward of 21 views and encompasses 5 clinical applications (cardiac, lung, FAST, aorta, and DVT) each with numerous nuances and pitfalls, difficult to master even for experienced clinicians. Moreover, patients in shock often present with mixed etiologies of shock (e.g. distributive, cardiogenic, and hypovolemic physiologies can co-present as septic shock). The regimented nature of the RUSH exam, can lead to delays in interventions (or even prolonged inappropriate interventions) while the sonographer attempts to complete the full RUSH exam. Moreover, a recent RCT found no mortality benefit in the group of patients randomly assigned to undergo the RUSH exam vs usual testing [3]. It is easy to see how such an elaborate exam might run counter to the spirit of retrieval medicine and rapid stabilization of the crashing patient in the field or other limited resource environment.

Fluid Administration Limited by Lung Sonography (FALLS) Protocol: Towards Sonography Driven Interventions

While the RUSH exam provides a conceptual framework to identify the physiology of shock, clinicians faced with a crashing, critically ill patient in an austere environment require immediate guidance on the most likely therapy to benefit the patient in front of them. In addition, it is important to rapidly limit therapies that are likely to harm the patient. In this section we will examine three categories of interventions potentially accessible to the austere environment clinician: Volume, Procedures, and Pressors (vasopressors and inotropes). These categories are summarized in Fig. 4. We will also discuss how POCUS (including elements of the RUSH exam) might aid in appropriate disposition for a patient.

Volume

The most common intervention accessible to the clinician capable of establishing IV access is rapid infusion of intravenous crystalloid solutions. This is typically the

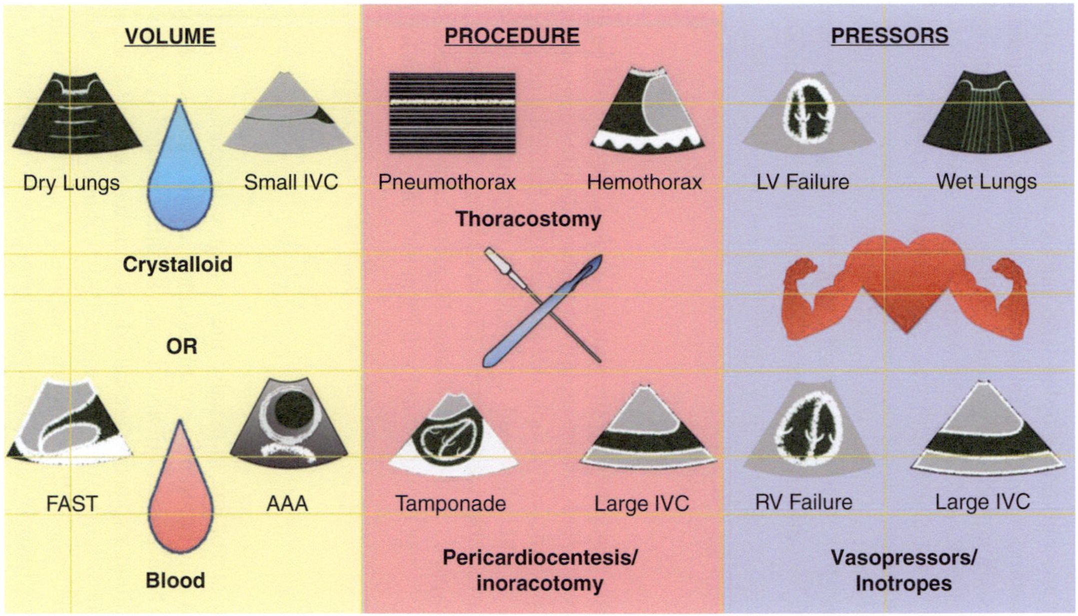

Fig. 4 Using sonography to drive interventions. Left: Features of volume tolerance includes A-lines suggesting dry lungs in anterior lung fields, small and collapsible IVC. Consider blood products if positive FAST or AAA if concern for hemorrhagic shock. Center: Findings of pneumothorax or hemothorax should prompt needle, finger, or tube thoracostomy depending on the capabilities of the clinician. Findings of pericardial tamponade should prompt pericardiocentesis or crash thoracotomy in a trauma patient. Right: findings of LV or RV failure or findings suggestive of volume intolerance (B-lines or plethoric IVC) should prompt initiation of vasopressors and inotropes as depending on the capabilities of the clinician

first step in the stabilization of the hypotensive patient. While it usually is an effective temporizing measure, how do we know if IV crystalloid infusion is going to benefit and not harm the patient? Moreover, how do we establish how much crystalloid to give? The FALLS (Fluid Administration Limited by Lung Sonography) exam [20] is one of the first protocols to apply sonography to specifically guide interventions of critically ill patients in shock. In this protocol, fluid administration is guided by lung ultrasonography coupled with cardiac views to determine serial response to IV fluids while monitoring for pulmonary edema. As discussed above, appearance of B-lines often predates respiratory failure and hemodynamically significant cardiogenic shock, and so transition to a B-line predominance should prompt the clinician to transition from treatment geared at treating hypovolemic shock, to treatment geared at treating cardiogenic shock (below).

In addition to crystalloid solutions, the clinician can also assess for signs of hemorrhagic shock via the eFAST views and AAA exam. Identification of hemorrhagic shock should prompt discontinuation of crystalloid solutions if blood products are available and rapid transfer to a trauma or vascular surgery capable center.

Procedures

During the sonographic assessment of the shocked patient, care should be given to address causes of shock, which can be rapidly reversed with lifesaving procedures. In the case of tension pneumothorax rapid decompression whether by needle, finger, or tube thoracostomy should be pursued. In the case of tamponade rapid pericardiocentesis is lifesaving even after cardiac arrest [5]. In addition, as the arsenal of pre-hospital procedures expands to include advanced endovascular procedures such as REBOA and ECMO, the use of ultrasound will be particularly important for proper cannulation.

Pressors

While administration of volume is usually the first step in managing a shocked patient, some patients may not improve with this intervention and a subset of those patients may actually be harmed. Patients who show improvement in cardiac output and perfusion with volume expansion are called "volume responsive". Patients who will not be harmed by volume expansion are called "volume tolerant". While the identification of patients who will be "volume responsive" can be very challenging, bedside ultrasound is extremely useful to identify patients who will not be "volume tolerant" by assessing for an overloaded "tank" and insufficient "pump" function. Patients with poor systolic function, plethoric/non collapsible IVCs, extensive bilateral B-lines, and venous congestion (ascites, pleural effusions) are at high risk of harm from further volume overload. These patients likely require medications to provide vasopressor and inotropic support with medications such as norepinephrine, epinephrine, or dobutamine.

From a practical standpoint, it is important to perform frequent reassessments during an ongoing resuscitation, especially during prolonged transports. If you note that the patient is not improving with fluids, serial ultrasound exams can help identify volume intolerance before extensive harm is done, and a prompt initiation of inotropes for cardiogenic shock and vasopressors for distributive shock can serve to temporize the patient to definitive therapy.

Transport and Disposition

Once the initial stabilization is complete, time can be spent in transport on the remaining pieces of the RUSH exam to communicate anticipated needs to the receiving center. The exact exams performed will be dictated by clinician expertise and resources available. If blood products are not available, this may be an appropriate time for the AAA and FAST exams. In the appropriate context, a DVT ultrasound may be appropriate to help mobilize resources at the receiving facility. If experienced and suggested by clinical history, biliary, renal and bowel exams may also be performed at this time to evaluate for an intraabdominal source of sepsis. Finally, repeat cardiopulmonary exams should always be performed to assess for patient response to interventions during transport.

Limitation of Current Knowledge and Future Opportunities

The use of ultrasound for diagnostic and therapeutic purposes has been steadily gaining acceptance in the emergency and in-hospital environment. Ultrasound use in the prehospital/limited resource environment is still in early stages, but has shown promise as an important adjunct to assist in determining etiology of shock and guiding resuscitation. Identification of the proper approach and application of this technology is essential to address and we think that the following three issues will be high yield to evaluate:

1. Validate the accuracy of austere/prehospital specific ultrasound. Several studies have demonstrated feasibility of ultrasound training of prehospital personnel [11, 21], however the exact test characteristics of prehospital POCUS vary widely from study to study. In addition, prehospital studies will often use protocols previously validated in the in-hospital environment. It is possible that time and ergonomic constraints (e.g. the back of an ambulance or helicopter) may dictate different exams or approaches, which may be specific to the out-of-hospital environment. For example, it is possible that a RUQ view only of the abdomen may be sufficient to guide resuscitation during a short transport, and it may not be necessary to perform the full "FAST" exam. Oftentimes, the equipment and training available to austere/prehospital providers are not equivalent to those available in tertiary hospital centers. The person performing the ultrasonography is also often the person with the highest level of medical training

responsible for interpreting and intervening upon the findings. However, there is no reason to think that adequate training cannot be provided to interested austere/prehospital providers. As we continue to improve our medical care and compact ultrasound technology continues to evolve, the quality of care will continuously be pushed outward from the main academic centers into the areas where it is often needed earliest. In order to do this, we need to expand the quality of evidence for prehospital ultrasound and develop a consistent approach to training and implementation.

2. Determine the utility of ultrasound as an adjunct to procedural interventions in limited resource environments. Ultrasound has become essential to many procedures including vascular access, pericardiocentesis, thoracentesis/thoracostomy, and CPR. Early studies have demonstrated promise in the prehospital environment for many of these procedures [5]. In addition to guiding procedures, ultrasound may also be very useful to rule out the need for an invasive procedure such as a chest tube [17]. Further optimization and validation of prehospital ultrasound exams is essential for our understanding of when to use this technology. In addition, the scope of ultrasound is constantly expanding. For example, recent studies have begun to evaluate ultrasound for prehospital endotracheal tube confirmation [25], nerve blocks for analgesia [7], and even confirmation of intraosseous needle position [31]. Finally, the procedural scope of critical care transport is expanding to include REBOA and ECMO, where ultrasound use will be essential to successful cannulation of vessels with relatively large catheters [16].
3. Define the downstream, patient-oriented consequences of ultrasound use for diagnostic and therapeutic guidance. Essentially – will this change patient outcomes? Obviously, this is a critical aspect of all medical research. In the austere/prehospital environment, interventions are often limited. However, many of the abnormalities appreciated upon the RUSH exam are amenable to (and in fact require) relatively simple, immediate interventions. While a recent RCT of the RUSH exam did not find a patient-oriented benefit to the RUSH exam [3], this study may have been limited, as the protocol did not give any guidance on how the findings ought to impact treatment. We hope that the intervention-centered approach as discussed in the FALLS protocol and sonography guided intervention as proposed above, may be more amenable to the study of patient-centered outcomes. Interventions (whether procedures such as finger thoracostomy or interventions like blood product transfusion or vasopressor initiation) can have enormous positive implications upon the patient's morbidity and mortality when appropriately applied [18]. Furthermore, we would be remiss not to consider one of the most important interventions—disposition. With an early diagnosis, it can be ensured that the patient is transferred to the appropriate facility by the appropriate team, thus substantially decreasing the time to definitive management. Further research is needed to clarify the optimal interventions as well as the integration of austere/prehospital into downstream medical care as a whole. We are confident that it will only lead to improved outcomes in our patients.

Conclusions

- POCUS and the RUSH exam can be an incredibly useful tool to guide the identification of the cause of shock.
- Specific sonographic features can be used to guide interventions including volume administration, procedures, and pressor administration.
- In the prehospital and austere environment, ultrasound can guide proper disposition and may decrease time to definitive management of life-threatening conditions.
- Serial ultrasound exams are useful to gauge response to resuscitation
- Each individual component of the RUSH exam must be understood deeply – not only the technical aspects of obtaining the images but also the physiology and management of the findings.
- Many patients can have multifactorial etiologies of shock, use the whole clinical picture and constellation of ultrasound findings to guide resuscitation and avoid anchoring bias.
- In patients with unclear past medical histories, the findings of the RUSH exam must be carefully interpreted in context of the patient's clinical picture to prevent misdiagnosis
- Often providers in the prehospital and austere environment will have limited interventions available, and so the interventions available must be kept in mind during the ultrasound evaluation

References

1. Adhikari S, et al. Isolated deep venous thrombosis: implications for 2-point compression ultrasonography of the lower extremity. Ann Emerg Med. 2015;66(3):262–6.
2. Alerhand S, Carter JM. What echocardiographic findings suggest a pericardial effusion is causing tamponade? Am J Emerg Med. 2018. https://doi.org/10.1016/j.ajem.2018.11.004.
3. Atkinson PR, et al. Does point-of-care ultrasonography improve clinical outcomes in emergency department patients with undifferentiated hypotension? An international randomized controlled trial from the SHoC-ED investigators. Ann Emerg Med. 2018;72(4):478–89.
4. Azhar B, et al. Misdiagnosis of ruptured abdominal aortic aneurysm: systematic review and meta-analysis. J Endovasc Ther. 2014;21(4):568–75.
5. Breitkreutz R, et al. Focused echocardiographic evaluation in life support and peri-resuscitation of emergency patients: a prospective trial. Resuscitation. 2010;81(11):1527–33.
6. Brennan JM, et al. Reappraisal of the use of inferior vena cava for estimating right atrial pressure. J Am Soc Echocardiogr. 2007;20(7):857–61.
7. Büttner B, et al. Prehospital ultrasound-guided nerve blocks improve reduction-feasibility of dislocated extremity injuries compared to systemic analgesia. A randomized controlled trial. PLoS One. 2018;13(7):e0199776.
8. Centers for Disease Control and Prevention. Underlying cause of death 1999–2016 on CDC WONDER online database, released 2015. Data are from the multiple cause of death files, 1999–2016, as compiled from data provided by the 57 Vital Statistics Jurisdictions through the Vital Statistics Cooperative Program. http://wonder.cdc.gov/ucd-icd10.html. Accessed 19 Feb 2018.

9. Chaikof EL, et al. The Care of Patients with an abdominal aortic aneurysm: the Society for Vascular Surgery Practice Guidelines. J Vasc Surg. 2009;50(4 Suppl):S2–49.
10. Hall MK, et al. Impact of point-of-care ultrasonography on ED time to disposition for patients with nontraumatic shock. Am J Emerg Med. 2016;34(6):1022–30.
11. Heegaard W, et al. Prehospital ultrasound by paramedics: results of field trial. Acad Emerg Med. June 2010;17(6):624–30.
12. Holler JG, et al. Nontraumatic hypotension and shock in the emergency department and the prehospital setting, prevalence, etiology, and mortality: a systematic review. PLoS One. 2015;10(3):e0119331.
13. Jones AE, Craddock PA, et al. Diagnostic accuracy of left ventricular function for identifying sepsis among emergency department patients with nontraumatic symptomatic undifferentiated hypotension. Shock. 2005;24(6):513–7.
14. Jones AE, Tayal VS, et al. Randomized, controlled trial of immediate versus delayed goal-directed ultrasound to identify the cause of nontraumatic hypotension in emergency department patients. Crit Care Med. 2004;32(8):1703–8.
15. Kent KC, et al. Analysis of risk factors for abdominal aortic aneurysm in a cohort of more than 3 million individuals. J Vasc Surg. 2010;52(3):539–48.
16. Ketelaars R, Reijnders G, et al. ABCDE of prehospital ultrasonography: a narrative review. Crit Ultrasound J. 2018;10(1):17.
17. Ketelaars R, Hoogerwerf N, et al. Prehospital chest ultrasound by a Dutch helicopter emergency medical service. J Emerg Med. 2013;44(4):811–7.
18. Ketelaars R, Beekers C, et al. Prehospital echocardiography during resuscitation impacts treatment in a physician-staffed helicopter emergency medical service: an observational study. Prehosp Emerg Care. 2018;22(4):406–13.
19. Lee CWC, et al. Corrigendum 'development of a fluid resuscitation protocol using inferior vena cava and lung ultrasound. J Crit Care. 2016;31:96–100. *Journal of Critical Care*, vol. 33, June 2016, p. 267.
20. Lichtenstein D. FALLS-protocol: lung ultrasound in hemodynamic assessment of shock. Heart Lung Vessels. 2013;5(3):142–7.
21. McCallum J, et al. Assessment of paramedic ultrasound curricula: a systematic review. Air Med J. 2015;34(6):360–8.
22. Mercé J, et al. Correlation between clinical and doppler echocardiographic findings in patients with moderate and large pericardial effusion: implications for the diagnosis of cardiac tamponade. Am Heart J. 1999;138(4):759–64.
23. Mok KL. Make it SIMPLE: enhanced shock management by focused cardiac ultrasound. J Intensive Care Med. 2016;4:51.
24. Nagdev AD, et al. Emergency department bedside ultrasonographic measurement of the caval index for noninvasive determination of low central venous pressure. Ann Emerg Med. 2010;55(3):290–5.
25. Nicholson B, et al. Feasibility of obtaining in-flight evaluation of endotracheal tube placement with ultrasound during helicopter transport. Air Med J. 2018;37(4):238.
26. Perera P, et al. The RUSH exam: rapid ultrasound in SHock in the evaluation of the critically Lll. Emerg Med Clin North Am. 2010;28(1):29–56, vii
27. Prekker ME, et al. Point-of-care ultrasound to estimate central venous pressure: a comparison of three techniques. Crit Care Med. 2013;41(3):833–41.
28. Roberts J, et al. Use of ultrasonography to avoid an unnecessary procedure in the prehospital combat environment: a case report. Prehosp Emerg Care. 2006;10(4):502–6.
29. Rudski LG, et al. Guidelines for the echocardiographic assessment of the right heart in adults: a report from the American Society of Echocardiography: endorsed by the European Association of Echocardiography, a registered branch of the European Society of Cardiology, and the Canadian Society of Echocardiography. J Am Soc Echocardiogr. 2010;23(7):685–713.
30. Shokoohi H, et al. Bedside ultrasound reduces diagnostic uncertainty and guides resuscitation in patients with undifferentiated hypotension. Crit Care Med. 2015;43(12):2562–9.

31. Tsung JW, et al. Feasibility of point-of-care colour doppler ultrasound confirmation of intraosseous needle placement during resuscitation. Resuscitation. 2009;80(6):665–8.
32. van Langevelde K, et al. Finding the origin of pulmonary emboli with a total-body magnetic resonance direct thrombus imaging technique. Haematologica. 2013;98(2):309–15.
33. Volpicelli G, et al. Point-of-care multiorgan ultrasonography for the evaluation of undifferentiated hypotension in the emergency department. Intens Care Med. 2013;39(7):1290–8.
34. Wanhainen A. How to define an abdominal aortic aneurysm–influence on epidemiology and clinical practice. Scand J Surg. 2008;97(2):105–9; discussion 109
35. Weingart, Scott. 'Original Rush Article.' *EMCrit Project*, http://emcrit.org/rush-exam/original-rush-article/. Accessed 18 Nov 2018.
36. Wilcox SR, et al. Pulmonary hypertension and right ventricular failure in emergency medicine. Ann Emerg Med. 2015;66(6):619–28.

Advanced Diagnostic Topic for Austere Providers: Abdominal Pain

Sean Burns and K. Meera Muruganandan

Abbreviations

AAA	Abdominal aortic aneurysm
CBD	Common bile duct
ED	Emergency department
IVC	Inferior vena cava
RUQ	Right upper quadrant
SBO	Small bowel obstruction
US	Ultrasound

Topic Discussion

Right Upper Quadrant/Gallbladder

Indication

Patients with severe right upper quadrant abdominal pain, epigastric pain, right sided flank pain or jaundice should be evaluated for possible gallbladder pathology including cholelithiasis (gallstones), cholecystitis (inflammation/infection of the gallbladder likely secondary to an obstructing stone), and choledocholithiasis (gallstones impacted in the common bile duct (CBD) which impair normal flow of bile resulting in infection/inflammation). Regardless of which of the three above pathologies is seen, all are potential surgical emergencies and require emergent care.

S. Burns (✉) · K. M. Muruganandan
Emergency Department, Boston Medical Center, Boston, MA, USA
e-mail: Sean.Burns@bmc.org; Meera.Muruganandan@bmc.org

B. D. Nicholson et al. (eds.), *Manual of Austere and Prehospital Ultrasound*,
https://doi.org/10.1007/978-3-030-64287-7_10

Image Acquisition

To best visualize the gallbladder, the patient can be lying flat or rolled on their left side which will use gravity to bring the gallbladder closer to the anterior abdominal wall. The gallbladder should be visualized in 2 planes, longitudinal and transverse. Start by scanning from midline to lateral along the inferior border of the ribs with the probe marker pointed towards the patient's head. Once the gallbladder is visualized, rotate the probe 90 degrees to visualize it in cross-section. Asking the patient to take a deep breath and hold their breath pushes the diaphragm along with the liver and the gallbladder down allowing better visualization of the gallbladder along the costal margin (below the ribs). The probe can also be held with probe marker towards the patient's right and with the probe held at a shallow or flattened angle to point the probe towards the patient's head in case the gallbladder is higher up under the ribs. The gallbladder is visualized as a large hypoechoic oval structure adjacent to the liver. Fanning through the gallbladder in transverse and longitudinal planes will help to visualize the whole structure as you look for stones or sludge. Most importantly, locate the neck where the gallbladder narrows to the cystic duct. If a stone is found here, it is likely the source of the patient's discomfort as it obstructs the outflow of the bile causing painful pressure on the gallbladder.

1. Position the patient flat on their back or on their left side
2. Scan along the right lower margin of the rib cage with the probe marker pointed to the patient's head. This will reveal the gallbladder as a dark oval structure behind the liver
3. Repeat this process with the probe maker to the patient's right side to get a cross-sectional view of the gallbladder
4. While holding the probe horizontal to the patient, fan up and down to find the gallbladder neck narrowing to the cystic duct.
5. Follow the cystic duct towards the porta hepatis, the region where the portal triad can be visualized (hepatic artery, CBD, and the portal vein). In cross section they resemble the "Mickey Mouse" face, with one large circle (portal vein) and two adjacent smaller circles (CBD and hepatic artery) (Figs. 10.1 and 10.2).

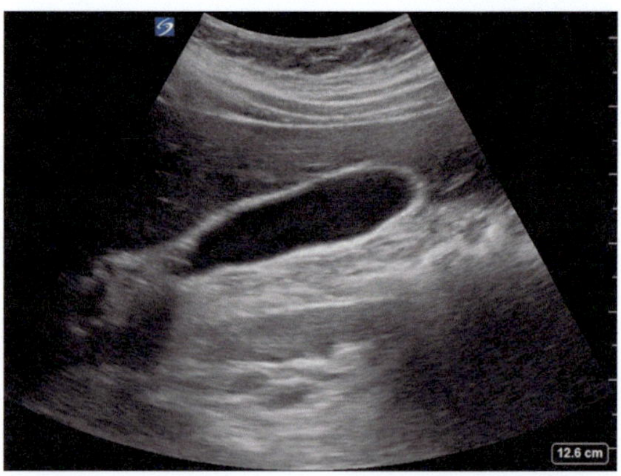

Fig. 10.1 Gallbladder in long axis: Gallbladder imaged in long axis

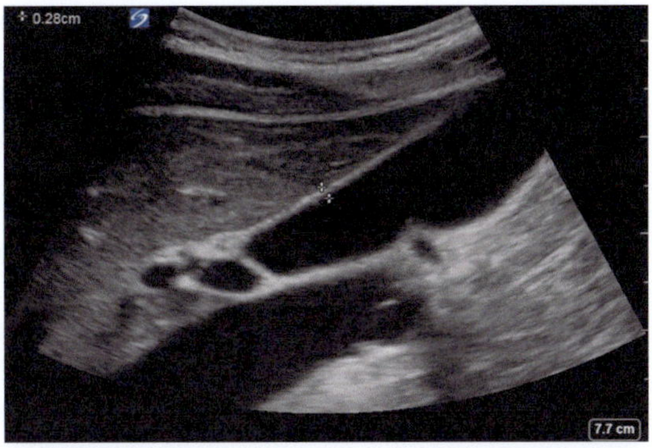

Fig. 10.2 Wall measurement in long axis: If unable to obtain an anterior wall measurement, measure the gallbladder wall that abuts against the liver in long axis at the thickest location

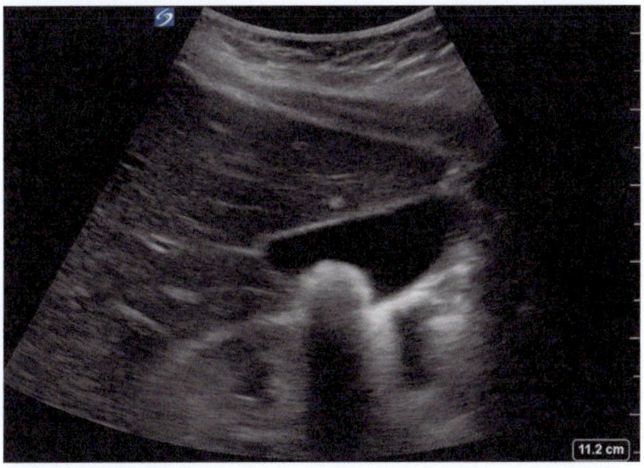

Fig. 10.3 Large Gallstone: Large gallstone with posterior acoustic shadowing

Pathology

Gallstones appear as hyperechoic semicircle structures with posterior shadowing, meaning that below their bright border, there will be a black shadow where the ultrasound beams cannot pass through the stones to visualize structures behind them. This is similar to imaging bony structures such as ribs which cause posterior shadowing as discussed previously in thoracic ultrasound. If a stone is visualized in the cystic duct or neck of the gallbladder, try rolling the patient to their left side and re-imaging the gallbladder to see if the stone moves out of the neck with the help of gravity. If the stone remains in the gallbladder neck with repositioning, this is concerning for an impacted stone (Fig. 10.3).

Cholecystitis is often a progression from cholelithiasis and is diagnosed by signs of inflammation. The ultrasound findings that may indicate cholecystitis include gallbladder wall edema, pericholecystic fluid, sonographic murphy's sign, and immobile gallstone (as discussed above) or presence of sludge. None of these signs in isolation is diagnostic of cholecystitis, but in the correct clinical context, these signs support the diagnosis. Gallbladder wall edema is determined if the anterior gallbladder wall is >3mm thick. However, this is nonspecific and can also occur in several other conditions including post prandial states, congestive heart failure, ascites, hepatitis, and protein wasting disease processes. Pericholecystic fluid can be visualized as a hypoechoic stripe in the space between the gallbladder and liver. We discussed the presence of an immobile stone in the gallbladder neck or cystic duct in the above paragraph. Finally, a Sonographic Murphy's sign is elicited when gentle pressure is applied with the probe directly over the gallbladder causing significant pain or guarding against the pressure. This is a particularly sensitive and useful sign, shown to be as sensitive as 86%, and when combined with other positive findings, is concerning for acute cholecystitis requiring emergent treatment [1] (Figs. 10.4 and 10.5).

Finally, choledocholithiasis is when a stone has descended through the cystic duct and now is obstructing the common bile duct preventing biliary drainage from both the gallbladder and the liver. The back pressure from the obstruction will dilate the common bile duct, and this can be measured in some scenarios. This is a difficult image to capture, and is often unattainable even in ideal conditions. However, as pathology increases in severity, such as in the case of a prolonged obstruction in choledocholithiasis, the CBD dilates more and may be more easily visualized. The CBD can be visualized by following the gallbladder neck to the portal triad. The CBD is visualized anterior to the portal vein. In a normal exam, the hepatic artery

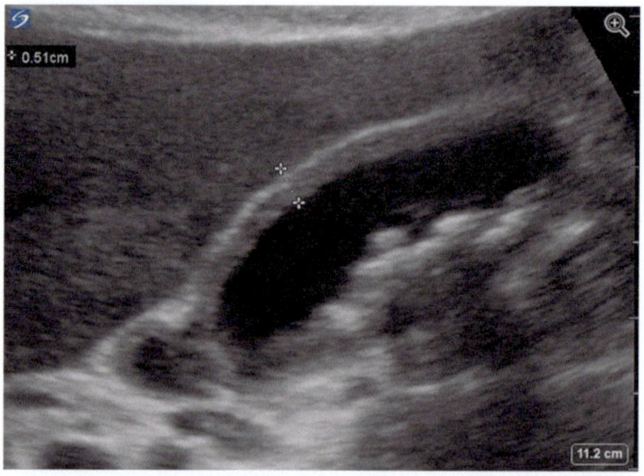

Fig. 10.4 Thickened wall in long axis: In long axis, the gallbladder wall is 5.1 mm consistent with thickened wall and concerning for acute cholecystitis

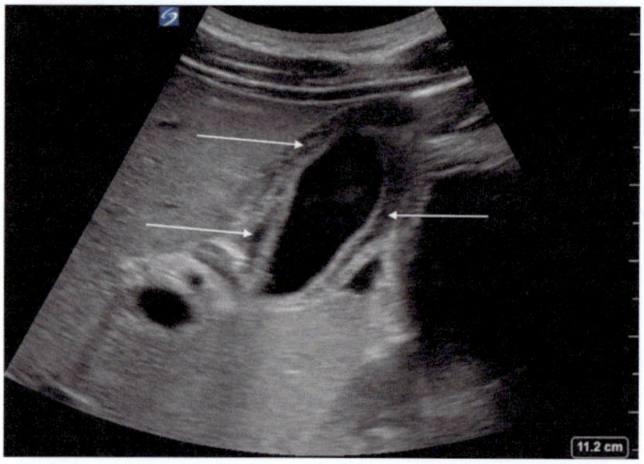

Fig. 10.5 Pericholecystic fluid: Pericholecystic fluid (arrows) is seen between the gallbladder and liver due to inflammation and likely acute cholecystitis

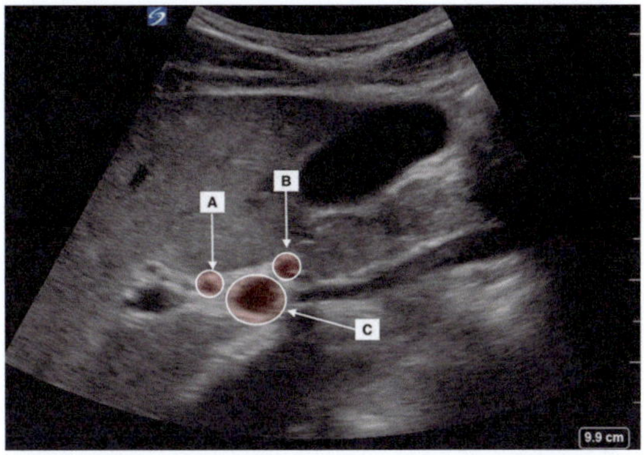

Fig. 10.6 Mickey Mouse sign: In cross section, the portal triad will appear as three hypoechoic circles, referred to as the Mickey mouse sign: common bile duct (**a**), hepatic artery (**b**) and the portal vein (**c**)

and CBD are smaller structures running in parallel to the larger portal vein, and the three are often compared to a "Mickey Mouse" face in cross-section (Fig. 10.6).

In the event of CBD dilation, the CBD may dilate to a size comparable to the portal vein. This is referred to as the "double barrel" sign. To differentiate the CBD from vascular structures, color doppler can be used to demonstrate the absence of flow in the CBD. Normally the CBD should be <6 mm but this upper limit increases with age. The general rule is that the normal upper limit of the CBD increases by an additional 1 mm for each decade of age greater than 50, so a 70-year-old should have a CBD <7 mm [2].

Key Literature

Several sources support the use of bedside ultrasound by emergency department (ED) physicians, often with competency demonstrated after as few as 25 completed studies [3]. While this has not been studied in the prehospital setting, it is conceivable that pre-hospital providers should be able to learn this focused skill under the appropriate training and supervision. In the hands of ED physicians, RUQ ultrasound was equally sensitive and specific when compared to formally obtained ultrasounds by US technicians and read by radiologists, with a sensitivity of 92% and specificity of 78% for cholelithiasis, and sensitivity 91% with specificity of 66% for cholecystitis [4]. Furthermore, Kendall et al. demonstrated that the majority of these ultrasounds take less than 10 minutes to complete [5].

Limitations of Current Knowledge and Opportunities for Further Research

The age adjusted cut offs for CBD measurement with age is up for debate. Wu et al. [2] proposed in 1984 that an additional 1 mm added for each decade over 50 years of age, but this is disputed in more recent studies [6, 7]. More studies are needed to determine if CBD diameter must be adjusted for age in order to achieve appropriate sensitivity/specificity.

Pearls and Pitfalls

- Rolling to the patient's left side may bring the gallbladder into better view
- The CBD is extremely difficult to visualize in most scenarios
- Polyps may mimic gallstones but do not cause posterior shadow

Kidney Stones (Nephrolithiasis)

Indication

Kidney stones are a frequent source of significant abdominal or flank pain that does not discriminate between healthy individuals and those with significant comorbidities. They should also be considered in patients complaining of back pain, lower abdominal pain or urinary symptoms. Renal stones are rarely visualized by ultrasound. More often clinicians rely on secondary signs of renal stones, such as hydronephrosis (dilation of the renal collecting system within the kidney). In the event there is access to point of care urinalysis, diagnosing a UTI in the setting of hydronephrosis is suggestive of an infected kidney stone causing pyelonephritis or renal abscess, which is a urologic emergency that may deteriorate rapidly to sepsis and death.

Image Acquisition

To visualize the kidneys, it is useful to use adjacent larger organs as guides. Similar imaging was discussed in the trauma chapter, as these views are largely extensions of the abdominal FAST views.

1. The right kidney can be found posterior to the liver. Place the probe over the lower ribs at the mid axillary line with the probe marker pointing towards the patient's head. Fan through the entire structure of the kidney.
2. Similarly, the left kidney can be found posterior to the spleen. The spleen is a smaller organ and thus provides a smaller acoustic window to visualize the left kidney. Place the probe over the lower ribs at the posterior axillary line with the probe marker pointing towards the patient's head. This position may require that the provider's knuckles graze the bed in order to visualize the kidney.
3. Both kidneys should be imaged in two planes, longitudinal and transverse. After the kidney is visualized in longitudinal, rotate the probe 90 degrees to visualize it in a transverse plane.
4. Finally, the bladder can be visualized by placing the probe above the pubic bone with the probe tilted towards the pelvis. Fan through the bladder in both planes, transverse and longitudinal (Fig. 10.7).

Pathology

While kidney stones cause significant pain, they often pass spontaneously with conservative treatment and rarely cause significant morbidity/mortality. However, ultrasound can help to differentiate between those that need for more immediate medical attention. Obstructing stones may cause a back pressure on the kidney due to lack of urinary outflow, ultimately resulting in hydronephrosis, or dilation of the collecting

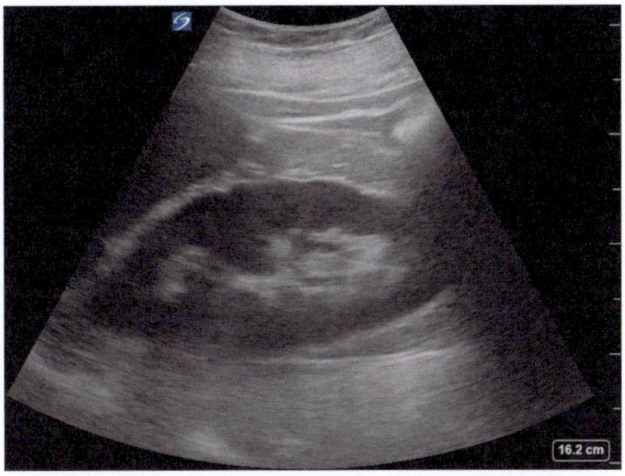

Fig. 10.7 Left kidney: The left kidney is visualized next to the spleen in long axis

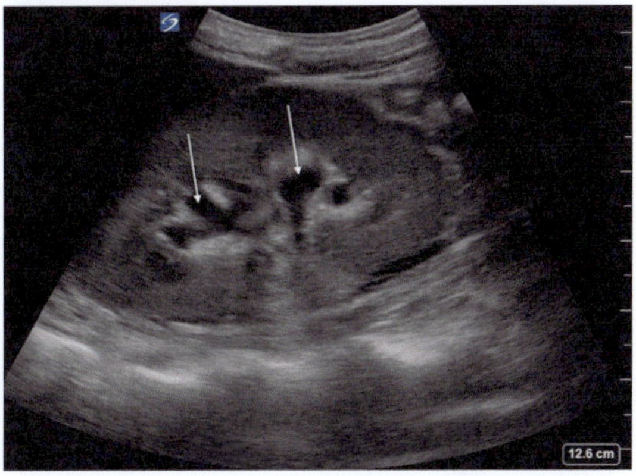

Fig. 10.8 Mild hydronephrosis: Mild dilation of the collecting system (arrows)

ducts within the kidney. Hydronephrosis is easily seen on ultrasound and is often compared to a head of broccoli given the appearance of the dilated medullary pyramids projecting from the central collecting system. It is very important to compare both kidneys. Bilateral hydronephrosis may be the result of congenital abnormalities, bladder outlet obstruction (such as severe benign prostatic hypertrophy or other causes of urinary retention), or pelvic masses. Color doppler can be used to differentiate hydronephrosis from pulsatile blood vessels in the renal pelvis. Another pathology that may be mistaken for hydronephrosis is renal cysts. Renal cysts, which also appear hypoechoic, are usually circular and located peripherally in the renal cortex as opposed to hydronephrosis which is centrally located (Figs. 10.8, 10.9 and 10.10).

Ultrasound can be used to measure bladder volume in cases where urinary retention is suspected. To measure the approximate volume of the bladder, measure the width and depth of the bladder in a horizontal plane (probe marker towards the patient's right) and the height of the bladder in a vertical view (probe marker facing patient's head). Multiplying these three measurements by 0.52 (or 0.5 for simplicity) estimates the volume in milliliters [8]. If enlarged (>300mL with the patient unable to void), a simple catheterization may provide significant relief.

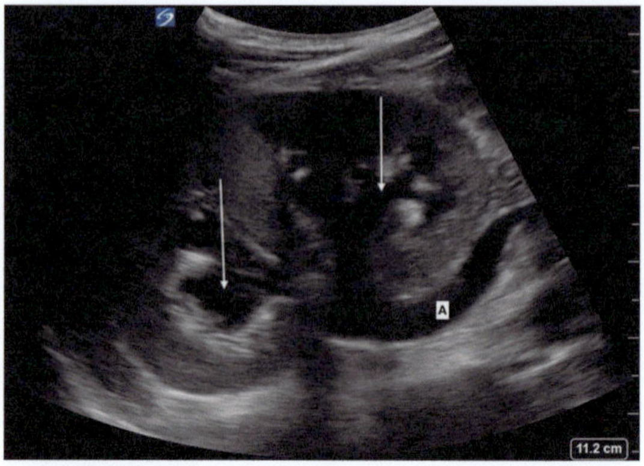

Fig. 10.9 Moderate hydronephrosis: Moderate dilation of the collecting system (arrows) with associated hydroureter (A)

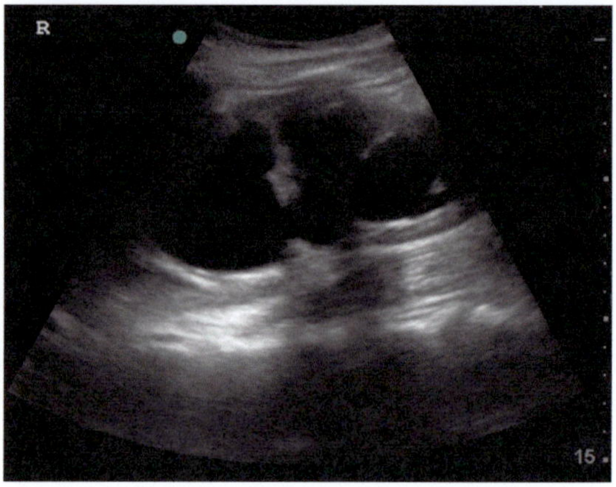

Fig. 10.10 Severe hydronephrosis: Significant dilation of the renal pelvis and collecting system with thinning of the renal cortex

Key Literature

Ultrasound demonstrated a sensitivity of 87% and specificity of 82% for diagnosing hydronephrosis in patients with flank pain when compared to CT as the gold standard [9]. Most importantly, Edmonds et al. determined that a normal bedside renal US predicted a less than 1% likelihood of urologic intervention in 90 days in patients with nephrolithiasis [10]. It is notable to add that ultrasound machines have improved in the past decade significantly, and that newer imaging may afford even better performance. Chan et al. demonstrated that US was highly accurate in predicting bladder volume when compared to the results after catheterization [11].

Limitations of Current Knowledge and Opportunities for Further Research

Since the kidney stones themselves are often not visualized, currently with ultrasound imaging alone, the operator is unable to predict the likelihood that the stone will pass spontaneously. Additionally, the presence of hydronephrosis alone may not predict a need for urologic intervention. Further studies could be performed to determine if ultrasound can delineate which patients will likely require hospital admission or surgical intervention versus outpatient medical management.

Pearls and Pitfalls

- Doppler flow can distinguish mild hydronephrosis from renal vasculature
- Always evaluate both kidneys to evaluate for bilateral hydronephrosis
- Consider AAA in all colic patients as this may present similarly with back/flank pain and carries a significant risk of death (see below)
- Point of care urinalysis pairs well with renal US if available

Abdominal Aortic Aneurysm

Indications

Abdominal aortic aneurysm (AAA) is one of the deadliest causes of abdominal pain and should be diagnosed as early as possible providing an excellent opportunity for pre-hospital ultrasound. Ultrasound is the first line diagnostic test of choice for this disease, and should be utilized broadly in elderly patients with hemodynamic instability and abdominal pain or back pain. Patients at risk include the elderly, males, smokers and those with connective tissue disorders. Again, as the pathology increases in severity, the results are more obvious on ultrasound imaging. A large 5 cm AAA is much easier to visualize than a normal 2 cm abdominal aorta.

Image Acquisition

1. To visualize the aorta, it is easiest to start subxiphoid (below the center of the ribcage) with the probe in transverse axis.
2. Gently increase your downward pressure on the probe to displace the intestines out of the way as the shadow from their intraluminal gas will obstruct views of the aorta.
3. Eventually with continued pressure, two circular structures will appear in the deep field. The two circles are the inferior vena cava (IVC) and aorta, and with the probe in the correct orientation (with probe marker to the patient's right), the IVC will be on the patient's right, and the aorta on the patient's left. Posterior to these structures should be a half crescent hyperechoic rim with posterior shadowing the thoracic vertebra. The IVC and aorta run just anteriorly to the vertebra, so this may serve as a guide to finding the vessels.
4. The aorta should be visualized from the subxiphoid area to the bifurcation in its entirety in transverse and longitudinal plane.
5. Color doppler can assist with identifying the pulsatile flow of the aorta compared with the venous flow of the IVC. It can differentiate other nonvascular structures such as vertebra or bowel (Fig. 10.11).

Pathology

The aortic diameter should be measured in four locations to rule out AAA including the proximal aorta, mid aorta, distal aorta and iliac vessels at the bifurcation. Measure the aorta diameter in cross-section at each location. Caliper placement

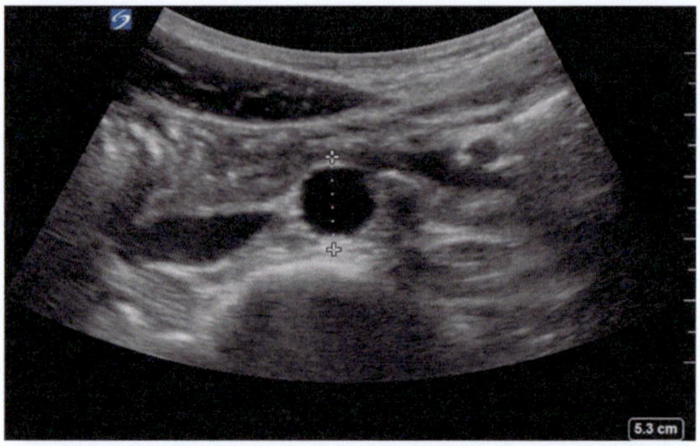

Fig. 10.11 Normal aorta measurement distal: Distal measurement of aorta from outer wall to outer wall

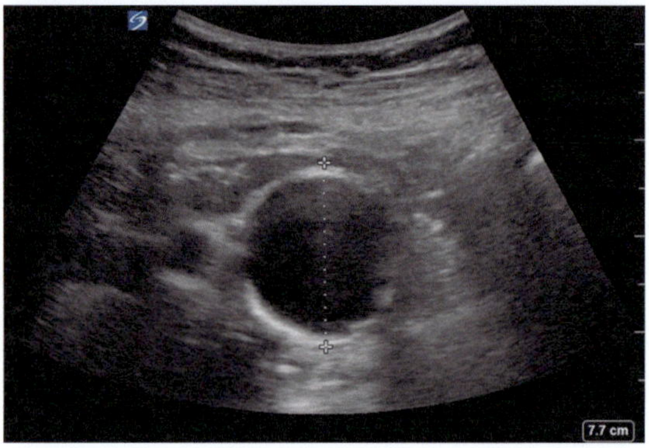

Fig. 10.12 Abdominal aortic aneurysm: Transverse view of a fusiform aneurysm measuring greater than 3.0 cm

should be outside the vessel wall in the anterior-posterior plane to ensure that any possible dissection or hematoma within the wall is included in the measurement. In symptomatic patients, aortic diameter >3 cm or iliac arteries >1.5 cm in diameter are considered abnormal and are concerning for aneurysm. Dissection flaps may be visualized in cases of aneurysms or normal caliber aortas [12] (Fig. 10.12).

Key Literature

The 2005 study by Knaue et al. confirmed that ultrasound in the hands of an ED physician accurately corresponds to the abdominal aorta visualized on CT [13]. In a study of ED residents in training who had completed 150 ultrasound studies of any type (with no requirement for number of AAA studies), ultrasound had a sensitivity of 0.94 (0.86–1.0 95% confidence interval [CI]) and specificity of 1 (0.98–1.0 95% CI) when compared to MRI/CT confirmed AAA in 238 at risk patients. Furthermore, as high as 6.7% of at-risk patients were incidentally found to have a AAA on presentation [14]. This study illustrates that this is not an infrequent disease process, and with the high mortality it carries, it is a crucial diagnosis to consider. Given the addition of ultrasound in the prehospital environment, there is a large opportunity to expedite resuscitation and transfer to a higher level of care based on the images alone.

Limitations of Current Knowledge and Opportunities for Further Research

There is no research at this point into the use of US in prehospital diagnosis of AAA. In the event this deadly disease is diagnosed in the prehospital setting, expedited transfer to a tertiary care center with appropriate surgical subspecialties could be lifesaving. The earlier the diagnosis is made, the higher the likelihood the patient may survive as it is all dependent on access to a higher level of care due to the medical and surgical complexity of management.

Pearls and Pitfalls

- The thoracic vertebra may be confused for a AAA given its circular contour and posterior shadowing that may mimic fluid. However, doppler color flow will not demonstrate any flow and can easily eliminate this error.
- Measure from outside wall to outside wall of the aorta/iliacs in order to not miss an intramural thrombus/hematoma which should be included in the diameter of the AAA
- Prolonged pressure with the probe will help to move the bowels aside to provide a clearer view of the IVC/aorta

Small Bowel Obstruction

Indications

Small bowel obstruction (SBO) is a more recent application of ultrasound with increasing support from the literature. Patients with small bowel obstructions are at risk for severe complications including bowel necrosis or perforation, making any tools of earlier diagnosis crucial to transferring patients to appropriate care for possible surgical intervention. This should be considered in patients complaining of abdominal pain, abdominal distension, bilious emesis, poor GI motility, and especially in patients with hernias or previous abdominal surgeries.

Image Acquisition

1. Utilize the curvilinear abdominal probe (or the linear probe in pediatrics or thin adults) and scan side to side across the abdomen, from the RLQ back and forth until ending in the LUQ (think of it like mowing a lawn)
2. This should be done twice, once with the probe held horizontally and second in the vertical plane. At regular intervals, apply gentle downward pressure to assess compressibility of bowel loops.
3. If a dilated loop of bowel is visualized (>3 cm) [15], hold the probe still, without moving, and assess for back and forth (bidirectional) flow of bowel contents indicating ineffective peristalsis
4. Do not confuse colon for small bowel, colon will have visible haustra which indent the outer border on the intestine wall. Small bowel that is distended may

have visible plicae circulares which appear as the "keyboard sign" where "keys" along the linear bowel wall are the plicae circulares.

Pathology

Dilated loops of bowel with lumen measuring greater than 3 cm in diameter measured from outer wall to outer wall is indicative of small bowel obstruction [15]. To confirm obstruction rather than ileus, dilated bowel must be followed by a transition point causing the obstruction where distally there is compressible bowel. A transition point is difficult to visual by ultrasound. However, in the clinical context of severe abdominal pain any incompressible dilated bowel is concerning. Additionally, SBO is characterized by ineffective or retrograde peristalsis, visualized as alternating back and forth flow of intestinal contents when watching a singular bowl loop over time. Thickening of the bowel wall >3 mm suggests edema and possible infarction of the affected loop of bowel [15]. Finally, free fluid surrounding the intestines is a very concerning finding indicative of possible strangulated bowel or bowel perforation (Fig. 10.13).

Key Literature

The 2018 article by A Pourmand et al. demonstrated that ED physicians can detect SBO by US with 93–100% sensitivity and 78–100% specificity based on multiple studies with differing levels of training [16]. In one of these studies, ED residents were provided with only 10 minutes of training on diagnosing SBO and then completed 5 ultrasounds on patients with SBOs to reach the above levels of sensitivity and specificity when compared to CT diagnosed SBO [17].

Limitations of Current Knowledge and Opportunities for Further Research

Differentiating between ileus and obstruction by ultrasound alone is difficult as it relies on finding a transition point after which the bowel is decompressed in order to diagnose true obstruction. There is not research into the ultrasound specificity of obstruction vs ileus in non-radiologists' hands. However, both diseases would likely require hospitalization until resolution, so this does not largely influence their prehospital care.

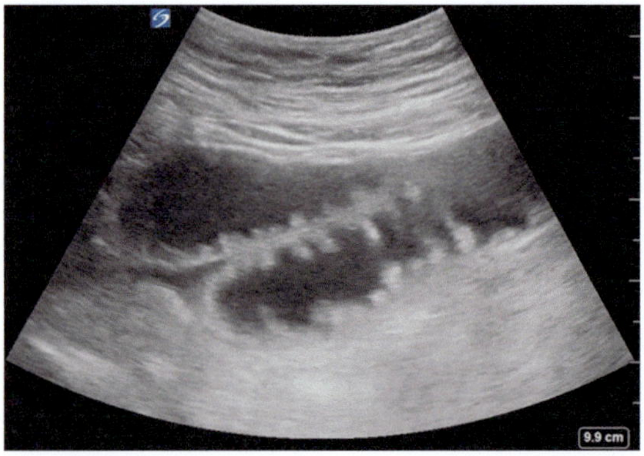

Fig. 10.13 Small bowel obstruction. Small bowel obstruction can be identified by dilated, noncompressible small bowel that is greater than 3 cm in diameter. There will typically be echogenic material within the lumen of the bowel exhibiting a to-and-fro whirling pattern

Pearls and Pitfalls

- Time is an important factor in SBO ultrasound, the bowels must be observed with the probe held constantly in place in order to catch diagnostic findings of SBO.
- Bowel loops filled with gas will obstruct visualization of the distal wall of the bowel and prevent measurement, so fluid filled loops are necessary for diagnosis

Appendicitis

Indications

While appendicitis is a very common cause of abdominal pain requiring hospitalization, historically diagnosis required a CT scan. However, ultrasound is now frequently used, particularly in pediatrics, as a first line screening test. A normal appendix is very difficult to locate by ultrasound whereas a dilated, painful appendix is easier for a patient and ultrasonographer to localize. Obese patients or those with significant colonic gas also pose a significant challenge in locating the appendix. This test should be considered in patients complaining of right sided abdominal pain or fever.

Image Acquisition

1. The appendix can be found often in the vicinity of the cecum in the RLQ. However, the easiest way to find an inflamed appendix to have the patient point to the area of maximal tenderness and ultrasound there
2. Apply gradual downward pressure in order to displace overlying bowel gas
3. Look for a tubular structure that originates at the cecum and comes to a closed end. The appendix's ending is what distinguishes it from the other continuous intestinal loops. It is often referred to as a "blind pouch" for this reason. A view of the distal tip is necessary to confirm it is indeed the appendix and to fully assess for possible appendicitis.
4. The patient can also be asked to turn on their left side for a few minutes to displace the overlying bowel, and then repeating the exam may provide a better view
5. There is significant anatomic variation to the location of the appendix, so sweep throughout the RLQ in an organized fashion to attempt to locate the appendix

Pathology

Findings suggestive of appendicitis include a non-compressible, dilated appendix measuring >6 mm in its outer diameter [18]. The presence of a hyperechoic appendicolith may also be detected. Periappendiceal fluid may indicate rupture, abscess formation, or surrounding edema. Color doppler may reveal a hyperemic wall suggesting inflammation. In a cross-section view of the appendix, the appearance is often described as a "target sign" due to visualizing concentric rings due to edema in the wall of the appendix from inflammation. Again, these findings are diagnostic

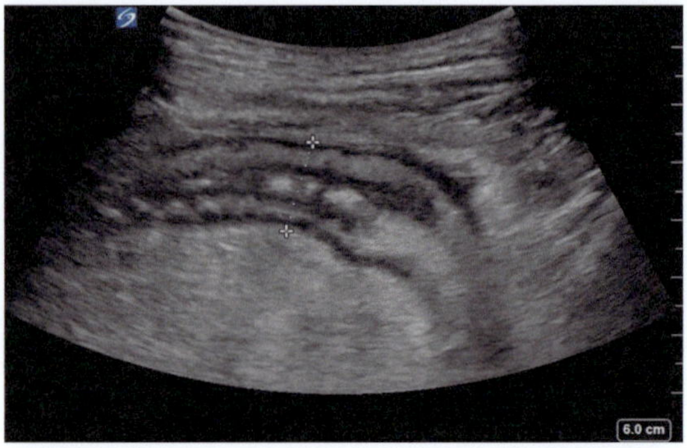

Fig. 10.14 Appendicitis with diameter measuring >6 mm. A diameter greater than 6 mm is indicative of acute appendicitis

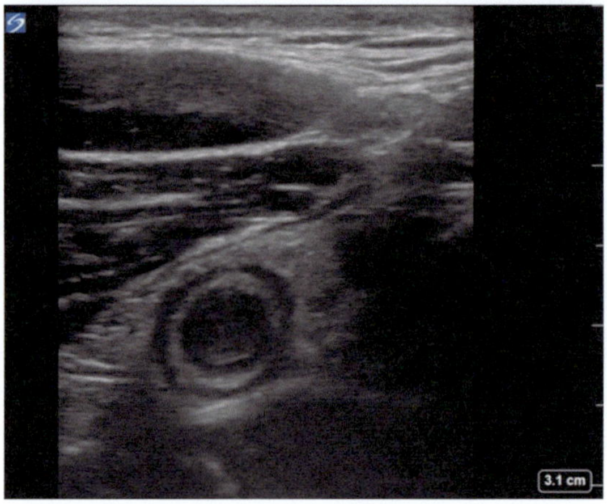

Fig. 10.15 Target sign. In short axis, acute appendicitis will often look similar to a target thereby earning the classic finding of "target sign"

of appendicitis, but the absence of finding the appendix or inability to visualize the appendix's tip does not rule out an appendicitis (Figs. 10.14 and 10.15).

Key Literature

Ultrasound has been rising in utility for appendicitis in recent years, however, much of the literature focuses on radiology obtained ultrasounds. In the hands of an experienced radiology ultrasonographer, a meta-analysis of 26 studies in children and 31 in adults demonstrated a pooled sensitivity of 88% in pediatrics, 83% in adults and specificity of 94% in pediatrics and 93% in adults [18]. Given this, many institutions are moving towards an ultrasound first in pediatric patients which may forgo a significant number of CTs while still maintaining appropriate sensitivity. This approach may miss appendicitis at rates of approximately 0.5% [19].

One study by Fox et al. found that ED physicians performed this study with sensitivity of 65% and specificity of 90% when compared to CT or OR diagnosed appendicitis [20]. Finally, 2012 Bachur et al showed significantly increased sensitivity of US with increased duration of symptoms whereas the sensitivity of CT was unchanged by duration, suggesting that early appendicitis is more difficult to assess by ultrasound [21].

Limitations of Current Knowledge and Opportunities for Further Research

There is not significant data about non-radiology generated ultrasounds for appendicitis. Given this is a newer application to be expanded to non-radiologists, it is expected that studies will follow that demonstrate the ability of other providers and experience required to gain proficiency in finding the appendix.

Pearls and Pitfalls

- Start the evaluation by scanning the location of maximal tenderness as identified by the patient.
- The normal appendix is very difficult to visualize, so ultrasound may prove an appendicitis is present, but is less likely to exclude it as a possibility
- An ultrasound alone may not adequately assess for rupture or abscess formation and a CT may be necessary despite a US demonstrating appendicitis

Conclusion

Given the many abdominal organs able to be visualized on ultrasound, it can provide early insight into the origin and severity of a patient's symptoms. Some applications, like the gallbladder ultrasound, are well established and easier to learn, while other applications like searching for an SBO or appendicitis are newer applications with ongoing studies and improvements. With this in mind, practice and broad use on a variety of patients will allow providers to become more comfortable with ultrasound as a means to triage and provide early diagnosis/management.

References

1. Bree RL. Further observations on the usefulness of the sonographic Murphy sign in the evaluation of suspected acute cholecystitis. J Clin Ultrasound. 1995;23(3):169–72.
2. Wu CC, Ho YH, Chen CY. Effect of aging on common bile duct diameter: a real-time ultrasonographic study. J Clin Ultrasound. 1984;12(8):473–8.
3. Gaspari RJ, Dickman E, Blehar D. Learning curve of bedside ultrasound of the gallbladder. J Emerg Med. 2009;37(1):51–6.
4. Rosen CL, Brown DF, Chang Y, et al. Ultrasonography by emergency physicians in patients with suspected cholecystitis. Am J Emerg Med. 2001;19(1):32–6.
5. Kendall JL, Shimp RJ. Performance and interpretation of focused right upper quadrant ultrasound by emergency physicians. J Emerg Med. 2001;21(1):7–13.
6. Karamanos E, Inaba K, Berg RJ, et al. The relationship between age, common bile duct diameter and diagnostic probability in suspected choledocholithiasis. Dig Surg. 2017;34(5):421–8.

7. Horrow MM, Horrow JC, Niakosari A, Kirby CL, Rosenberg HK. Is age associated with size of adult extrahepatic bile duct: sonographic study. Radiology. 2001;221(2):411–4.
8. Dicuio M, Pomara G, Menchini fabris F, Ales V, Dahlstrand C, Morelli G. Measurements of urinary bladder volume: comparison of five ultrasound calculation methods in volunteers. Arch Ital Urol Androl. 2005;77(1):60–2.
9. Gaspari RJ, Horst K. Emergency ultrasound and urinalysis in the evaluation of flank pain. Acad Emerg Med. 2005;12(12):1180–4.
10. Edmonds ML, Yan JW, Sedran RJ, Mcleod SL, Theakston KD. The utility of renal ultrasonography in the diagnosis of renal colic in emergency department patients. CJEM. 2010;12(3):201–6.
11. Chan H. Noninvasive bladder volume measurement. J Neurosci Nurs. 1993;25(5):309–12.
12. Ultrasound screening for abdominal aortic aneurysm an evidence-based analysis health quality ontario. Ont Health Technol Assess Ser. 2006;6(2):1–67. 006 Jan 1. PMID: 23074490.
13. Knaut AL, Kendall JL, Patten R, Ray C. Ultrasonographic measurement of aortic diameter by emergency physicians approximates results obtained by computed tomography. J Emerg Med. 2005;28(2):119–26.
14. Moore CL, Holliday RS, Hwang JQ, Osborne MR. Screening for abdominal aortic aneurysm in asymptomatic at-risk patients using emergency ultrasound. Am J Emerg Med. 2008;26(8):883–7.
15. Silva AC, Pimenta M, Guimarães LS. Small bowel obstruction: what to look for. Radiographics. 2009;29(2):423–39.
16. Pourmand A, Dimbil U, Drake A, Shokoohi H. The accuracy of point-of-care ultrasound in detecting small bowel obstruction in emergency department. Emerg Med Int. 2018;2018:3684081.
17. Jang TB, Schindler D, Kaji AH. Bedside ultrasonography for the detection of small bowel obstruction in the emergency department. Emerg Med J. 2011;28(8):676–8.
18. Doria AS, Moineddin R, Kellenberger CJ, et al. US or CT for diagnosis of appendicitis in children and adults? A meta-analysis. Radiology. 2006;241(1):83–94.
19. Ramarajan N, Krishnamoorthi R, Barth R, et al. An interdisciplinary initiative to reduce radiation exposure: evaluation of appendicitis in a pediatric emergency department with clinical assessment supported by a staged ultrasound and computed tomography pathway. Acad Emerg Med. 2009;16(11):1258–65.
20. Fox JC, Solley M, Anderson CL, Zlidenny A, Lahham S, Maasumi K. Prospective evaluation of emergency physician performed bedside ultrasound to detect acute appendicitis. Eur J Emerg Med. 2008;15(2):80–5.
21. Bachur RG, Dayan PS, Bajaj L, et al. The effect of abdominal pain duration on the accuracy of diagnostic imaging for pediatric appendicitis. Ann Emerg Med. 2012;60(5):582–590.e3.

Advanced Diagnostic Topic for Austere Providers: Ocular

Nicholas E. Weinberg and Zachary P. Soucy

Introduction

Point of care ultrasound (POCUS) has been used by ophthalmologists for many years with numerous applications. Today's typical B-mode POCUS has been found to be highly sensitive and specific in the evaluation of various types of ocular pathology which often present similarly and previously required detailed fundoscopic exam by an ophthalmologist to differentiate [1, 2]. In recent years emergency physicians have increasingly used ultrasound at the bedside to diagnose ocular emergencies as an adjunct to a traditional dilated fundoscopic exam which has limitations in the emergency department setting given skill and time requirements [2–5]. POCUS also appears to have significant potential in its application in pre-hospital and resource-poor settings where advanced imaging and/or an ophthalmologist capable of completing a full fundoscopic exam may not be available. In this chapter we will review the technique used for ocular POCUS, the application of ultrasound to diagnose certain types of acute traumatic and non-traumatic ocular emergencies, including some of its limitations, and review literature to support its use.

N. E. Weinberg · Z. P. Soucy (✉)
Department of Emergency Medicine, Dartmouth Hitchcock Medical Center, Lebanon, NH, USA
e-mail: Zachary.P.Soucy@hitchcock.org

B. D. Nicholson et al. (eds.), *Manual of Austere and Prehospital Ultrasound*,
https://doi.org/10.1007/978-3-030-64287-7_11

Topic Discussion

General Strategy

Anatomy

The normal eye predominantly contains anechoic vitreous humor – a gelatinous substance which fills the anterior and posterior chambers. The anterior chamber is bordered anteriorly by the cornea which may be visible as a thin hyper-echoic sliver, and posteriorly by the lens, iris, and uvea. Deep to these latter structures is the posterior chamber – a large round vitreous-filled cavity which is lined by the retina, choroid, sclera, macula, and optic vessels (Fig. 1). The optic nerve is a linear hypoechoic structure which lies slightly medial and deep to the posterior globe.

Under normal gain settings the vitreous should not appear significantly echoic, however, if over gained, the vitreous may demonstrate hyper-echoic streaks of collagen fibers which may be normal, and the vitreous of elderly patients may demonstrate diffuse evenly scattered echoes [5]. These non-pathologic findings can be mis-interpreted as vitreous hemorrhage; if uncertain about this finding, it can be useful to compare the contra-lateral eye for similar findings which would suggest against hemorrhage.

POCUS Evaluation of the Eye

Compared with other POCUS applications such as abdominal and cardiac ultrasound which may pose image acquisition challenges due to body habitus, anatomical variation and bowel gas; ocular ultrasound is unique in that the eye and surrounding components are superficial, easily accessible with the ultrasound probe, and rarely obscured by other tissue or gas. Additionally, many practitioners new to POCUS find the ease of ocular image acquisition gratifying. Ultrasound has a niche application when the eye may be obscured on physical exam by overlying edema or blood, such as in trauma, or when pathology opacifies the cornea, lens or fundus since a traditional visual exam may not be possible.

Ophthalmologists have long used specialized smaller high frequency ocular probes which are often placed on the cornea itself, employing both A-mode and B-mode [1]. For the purposes of this book, given that the typical emergency and

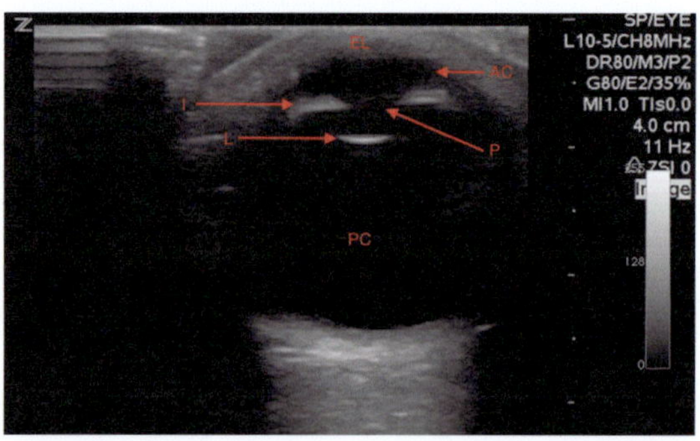

Fig. 1 Normal ocular anatomy including: eye lid (EL), anterior chamber (AC), iris (I), posterior chamber (PC), lens (L), pupil (P), optic nerve see Fig. 4, 5, and 6. Note, vitreous membrane and retina line the posterior 2/3 of the globe

pre-hospital provider will not have access to these probes they will not be discussed. Most emergency providers currently use whichever high frequency (12-7 MHz) linear probe is readily available on their bedside machine when performing an ocular exam. This probe type is appropriate for most emergency ophthalmologic applications since ocular structures and pathology are usually superficial and require high resolution imaging to evaluate subtle structures [6]. Some ultrasound machines will have an ocular preset which may optimize structures and pathology. If no linear array probe is available a curvilinear or phased array probe set to its highest frequency will provide less detailed imaging of the eye but may be able to identify significant structural defects. The phased array probe may be easier to acquire images given its flat contact surface though movement in the long axis of the probe may be required to image the entire eye.

There are two methods to apply gel to the closed eyelid. In a resource limited setting it may be preferred to apply gel directly to the closed eyelid. Technically, this optimizes imaging of underlying structures by minimizing trapped air between the probe and skin surrounding the eye. It is safe, as standard US gel is non-toxic, and minimizes additional supplies needed. Use caution if another coupling agent is used which may be toxic to the eye. Alternatively, a large transparent adhesive film dressing such as a Tegaderm can be applied to the eyelid and orbit to keep gel out of the spaces of the eye. Gently press the dressing into the indentations of the eye and orbit to remove any air pockets and take care to avoid pulling hair out by removing it gently when finished [7].

Given the irregular shape of the eye and surrounding orbit, ocular POCUS generally requires more gel than other ultrasound studies on flatter surfaces such as lungs and abdomen however, the exact amount of gel required may vary based on the clinical scenario. When scanning, the extra fingers not holding the probe should be used to support the probe on either the bridge of the nose or the forehead (Fig. 2). This has a dual advantage of increasing patient comfort since excessive pressure on the globe is unpleasant, and avoiding exacerbating existing trauma if globe rupture is present; ideally, the probe should be lightly "floating" on a thick cushion of gel. In contrast to other studies where warm gel is welcomed, cool or cold gel will maintain its shape and allow the operator to contact the gel without directly contacting the eyelid.

Vitreous Hemorrhage (VH)

VH may occur spontaneously secondary to diabetic retinopathy, age-related macular degeneration, retinal vein occlusion, retinal tears, subarachnoid hemorrhage or anti-coagulant use [8]. It may also happen secondary to trauma including shaken-baby syndrome, direct ocular insult, or head or facial blow [5]. It is usually described as a painless sudden change of vision, sometimes associated with dark streaks or floaters in the visual field.

Ultrasound findings vary based on the size and age of the hemorrhage. Care should be taken not to misdiagnose normal findings in the over-gained vitreous for hemorrhage (as stated above), thereby missing the actual cause of the visual complaint. Initial hemorrhage may be visualized as small echogenic dots or short lines (Fig. 3). A large, severe, acute hemorrhage may demonstrate highly echogenic clots in the vitreous, while more chronic hemorrhage may demonstrate dependent

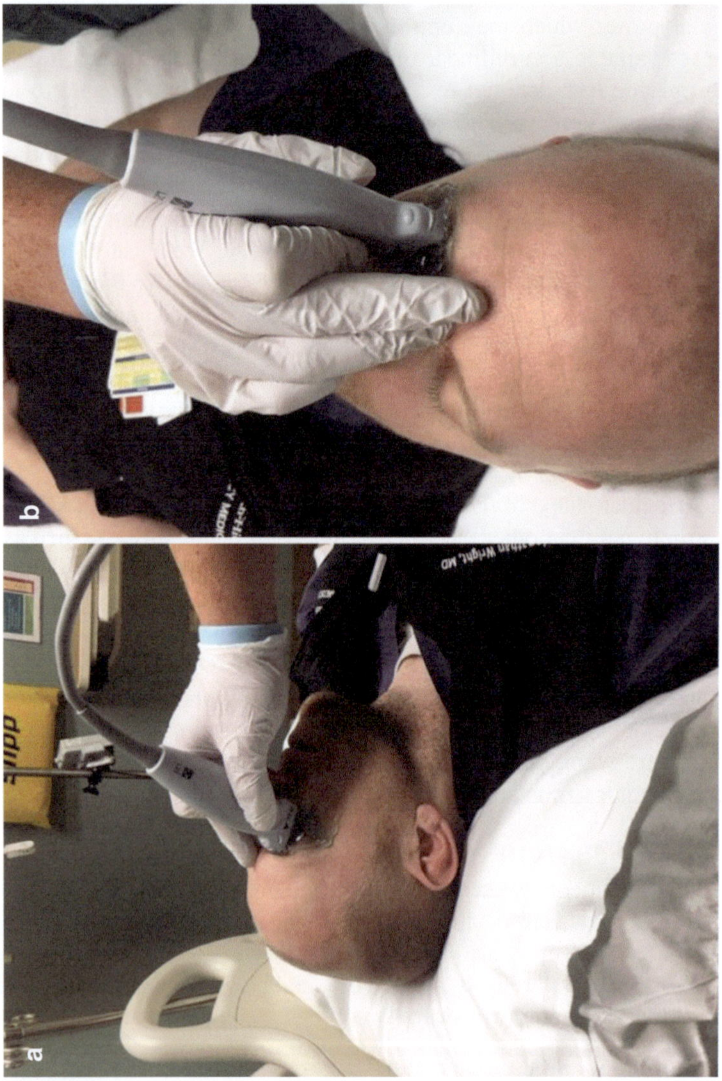

Fig. 2 (**a**, **b**) Appropriate sagittal probe position including anchoring on nasal bridge and forehead with use of gel pillow

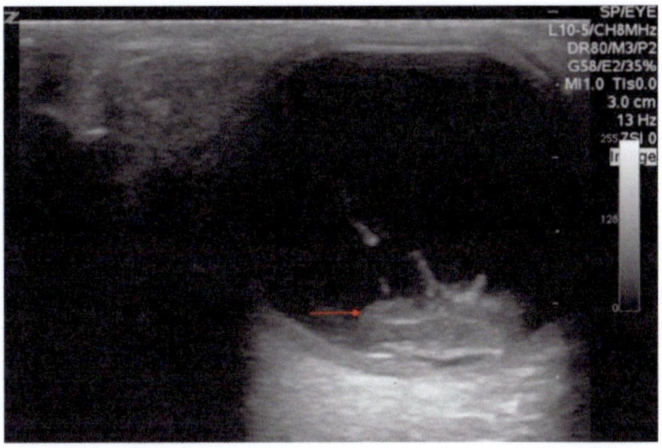

Fig. 3 Classic starry sky with speckled clot floating in vitreous humor. Arrow indicates large clot layering out in the posterior globe

layering, less echogenic clot, or a "pseudomembrane" which may resemble a retinal detachment [5, 9].

Early evaluation by an ophthalmologist is recommended in cases of trauma, severe coagulopathy, or when retinal tear is suspected, while urgent (24 hr) evaluation is recommended in all other cases. Patients should be instructed to keep their heads elevated at 30–45 degrees to allow blood to settle inferiorly.

Posterior Vitreous Detachment (PVD)

PVD results when the vitreous pulls away from the surrounding retina and commonly occurs secondary to normal aging of the eye, but can also be caused by any type of ocular inflammation, hemorrhage, or trauma, and may occur concomitantly with VH [8]. Patient's classically present with painless "flashes and floaters" as the vitreous pulls away from the retina and may have decreased visual acuity if associated with hemorrhage or retinal tears [2, 5].

PVD is usually well visualized on ultrasound as a thin, smooth, and mobile membrane running adjacent to the posterior globe. This membrane is highly mobile with eye movements – commonly described as a "jiggly" appearance and is not anchored posteriorly at the optic nerve (Fig. 4) [5]. These can be differentiated from a retinal detachment which is thicker, less mobile, and may be tethered to the optic nerve posteriorly or ora serrata anteriorly. PVD is usually a benign finding that resolves spontaneously, however, patients should be referred to ophthalmology urgently as this may predispose them to retinal tears which cannot be visualized on US.

Retinal Tear and Detachment (RD)

Retinal tears and detachments result when the retina tears and separates from the surrounding sclera and are a potentially vision threatening condition which can often be rapidly diagnosed by a practitioner trained in POCUS. Causes include diabetic retinopathy, tumors, uveitis, remote trauma, ocular surgery, and acute trauma. They can also take place spontaneously in near sighted individuals [5]. Similar to PVD, patients may complain of "flashes and floaters" initially, however, as the tear progresses they may complain of the hallmark "curtain" or "veil" covering part of

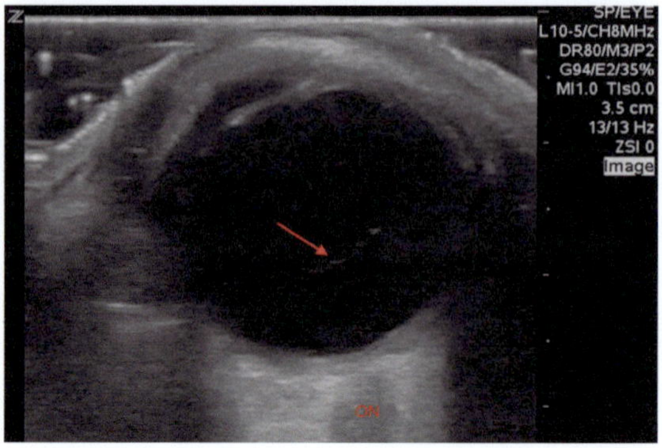

Fig. 4 PVD pictured is thinner than RD, not anchored to ON, and more mobile on oculokinetics

their visual field. Visual acuity may be significantly affected if the tear includes the macula – the portion of the retina lateral to the optic nerve critical for vision.

POCUS has been found to be highly useful in the diagnosis of RD with sensitivities reported as high as 96–100% in those with formal ultrasound training [10–12]. This is visualized sonographically as a thicker, less mobile membrane that is tethered posteriorly at the optic nerve. The detached retina may appear as a distinctive V-shaped hyper-echoic structure with the point of the V indicating the location that the retina is tethered to the optic nerve – again helping to differentiate it from a PVD (Fig. 5) [7]. If a thick minimally mobile flap without tethering to the optic nerve is identified RD should still be strongly considered as the RD may not have yet progressed to the optic nerve. Concomitant VH may also be associated with retinal tears and detachments so careful attention must be paid to imaging the entire globe.

RD is considered a time sensitive ophthalmologic emergency and requires emergent ophthalmologic consultation – especially if the macula is not detached since there is still a chance of preserving visual acuity. If the macula is already detached consultation for surgical repair is required but vision loss may be irreversable.

Optic Nerve Edema/Elevated Intracranial Pressure

There has been much recent interest in the use of ultrasound to assess for elevations in intracranial pressure (ICP). Of particular interest are the patients with concern for idiopathic intracranial hypertension or the hemodynamically unstable trauma patient with concern for intracranial hemorrhage, in whom CT imaging would like to be avoided. There is also potential use in its ability to asses for increased ICP in austere and wilderness settings in which CT and MRI imaging as well as neurosurgical consultation are not available. There have been various studies assessing optic nerve sheath diameter (ONSD) as a proxy for intracranial pressure, demonstrating a correlation between ONSD and ICP [13–15]. Kimberly et al reported sensitivity and specificity of 88% and 93% respectively for an optic nerve sheath diameter of >5 mm (measured 3 mm from the back of the globe), to detect ICP of >20 cm H_2O in adults (Fig. 6) [15]. In pre-hospital or austere setting these measurements can be used to increase suspicion for increased ICP and expedite evacuation to definitive medical care but is not sensitive enough to rule out this condition.

There are additional studies suggesting that ONSD can be elevated in patients with acute mountain sickness, high altitude cerebral edema, and high altitude

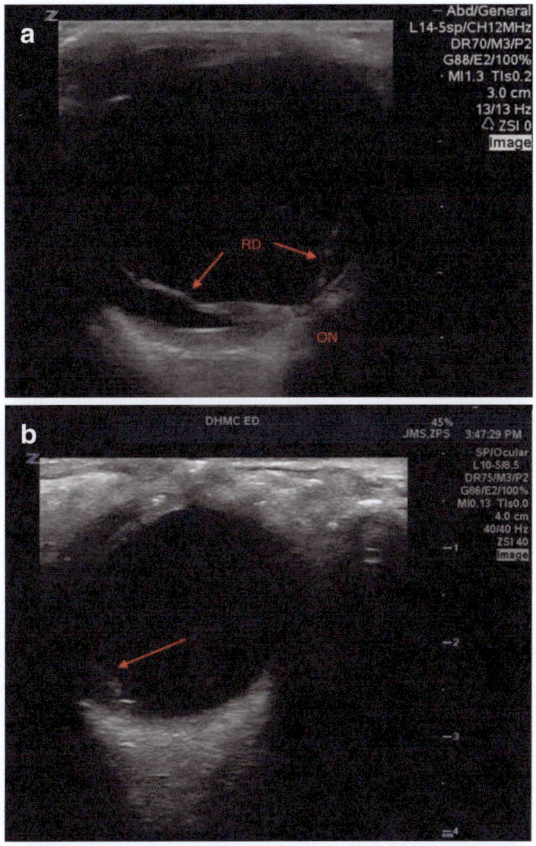

Fig. 5 (**a**) Classic V shaped RD anchored to ON, (**b**) far anterior lateral RD visualized on POCUS unable to be visualized by ophthalmology in emergency department without specialized equipment from clinic

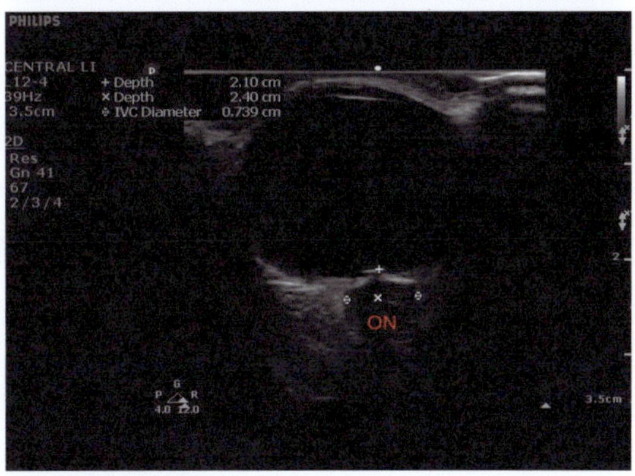

Fig. 6 Intubated pt too unstable to get CT scan revealed ONSD of 7.39 mm. Patient found to have uncal herniation

pulmonary edema [16, 17]. However, these diseases are usually clinically diagnosed and do not usually require advanced brain imaging or neurosurgical intervention; this in conjunction with its sensitivity noted above limit the use of ultrasound in these scenarios.

Globe Rupture

Globe injury and rupture may result from either blunt or penetrating traumatic injury and is considered an ophthalmologic emergency. Despite CT imaging traditionally being the definitive diagnostic modality for this condition, POCUS can be useful in a very limited number of situations, including austere settings without CT, or in the hemodynamically unstable patient who's globe cannot be directly visualized or who cannot safely undergo CT imaging. In this situation it is useful to have a diagnosis for early ophthalmologic consultation. Patients may present with significant pain, swelling, decreased extra-ocular movements (entrapment), or obvious disruption of ocular anatomy such as extruding tissue, leaking vitreous, or a tear-shaped pupil. If findings of globe rupture or perforation are present on direct visualization ocular US should be conducted only at the discretion of the ophthalmology consultant.

At times globe rupture or leak may be an unexpected finding. Operators should be aware of this sonographic appearance which includes gross distortion of ocular structures – specifically folding of the sclera instead of a consistent round shape, as well as flattening of the anterior chamber [5]. Associated retinal detachments, VH, or foreign body in the case of penetrating injury may also be seen (Fig. 7). Extreme care must be taken to use copious amount of cold gel, rest the scanning hand on surrounding facial bones and eliminate any ocular probe pressure, as even minimal pressure on a ruptured globe can exacerbate the injury causing extrusion of internal globe contents. This is another time-sensitive ophthalmologic emergency requiring immediate consultation for surgical repair.

Penetrating Foreign Body

POCUS has been increasingly used to evaluate for cutaneous foreign bodies due to its ease of use and ability to identify radiolucent foreign bodies such as certain types of glass or wood splinters, and can also be useful in the evaluation of the eye. One study suggests that ultrasound may be more sensitive than CT imaging for evaluation of foreign bodies [18]. Patients symptoms may vary from mild redness and

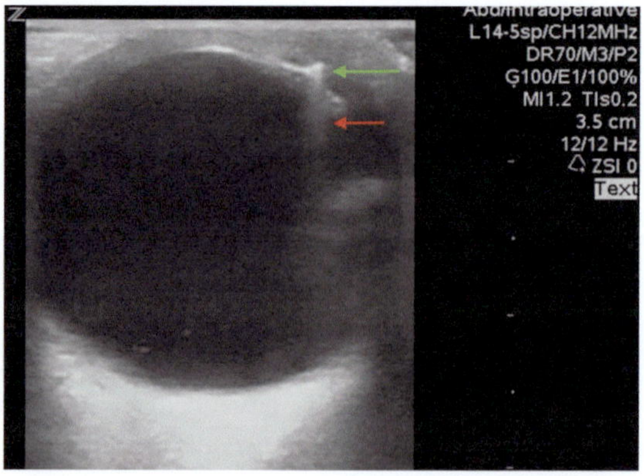

Fig. 7 Metal foreign body lodged in the lateral anterior chamber (green arrow) with ringdown artifact (red arrow)

irritation from small and superficial foreign bodies to severe pain and or vision loss due to globe rupture or VH from larger objects.

The sonographic appearance of objects in the eye varies as a function of their size and material. Small objects may only be represented by a hemorrhage tract within the vitreous, while large dense metal or plastic objects will be highly visible as hyper-echoic objects with posterior shadowing (Fig. 7). Wood and glass may be more challenging to visualize, and obtaining views from multiple angles around the globe and examining carefully for posterior shadowing may be helpful [5]. Color doppler may demonstrate an otherwise difficult to image foreign body by "twinkle artifact" a flashing colored image [18].

Lens Dislocation or Subluxation

Blunt trauma may result in partial (subluxation) or complete dislocation of the lens from its position between the anterior and posterior chambers. Patients will generally complain of varying visual acuity deficits depending on the degree of dislocation.

Sonographically, subluxation will be visualized as a lens that is out of alignment and may be displaced anteriorly, posteriorly, or laterally (Fig. 8). Complete dislocation will be demonstrated by absence of the hyperechoic lens in its normal anatomical position. Instead it may be positionally dependent, usually within the vitreous or along the posterior floor of the globe. This condition requires emergent ophthalmological consultation for surgical repair. POCUS may not be sensitive for subtle lens dislocations, so if significant clinical suspicion exists consider ophthalmologic consultation even in the presence of a perceived normal ultrasound study. Despite a somewhat limited sensitivity for this condition, POCUS has been found to be highly specific, suggesting that it can be effectively ruled in by ultrasound [19].

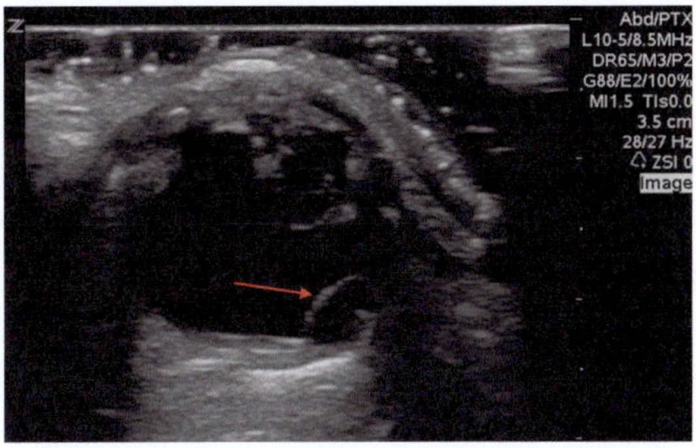

Fig. 8 Pt with massive ocular trauma demonstrating lens dislocation positioned in the posterior globe

Pearls and Pitfalls

- POCUS is user dependent requiring significant training to master and increase confidence in diagnosis.
- POCUS can diagnose numerous traumatic and non-traumatic conditions safely, quickly and effectively but sensitivity and specificity are pathology specific and user dependent.
- Ocular POCUS is generally more specific than sensitive and should be used to rule in suspected pathology rather than definitively rule out.
- POCUS can be useful in the evaluation of an acutely swollen eye or in other situations when a direct funduscopic examination is limited.
- Always confirm findings in a long and short axis. Oculo-kinetics, having the patient slowly move their eye can be helpful to highlight pathology.
- Be aware that although POCUS is highly sensitive for RD it may miss small retinal tears which may be vision threatening.
- POCUS can be useful in expediting definitive diagnosis and consultation in the pre-hospital setting as well as confirming diagnosis of RD definitively in austere settings with high sensitivity and specificity.
- Take care not to confuse PVD with RD since the former is relatively benign while the latter can be vision threatening.
- Take care to minimize pressure on globe with ultrasound probe if any concern for globe rupture exists as this can exacerbate an injury.
- Be sure to use copious amounts of cool or cold gel to fill air spaces and keep the probe floating above the eye to better visualize superficial anatomy.

Discussion of the Literature

There is a significant body of literature supporting the use of POCUS to diagnose ocular emergencies. Particular areas in which POCUS has been shown to be effective is in the diagnosis of RD, demonstrating both high sensitivity and specificity [10, 11]. One study showed decreased sensitivity (75%) for RD in emergency physicians compared to ophthalmologists; yet emergency medicine residents and fellows demonstrated sensitivities approaching 100% suggesting that those with formal POCUS training were effective in diagnosing this condition [12]. The high specificity of these evaluations demonstrates a significant utility for ultrasound in resource-poor settings where disposition decisions could be definitively made with the use of ultrasound. For example a patient diagnosed with a RD might be evacuated emergently, while one with a PVD might not be evacuated at all. This philosophy can be applied to various settings and multiple applications for the eye and at other sites in the body; essentially using ultrasound to help with triage.

Limitations of the Current Literature

While there is a significant body of literature describing use of ocular ultrasound, the majority of studies are in the ophthalmology and radiology literature. There are fewer studies in the field of emergency medicine and even fewer in the pre-hospital medicine and austere medicine specialties. Further study in these two latter fields would be useful to demonstrate utility in these patient populations. Specific research in the area of ONSD to evaluate for elevated ICP in pre-hospital and austere settings would be particularly useful since there are still numerous practice areas in both developed and undeveloped countries without access to definitive brain imaging and neurosurgical care.

Additional areas of controversy requiring further research include the evaluation of foreign bodies. While some studies suggest ultrasound is more sensitive than CT, others suggest that CT has superior sensitivity [15, 20]. Additionally, although there is excellent data demonstrating high sensitivities and specificities using ultrasound to diagnose RD, there is significantly less research documenting the accuracy of ultrasound in diagnosing VH and PVD. Although many practitioners infer that ultrasound has high accuracy in diagnosing these latter diseases additional research would be valuable.

References

1. Abdulrahman H, Kozak I. Clinical atlas of ophthalmic ultrasound. New York: Springer; 2019.
2. Fielding J. Ultrasound imaging of the eye through the closed lid a non-dedicated scanner. Clin Radiol. 1987;38:131–5.
3. Blaivas M. Bedside emergency department ultrasonography in the evaluation of ocular pathology. Acad Emerg Med. 2000;7:947–50.
4. Blaivas M, Theodoro D, Sierzenski P. A study of bedside ocular ultrasonography in the emergency department. Acad Emerg Med. 2002;9:791–9.
5. Jehle D, Bouvet S, Braden B, et al. Emergency ultrasound of the eye and orbit. Buffalo: Grover Cleveland Press; 2011.
6. Noble V, Nelson B. Manual of emergency and critical care ultrasound. 2nd ed. Cambridge, UK: Cambridge University Press; 2011.
7. Ma O, Matter J, Reardon R, Joing S. Ma & Mateer's emergency ultrasound. 3rd ed. New York: McGraw Hill; 2008.
8. Phillpotts B, et al. Vitreous hemorrhage. www.emedicine.com. 2005
9. De La Hoz Polo M, Torramilans Lluís A, Pozuelo Segura O, Anguera Bosque A, Esmerado Appiani C, Caminal Mitjana JM. Ocular ultrasonography focused on the posterior eye segment: what radiologists should know. Insights Imaging. 2016;7(3):351–64.
10. Kuzmanović Elabjer B, Bušić M, Biščan Tvrdi A, Miletić D, Bosnar D, Bjeloš M. Ultrasound reliability in detection of retinal tear in acute symptomatic posterior vitreous detachment with vitreous hemorrhage. Int J Ophthalmol. 2017;10(12):1922–4.
11. Lorenzo-Carrero J, Perez-Flores I, Cid-Galano M, Fernandez-Fernandez M, Heras-Raposo F, Vazquez-Nuñez R, Lopez-Fuentes M. Ophthalmology. 2009;116(1):94–9.
12. Kim DJ, et al. Test characteristics of point of care ultrasound for the diagnosis of retinal detachment in the emergency department. Acad Emerg Med. 2019;26:16.
13. Galetta S, Burne SF, Smith JL. Echographic correlation of optic nerve sheath size and cerebral spinal fluid pressure. J Clin Neuroopthalmol. 1989;9:79–82.

14. Newman WD, Hollman AS, Dutton GN, Karachi R. Measurement of optic nerve sheath diameter by ultrasound: a means of detecting acute raised intracranial pressure in hydrocephalus. Br J Opthalmol. 86:1109–13.
15. Kimberly HH, Shah S, Marill K, Noble V. Correlation of optic nerve sheath diameter with direct measurement of intracranial pressure. Acad Emerg Med. 2008;15:201–4.
16. Fagenholz PG, Gutman JA, Murray AF, Noble VE, Camargo CA, Harris NS. High Alt Med Biol. 2007;8(4):331–6.
17. Lochner P, Falla M, Pohl M, Strapazzon G. High Alt Med Biol. 2015;16(3):195–203. https://doi.org/10.1089/ham.2014.1127. Epub 2015 May 28
18. McNicholas MM, Trophy DP, Power WJ, et al. Ocular trauma: evaluation with ultrasound. Radiology. 1995;195:423–7.
19. Ojaghi Haghighi SH, Morteza Begi HR, Sorkhabi R, et al. Diagnostic accuracy of ultrasound in detection of traumatic lens dislocation. Emerg (Tehran). 2014;2(3):121–4.
20. Clinical application of X-ray. B-scan, and CT in the diagnosis of ocular foreign bodies. Eye Sci. 2013;28(1):11–4.

Advanced Diagnostic Topic for Austere Providers: Obstetric

Sarah C. Crockett and Zachary P. Soucy

Introduction

Obstetrical and gynecological emergencies in an austere setting can be challenging for the provider and patient alike. Gravid patients may need management of traumatic injuries, abdominal pain, vaginal bleeding, and complications of pregnancy, among other complaints. This chapter describes the ultrasound techniques used to identify an intrauterine pregnancy (IUP) and how to evaluate fetal condition by identifying fetal heart tones (FHTs). If the gestational age of the fetus is advanced (e.g. suspected to be greater than 20 weeks,) US can also be used to identify the fetal head position. When appropriate in the trauma setting, FAST exam for pregnant patients is recommended and guidelines described in the Trauma Section should be followed. In addition, if no IUP is identified in a patient known or suspected to be pregnant, US can be used to assess for signs of ectopic pregnancy, a potentially life threatening condition. The literature is sparse regarding use of point of care ultrasound (POCUS) in the prehospital setting to evaluate obstetrical and gynecologic emergencies. However, based on the review of curricula used to train prehospital providers in the use of POCUS, it is reasonable to include limited transabdominal obstetric pelvic US, referred to as pelvic POCUS throughout this chapter, in the toolkit of skills available to EMS providers and health care providers in austere settings [1, 2].

S. C. Crockett · Z. P. Soucy (✉)
Department of Emergency Medicine, Dartmouth Hitchcock Medical Center, Lebanon, NH, USA
e-mail: Zachary.P.Soucy@hitchcock.org

B. D. Nicholson et al. (eds.), *Manual of Austere and Prehospital Ultrasound*,
https://doi.org/10.1007/978-3-030-64287-7_12

Topic Discussion

General Strategy

Prehospital pelvic POCUS is most useful to determine if the patient is pregnant, identify basic signs of fetal distress, and presentation if beyond 20 weeks. Pregnancy should be considered in any female between the ages of 10–55. We recommend the following systematic approach to using pelvic POCUS in evaluating a patient in the prehospital or austere setting:

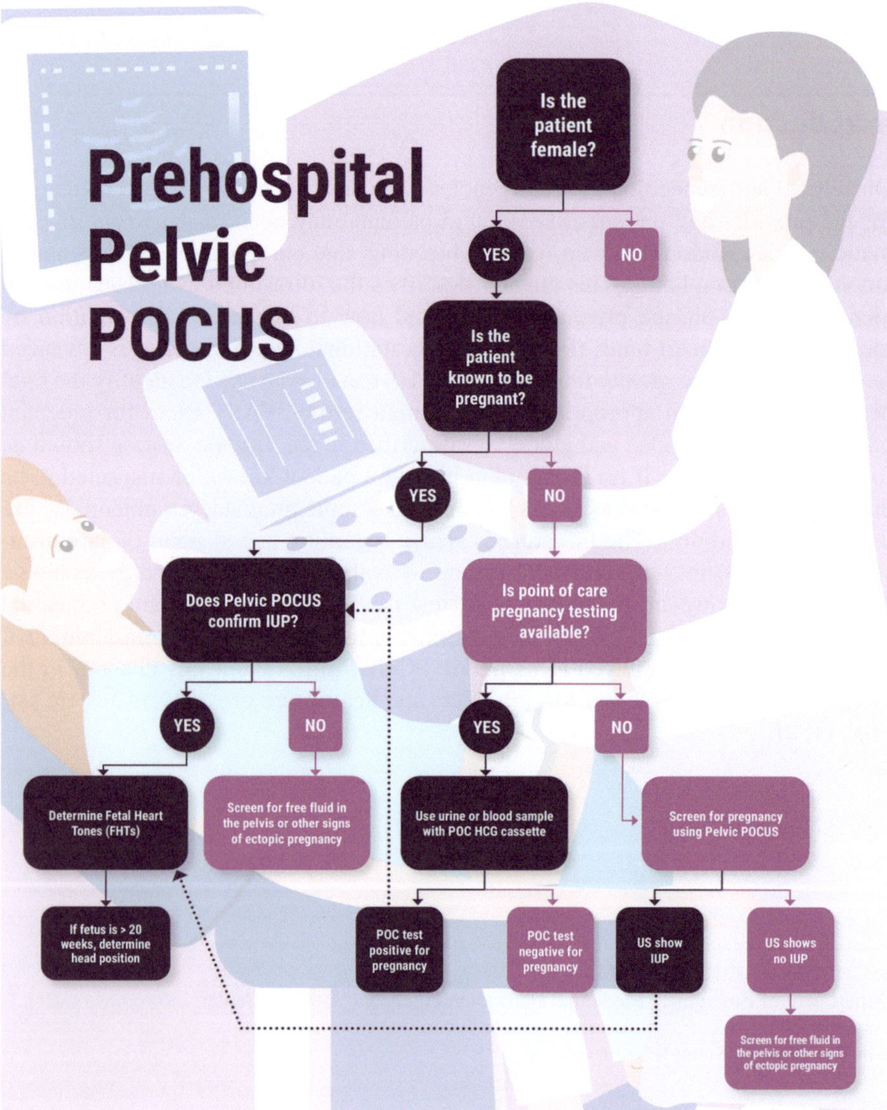

If a female patient is known to be pregnant either by history or by point of care testing, pelvic POCUS can be used to confirm IUP. If no IUP is identified, consideration should be given to a possible diagnosis of ectopic pregnancy. This obstetrical complication typically develops in the first trimester and epidemiologic studies report an incidence somewhere between 6.4 and 20.7 out of 1000 pregnancies [3, 4]. Risk factors such as prior history of PID, prior ectopic pregnancy, IUD use, and a history of infertility can significantly increase the patient's risk of ectopic pregnancy [5]. In addition, a history of having undergone infertility treatments in order to achieve the current pregnancy significantly increases a patient's risk for heterotopic pregnancy, a condition where there is simultaneously an IUP and an ectopic pregnancy.

Definitive identification of ectopic pregnancy may not be possible by transabdominal US, and transvaginal US in the prehospital setting is not recommended. However, a scan for free fluid in the pelvis can be used to risk stratify the patient for likelihood of ruptured ectopic pregnancy. If a pregnant patient with abdominal pain or vaginal bleeding in the first trimester is found to have no clear evidence of IUP and has significant amounts of free fluid in the pelvis or abdomen, ectopic pregnancy should be considered high on the differential, and immediate stabilization and treatment in the hospital setting should be sought.

While the clinical scenario is exceedingly rare, US may also have a role in maternal and fetal monitoring in the case of cardiac arrest in the gravid patient. For maternal resuscitation, ACLS or ATLS guidelines should be followed with appropriate modifications for gravid women of greater than 20 weeks gestation. Recommendations for prehospital resuscitative hysterotomy/peri-mortem C-Section (RH/PMCS) have been published, however, we recommend consulting with local medical directors to determine local protocols appropriate to your specific situation. US may be used to monitor cardiac status of the mother and/or the fetus [6].

In women in whom pregnancy is identified, POCUS may be used to assess the status of the fetus by measuring fetal heart tones. Fetal cardiac activity is generally present at 6–6.5 weeks of gestation, however, it may be difficult to obtain adequate images using transabdominal US at this early stage. Transabdominal pelvic US is most likely to visualize an intrauterine embryo by 8 weeks of gestational age or later. Cardiac activity at this stage can be visualized as a flickering within the thorax of the embryo. We recommend measuring fetal heart rate (FHR) using M-Mode. Typical embryonic and fetal heart rates are as follows:

- 6 weeks: 100–115 beats/minute.
- 8 weeks: 145–170 beats/minute.
- 9 weeks and greater: 137–144 beats/minute.

If the level of the uterus is palpated to be at or above the level of the umbilicus of the patient, then the gestational age is estimated to be 20 weeks or greater. In this case, POCUS can be useful to determine fetal head presentation.

Anatomy

The non-gravid female pelvis includes many important structures which can be often be identified by pelvic POCUS though image quality can vary greatly, depending on operator experience and the patient's body habitus. The pelvic cavity is the space enclosed by the bony pelvis and extends from the iliac crests superiorly to the pelvic floor inferiorly. The female pelvis contains the following structures: uterus, vagina, fallopian tubes, ovaries, urinary bladder, rectum, intestines as well as major blood vessels, muscles and ligaments. The uterus is a pear-shaped muscular structure that lies posterior to the urinary bladder. In a post-pubertal adult female, the non-gravid uterus typically measures 8 cm long, 5 cm wide and 3 cm deep [14].

Understanding the peritoneal spaces within the pelvis will help the health care provider to identify normal and abnormal fluid within the pelvis. The posterior cul-de-sac, or Pouch of Douglas, is the space posterior to the uterus and anterior to the rectum. If the patient is in the supine position, it is the most dependent intraperitoneal space and the most likely space for intraperitoneal fluid to accumulate. A small amount of free fluid in the posterior cul-de-sac, 5–21 ml, can be physiologically normal, especially in menstruating females, and can often be seen on ultrasound [7]. A full bladder helps to create a good acoustic window for visualization of the uterus and posterior cul-de-sac, and image visualization may be more challenging in a patient with an empty bladder (Fig. 1).

The anterior cul-de-sac, or vesicouterine pouch, is the space anterior to the uterus and posterior the urinary bladder. Ultrasonic visualization of fluid within this space in a supine patient should be considered abnormal and could represent intra-abdominal hemorrhage (Fig. 2).

The uterus is a remarkable organ which during pregnancy can increase to 20 times its original weight. Before 12 weeks, the uterus remains an intrapelvic organ, being contained below the pelvic brim. By 20 weeks, it reaches the umbilicus and at 34–36 weeks is at the level of the costal margins. At term, the uterus has often enlarged from 6 to 8 cm in length to over 30 cm which alters the normal anatomic

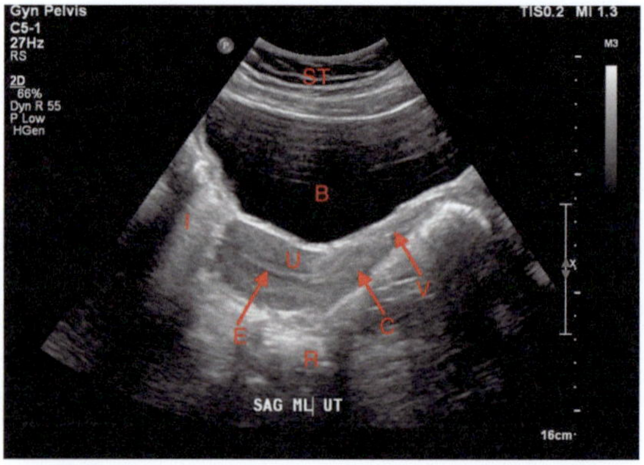

Fig. 1 Normal non-gravid sonographic anatomy in sagittal plane highlighting: subcutaneous tissue (ST), bladder (B), intestines (I), uterus (U), endometrial stripe (E), cervix (C), vaginal stripe (V), rectum (R)

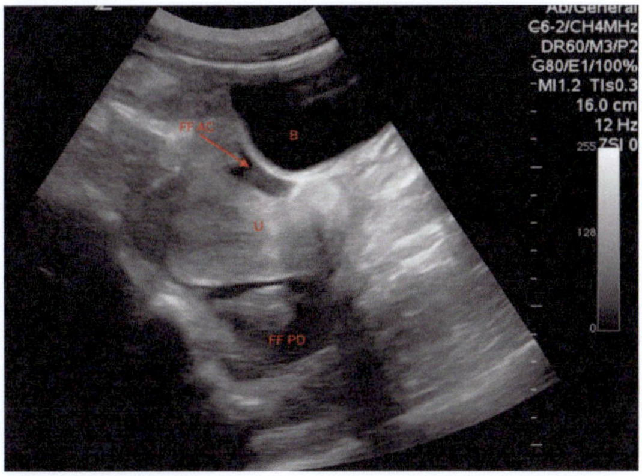

Fig. 2 Long axis view of a pelvis with large free fluid (FF) pooling in the anterior cul-de-sac (AC), Pouch of Douglas (PD) with uterus (U) and bladder (B) highlighted

location and function of multiple structures including the bladder, abdominal viscera, and diaphragm. These changes are particularly important to consider when evaluating the pregnant trauma patient, but are pertinent in medical and obstetrical considerations as well [30].

Ultrasound Evaluation for Intrauterine Pregnancy (IUP)

Transabdominal pelvic US is best performed using a low frequency curvilinear probe (5–2 MHz). Many ultrasound machines have an obstetrical preset that can be selected for this exam. The ability to identify IUP depends on both the gestational age of the fetus, discussed above, and the mother's body habitus. Prior to scanning, place an adequate amount of ultrasound gel directly onto the patient's lower abdomen. The probe is positioned above the pubic symphysis in the midline. Begin with the longitudinal view by positioning the probe marker toward the patient's head. The bladder, when full, will be noted as a dark, anechoic structure with the relatively hyperechoic uterus lying posteriorly. Be sure to decrease the gain to such that the fluid in the bladder appears black. If the gain is too high, there may be posterior acoustic enhancement which could hide free fluid or distort the operator's ability to identify an IUP.

Fan or translate the probe from the iliac fossa on the right to the one on the left to visualize the entire pelvis. Look first at the hyperechoic endometrial stripes and then for signs of IUP such as a gestational sac and yoke sac. Then place the probe in the transverse plane with the probe marker toward the patient's right and fan through the entire length of the uterus inferiorly to superiorly. The earliest definitive sign of IUP is the presence of a gestational sac with a yolk sac within the endometrium of the uterus which occurs around 5 weeks gestation (Fig. 3). After 6 weeks, the formation of a fetal pole adjacent to the yolk sac can be identified with a flickering of cardiac activity indicating a viable IUP.

Identification of an IUP excludes the diagnosis of ectopic pregnancy in most cases. An exception to this is in the case of patients undergoing fertility treatments.

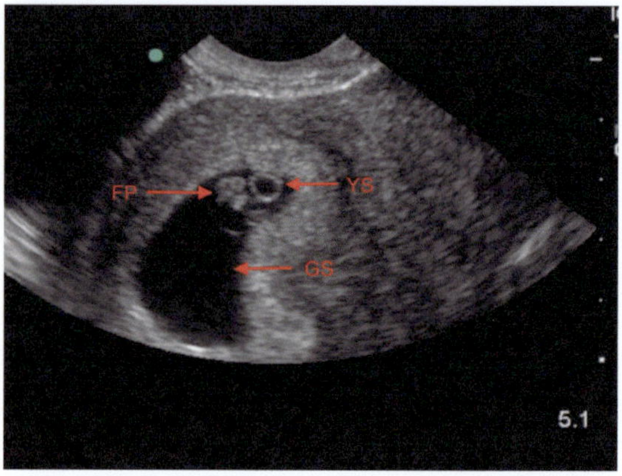

Fig. 3 A gravid uterus with pregnancy including gestational sac (GS), yolk sac (YS), fetal pole (FP)

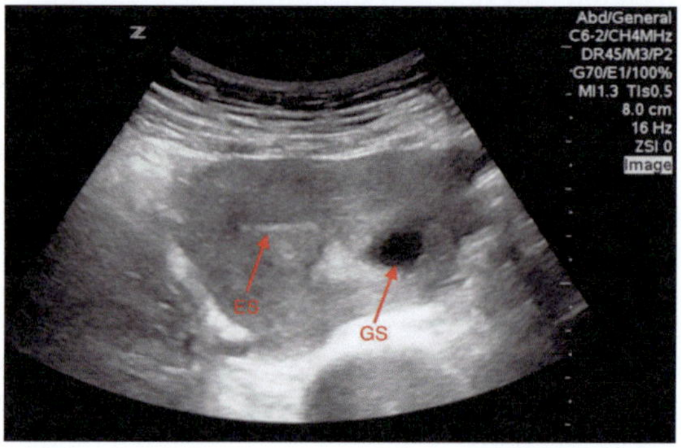

Fig. 4 Interstitial pregnancy demonstrating a gestational sac (GS) imbedded in the myometrium outside the endometrial stripe (ES)

These patients are at significantly increased risk for heterotopic pregnancy where there is simultaneously both an IUP and an ectopic pregnancy. Be sure to ask any symptomatic patient in the first trimester if they have undergone fertility treatments, and have an increased level of concern if they are experiencing symptoms of abdominal pain, vaginal bleeding or shock. Another rare complication of early pregnancy is intramural (or interstitial) ectopic pregnancy where the embryo implants into the uterine wall (Fig. 4). In these cases, the ultrasound can appear to confirm IUP, yet the patient is at risk for uterine rupture, hemorrhage and death if the problem is not detected and treated. The diagnosis of intramural ectopic pregnancy by ultrasound is beyond the scope of this chapter. However, by being aware of this rare diagnosis, the health care provider can use ultrasound to screen for free intraperitoneal fluid in symptomatic patients, even if a previously normal US is reported [8, 9].

Ultrasound Evaluation of Free Fluid in the Pelvis and Abdomen

In addition to looking for evidence of IUP, transabdominal US can also be used to identify free fluid in the pelvis or abdomen which can be associated with life threatening diagnoses. In the case of a female patient involved in trauma, any evidence of fluid in the abdomen or pelvis should be considered abnormal as the presence of

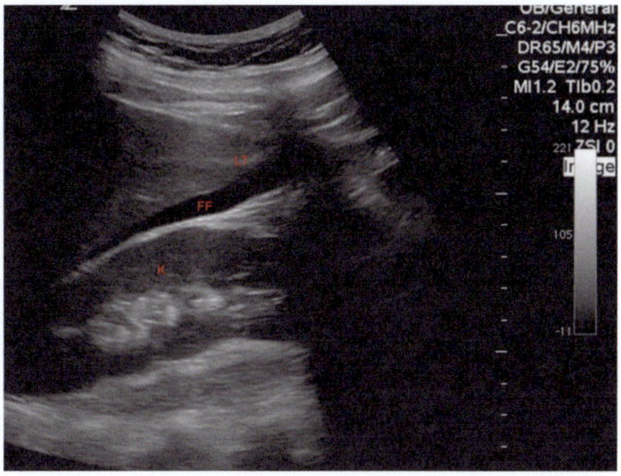

Fig. 5 Free fluid (FF) in Morrisons Pouch between kidney (K) and liver tip (LT)

fluid within the abdomen or pelvis after trauma is associated with significantly higher rates of intra-abdominal injury [7]. In the non-traumatic female patient, a small amount of free fluid in the pelvis may be considered physiologic or "normal." The fluid level, as it tracks along the posterior cul-de-sac, can be measured in comparison to the fundal height of the anteverted uterus. Fluid measuring one third the height of the uterus is considered small, two thirds is moderate, and fluid reaching more than two thirds the height of the uterine wall is considered large (Fig. 5). The likelihood of ectopic pregnancy increases significantly in the presence of moderate or large free fluid [13].

When evaluating for free fluid in the setting of suspected ectopic pregnancy, a scan for intraperitoneal fluid should also be performed by looking at the hepatorenal space (Morrison's Pouch) (Fig. 5). This is done using the same technique described in the FAST exam. The presence of free fluid in the hepatorenal space of a symptomatic pregnant patient without an IUP is virtually diagnostic of a ruptured ectopic pregnancy [10, 11].

Obtaining Fetal Heart Tones (FHTs)

To monitor the fetal heart rate, the ultrasound machine should be placed in M-mode with probe situated such that the fetal cardiac activity is consistently visualized. While in M-mode, the marker should be placed directly over the flicker of cardiac activity within the fetus. The alternating black and gray bands represent cardiac chamber movement over time. Using the measurement function while in the obstetrics mode, two lines are situated to mark a cardiac cycle, and the machine will then calculate the heart rate (Fig. 6) [13, 14]. A video clip documenting fetal cardiac activity can also be recorded in B-mode.

Ultrasound for Determination of Fetal Presentation

Evaluation of the fetal presentation in patients with a gestational age greater than 20 weeks can be useful in prehospital and austere settings, particularly in the setting

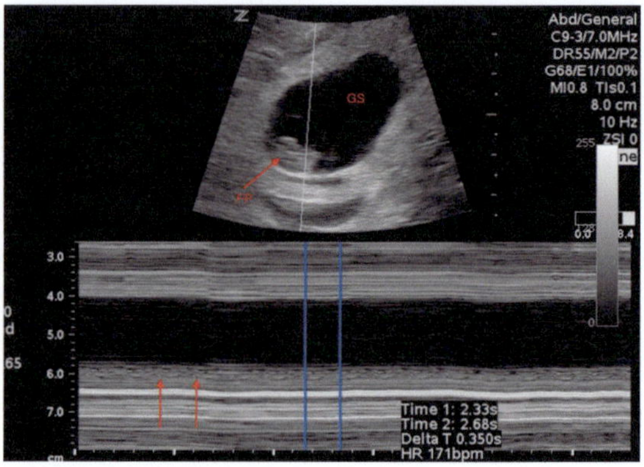

Fig. 6 M-Mode measuring fetal heart rate. Two red arrows indicating heartbeats used for measurement. Gestational sac (GS) and fetal pole (FP) highlighted

of a patient suspected to be in labor. Fetal presentation refers to the way the fetus is positioned within the uterus presenting to the birth canal and includes cephalic (head), breech, and shoulder presentations. Fetal lie refers to the longitudinal orientation of the fetus in relation to the long axis of the mother and can be longitudinal, oblique or transverse. Fetal position describes the rotational orientation of the head inside the mother's pelvis and can be occiput anterior (OA), occiput posterior (OP) and many different angles in between. If the uterus can be palpated at or above the umbilicus, then the gestational age of the fetus can be estimated to be greater than 20 weeks. If the health care provider suspects that a mother with a potentially viable fetus is showing signs of labor including regular, frequent uterine contractions or passage of amniotic fluid per the vagina, then pelvic POCUS can be used to determine the presentation of the fetus within the uterus. The most common location of a fetus during labor is to be aligned longitudinally within the uterus with the fetal head as the presenting part. Any other position such as breech or transverse fetal lie is considered a malpresentation. These malpresentations can result in increased perinatal morbidity and mortality during delivery and are important to know if managing delivery in the field or giving report to providers administering definitive care.

To determine fetal presentation, a low frequency curvilinear probe should again be used (5–2 MHz). The probe should be first placed transversely on the maternal abdomen with the probe marker oriented to the patient's right side. In normal cephalic or "head first" fetal positioning, an axial view of the fetus within the uterus should show evidence of the hyperechoic fetal spine (Fig. 7). By sliding down to the maternal suprapubic region, the fetal head should then be visualized by noting the circular hyperechoic skull, isoechoic brain with anechoic ventricles (Fig. 8). Repeating the transabdominal scan in the longitudinal plane should again reveal the fetal head in the maternal pelvis [17]. If the head is not identified in the pelvis, the entire uterus should be evaluated to determine if the fetus is in a breech or transverse fetal lie.

Studies have demonstrated that US is useful in determining if the fetal head position is occiput anterior (normal position) or occiput posterior (malposition) during the second and third stages of labor, however, that degree of detail is beyond the scope of this text to teach adequately [15].

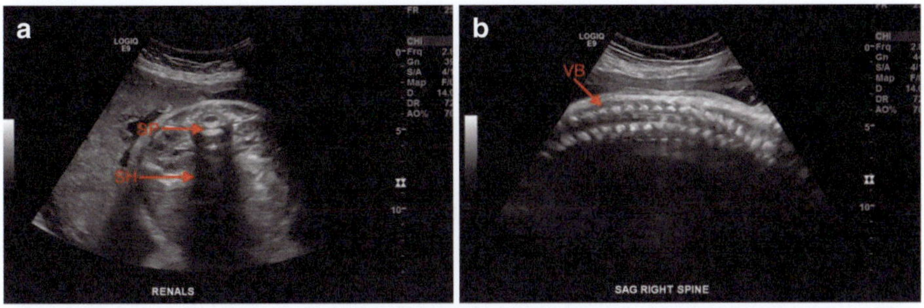

Fig. 7 (**a**) Transverse of 36wk fetus mid abdomen demonstrating fetal spine (SP) anteriorly with shadowing (SH). (**b**) Sagittal of same fetal spine with vertebral body (VB) indicated. The spine can be followed to the head to determine presentation

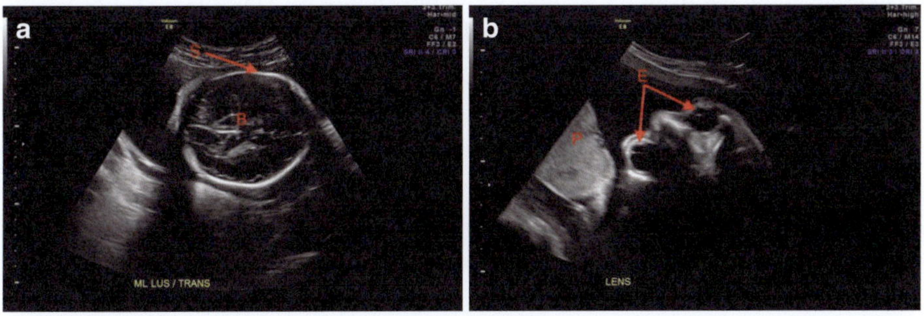

Fig. 8 (**a**) Transverse of 28 wk fetal head highlighting skull (S) and brain (B) demonstrating longitudinal lie, head presentation. (**b**) Transverse of a 30 wk fetus demonstrating eye sockets (E) anterior and occiput posterior with placenta (P) highlighted

Key Literature Reviewed

Research on the use of prehospital pelvic ultrasound for obstetrical evaluation is extremely limited at this time. However, pelvic ultrasound, particularly for the purpose of ruling out ectopic pregnancy in the first trimester in patients presenting to emergency departments, has be studied extensively [10–12, 16, 29].

In the pre-hospital setting, Galisnki et al. reported an exceptional case report of a ruptured ectopic pregnancy diagnosed by prehospital US. The patient reported having a prior pelvic ultrasound which had been interpreted to be a "normal" 11 week pregnancy. However, while under evaluation by EMS, the patient became hypotensive and dizzy. Transabdominal US showed free intraperitoneal fluid. The patient had actually experienced a very rare intramural ectopic pregnancy resulting in uterine rupture. The prehospital diagnosis of hemoperitoneum resulted in prompt intervention with the patient undergoing to emergent laparotomy immediately upon arrival to the hospital [9].

In 2004, Polk et al. published a case series of 3 obstetrical cases managed by and air medical team using prehospital US. In each case, US findings changed the course of patient management. The authors proposed the use of US evaluation they termed

Fetal Evaluation for Transport by Ultrasound (FETUS). FETUS examination performed by the flight team included a direct assessment of fetal heart rate, fetal movement, fetal position, presence of amniotic fluid, and general condition of the placenta [18].

Limitations of Current Knowledge and Opportunities for Future Research

Virtually no studies have looked at the systematic use of pelvic US in the prehospital setting. Many studies have shown that health care providers including paramedics, EMTs, and first responders can acquire the skills needed for ultrasound evaluation of patients in austere and prehospital settings [19–28]. The most common prehospital applications include using ultrasound for FAST and eFAST exams and cardiac evaluation. Given the similarities in technique between these types of studies, the next logical step is to develop curricula and to research the utility of pelvic POCUS in austere settings.

Pearls and Pitfalls

- Transabdominal US can be used to rule out ectopic pregnancy by identifying an intrauterine pregnancy with exception in special populations.
- An empty or inadequately filled bladder can make transabdominal pelvic US more difficult while a full bladder provides an excellent acoustic window for viewing of pelvic structures.
- A full bladder may cause posterior acoustic enhancement which may hide free fluid or distort the operator's ability to identify an IUP. Decrease the gain posterior to the bladder to improve imaging.
- When fanning or translating the probe through the pelvic organs, care should be taken to visualize the entire space from iliac fossa on the right to the one on the left. The same philosophy should be applied to the caudal and cephalad scanning in transverse axis.
- All findings should be confirmed on imagine in two perpendicular planes.
- The earliest definitive sign of an IUP is the presence of a gestational sac with a yolk sac within the endometrium of the uterus, often visible on transabdominal pelvic POCUS at 6–8 weeks gestation.
- Identification of an IUP with cardiac activity reliably rules out ectopic pregnancy with rare exceptions.
- Heterotopic pregnancy (presence of ectopic pregnancy IN ADDITION to an IUP) should be considered in any symptomatic pregnant patient who has undergone fertility treatments to achieve their current pregnancy.
- Fetal Heart Rate (FHR) can be calculated using M-Mode.
- Fluid in the anterior cul-de-sac, or vesicouterine pouch should be considered abnormal and may represent intra-abdominal hemorrhage.

- Moderate or large amounts of free fluid seen in the posterior cul-de-sac (>1/3 the fundal height of the uterus) should be considered abnormal.
- Fluid in the right upper quadrant in a non-traumatic patient in the first trimester of pregnancy is highly concerning for ruptured ectopic pregnancy.
- Any fluid in the pelvis after blunt trauma should be concerning for possible intra-abdominal injury.
- Fetal position can be established by using US to locate the fetal head within the uterus.

References

1. Meadley B, Olaussen A, Delorenzo A, et al. Educational standards for training paramedics in ultrasound: a scoping review. BMC Emerg Med. 2017;17(1):18 . Published 2017 Jun 17. https://doi.org/10.1186/s12873-017-0131-8.
2. McCallum J, Vu E, Sweet D, Kanji HD. Assessment of paramedic ultrasound curricula: a systematic review. Air Med J. 2015;34(6):360–8. https://doi.org/10.1016/j.amj.2015.07.002.
3. Van Den Eeden SK, Shan J, Bruce C, et al. Ectopic pregnancy rate and treatment utilization in a large managed care organization. Obstet Gynecol. 2005;105(5 Pt 1):1052–7.
4. Hoover KW, Tao G, Kent CK. Trends in the diagnosis and treatment of ectopic pregnancy in the United States. Obstet Gynecol. 2010;115:495–502.
5. Bouyer J, Coste J, Shojaei T, et al. Risk factors for ectopic pregnancy: a comprehensive analysis based on a large case-control, population-based study in France. Am J Epidemiol. 2003;157:185–94.
6. Battaloglu E, Porter K. Management of pregnancy and obstetric complications in prehospital trauma care: prehospital resuscitative hysterotomy/perimortem caesarean section. Emerg Med J. 2017;34:326–30.
7. Ormsby EL, Geng J, Mcgahan JP, Rıchards JR. Pelvic free fluid: clinical importance for reproductive age women with blunt abdominal trauma. Ultras Obstet Gynaecol. 2005;26:271–8.
8. Lewiss RE, Shaukat NM, Saul T. The endomyometrial thickness measurement for abnormal implantation evaluation by pelvic sonography. J Ultrasound Med. 2014;33:1143–6. https://doi.org/10.7863/ultra.33.7.1143.
9. Galinski M, Petrovic T, Rodrigues A, Hermann M, Catineau J, Adnet F, Lapostolle F. Out-of-hospital diagnosis of a ruptured ectopic pregnancy: myometrial embryo implantation, an exceptional diagnosis. Prehosp Emerg Care. 2010;14(4):496–8. https://doi.org/10.3109/10903127.2010.493984.
10. Nyberg DA, Hughes MP, Mack LA, Wang KY. Extrauterine findings of ectopic pregnancy of transvaginal US: importance of echogenic fluid. Radiology. 1991;178:823–6.
11. Moore C, Todd WM, O'Brien E, Lin H. Free fluid in Morison's pouch on bedside ultrasound predicts need for operative intervention in suspected ectopic pregnancy. Acad Emerg Med. 2007;14:755–8. https://doi.org/10.1197/j.aem.2007.04.010.
12. Rodgerson JD, Heegaard WG, Plummer D, Hicks J, Clinton J, Sterner S. Emergency department right upper quadrant ultrasound is associated with a reduced time to diagnosis and treatment of ruptured ectopic pregnancies. Acad Emerg Med. 2001;8:331–6. https://doi.org/10.1111/j.1553-2712.2001.tb02110.x.
13. Soni N, Arntfield R, Kory P. Point-of-care ultrasound. Philadelphia: Elsevier; 2014.
14. Noble VE, Nelson B, Sutingco AN. Manual of emergency and critical care ultrasound. Manual Emerg Crit Care Ultras. 2007:1–249. https://doi.org/10.1017/CBO9780511547249.

15. Merz E, Mirio-Tesanic D, Bahlmann F, et al. Sonographic size of uterus and ovaries in pre- and postmenopausal women. Ultrasound Obstet Gynecol. 1996;7:38–42.
16. Ghi T, Eggebø T, Lees C, Kalache K, Rozenberg P, Youssef A, Salomon LJ, Tutschek B. ISUOG practice guidelines: intrapartum ultrasound. Ultrasound Obstet Gynecol. 2018;52:128–39. https://doi.org/10.1002/uog.19072.
17. Akmal S, Tsoi E, Kametas N, et al. Intrapartum sonography to determine the fetal head position. J Matern Fetal Neonatal Med. 2002;12:172–7.
18. Youssef A, Ghi T, Pilu G. How to perform ultrasound in labor: assessment of fetal occiput position. Ultrasound Obstet Gynecol. 2013;41:476–8. https://doi.org/10.1002/uog.12439.
19. Polk JD, Merlino JI, Kovach BL, Mancuso C, Fallon WF Jr. Fetal evaluation for transport by ultrasound performed by air medical teams: a case series. Air Med J. 2004;23(4):32–3. https://doi.org/10.1016/j.amj.2004.04.005.
20. Workman A, Hecht C, Callie C, Sewell B, Rippy W, Palla D, Rajesh G. Can firefighters be taught ultrasound? Am Surg. 2018;84(6):E192–8.
21. Rudolph SS, Sorensen MK, Svane C, Hesselfeldt R, Steinmetz J. Effect of prehospital ultrasound on clinical outcomes of non-trauma patients—a systematic review. Resuscitation. 2014;85(1):21–30.
22. O'Dochartaigh D, Douma M. Prehospital ultrasound of the abdomen and thorax changes trauma patient management: a systematic review. Injury. 2015;46(11):2093–102.
23. Heegaard W, Hildebrandt D, Spear D, Chason K, Nelson B, Ho J. Prehospital ultrasound by paramedics: results of field trial. Acad Emerg Med. 2010;17(6):624–30.
24. El Sayed MJ, Zaghrini E. Prehospital emergency ultrasound: a review of current clinical applications, challenges, and future implications. Emerg Med Int. 2013;2013:531674.
25. Scharonow M, Weilbach C. Prehospital point-of-care emergency ultrasound: a cohort study. Scand J Trauma Resusc Emerg Med. 2018;26:49. https://doi.org/10.1186/s13049-018-0519-9.
26. Chin EJ, Chan CH, Mortazavi R, Anderson CL, Kahn CA, Summers S, Fox JC. A pilot study examining the viability of a Prehospital Assessment with UltraSound for Emergencies (PAUSE) protocol. J Emerg Med. 2013;44(1):142–9. https://doi.org/10.1016/j.jemermed.2012.02.032.
27. Bøtker MT, Jacobsen L, Rudolph SS, Knudsen L. The role of point of care ultrasound in prehospital critical care: a systematic review. Scand J Trauma Resusc Emerg Med. 2018;26(1):51 . Published 2018 Jun 26. https://doi.org/10.1186/s13049-018-0518-x.
28. Lapostolle F, Petrovic T, Lenoir G. Usefulness of hand-held ultrasound devices in out-of-hospital diagnosis performed by emergency physicians. Am J Emerg Med. 2006;24:237–42.
29. Wong TW, Lau CC, Yeung A, Lo L, Tai CM. Efficacy of transabdominal ultrasound examination in the diagnosis of early pregnancy complications in an emergency department. J Accid Emerg Med. 1998;15(3):155–8.
30. Marx JA, Rosen P. Rosen's emergency medicine: concepts and clinical practice. 8th ed. Philadelphia: Elsevier/Saunders; 2014.

Advanced Diagnostic Topic for Austere Providers: Skin and Soft Tissue

Justin Grisham and Michael D. Perreault

Introduction

Soft tissue injuries and infections account for 80% of injuries sustained in a wilderness or austere setting [1]. Ultrasonography provides an excellent means to evaluate for and identify many of these soft tissue injuries including cellulitis, abscesses, and foreign bodies. The skilled practitioner can also use ultrasound to provide procedural guidance for abscess drainage and the removal of foreign bodies.

Equipment Considerations

A high frequency linear array probe of 7.5 MHz or higher is ideal for the evaluation of the soft tissue (*see* Fig. 1). Deep penetration of the tissue is usually not required, and the higher frequency probe offers the resolution required to identify minimal areas of fluid and small foreign bodies. In general, most high frequency linear arrays will penetrate to a depth of up to 6 cm or so. There are rare cases in which a low frequency curvilinear (1–5 MHz) or phased array (2–5 MHz) probe may be required to achieve the adequate penetration to clearly identify the back wall of an abscess (see Figs. 2 and 3). This is particularly important when scanning thoracic or abdominal abscesses that may communicate with the thoracic or peritoneal cavities respectively. The lower frequency probes may also be necessary to adequately evaluate obese patients.

Probe size and thus footprint varies, but a larger probe is generally utilized in order to facilitate the evaluation of a greater amount of soft tissue. Smaller probes may be useful in procedural guidance or when evaluating smaller anatomical structures such as digits.

J. Grisham (✉) · M. D. Perreault
Department of Emergency Medicine, Madigan Army Medical Center, Tacoma, WA, USA
e-mail: Justin.d.grisham.mil@mail.mil; michael.d.perreault.mil@mail.mil

B. D. Nicholson et al. (eds.), *Manual of Austere and Prehospital Ultrasound*,
https://doi.org/10.1007/978-3-030-64287-7_13

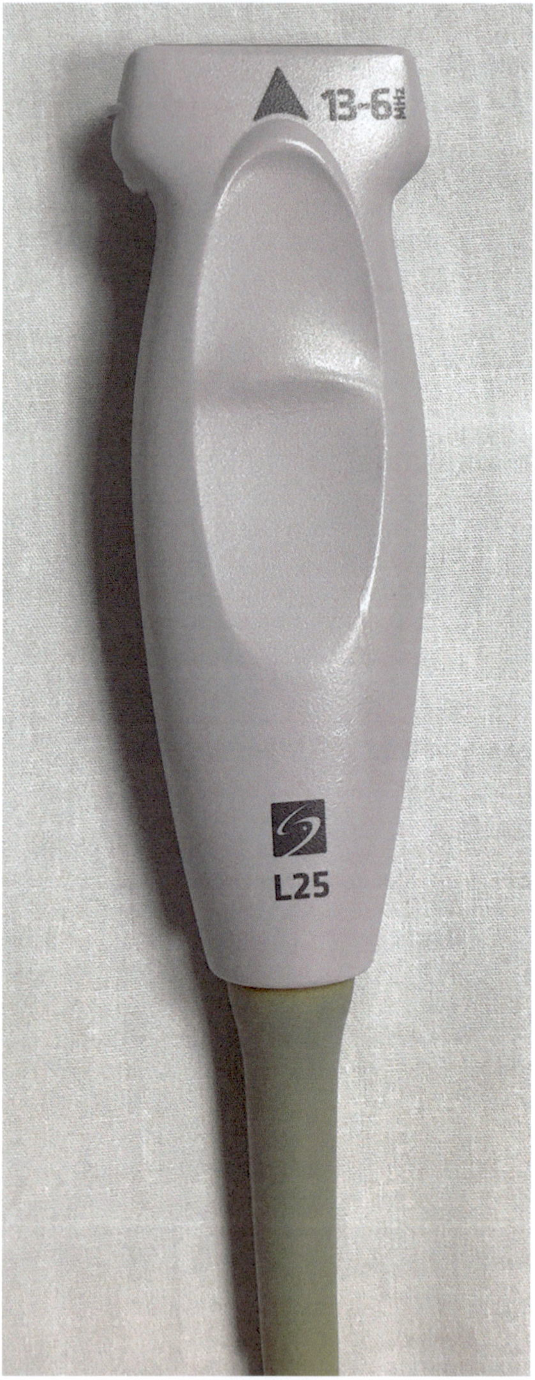

Fig. 1 Linear transducer: Linear transducers produce rectangular images using high frequency

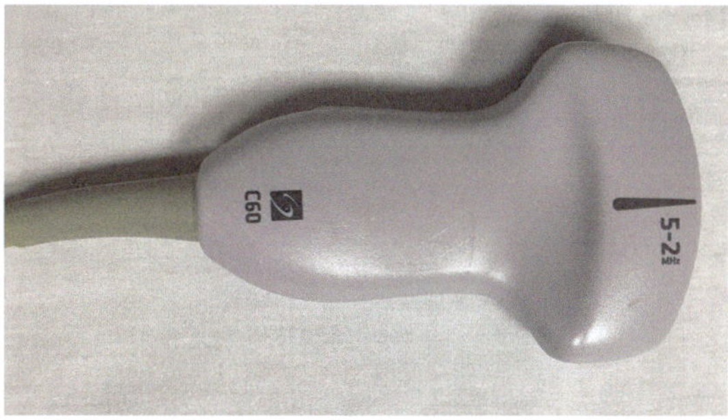

Fig. 2 Curvilinear transducer: Curvilinear transducers exhibit low frequency and a wide field of view

Ultrasound resolution (and corresponding image quality) is normally greatest at a point where the ultrasound beam narrows to its minimum size. This is known as the focal zone. For any given probe, there is a minimum distance from the surface of the probe to the focal zone. For this reason, the resolution of superficial structures closest to the ultrasound probe (before the focal zone is reached) can be limited. Utilizing a water bath to increase the standoff distance between the probe and the anatomical structure in question can improve visualization by placing the area of interest within the focal zone of the probe [2] (*see* Fig. 4). This technique can also aid in the evaluation of small structures such as fingers or toes that may be difficult to maintain probe contact with due to their small and spherical nature (*see* Fig. 5).

Technique

Soft tissue structures of interest should be evaluated in the transverse and longitudinal axis. Traditionally the probe marker is placed towards the patient's head or to the patient's right. However, if the ultrasound images will be used for procedural guidance, the probe should be oriented so that the directionality of the images seen matches the surface alignment of the patient. Scanning with the ultrasound probe in a dedicated fashion such as from distal to proximal or lateral to medial and labeling images as such will prevent confusion during future review.

Cellulitis

Cellulitis accounts for 25% of all soft tissue injuries in the austere environment [3]. It may accompany abscesses and in rare cases lead to necrotizing soft tissue infections. Ultrasound identification of cellulitis is nonspecific and requires the correct clinical picture of erythematous, warm, and painful skin, usually in a limited and unilateral distribution.

Soft tissue is expected to have well-delineated tissue planes. Cellulitis can be identified as anechoic layering of fluids between and among soft tissue planes. This is often described as a "cobblestone" like appearance (*see* Figs. 6 and 7). A "cobblestone" appearance is not specific for cellulitis, as many other conditions may lead to

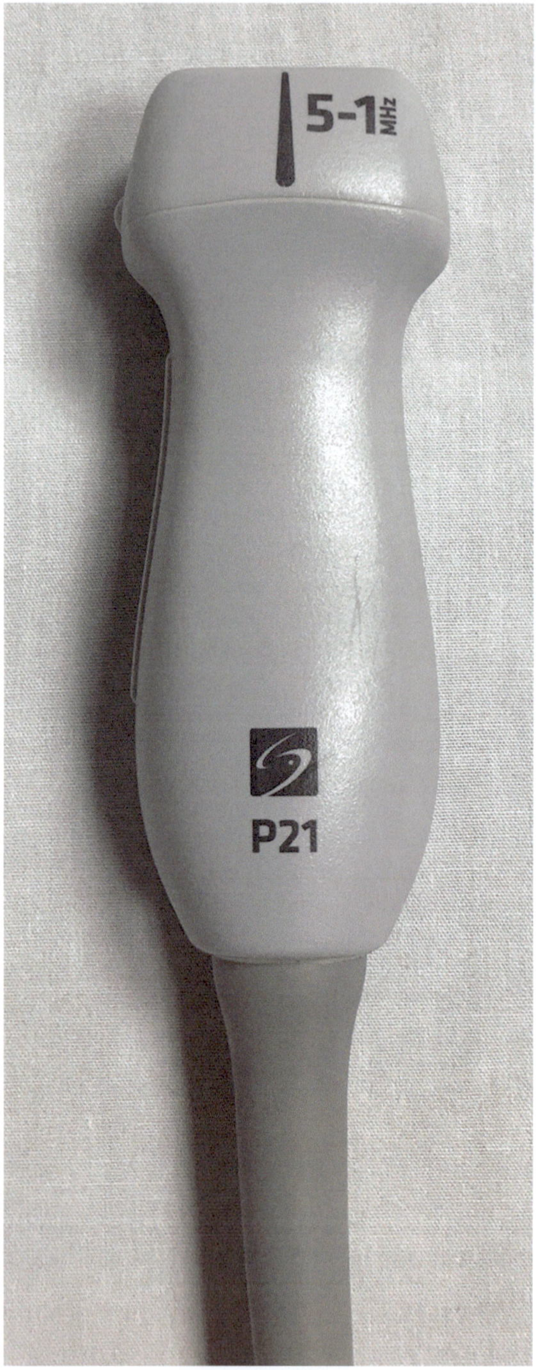

Fig. 3 Phased array transducer: Phased array transducers have smaller flat footprints and exhibit a pie-shaped field of view

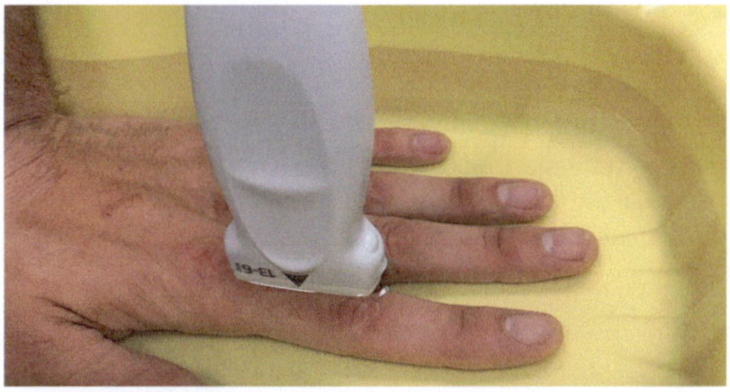

Fig. 4 Water bath positioning. To facilitate visualization of small parts, have the patient place the affected area in a container of water, and hover the probe over the area of interest

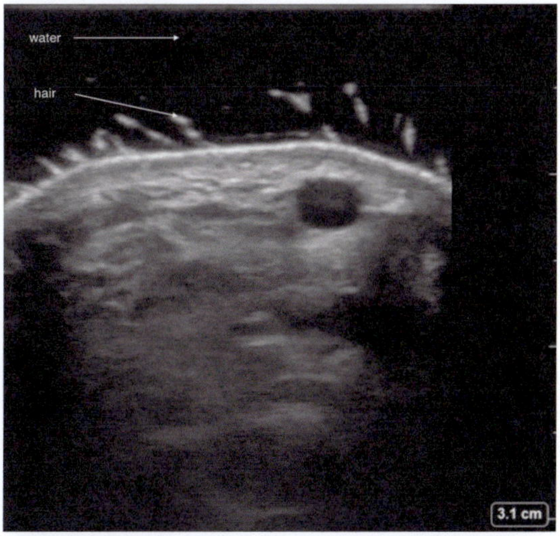

Fig. 5 Water bath ultrasound. Dorsal hand ultrasound using a water bath showing separation of transducer from the tissue of interest

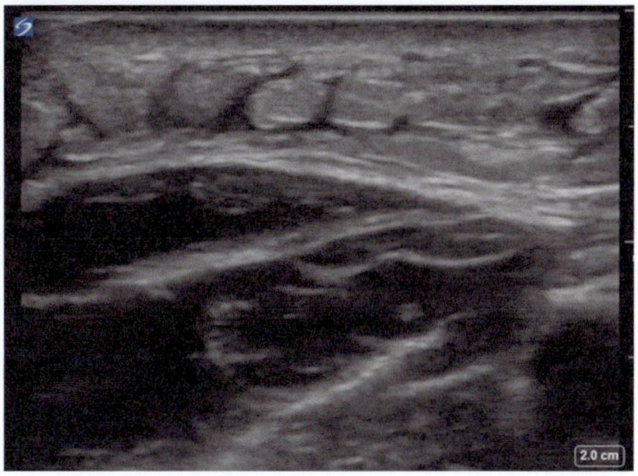

Fig. 6 Cellulitis. Cellulitis typically appears as cobblestoning of the subcutaneous tissue with associated thickening of the dermal layers

fluid accumulation in soft tissue (any cause of peripheral edema or localized inflammation). Cellulitis may also be identified by a loss of the usually well-delineated tissue planes which is thought to occur due to tissue thickening and inflammation. Air that is identified within soft tissue planes or obstructs images should raise the clinical suspicion for a necrotizing soft tissue infection in the correct clinical

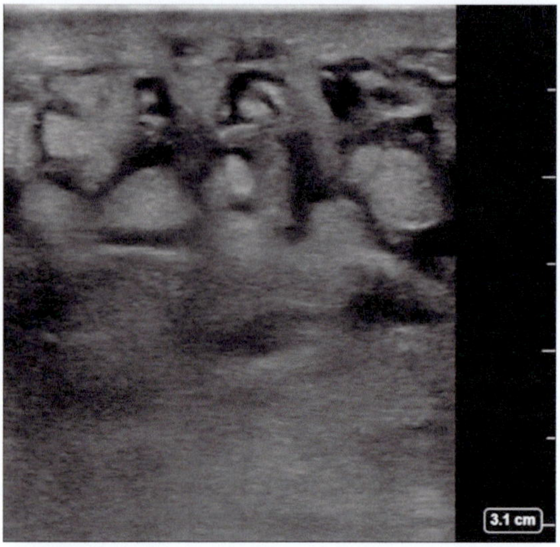

Fig. 7 Cellulitis with increased soft tissue edema. As cellulitis becomes more severe or with concomitant edema, there will be increased fluid within the subcutaneous tissue visualized by thicker anechoic pockets

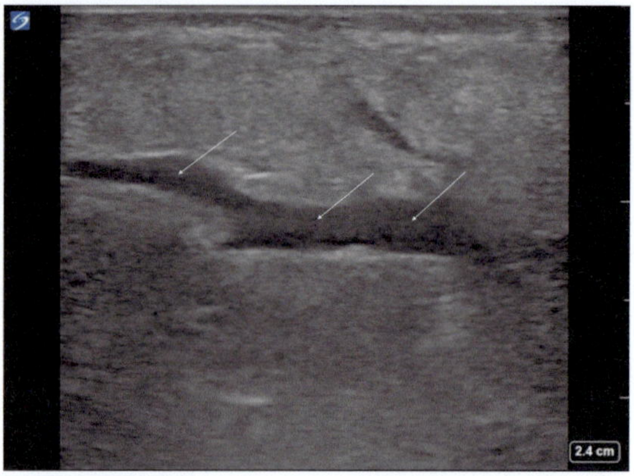

Fig. 8 Necrotizing fasciitis with perifascial fluid. Fluid tracking along the fascial plane with thickened subcutaneous tissue and a loss of normal architecture. Perifascial fluid greater than 4 mm likely indicates a diagnosis of necrotizing fasciitis

context (*see* Fig. 8). Sonographic findings of necrotizing soft tissue infection include distorted and thickened fascial planes with turbid fluid accumulation in both the fascial layers and subcutaneous edema [4].

The soft tissue in question should be systematically scanned in both transverse and longitudinal axis while looking for the nonspecific signs of cellulitis and examining for such complicating features as abscesses or foreign bodies. Examine the affected tissue completely to the margins to visualize the return of normal well-delineated tissue planes. If there is doubt about the diagnosis, compare the affected tissue to the tissue on the contralateral side or tissue elsewhere on the body that is thought to be normal.

Abscess

Ultrasound greatly improves the identification of abscess when compared to palpation. Physical exam has an accuracy of 86% while utilization of ultrasound improves that accuracy to 98% [5]. Further, ultrasound can be used to measure the size of the abscess to evaluate if drainage is required, as abscesses under 1 cm are unlikely to require drainage [6]. Color Doppler (if available) may also be used to better identify vascular structures and ensure no vascular flow exists within a suspected abscess cavity. Prior to drainage, the tissue around the abscess can be examined for communication to deeper structures that may require more advanced intervention, neurovascular structures and tendons that should be avoided during incision, and foreign bodies that may injure the provider and cause recurrent infection in the patient [7].

An abscess can be identified by an irregularly shaped to round anechoic or hypoechoic structure that may contain echogenic material. The soft tissue in question should be systemically scanned in both transverse and longitudinal axis while looking for the suspected abscess. Light pressure applied from the probe to the abscess may result in movement of the echogenic purulent material within the abscess and aid in identification. Once the abscess has been identified, measure its dimensions in short and long axis to determine the need for drainage. Visualize the complete margins of the abscess and look specifically for any deeper tracts or connections to deep structures. Consider more advanced surgical management if either is found. If point of care drainage is appropriate, the depth of the abscess should be measured from the skin surface and the surrounding tissue examined for neurovascular structures and tendons that should be avoided during drainage. Find the most superficial portion of the abscess and mark the corresponding skin (Fig. 9).

Abscess drainage is rarely performed with live ultrasound guidance. As previously mentioned, utilize the ultrasound to mark the most superficial portion of the abscess, clean and anesthetize the skin around this mark, and perform an incision

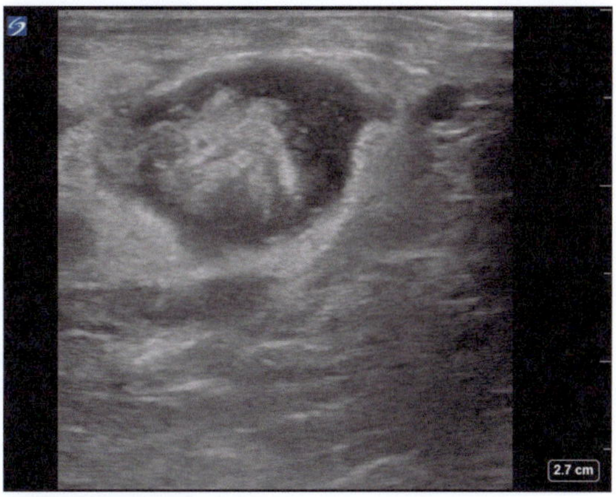

Fig. 9 Abscess. Hypoechoic fluid collection with thick echogenic material representing a small abscess

and drainage of the abscess. Examine the area of the abscess after incision and drainage with the ultrasound to ensure there are no missed pockets of purulent material or loculations.

Foreign Body

Foreign bodies such as wood, glass, metal, plastic, and organic material in soft tissue account for about 2% of soft tissue injuries in the austere environment [8]. Given the potential for delayed treatment in these environments, early identification of foreign bodies is important to reduce infection, pain, and inflammation. Patients with foreign bodies in their feet or hands may not be able to ambulate or perform work duties. Ultrasonography has been proven in the identification of foreign bodies as well as in procedural guidance for their removal [9, 10]. Ultrasonography is more sensitive than plain film radiography and can identify between 94% to 98% of foreign bodies [11, 12]. In addition, ultrasound can be used to identify injuries to neurovascular structures while evaluating for foreign bodies or after their identification.

Identification of a foreign body is made through direct visualization of an echogenic structure in the area of suspicion or by identification of secondary signs such as reverberation artifact, shadowing, or fluid collection (Figs. 10 and 11).

Reverberation artifact occurs when an ultrasound beam encounters two strong parallel reflectors. It is often seen with metallic or glass objects such as a needle or shrapnel when viewed in a long axis or short axis. If these objects are small or in the superficial skin, the artifact may aid in their identification [13]. A foreign body that has been retained for greater than 24 hours may have a surrounding hypoechoic rim of fluid. Such a finding increases the sensitivity and specificity of foreign body identification [14]. Foreign bodies with smooth and flat surfaces tend to produce

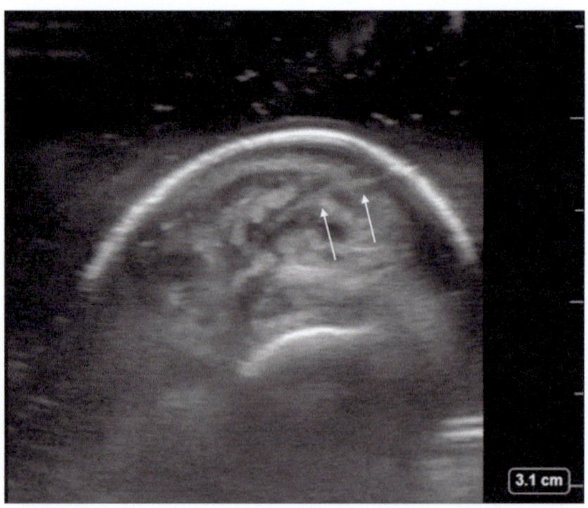

Fig. 10 Foreign body. Finger ultrasound in water bath with embedded foreign body (arrows)

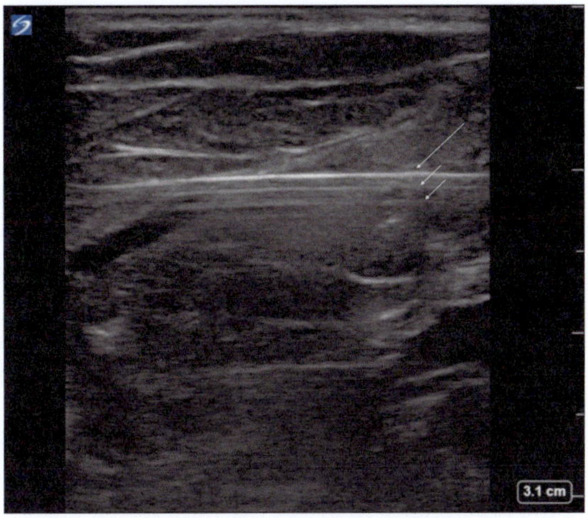

Fig. 11 Metal foreign body. Brightly echogenic foreign body represents a broken needle within the neck of a patient from intravenous drug abuse

clean shadowing deep to the foreign body while objects with irregular surfaces usually demonstrate dirty shadowing [15].

Before using ultrasound to scan for foreign bodies, evaluate the patient for entrance wounds and estimate the trajectory and path of any foreign bodies. Palpation may be useful. Then place the probe over the entrance wound and evaluate a wide margin of tissue in the suspected trajectory of the foreign body. Evaluate the tissue in both transverse and longitudinal axis while looking for the hyperechoic foreign body or secondary signs such as fluid collection, artifact, or shadowing. Once the foreign body has been identified, examine the surrounding tissue for damage to other structures such as nerves, vasculature, or tendons. Measure the size of the foreign body in both the short and long axis as well as its depth. Mark the location of the foreign body on the skin.

Once a foreign body has been recognized, ultrasound is a useful modality to guide its removal. Using ultrasound in this fashion decreases complications [12]. The size and position of a foreign body can be accurately identified with ultrasonography, and the surgical incision required to remove the foreign body can be smaller and more accurate [16].

Ultrasound can be used to guide foreign body removal in a similar fashion to ultrasound guidance for vascular access or a peripheral nerve blocks (see chapters "Initial Training, Credentialing, and Quality Assurance/Quality Improvement Processes", "Care of Equipment", 30 and 31). Estimate the surgical path by evaluating the skin around the foreign body. Identify any nerves, tendons, or vascular structures that should be avoided. Clean the skin at the planned incision site and anesthetize the superficial skin and deeper structures along the surgical path while using the ultrasound for direct visualization. Make a small incision in the skin and perform a blunt dissection with forceps while maintaining visualization of the foreign body and any structures along the dissection path that should be avoided. Capture and remove the foreign body, irrigate the site, and then close or allow the wound to heal by secondary intention.

Limitations of Current Knowledge and Opportunities for Future Research

Ultrasound examination of soft tissue has been used successfully for decades to identify cellulitis, abscesses, and foreign bodies. Nevertheless, there are plenty of opportunities for research in this application of ultrasound. As small, portable ultrasound devices become more readily available, there will likely be questions raised regarding validation of image quality in relation to more standardly used cart-based systems. This is certainly relevant in the austere environment. Additionally, as the "democratization" of ultrasound continues, ultrasound capabilities will be increasingly available to medical providers at diverse levels of experience and expertise, and will likely include advanced practice practitioners, nurses, paramedics, and other paraprofessionals. Research into the optimal model for initial training and skills sustainment for these varied groups will be needed. Some of this is already being done, particularly in the military.

Pearls

Use a linear high frequency array for most soft tissue scanning.

Be thorough and systematic when scanning soft tissue to avoid missing subtle findings.

Orient the screen image to the surface features of your patient.

Whenever possible, scan in two planes.

Use water baths or other methods to achieve stand-off from the surface of the probe in order to better image superficial structures.

Use color Doppler when available to delineate vascular structures.

Use ultrasound in conjunction with physical exam to improve the sensitivity of your clinical assessments.

If you are uncertain about what you are seeing, compare it to an unaffected side or region.

Pitfalls

You may need to use a lower frequency probe in order to adequately image deeper structures.

Not all that "cobblestones" is cellulitis – use clinical judgement and be alert for other causes of soft tissue edema.

If you can't clearly see the back wall of an abscess, beware extension or tracking into deeper tissue or cavities.

Failure to recognize subtle artifacts may lead to missed recognition of more serious soft tissue infections or foreign bodies.

Failure to completely scan through the entire area of interest into normal appearing surrounding tissue may lead to misdiagnosis.

Key Literature Reviewed

1. Gentile DA. Wilderness injuries and illnesses. Ann Emerg Med. 1992;21:853–61.
2. Blaivas M. Water bath evaluation technique for emergency ultrasound of painful superficial structures. Am J Emerg Med. 2004;22:589–93.
3. Stanford KA. Trends in skin and soft tissue-related injuries in NOLS wilderness expeditions from 1984 to 2012. Wilderness Environ Med. 2017;28:307–12.
4. Fugitt JB. Necrotizing fasciitis. Radiographics. 2004;24:1472–6.
5. Squire BT. ABSCESS: applied bedside sonography for convenient evaluation of superficial soft tissue infections. Acad Emerg Med. 2005;12:601–6.
6. Adhikari S. Sonography first for subcutaneous abscess and cellulitis evaluation. J Ultrasound Med. 2012;31:1509–12.
7. Tayal VS. The effect of soft-tissue ultrasound on the management of cellulitis in the emergency department. Acad Emerg Med. 2006;13:384–8.
8. Montalvo R. Morbidity and mortality in the wilderness. West J Med. 1998;168:248–54.
9. Shrestha D. The role of ultrasonography in detection and localization of radiolucent foreign body in soft tissues of extremities. JNMA J Nepal Med Assoc. 2009;48:5–9.
10. Graham DD. Ultrasound in the emergency department: detection of wooden foreign bodies in the soft tissues. J Emerg Med. 2002;22:75–9.
11. Horton LK. Sonography and radiography of soft- tissue foreign bodies. AJR Am J Roentgenol. 2001;176:1155–9.
12. Soudack M. Clinically unsuspected foreign bodies: the importance of sonography. J Ultrasound Med. 2003;22:1381–5.
13. Feldman MK. US artifacts. Radiographics. 2009;29:1179–89.
14. Jacobson JA. Wooden foreign bodies in soft tissue: detection at US. Radiology. 1998;206:45–8.
15. Rubin JA. Clean and dirty shadowing at US: a reappraisal. Radiology. 1991;181:231–6.
16. Paziana K. Soft tissue foreign body removal technique using portable ultrasonography. Wilderness Environ Med. 2012;23:343–8.

Advanced Diagnostic Topic for Austere Providers: Skeletal Trauma

Laurel O'Connor and Ricky C. Kue

Introduction

Musculoskeletal trauma and injury is a common peril in the austere and wilderness environment. Proficiency in identifying skeletal injuries, chief among them bony fractures, muscle and tendon injuries, and joint dislocation, is essential. Such injuries must be managed immediately either with temporizing measures, such as an improvised splint, or definitively with joint reduction in order to promote optimal healing and facilitate the evacuation of the patient and his or her medical providers. The timely identification and management of skeletal injuries is of particular importance in the austere environment because such injuries may present a barrier to the mobility of a patient when safety or the need for definitive management is a concern. Skeletal injury is also a common life and limb threatening condition associated with polytrauma. Sonography has already been integrated into use for acute triage and initial survey in the trauma patient. The additional of skeletal ultrasound to the initial sonographical assessment after trauma is a valuable adjunct to this exam and facilitates the injury management of critical patients.

Point of care ultrasonography is portable and relatively easy to operate, and it affords providers with the ability to quickly assess and manage injuries accurately, with no radiation exposure to patient or provider. There is no need for extensive equipment or a specialized building. It is capable of transmitting images in real time and displaying dynamic changes with position, which is of particular interest in the musculoskeletal system. While not a definitive imaging modality for all skeletal injuries, for both bone and soft tissue injuries, its sensitivity rivals more conventional imaging types such as x-ray or MRI.

L. O'Connor (✉)
Department of Emergency Medicine, University of Massachusetts Medical School, Worcester, MA, USA

R. C. Kue
Massachusetts Urban Search and Rescue Task Force-1 (MA-TF1), Beverly, MA, USA

B. D. Nicholson et al. (eds.), *Manual of Austere and Prehospital Ultrasound*,
https://doi.org/10.1007/978-3-030-64287-7_14

In this chapter the emphasis will be on the sonographic identification of long bone fracture, joint effusion, and tendon injury, as well as the diagnosis and management of shoulder dislocation and reduction.

Topic Discussion

Basic Musculoskeletal Sonographic Technique

Most musculoskeletal ultrasound can be performed using a high-frequency linear array transducer, as the desired images will typically be closer to the skin surface, although a curvilinear probe can be used for very large patients or deeper structures [1]. Because of the relatively superficiality of these structures, ensuring an adequate volume of medium for good transduction is essential; this can be accomplished with a copious layer of ultrasound gel. Alternatively, operators may use a premade medium tool such as a commercial gel pad, or a water bath; the latter may be more practical in the austere setting. A large bag of saline or other liquid will suffice for this purpose. Alternatively, the tissue of interest can be submerged in a tub of water and the tip of the probe immersed. With this technique, the probe need not be touching the structure being examined and in fact can be placed just underneath the surface of the water to transmit an excellent image. Regardless of the medium used, the depth of the image may need to be adjusted upon initial examination to adequately capture the structure being scanned depending on the size of the patient, depth of the transduction medium and the probe being used.

All imaged tissues should be viewed in both the transverse and longitudinal plane to ensure that a comprehensive and diagnostically accurate picture is obtained; the approach and technique for different structures vary and are discussed in more detail individually. In some instances, the dynamic nature of tissue (such contraction and relaxation in the diagnoses of muscular and tendon pathology) is important to identifying abnormal findings and so patients may be instructed to flex or extend the structure of interest.

Finally, as is the case in many types of point of care ultrasound but of particular relevance in musculoskeletal ultrasound, it is important to be vigilant to control for artifact when obtaining images, as it can interfere with the correct identification and diagnosis of pathology. A common culprit is anisotropy, when the echogenicity of a structure changes based on the angle of the probe. The same structure may appear more hyper- or hypo- echoic depending on the angle of the probe and cause a false positive pathological finding. A similar false positive can result from bone pseudodefect, which occurs when the transmitted beam impacts the bone in a semi tangential angle, resulting in the deflection of the reflected beams and causing a false disruption (dark space in the image). This can create the illusion of a cortical disruption [2]. These hazards can be identified and avoided by slowly changing the angle of the probe during transduction, "fanning" through the image to see if the echogenicity varies with position. A truly abnormal finding will remain visible with stable echogenicity even when the probe's angle is changed whereas if the effect is due to anisotropy, the echogenicity will change with the angle of the transducer. Also consider the immediately adjacent images, the corresponding image on the contralateral side, if applicable, and the all-important clinical correlation.

Anatomy

When orienting oneself for musculoskeletal ultrasound, begin by identifying the three major hyperechoic (bright white) layers visible upon initial probe placement. In general, it is easiest to begin in the transverse axis. The most superficial layer is skin and dermis; this will appear closest to the transducer, followed by the slightly deeper fascia. The more anechoic subcutaneous fat lays between dermis and the fascia. Deep to the fascia but superficial to the cortical surface is muscle and connective tissue, which tends to form an echogenic, tight fibrillar matrix in the long access view and a speckled appearance in transverse axis [1]. When uninjured, this layer is typical regular and symmetrical; the striated muscle fibers lie close to each other. The final layer, which should appear bright white and smooth, is the line of the bony cortex [1]. When healthy, this layer should appear as a straight uninterrupted surface. Once the cortex has been identified it can be positively confirmed by then rotating the transducer into the longitudinal plane, which will yield an acoustic shadow in the deep aspect of the image. The operator will observe darkness deep to the cortex because ultrasound doesn't penetrate the bone well.

Diagnosis of Bony Fracture

When imaging a long bone for fracture, begin in the transverse plane. Orient the depth to optimize the bony cortex relative to other structures on the viewing device. Once orientation has been accomplished, the probe can be rotated to the longitudinal plane and the length of the bone can be scanned to evaluate for cortical disruptions. Bony fracture is identified on sonographic image by a hypoechoic (dark) break in the smooth, hyperechoic line of the cortex or periosteal elevations, which has the appearance of one edge of the cortical surface rising above an adjacent edge with a step-off between them [1]. Other anatomical abnormalities such as surrounding hypoechoic effusion or hematoma superficial to the cortex can hint at an occult fracture; in general this will appear as a dark heterogeneous region around the cortical surface. In some studies, the, longitudinal view has been shown to be more accurate in identifying long bone fracture but they are frequently visible in both planes [3]. This technique has been validated for long bone fracture in both the hospital and out-of-hospital setting [4, 5]. In addition, similar technique, in combination with the clinical presentation can be used on the thorax to identify rib fractures [6] and sternal fractures [7] (Figs. 1 and 2).

Beyond its utility when specific isolated injuries are suspected, the addition of long bone ultrasonography in screening point of care ultrasound after polytrauma, dubbed "CAVEAT" has been proposed as an addition to the more traditional "FAST"

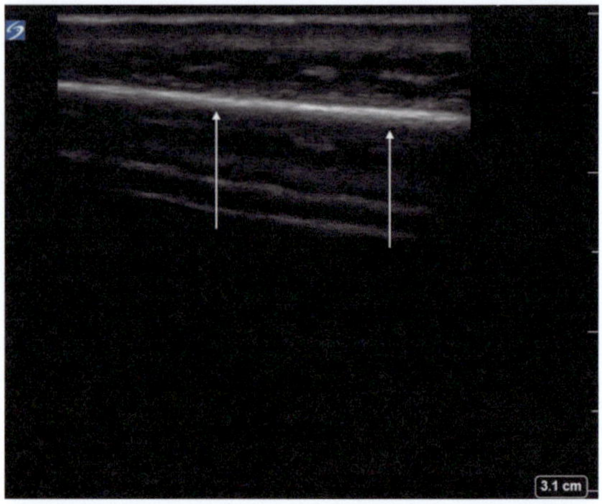

Fig. 1 Normal bone: Normal bone is hyperechoic with posterior shadowing

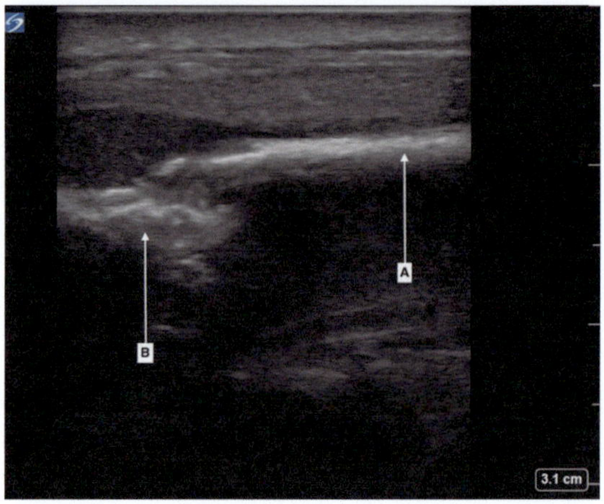

Fig. 2 Fracture: Bone (**a**) loses its typical appearance and will be seen as a disruption of the bony cortex at the site of the fracture (**b**)

or "RUSH" exam [1]. CAVEAT, which stands for ultrasound-assisted Chest, Abdomen, Vena Cava, and Extremities for Acute Triage is intended to enable a expeditious and accurate diagnosis of major long bone fractures in order to facilitate quick stabilization and prioritized advanced radiographical studies and subspecialist care [8]. After imaging the thorax, the operator performing a CAVEAT exam scans both upper and lower extremities in the transverse and longitudinal plane to evaluate for significant long bone fracture. Obviously this screening scan should not replace re-evaluation and more advanced imaging. Additionally, the operator should be vigilant that the integration of standardized CAVEAT sonography should not disrupt other validated trauma procedural algorithms intended to identify and stabilize life-threatening injuries.

Diagnosis of Muscle/Tendon Injury

Like long-bone ultrasonography, the typical approach to tendon ultrasonography is to begin in the transverse position in order to orient the operator and identify landmarks; when the tendon of interest is identified, it should be scanned through the entire structure in the transverse plan and subsequently the longitudinal plane.

Whereas normal connective tissue is sonographically visualized as a well-organized matrix, an injured tendon will appear irregular and asymmetric. The fibrillar matrix will be disrupted at the site of insult. This may manifest with hypoechoic edema or heterogeneous hematoma between strands that differs from the regularity of surrounding healthy tendon [1, 9]. Anisotropy is of particular concern when using sonography for tendon injuries so upon the identification of hypoechoic irregularities in the tissue, it important to adjust the angle of the probe on the skin; if the hypoechoic change remains, it is more likely to be true injury, whereas if the echogenicity varies, one should suspect artifact [9]. Tendon tears are also readily identifiable on ultrasound. In this situation the regular network of fibers will be completely disrupted; often a hematoma will sit between the two ragged ends of the tendon, which will likely both have an edematous irregular appearance. With dynamic movement of the flexion and extension the two ends may separate even further, confirming the suspected diagnosis (Figs. 3 and 4).

Diagnosis of Joint Effusions

A joint effusion, or abnormal fluid in the joint capsule, can be indicative of multiple different insults to the surrounding muscular and skeletal structure as well as the joint itself. In the setting of trauma, a joint effusion visualized on ultrasound may be the result of injury to local structures including ligaments, cartilage or occult bony fracture [10, 11]. Currently the most widely imaged joint for effusion is the knee, but hips, elbows, shoulder and ankles are routinely imaged to evaluate for effusions indicative

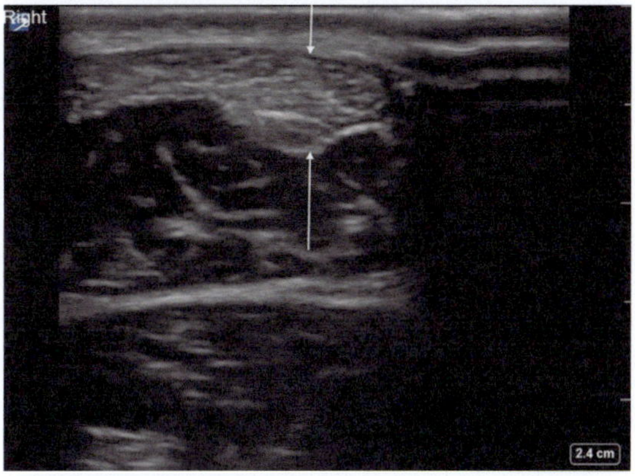

Fig. 3 Tendon in cross section: In cross section, tendons will have hyperechoic punctate structures

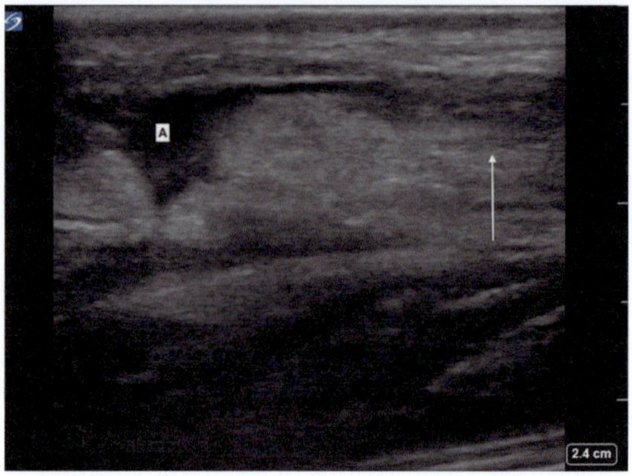

Fig. 4 Partial tendon rupture: The normal tendon (arrow) becomes edematous then has a noticeable defect (A) where it is torn. The hypoechoic area is blood filling the defect

of pathology [2]. Sonographically, joint effusions present as an anechoic intra-articular fluid collection. Particulate material indicative of blood or purulence may make the effusion appear echogenic; sometimes variations in the amount of pressure put on the probe will make the intra-articular debris "swirl" around the capsule [12].

As with all muscular ultrasound, it is important to completely scan in both the transverse and longitudinal planes to detect joint effusion, and the contralateral joint should also be imaged for comparison. It should be noted that while being indicative of skeletal injury in the setting of trauma, an effusion identified in isolation is not diagnostic of a specific injury. It should also be noted that joint effusion can be caused by atraumatic etiologies such as inflammatory arthritis (rheumatoid arthritis, gout etc.) and infection (septic arthritis) so clinical correlation is key. Although uncommonly performed in the out-of-hospital setting arthrocentesis under direct ultrasound guidance is an efficient way to ensure first attempt success and avoid vessel injury.

Diagnosis and Reduction of Joint Dislocation

The joint pathology most frequently diagnosed and reduced with ultrasound guidance is shoulder dislocation. This pathology is commonly implicated in trauma and therein is a frequent injury the austere setting. The use of ultrasound for the identification of shoulder dislocation in the acute setting is both highly sensitive and specific [13]. It is of particular utility because it can be used primarily to diagnosis a dislocation and then subsequently after attempted reduction, to confirm the success of the procedure. The shoulder is a deeper structure and may require the curvilinear probe for evaluation but in smaller patients, the linear probe may be used (Fig. 5).

Basic Technique

The operator should begin in the transverse orientation behind the shoulder, over the scapular spine. The probe should then be moved laterally until the hyperechoic, curved glenoid is visualized. Once the operator has identified the glenoid, she/he

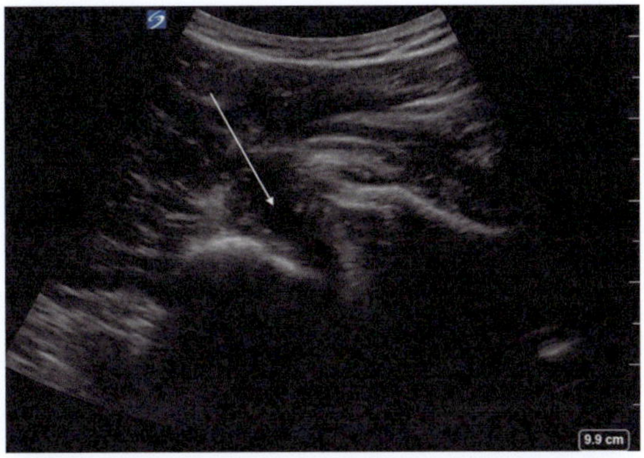

Fig. 5 Shoulder effusion: A shoulder effusion can be visualized as a hypoechoic area between the humeral head and scapula. Heterogeneous material may sometimes be visualized if blood has started to clot

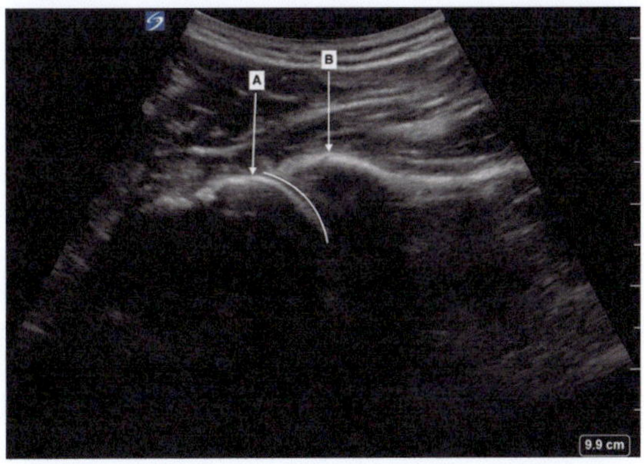

Fig. 6 Normal shoulder on ultrasound: In the normal shoulder, you can see the humeral head (**a**) sitting in the glenoid joint fossa (curved line) created by the scapula (**b**)

should continue to move the probe laterally until the bright, round cortical surface of the humeral head is visualized. If the shoulder joint is in proper anatomic position, then the humeral head should be directly adjacent to the glenoid. A radial head that is above the glenoid, proximal in the image to the glenoid (which will appear closer to the probe on the image) suggests a posterior shoulder dislocation. A humeral head below the glenoid, more distal in the image (further from the probe) suggests an anterior dislocation [14]. A hyperechoic hemarthrosis may also seen between the glenoid and the humerus when the joint is dislocated (Figs. 6 and 7).

Intra-articular Nerve Block

Intra-articular nerve block in shoulder dislocation has the advantage of providing significant analgesia to patient with a dislocated shoulder and permitting them to tolerate a reduction attempt with the benefit of avoiding sedating medications and a prolonged recovery period. In the hospital setting it has been shown to be non-inferior to procedural sedation in terms of patient satisfaction and pain scores while decreasing the time and resources required for a procedural sedation [15]. It also negates the need for a monitored setting [15].

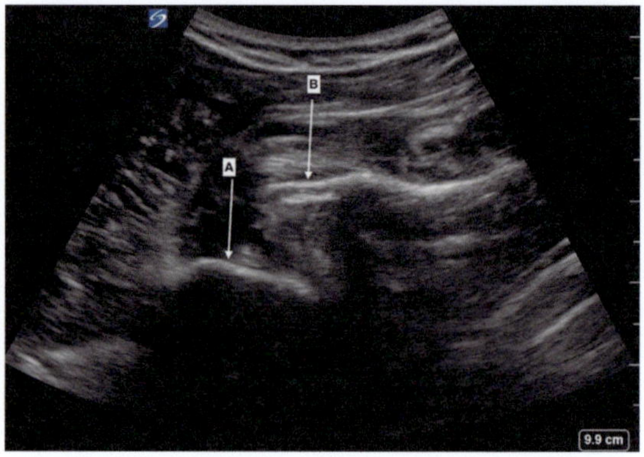

Fig. 7 Anterior shoulder dislocation: With an anterior dislocation, the humeral head (**a**) will be displaced anteriorly away from the scapula (**b**)

Like the evaluation of a dislocated shoulder, intra-articular nerve block under ultrasound guidance can be performed with either the linear or curvilinear probe depending on the size of the patient. In additional to the ultrasound, required tools include a 20 CC syringe, 1% lidocaine without epinephrine, a long (at least 3.5 cm, spinal needles work well) 18 gauge needle, sterile gloves, sterile ultrasound cover, and antiseptic. The lateral aspect of the effected shoulder should be sterilized and syringe prepared with 20 ml of lidocaine. The patient should be positioned in the sitting or semirecumbant position. The provider should take a posterior-lateral approach to the shoulder (lateral deltoid, underneath the acromion) and begin by anesthetizing the skin at the insertion site by injecting a subcutaneous wheel of lidocaine. The covered ultrasound probe should be placed in plane (longitudinally parallel to the needle). The needle should then by advanced under direct visualization towards the glenoid fossa (space between radial head and glenoid) until the needle appears to be in the joint capsule. Intermittently, the operator should stop, aspirate to ensure that there is no blood in the syringe, and inject 1–2 cc of lidocaine to anesthetize deeper tissue. When the needle is visualized within the hemarthrosis, aspiration should again be attempted; at this point blood return is appropriate as this is indicative that the needle has penetrated the hematoma in the joint capsule. The remaining lidocaine should be injected into the joint capsule; a "swirling" pattern will be visible on the ultrasound as the lidocaine is instilled. Full onset of analgesia should be accomplished within 15 minutes. Shoulder reduction can then proceed. There are multiple methodologies for this procedure, which will not be discussed in detail in this manual. Once reduction has been attempted, confirmation can be accomplished by direct ultrasound imaging as discussed above; a radial head immediately adjacent to the glenoid, when correlated clinically with improvement in pain and range of motion of the extremity, indicates a successful reduction [16].

Key Literature Reviewed

Prior studies have shown promising sensitivity and specificity in sonographic diagnosis of connective tissue, muscle, and long bone fractures in the emergency department [5, 9, 17]. Similar success has also been demonstrated specifically in the austere setting [4, 18].

Sonographic diagnosis of long bone fracture has been validated as having similar sensitivity to x-ray [5, 19] and the added benefit of avoiding radiation. Frouzan et al., which examined ultrasound diagnosis of upper and lower limb trauma demonstrated an overall sensitivity and specificity of 95.3% and 87.7% respectively for radiographically identified upper arm fracture with a positive predictive value of 87.2%. In the lower extremity sensitivity and specificity were 98.6% and 83% with a positive predictive value of 65.4% [19]. Dossing et al., in a study also examining upper and lower extremity fractures demonstrated overall sonographical sensitivity of 92%, a specificity of 94%, and a positive predictive value of 85% [5].

Besides long bone fractures, a study by Griffith et al. that compared evaluation of rib fractures with ultrasonography to conventional chest radiography noted that ultrasound was superior; Sonography had 78% sensitivity as opposed to 12% sensitivity for radiographs [6]. Most fractures identified by sonography were located in the rib as opposed to in the costochondral junction, or costal cartilage [6]. Three weeks later, repeat sonography reveal changes consistent with healing in all previously detected fractures [6].

Although not discussed in detail here, ultrasound guidance has also been shown to be effective for guiding fracture reduction. A 2016 study by Sabzghabaei et al. showed that ultrasound guided distal radius reduction reduced the need for repeat reduction or operative management as compared to blind reduction group (9.2% versus 24.6% when ultrasound guidance was not use; $P = .019$) with similar post reduction indices [20]. A comparable study by Chinnock et al. demonstrated similar outcomes, which showed both that ultrasound guided reduction was as successful as the control group, and that the participating physicians' interpretation of sonographic assessment of each reduction was highly sensitive for successful reduction when compared to x-ray assessment of reduction [21].

Ultrasound guided diagnosis of shoulder dislocation with ultrasound-guided nerve block and confirmation of successful reduction has also performed well when compared to more conventional imaging studies. It has been shown to be especially strong in diagnosing posterior shoulder dislocations, which can be particularly difficulty to diagnosis on plain films [22].

A Systemic review by Gottleib et al. showed a range of sensitivity but 100% specificity for diagnosis of shoulder dislocation. This review, which included 531 assessments and 202 dislocations showed that most studies had a sensitivity of 100% for detecting dislocation (a lone study had a sensitivity of 54%, and another had only one dislocation that was misidentified. All reviewed studies demonstrated 100% specificity for dislocation) [13].

Limitations of Current Knowledge and Opportunities for Future Research

While the identification of long bone and rib fracture by ultrasound has shown promising results, use of ultrasound for diagnosis of smaller bone fractures such as those in the ankle, wrist and hand have yet to be validated. Currently, for such small bones with irregular shapes or ends, ultrasound is not recommended for diagnostic use in isolation however, it may have value as an adjunct to the diagnosis of occult fractures that are not radiographically apparent [1].

Ultrasound guided fracture reduction is also a niche where little literature exists beyond forearm fracture; ultrasound guided reduction of displaced lower extremity fractures and other long bones would certainly prove valuable but is not validated in larger studies. There is also relatively little literature on ultrasound guided nerve blocks and reductions of other large joints beyond the shoulder, especially in the out of hospital setting. A small study completed by Buttner at al demonstrated potential for nerve block as a superior means of pain management in a head to head comparison of peripheral nerve block (sites included femoral nerve block, sciatic nerve block, interscalene brachial plexus block, and intraclavicular nerve blocks depending on the injured extremity) when compared to intravenous sedation for isolated out of hospital extremity injuries [23]. Larger scale prehospital and austere studies may demonstrate widespread success with ultrasound guided peripheral nerve block. Such blocks are relatively safe and extremely efficacious for analgesia in extremity trauma.

The majority of existing studies that have demonstrated sonographical success in musculoskeletal ultrasounds have been completed by experienced operators whereas the literature on more novice operators or those with more condensed training on specific point of care procedures is more limited. While the use of ultrasound for the diagnosis of skeletal injury in the acute care setting is well validated, there is a relative paucity of validated literature demonstrating equal efficacy in the truly austere setting. Some small studies regarding long bone fracture identification exist [4] but there is much less information available about out of hospital nerve blocks, joint reduction and fracture reduction.

As the scope of practice of the austere provider becomes more sophisticated, so will the capacity of ultrasound utility. More advanced, invasive orthopedics procedures that may become necessary in the austere environment are being studied in simulated settings. For example, the placement of Schanz pin for external fixation of long bone fractures [24–26] has been described in educational literature, generally as a physician-performed procedure. If introduced to the field, this will make an important contribution to the ability of out of hospital providers to provide more definitive orthopedic injury management.

In the future, when point of care ultrasound becomes a more standard tool for providers in out-of-hospital environments, outcomes from ultrasound guided diagnosis and management of musculoskeletal injury outside of the hospital setting will be better described. Musculoskeletal ultrasound for trauma has a wide breadth of utility and is ideal for the austere setting due to its versatility and portability. Skeletal trauma is of particular interest because it is so ubiquitous in the out-of-hospital setting. While not a comprehensive substitute for other imaging modalities, ultrasound has demonstrated outstanding performance in aiding the diagnosis and management of acute injury, and proficiency in musculoskeletal sonography is an essential skill for any provider who practices in the austere environment.

Pearls and Pitfalls

- When evaluating for long bone fracture, scan in both planes for evidence of cortical disruption, hematoma or effusion. Also note any interruption in the fibrillar matrix of connective tissue, which could indicate soft tissue injury or occult fracture.
- Be aware of the hazard of anisotropy and other angle dependent artifact that could result in a false positive image. Always scan through both planes and fan over multiple angles when examining a perceived pathological finding. A true finding will be visible at multiple angles. Also consider comparing the image with adjacent structures or the uninjured limb.
- For very superficial structures a standoff pad or water bath will greatly improve transmitted images. A bag of normal saline will suffice for this purpose, or alternatively, submerse the limb of interest in water. The transducer need not touch the limb in a water bath to transmit a high quality image.
- Clinical correlation is absolutely crucial in diagnosing musculoskeletal pathology so always compare the images obtained with superficial injuries, localized tenderness, and the mechanism of injury.

References

1. Chen KC, Lin AC, Chong CF, Wang TL. An overview of point-of-care ultrasound for soft tissue and musculoskeletal applications in the emergency department. J Intensive Care. 2016;4:55. https://doi.org/10.1186/s40560-016-0173-0.
2. Vlad VM. Pitfalls in muscularskeletal ultrasound. In: Miedany YM, editor. Musculoskeletal ultrasonography in rheumatic diseases. Cham: Springer; 2016. p. 21–55.
3. Farahmand S, Arshadi A, Bagheri-Hariri S, Shahriarian S, Arbab M, Mojftaba S. Extremity fracture diagnosis using bedside ultrasound in pediatric trauma patients referring to emergency department; a diagnaostic study. Int Ped. 2017;5(10):5959–43.
4. McNeil CR, McManus J, Mehta S. The accuracy of portable ultrasonography to diagnose fractures in an austere environment. Prehosp Emerg Care. 2009;13(1):50–2. https://doi.org/10.1080/10903120802474513.
5. Døssing K, Mechlenburg I, Hansen LB, Søballe K, Østergaard H. The use of ultrasound to exclude extremity fractures in adults. J Bone Joint Surg. 2017;2(3):e0007. https://doi.org/10.2106/JBJS.OA.17.00007.
6. Griffith JF, Rainer TH, Ching AS, Law KL, Cocks RA, Metreweli C. Sonography compared with radiography in revealing acute rib fracture. Am J Roentgenol. 1999;173(6):1603–9.
7. Engin G, Yekeler E, Gulogolu R, Acunas B, Acunas G. US versus conventional radiography in the diagnosis of sternal fractures. Acta Radiol. 2000;41(3):296–9.
8. Stawicki SP, Howard JM, Pryor JP, Bahner DP, Whitmill ML, Dean AJ. Portable ultrasonography in mass casualty incidents: the CAVEAT examination. World J Orthop. 2010;18:10–9.
9. Robinson P. Sonography of common tendon injuries. Am J Roentgenol. 2009;193:607–18. https://doi.org/10.2214/AJR.09.2808.
10. Pavić R, Margetić P, Hnatešen D. Diagnosis of occult radial head and neck fracture in adults. Injury. 2015;46(Suppl 6):S119–24.

11. Guillodo Y, Riban P, Guennoc X, Dubrana F, Saraux A. Usefulness of ultrasonographic detection of talocrucial effusion in ankle sprains. J Ultrasound Med. 2007;26:831–6.
12. Rippey J. Ultrasound for knee effusion: lipohaemarthrosis and tibial plateau fracture. Aust J Ultrasound Med. 2014;17:159–66.
13. Gottlieb M, Russell F. Diagnostic accuracy of ultrasound for identifying shoulder dislocations and reductions: a systematic review of the literature. Western J Emerg Med. 2017;18(5):937–42. https://doi.org/10.5811/westjem.2017.5.34432.
14. Meer J, Beck MD, Taylor T. Emergency ultrasound: musculoskeletal shoulder dislocation. Emerg Med. 2016;48(3):128–9.
15. Blaivas M, Adhikaria S, Lander L. A prospective comparison of procedural sedation and ultrasound-guided interscalene nerve block for shoulder reduction in the emergency department. Acad Emerg Med. 2011;18(9):922–7. https://doi.org/10.1111/j.1553-2712.2011.01140.x.
16. JoVE Science Education Database. Emergency medicine and critical care. Intra-articular shoulder injection for reduction following shoulder dislocation. JoVE, Cambridge, MA. https://www.jove.com/science-education. Accessed 10 Oct 2018.
17. Douma-den Hamer D, Blanker MH, Edens MA, et al. Ultrasound for distal forearm fracture: a systematic review and diagnostic meta-analysis. PLoS One. 2016;11(5):e0155659. https://doi.org/10.1371/journal.pone.0155659.
18. Russell TC, Crawford PF. Ultrasound in the austere environment: a review of the history, indications, and specifications. Mil Med. 2013;178(1):21–8.
19. Frouzan A, Masoumi K, Delirroyfard A, Mazdaie B, Bagherzadegan E. Diagnostic accuracy of ultrasound in upper and lower extremity long bone fractures of emergency department trauma patients. Electron Physician. 2017;9(8):5092–7. https://doi.org/10.19082/5092.
20. Sabzghabaei A, Shojaee M, Arhami Dolatabadi A, Manouchehrifar M, Asadi M. Ultrasound-guided reduction of distal radius fractures. Emergency. 2016;4(3):132–5.
21. Chinnock B, Khaletskiy A, Kuo K, Hendey GW. Ultrasound-guided reduction of distal radial fractures. J Emerg Med. 2011;40(3):308–12. https://doi.org/10.1016/j.jemermed.2009.09.019.
22. Abbasi S, Molaie H, Hafezimoghadam P, et al. Diagnostic accuracy of ultrasonographic examination in the management of shoulder dislocation in the emergency department. Ann Emerg Med. 2013;62(2):170–5. https://doi.org/10.1016/j.annemergmed.2013.01.022.
23. Buttner B, Mansur A, Kalmbach M, Hinz J, Volk T, Szalai K, Roessler M, Bergmann I. Prehospital ultrasound-guided nerve blocks improve reduction-feasibility of dislocated extremity injuries compared to system analgesia. A randomized control trial. Plos One. 2018;13(7):e0199776. https://doi.org/10.1371/journal.pone.0199776.
24. Nelson BP, Melnick ER, Li J. Portable ultrasound for remote environments, part II: current indications. J Emerg Med. 2011;40(3):313–21. https://doi.org/10.1016/j.jemermed.2009.11.028. Epub 2010 Jan 25
25. Dahl BP, Pemberton AJ, Beck RT, Cetindag B, Wohltmann CD, McAndrew M. Is portable ultrasonography accurate in the evaluation of Schanz pin placement during extremity fracture fixation in austere environments? Am J Disaster Med. 2013;8(2):91–6. https://doi.org/10.5055/ajdm.2013.0115.
26. Talbot M, Harbey EJ, Reindl R, Martineau P, Schneider P. Ultrasound-assisted external fixation: a technique for austere environments. J R Army Med Corps. 2016;162(6):456–9. https://doi.org/10.1136/jramc-2015-000550.

Part IV

Introduction to Monitoring

Monitoring studies are used serially to track changes in patient conditions beyond what typical vital sign parameters indicate. These studies may be used intermittently during patient transport, such as at rest stops when patients are being carried over long distances or to monitor the response to interventions.

Ultrasound Guidance of Resuscitation in Shock

Konrad Karasek and Megan Leo

Introduction

Shock is an abnormal physiologic state of the circulatory system that results in inadequate organ perfusion and tissue oxygenation, leading to the dysfunction of one or multiple organ systems. There are several types of shock. Most critically ill and injured patients in shock have some element of hypovolemia but must be evaluated for other causes, such as cardiogenic, obstructive, neurogenic, and septic shock (a form of distributive shock). In injured trauma patients, hemorrhage is still the second most common cause of death, representing 30–40% of trauma mortality [1].

When initially evaluating a patient in shock while in a resource-limited environment, it is important to consider the volume status of the patient. Many patients have had prolonged exposure to extreme environments and are dehydrated from inadequate oral intake. Physical examination has been shown to be unreliable in estimating the volume status and fluid responsiveness of patients. Studies have shown that inconsistent sensitivities and specificities of various physical exam findings and maneuvers do not allow for the definitive assessment of a patient's volume status [2, 3]. This has also been found to be true in studies specifically evaluating shock in trauma patients [4].

This challenging assessment is particularly important in the pre-hospital setting, where the initial appraisal of the patient will take place and the demands of the care are recognized. The overall goal of pre-hospital triage and transport is to match appropriate available medical resources and interventions with the needs of a critically ill patient. It is important to avoid under-triage, which mis-categorizes patients that would benefit from more aggressive trauma and/or medical care and transport [5]. Differentiating the causes of shock and determining which patients will be fluid tolerant or fluid responsive can be challenging. Please reference chapter "Advanced

K. Karasek (✉) · M. Leo
Department of Emergency Medicine, Boston Medical Center, Boston, MA, USA
e-mail: kkarasek@bu.edu; megan.leo@bmc.org

B. D. Nicholson et al. (eds.), *Manual of Austere and Prehospital Ultrasound*,
https://doi.org/10.1007/978-3-030-64287-7_15

Diagnostic Topic for Austere Providers: Skeletal Trauma": *Undifferentiated Shock* on point-of-care ultrasound (POCUS) in shock for a more comprehensive explanation of this evaluation. POCUS can make a large impact on delivering appropriate care to these patients while guiding resuscitation efforts and aiding the provider in efficient resource utilization and management.

Discussion

When evaluating a critically ill patient with hemodynamic instability, it is crucial to identify potential time-sensitive interventions. Prolonged hypotension and shock have serious implications. These patients are often ill and have a high mortality. For example, one study found an 18% in-hospital mortality rate in patients with symptomatic hypotension [6]. In another study, the identification of hypotension (<100 mmHg) in the pre-hospital setting conferred a highly specific increased mortality rate of 32%, versus 11% in the non-hypotensive cohort [7].

Aside from the Focused Assessment with Sonography in Trauma (FAST), current care models like Advanced Trauma Life Support (ATLS) and Advanced Cardiac Life Support (ACLS) have not formally incorporated aspects of point-of-care ultrasound (POCUS) to more comprehensively assess the volume status and guide resuscitation, but rather recommend only a broad and generalized approach. POCUS could impact outcomes in these patients by guiding intravenous fluid (IVF) resuscitation and provide the information pre-hospital providers need to transition to vasoactive pressor medications. For example, the ninth edition of ATLS recommends universal warmed isotonic electrolyte solutions, such as lactated Ringer's or normal saline, for initial IVF resuscitation. The fluid is thought to provide transient intravascular expansion and replaces the fluid losses that occur into the interstitial space [8]. The recommended initial volume of administration is 1–2 L for adults and 20 mL/kg for children. Generally, providers must assess the response to IVF resuscitation by evaluating different clinical features such as vital signs, urinary output, level of consciousness, capillary refill, and skin perfusion. The total volumes administered should be based on clinical presentation and the patient's response to the initial intervention, with the goal of restoring end-organ perfusion. However, as mentioned previously, clinical findings are often unreliable and imprecise in assessing these end points. This method of *uninformed* resuscitation can cause complications, both from under- or over-resuscitation. For example, excessive IVF administration can exacerbate the coagulopathy, acidosis, and hypothermia (the so-called *Triad of Death*) that are often associated with increased mortality in critically ill trauma patients [1]. Fluid administration may also contribute to pulmonary edema in patients with acute respiratory distress syndrome (ARDS), whose alveolar-capillary permeability is increased [9]. Additionally, both medical and trauma patients have been shown to have unintended complications secondary to over-aggressive resuscitation including, but not limited to, increased morbidity, prolonged ICU and hospital length of stay, respiratory compromise, and increased mortality [8, 10]. Therefore, optimizing pre-hospital and in-hospital resuscitation by assessing the volume status and/or volume responsiveness of these patients is of utmost importance. This is where POCUS can have a positive impact in patient care by implementing an *ultrasound-informed* resuscitation early in the initial pre-hospital encounter and providing the most benefit when care includes prolonged transport times to definitive treatment.

POCUS in the hands of a knowledgeable provider can offer a safe, rapid, and non-invasive investigative technique that can help resolve diagnostic dilemmas and potentially guide time-sensitive interventions [11, 12]. It is commonplace for Emergency Physicians (EPs) to utilize POCUS to evaluate critically ill patients. Furthermore, the same techniques have proven to be teachable to non-EPs [13–15]. Multiple studies have shown that the limited transthoracic echocardiogram provides a teachable and immediately accessible tool for volume status evaluation in critically ill patients for trauma providers and can be performed by non-EP providers as well [13–15]. POCUS offers several advantages over traditional techniques of assessing shock, volume status, hypotension, and fluid responsiveness. It can be performed in real-time, is dynamic, reproducible, teachable, and non-invasive. It utilizes more objective data and measurements to help determine the underlying cardiac function/dysfunction, intravascular volume status, pulmonary compromise, and can evaluate the response to time-sensitive medications, interventions, and resuscitation. This approach has been evaluated for both medical and trauma patients [16, 17]. Many protocols consisting of *goal-directed* ultrasonographic evaluations for the diagnosis of shock that integrate cardiac, abdominal, pulmonary, and vascular examinations have already been proposed and validated [11, 12, 18]. Additionally, chapter "Advanced Diagnostic Topic for Austere Providers: Skeletal Trauma": *Undifferentiated Shock*, discusses these protocols in more detail.

The idea of pre-hospital POCUS is not new and a meta-analysis from 2005 found approximately 1000 references for its feasibility and use [19]. In the early-to-mid 2000s, POCUS was introduced into the pre-hospital arena on multiple continents, including Europe, Australia, and North America. Despite this, a recent survey of EMS medical directors in the United States and Canada found that pre-hospital POCUS was used in only 4.1% of services, but that an additional 21% of services were considering implementation [20].

Unlike the FAST exam, there is less uniformity and consensus about the best practices of POCUS use to guide the resuscitation of shock in the pre-hospital setting. In this chapter, we will briefly review the fundamentals of assessing volume status to guide IVF resuscitation, and explore the integration of limited cardiac, vascular, and thoracic ultrasound into the management of critically ill patients. This will help providers deliver *ultrasound-informed resuscitation* instead of guiding therapy with unreliable parameters and avoid subjecting sick patients to a trial-and-error treatment model.

Brief Review of POCUS Protocols Used to Determine the Etiology of Shock

It is important to identify shock early, as studies have shown a mortality increase associated with prolonged hypotension. One study found that symptomatic patients with a systolic blood pressure <100 mm Hg measured during ambulance transport, or in the pre-hospital setting, had an in-hospital mortality rate of 25% [7].

Studies looking at immediate versus delayed POCUS to identify the cause of nontraumatic hypotension demonstrated that *a goal-directed ultrasound protocol* can positively affect the differential diagnosis for an undifferentiated, but life-threatening, condition. Access to this information allowed providers to shorten their differential diagnosis rank-list by 50% and diagnose with 30% more accuracy [11].

The first ultrasound-directed protocol for shock management was published in 2001 as the *Undifferentiated Hypotension Protocol* (UHP) [12]. While the ***R**apid **U**ltrasound in **SH**ock* (RUSH) protocol is among the most well-known, there are at least 15 other published protocols for the evaluation of hypotension and shock [12, 21–27]. Certain protocols have been promoted as helpful for providers with limited or minimal experience in integrating POCUS into their shock management. For example, the *Echo-Guided Life Support* (EGLS) protocol is structured to answer a series of five *"yes/no"* questions, in a binary fashion, to identify one type of shock at a time [28]. This can help *cognitively off-load* pre-hospital providers and simplify their approach to POCUS.

The RUSH protocol breaks down the evaluation into three distinct areas: *Pump* (Cardiac), *Tank* (IVC, Abdomen, Thorax), and *Pipes* (Vascular) [22]. *Weingart et al* also developed a mnemonic to help providers work through the protocol in a systematic way: **HI-MAP** - **H**eart, **I**VC, **M**orison's (FAST with thoracic views), **A**orta, **P**neumothorax [29]. This approach is discussed in further detail in chapter "Advanced Diagnostic Topic for Austere Providers: Skeletal Trauma": *Undifferentiated Shock.* However, some of steps in evaluating a patient with undifferentiated shock are also integral to determining a patient's fluid tolerance or fluid responsiveness.

POCUS for *Ultrasound-Informed Resuscitation*

There are three components to an *ultrasound-informed* resuscitation. These include a limited cardiac ultrasound, IVC assessment, and a limited thoracic/pulmonary assessment. By focusing on these three components, the pre-hospital provider can determine if the patient will be fluid tolerant and a candidate for initial resuscitation with IVF or if they have features of suspected fluid intolerance. The later requires more careful thought in administering IVF for initial resuscitation and will identify patients that will likely benefit from earlier adjunctive therapies such as vasoactive medications.

Limited Cardiac Ultrasound Assessment and Management

The heart should be the focal point of the POCUS assessment in shock, as many cardiac findings can affect the plan for resuscitation of the patient. Assessment of the general contractility (left ventricular systolic function/dysfunction/dilation), right heart dysfunction/dilation, pericardial effusions, cardiac tamponade, or standstill can dramatically change the course of management. Studies have shown that pre-hospital and EMS providers can reliably integrate POCUS into their cardiac assessments of critically ill patients and out-of-hospital cardiac arrests [30, 31].

Cardiac function can be distilled to the assessment of global left ventricular ejection fraction (LVEF) and is integral in gleaning an overall impression of the patient's cardiac output (CO). CO is defined as the volume of blood pumped by the heart per minute. CO can be determined by multiplying the heart rate (HR) and the stroke volume (SV). The resulting equation is $\boldsymbol{CO = HR \times SV}$. The SV, which is the volume of blood pumped with each cardiac contraction/cycle, can be modified by multiple variables including preload, myocardial contractility/systolic function, and afterload. Changes in any of these variables will accordingly modify the SV, and thus the CO.

The use of POCUS for cardiac assessment during resuscitative efforts can be simplified to include a subjective global assessment of LVEF (which can be applied to the overall impression of the CO). LVEF can be designated as *normal*, *depressed*, or *severely depressed*. This classification as performed by EPs has been shown to be equivalent to a formal cardiology measurement of LVEF [6].

The cardiac status should be evaluated using a low frequency probe, preferably a phased-array probe, but a curvilinear probe can be used depending on availability. The four standard echocardiography views of the heart include the parasternal long (PSL) view, parasternal short (PSS) view, apical four chamber (A4C) view, and the subxiphoid (SX) view. This should always be followed by imaging the inferior vena cava (IVC) to determine right sided heart pressures, often assumed to be an estimate of overall intravascular volume status for the patient. An existing protocol has been coined the *5-Es of Emergency Echo*, evaluating *Effusion* (pericardial effusion), *Ejection* (global LVEF), *Equality* (right heart strain assessment), *Exit* (thoracic aortic aneurysm assessment), and *Entrance* (IVC assessment) [32]. These 5 views will help the provider determine the best approach to IVF resuscitation in shock or alternative interventions.

Pericardial Effusion Assessment and Management

Studies have shown that cardiac tamponade can be easily and reliably identified by pre-hospital and EMS providers [30]. When performing a cardiac POCUS in a patient with shock, an evaluation for the presence or absence of a pericardial effusion (PCE) and cardiac tamponade should be included [33, 34]. The views that can be helpful in diagnosing a PCE are the subxiphoid (SX) view and the parasternal long (PSL) axis view. The SX view can be obtained just inferior to the xyphoid process, aiming up into the thoracic cavity towards the heart and left shoulder (Fig. 1).

The effusion, if present, is visible as an anechoic (black) strip of fluid partially or circumferentially surrounding the myocardium, between the heart and the stiff, echogenic pericardium. The size of the pericardial effusion can be classified by locating the largest pocket of fluid during end-diastole and measuring orthogonally to the surface of the heart. These can be graded as small (<1 cm), medium (1–2 cm), or large (>2 cm) [35]. Alternatively, the PSL view is obtained at approximately the fourth or fifth intercostal space adjacent to the patient's left lower sternal border. The effusion tends to accumulate dependently, or in the far field of the image, but can also be loculated or circumferential (Fig. 2).

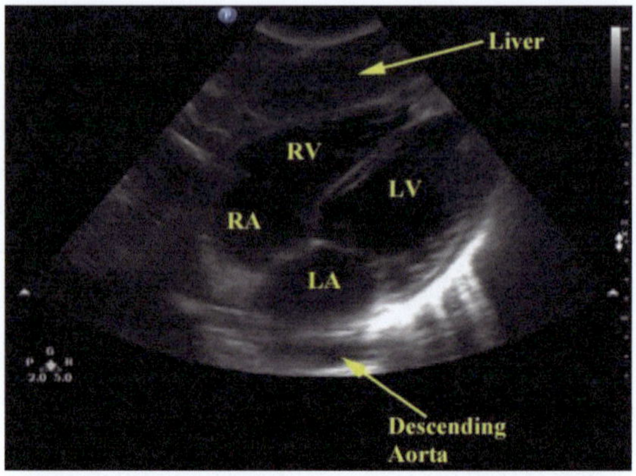

Fig. 1 Subxiphoid Cardiac View. Liver in the upper portion of the image. RV right ventricle, RA right atrium, LV left ventricle, LA left atrium

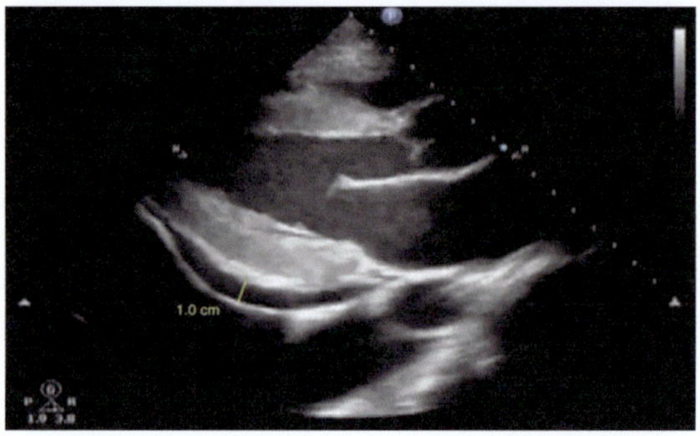

Fig. 2 Parasternal Long Axis Cardiac View demonstrating a 1.0 cm effusion posterior to the Left Ventricle

Additional characteristics to describe PCEs include circumferential (typically in moderate to large PCE), loculated, complex/echogenic, simple/anechoic, and presence of tamponade physiology. A change in the amount of fluid, whether acute or acute-on-chronic can negatively impact cardiac function by inhibiting preload, decreasing SV and CO, and therefore, end-organ perfusion.

The size of the effusion is not always the important feature, but rather attention should be paid to its hemodynamic implications. For example, large chronic effusions may be less hemodynamically significant than new, rapidly accumulating, small effusions, which may quickly lead to cardiovascular collapse. This is thought to be due to the thick, fibrous pericardial sac not having time to stretch and accommodate the increase in fluid, causing compression of the heart [34, 36, 37]. Once intra-*pericardial* pressure exceeds the intra-*cardiac* pressure, the patient will develop tamponade physiology. This process is a spectrum and it first develops on the low pressure side of the heart, specifically the right atrium and right ventricle. In general, paradoxical movement of heart chambers is concerning for altered physiology. For example, right atrial collapse during systole is the earliest sign of tamponade (most *sensitive* finding). Similarly, collapse of the right ventricle in diastole is less sensitive, but more *specific* for cardiac tamponade, and a marker of impending hemodynamic collapse (Fig. 3). Furthermore, the increased pericardial pressures will increase right sided circulatory pressure causing distention of the IVC [34, 36].

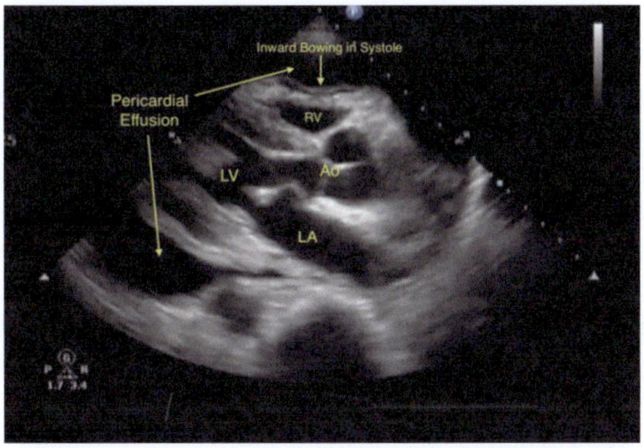

Fig. 3 Parasternal Long Axis Cardiac View demonstrating a pericardial effusion with signs of cardiac tamponade – namely, inward bowing of the Right Ventricle in Systole. The pericardial effusion tracks anterior to the descending thoracic aorta posteriorly, helping to differentiate it from a pleural effusion (which tracks posterior to the descending thoracic aorta). RV right ventricle, LV left ventricle, LA left atrium, Ao aorta

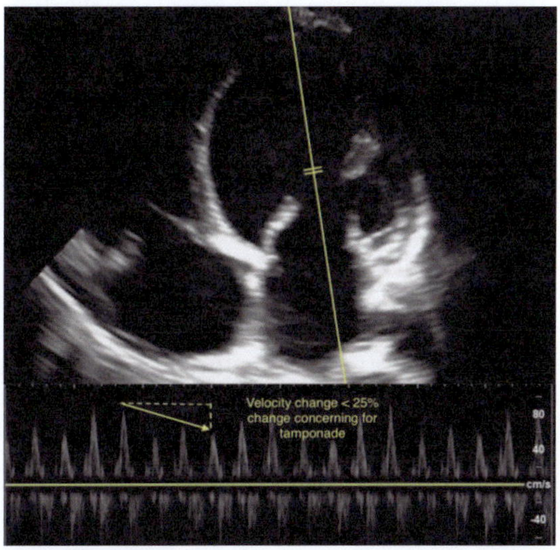

Fig. 4 Apical 4 Chamber Cardiac View with pulsed wave doppler gate positioned above the mitral valve measuring the respiratory change in flow velocities across the valve. A velocity change of less than 25%, as in this case, is concerning for tamponade physiology.

Another technique to assess for echocardiographic signs of tamponade is to measure the respiratory variation of the peak *E*-wave inflow velocities over the mitral or tricuspid valves using pulsed wave doppler. In the A4C view, the doppler gate can be placed just within the valvular inflow, at the tips of the valves. A respiratory change of less than 25% in the measured velocities across the mitral valve between inspiration and expiration, or less than a 40% change in the measured velocities across the tricuspid valve are suggestive of tamponade physiology (Fig. 4) [38]. Identification of this pathology can prompt immediate intervention in the pre-hospital setting with emergent pericardiocentesis and more aggressive IVF resuscitation to improve preload. The diagnosis of a PCE with hemodynamic changes can also help appropriately triage patients for a rapid transport to an adequately-resourced medical center [39, 40].

Left Ventricular Ejection Function (LVEF) Assessment and Management
This portion of the examination focuses on evaluating motion of the left ventricular endocardial walls, as judged by a visual calculation of the percentage volume change from diastole to systole [41]. Utilizing the PSL and PSS views can help assess the function of the left ventricle, which is directly related to the cardiac output and relevant for resuscitation assessment in shock. Studies have been conducted to evaluate the ability of non-cardiologists to perform accurate assessments of LVEF, and showed that EPs are able to evaluate LVEF with good accuracy and reliability [6, 42]. Various grades of LVEF are distinguished as follows: a *normal* LVEF of approximately 50%, a *moderately depressed* LVEF of 30–50%, and *severely depressed* LVEF of <30% [43]. At the time of publication, there were no studies looking specifically at whether pre-hospital and EMS providers would be able to reliably determine LVEF. However, one can suspect that if these providers received dedicated training, they would also be able to perform similar assessments, as has been shown to be the case in other POCUS applications [30, 31].

This exam is performed by placing the probe in the fourth or fifth intercostal space on the anterior chest adjacent to the left lower sternal border of the patient, with the probe marker to the patient's right shoulder. The PSL view will provide a long axis view of the left ventricle (LV) (Fig. 5).

To obtain the PSS view, simply rotate the head of the probe 90° clockwise, to visualize the smaller, thin-walled, right ventricle (RV), sitting on top of the larger, thicker-walled LV. This view should be obtained at approximately the level of the mid-ventricle, which is identified by the papillary muscles (the prominences in the endocardium noted in Fig. 6). In the parasternal short-axis view, a < 30% change between the size of the LV in systole and diastole indicates a severely decreased LVEF (*(end diastolic size - end systolic size)/end diastolic size)* [6].

Motion of the anterior leaflet of the mitral valve can also be used to assess contractility in the PSL view (Fig. 7). This is defined as the *end-point septal separation* (EPSS). In a normal contractile state, the anterior leaflet will vigorously approximate and sometimes touch the wall of the septum during ventricular filling when examined using the PSL view [37]. A cutoff of 6 mm or less between the mitral

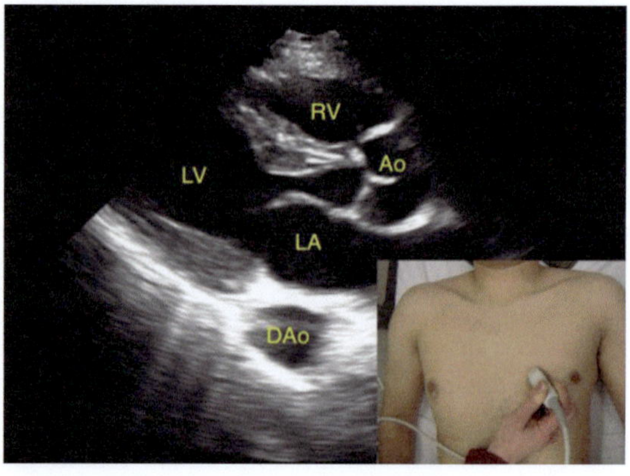

Fig. 5 Parasternal Long Axis Cardiac View as demonstrated here is helpful in estimating a patient's ejection fraction. Probe position, with marker towards the right shoulder is shown in insert. RV right ventricle, LV left ventricle, LA left atrium, DAo descending thoracic aorta

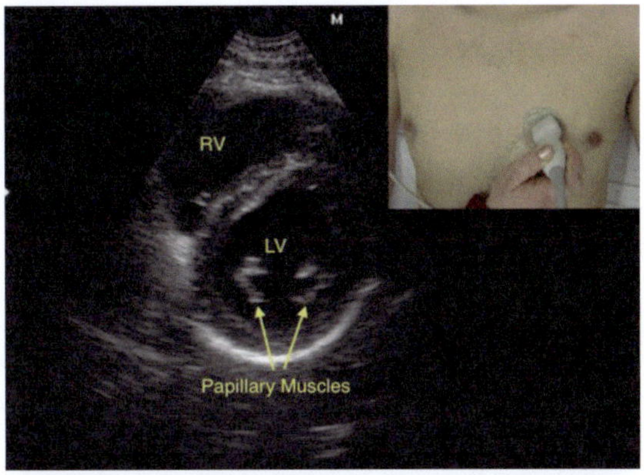

Fig. 6 Parasternal Short Axis Cardiac View as demonstrated here is helpful for determining a patient's ejection fraction and RV:LV ratio. Probe position, with marker towards the left shoulder (90° from PSL View) is shown in insert. LV left ventricle, RV right ventricle

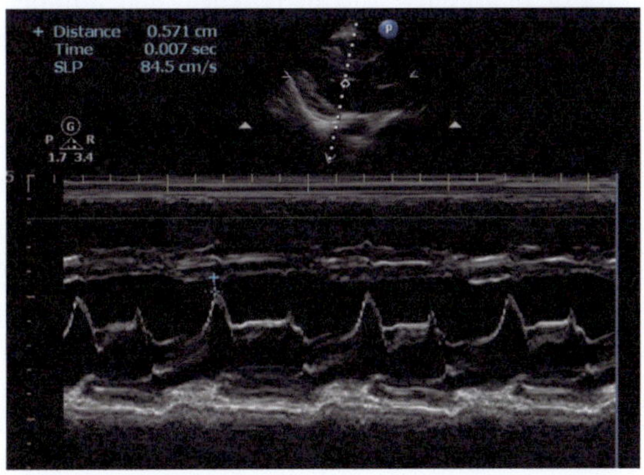

Fig. 7 Parasternal Long Axis Cardiac View demonstrating the End Point Septal Separation (EPSS), with the measurement of the distance between the anterior mitral valve leaflet and the interventricular septum

valve and the septum suggests a normal LVEF. If there is reduced or little movement of the anterior leaflet (>7 mm), one can suspect decreased LVEF. This method of measuring EPSS has been shown to be achievable in novice POCUS users [44].

Cardiac contractility is important to consider when assessing for fluid tolerance and responsiveness. Patients with noted poor contractility will likely not benefit from additional fluid boluses. A patient with moderate or severely depressed LVEF should prompt the provider to use caution in administering aggressive volumes of IVF given the heart's inability to adjust to rapid increases in preload. Rather, these patients may benefit from inotropes or other vasoactive agents, which may or may not be within the scope of practice of pre-hospital providers, and should be guided by local guidelines and regional practice. This information should be combined with other ultrasonographic data including IVC size and respirophasic variation, as well as intrathoracic lung evaluation (both to be discussed later).

Increased contractility, on the other hand, to the point where the walls of the LV are nearly touching, would indicate a *hyperdynamic* heart. This is defined as an LVEF >75% and is described as a complete or near complete obliteration of the LV cavity during systole. This condition is commonly found in cases of sepsis and hypovolemia (most common), as well as other medical conditions like drug ingestions, high-output heart failure, anemia, thyroid disease, among others [37]. These patients generally need aggressive IVF resuscitation [45]. The provider should be careful to assess the true contractility of the heart, as tachycardia itself can often be mistaken as a *hyperdynamic* heart. In other words, hyperdynamic hearts are generally tachycardic, but tachycardic hearts are *not* always hyperdynamic.

Right Heart Strain and Management

The right heart is a thin-walled structure that is extremely sensitive to changes in volume status and intravascular pressure. Thus, the right heart can also give the provider information regarding a patient's volume status, or potential volume responsiveness. Images of the right heart are best obtained in the A4C view or the PSS view. The A4C view is obtained by placing a phased-array probe (or similar low frequency probe) near the apex of heart, generally adjacent to the left nipple in males, or in the inferior mammary fold in females, and aiming the ultrasound beam towards the patient's midline, right shoulder, or base of the heart (Fig. 8). This view attempts to visualize all four chambers of the heart simultaneously. Alternatively, the PSS view can be obtained as previously described above. Visualizing a *D*-shaped septum (*D-sign*) is an indicator of right heart strain on the PSS view (Fig. 9).

In a normal heart, the LV is larger than the RV. The LV:RV ratio is generally cited as approximately 1:0.6 [37, 46, 47]. Because the right ventricle has thinner myocardium, it is more susceptible to pressure and volume changes, especially in the acute setting. RV dilation in the A4C view can indicate an increase of pressure in the pulmonary circulation/vasculature or right ventricular failure as one of the contributors to the patient's shock state. Shock and hypotension occur because RV failure decreases the preload to the LV, and as a result, decreases the SV and CO. RV failure has many causes, but in the acute setting the most likely diagnoses are massive pulmonary embolism and/or right ventricular infarction [25, 37, 46]. This finding should prompt the provider to initiate more aggressive IVF resuscitation during transport to temporize the preload mismatch and maintain adequate CO.

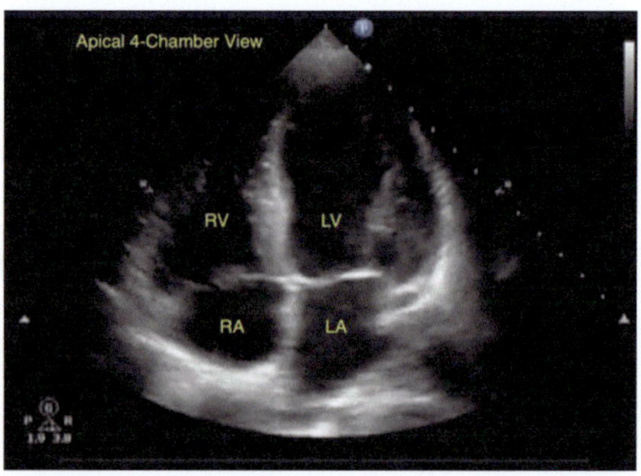

Fig. 8 Apical 4 Chamber Cardiac View demonstrating all four chambers of the heart including their respective atrio-ventricular valves. RV right ventricle, RA right atrium, LV left ventricle, LA left atrium

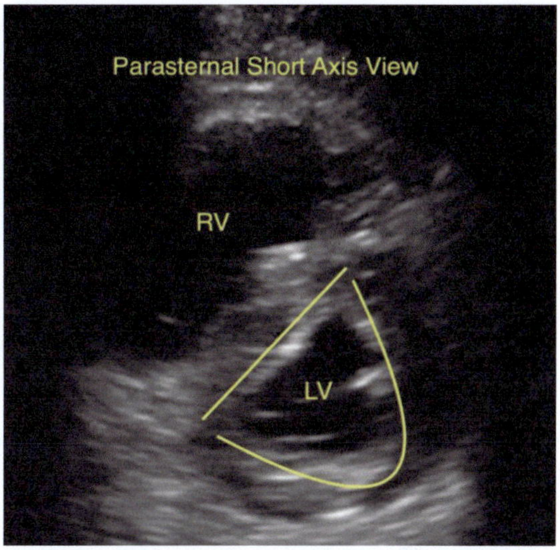

Fig. 9 Parasternal Short Axis Cardiac View demonstrating the "D-Sign" which can be a marker of increased right sided circulatory pressure and/or interventricular dependence. This view is also helpful to compare the LV:RV ratio. RV right ventricle, LV left ventricle

Inferior Vena Cava (IVC) Assessment and Management

After examining the heart, the evaluation of the IVC should always be included prior to forming a plan for initial resuscitation. IVC indices in isolation should never be used to determine intravascular fluid status. It is best to do an assessment of the heart, IVC, and lungs concurrently to gain a sense of the overall cardiopulmonary status of the patient. Cardiac Output (CO) is the product of the Heart Rate (HR) and Stroke Volume (SV), yielding the following equation: $\boldsymbol{CO = HR \times SV}$. In the pre-hospital setting, the most easily modifiable variable of CO is the SV. *Preload*, the volume of blood returning through the venous system to the heart, is determined by the patient's volume status, the capacitance of the venous system, and the difference between the mean venous systemic pressure and right atrial pressure. Many studies have attempted to evaluate the use of POCUS to determine the relationship between inferior vena cava indices as a correlate to right sided pressures, central venous pressure (CVP), hydration status, and for intravenous fluid resuscitation guidance [9, 48–52].

The IVC runs along the vertebral column and can be imaged utilizing a low frequency probe, such as the curvilinear or phased-array probes [37, 53]. The probe should be placed in the patient's subxiphoid region and to the right of midline, in a cranio-caudal orientation. This way, one can assess the IVC in the longitudinal/sagittal view. The IVC can be seen passing through the liver, proceeding cephalad past the confluence of the hepatic veins, until it reaches the right atrium (Fig. 10). Careful attention should be paid to ensure that the tubular structure being visualized is in fact the IVC and not the aorta, which runs in parallel, adjacent, and medial to the IVC. This can be confirmed by visualizing the IVC emptying directly into the right atrium, or alternatively utilizing pulse waved doppler and/or color doppler to differentiate between monophasic venous flow or pulsatile arterial flow [54]. Visualized pulsations on plain 2D imaging are not sufficiently reliable to differentiate between

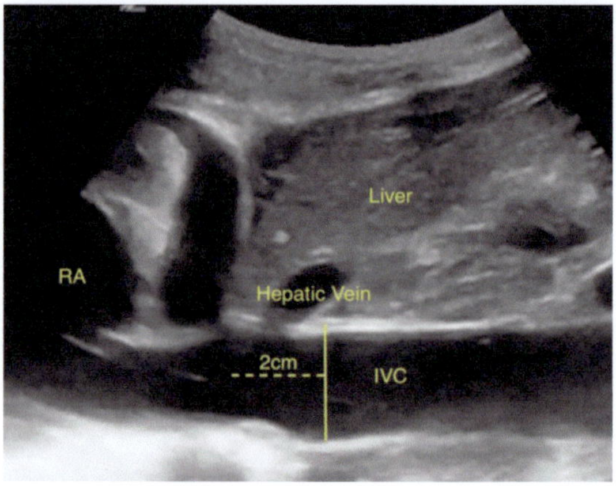

Fig. 10 Parasagittal subcostal view demonstrating a plethoric and enlarged IVC and its entry into the RA. Measurement of the IVC diameter should take place approximately 2 cm caudal from the diaphragm as noted in the image. IVC inferior vena cava, RA right atrium

the IVC and the aorta, as pulsations can be transmitted between the two. In this view, one should measure the IVC diameter at approximately 2 cm distal to the right atrium and diaphragm (Fig. 10) [55]. Additionally, it is important not to mistake lateral translation of the IVC during the respiratory cycle as collapse.

The walls of the IVC can be measured in *static* and *dynamic* views to determine the size and compliance of the vessel with respirations, which can be a surrogate for right sided circulatory pressures, or central venous pressure (CVP). Historically, many studies have attempted to evaluate the use of POCUS to determine the relation between IVC indices and right sided circulatory pressures, (CVP), hydration status, and for IVF resuscitation guidance [9, 48–52]. Most of the studies evaluating the IVC and caval indices as a proxy for CVP were performed in patients who were on ventilators, which is different than the spontaneously breathing patients that most pre-hospital providers will encounter. However, more general and subjective assessments of IVC size and compliance can be useful in this patient population and can guide resuscitation in shock. Subjective assessments of the IVC and global cardiac function have been shown to be reliable compared to formal measurements [56]. This approach is undoubtedly more practical in the pre-hospital setting and for more novice users of POCUS. In a spontaneously breathing patient, the negative pressure that is generated between the pleura and airways during inspiration, secondary to the downward movement of the diaphragm, increases the venous return to the right side of the heart. This generally causes a decrease in the diameter of the IVC with inspiration [48, 54]. Conversely, the normalization of intrathoracic pressure during exhalation generally causes the IVC to return to its normal diameter or dilate. This can be used to determine the minimum and maximum diameters of the IVC (known as *respirophasic variation*) over the course of the respiratory cycle [57]. IVC diameters at end-expiration and the degree of inspiratory change, sometimes referred to as *IVC collapsibility index* (IVCCI), have been shown correlate well with CVP. Although this measurement can be performed in a single recorded image using M-mode (motion mode), we do *not* encourage this method as lateral translation or displacement of the IVC itself relative to the probe can be mistaken for collapsibility [54, 58]. It is also important to realize that if the patient is intubated (or on any form of non-invasive positive pressure ventilations like BPAP/CPAP) in the pre-hospital setting, the IVC dynamics will be the *opposite* of a spontaneously breathing patient. Positive pressure (breath delivered/inhalation), will increase the intrathoracic pressure, decreasing the amount of venous return, distending the IVC. This effectively reverses the wave form seen on M-mode.

Low IVC diameters (<1.5 cm) with high respiratory variation (high IVCCI, >50%) are generally associated with low CVP states [51, 59]. These patients are generally fluid tolerant/fluid responsive, and would be better candidates for initial IVF resuscitation. Conversely, patients with distended IVCs, generally greater than 2.0–2.5 cm and/or with little to no respirophasic variation (low IVCCI, <50%), are likely to have an elevated CVP (Fig. 11) [60]. These patients are likely to be fluid intolerant and would benefit from interventions that would improve their forward-flow cardiac mechanics, like positive inotropy and afterload reduction [51, 60, 61].

There is some evidence-based research to support the use of IVC ultrasound to guide IVF resuscitation. One study found that a 12% increase in inferior vena cava diameter during lung inflation allowed discrimination between responders and non-responders to volume loading, with a positive predictive value of 93% and a negative predictive value of 92% [62]. Another study demonstrated that in mechanically ventilated patients, an IVC that distends >18% in diameter during respirations is likely to respond to a fluid challenge [63]. Correspondingly, in hypotensive emergency room patients, volume resuscitation was associated with increases in the IVC diameter and less inspiratory collapsibility [56]. Additionally, another study showed that inadequate dilation of the IVC after a fluid challenge was more sensitive than blood pressure for identification of hypovolemia in trauma patients [64]. Serial IVC exams after each IVF bolus, along with a repeated cardiac and lung ultrasound may be a good approach to assess the effectiveness of the treatment and to ensure the patient does not develop signs of over-resuscitation.

However, this issue is far from one-sided as there is conflicting evidence regarding the utility of evaluating the IVC in isolation as it relates to the CVP and fluid responsiveness. One prominent systematic review from 2008 demonstrated a very poor relationship between CVP and blood volume, as well as the inability to predict response to a fluid challenge [65]. The same group published an updated meta-analysis in 2013 with similar results and encouraged providers to discontinue the practice of using CVP to guide fluid resuscitation [66]. Therefore, given the lack of correlation of IVC indices with CVP, one could argue that there is limited utility in using these values to assess for volume status and fluid responsiveness. Another study of undifferentiated ED patients showed that the IVCCI did not predict fluid responsiveness [67]. Moreover, in patients with acute circulatory failure, another study showed that respiratory variation of the IVC is not a reliable predictor of fluid responsiveness [68].

This supports the argument that evaluation of the IVC should not be used in isolation to guide fluid resuscitation. But rather, it should be combined with the additional components of cardiac and lung POCUS to help evaluate whether the transmitted right atrial pressures/CVP are secondary to issues in the right heart, pulmonary vasculature, left side of the heart, or intravascular volume loss/overload.

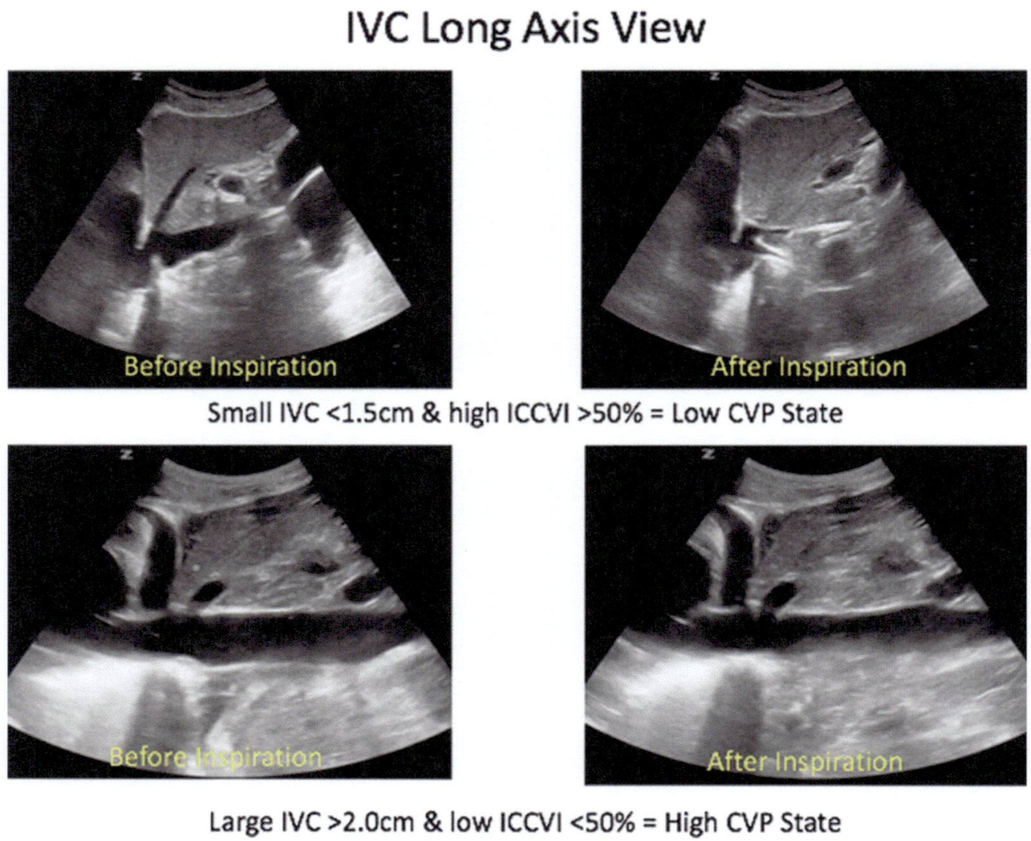

Fig. 11 Top; Parasagittal subcostal view demonstrating small IVC and increased respirophasic variation (before and after inspiration). Bottom; Parasagittal subcostal view demonstrating a large IVC and decreased respirophasic variation (before and after inspiration). IVC inferior vena cava

Additionally, rather than relying on a single measurement of the IVC, it is better to follow changes in size and respiratory dynamics over time with fluid resuscitation.

Lung Assessment and Management

For the complete evaluation of a patient's volume status and to help determine fluid tolerance/responsiveness, the provider must also evaluate the lungs and thorax. POCUS integrated with a clinical exam has been shown to be more accurate for the diagnosis of acute decompensated heart failure than an exam with chest radiography [69]. This means that with POCUS, the pre-hospital provider has the tools to diagnose pulmonary edema and heart failure just as well as an in-hospital provider. This information is important for guiding the use of IVF for initial resuscitation or to move forward with other therapies.

Each hemithorax is divided into four distinct areas, for a combined eight zones on the antero-lateral chest (Fig. 12). The lung assessment should be performed using a low frequency probe, either curvilinear or phased array, in a systematic and comprehensive manner, when time and resources permit. With the patient supine or in a 45-degree semi-recumbent position, each hemithorax should be imaged in a longitudinal/sagittal orientation, with the probe marker toward the patient's head. Landmarks including the pleural line and lung field between the rib spaces should be identified while manipulating the angle of insonation in a fanning motion to optimize the clarity of the pleural line (Fig. 13).

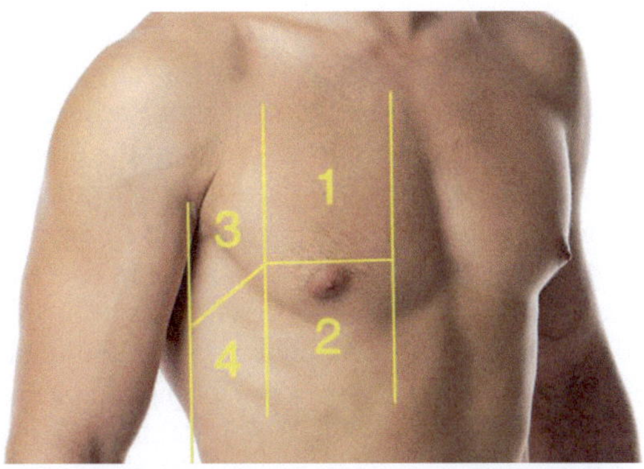

Fig. 12 Diagram depicting the four thoracic fields required in an ultrasonographic lung assessment. This should be performed on both hemi-thoraces

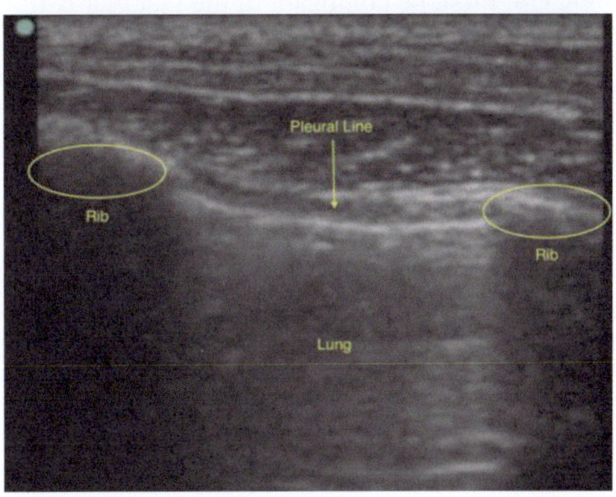

Fig. 13 Linear ultrasound image showing the pleural interface between thoracic ribs as indicated

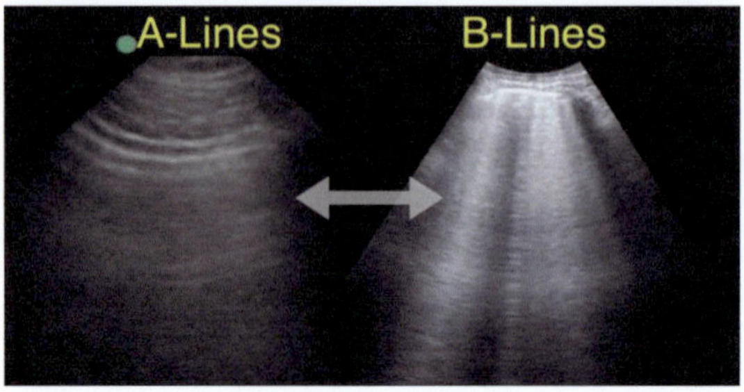

Fig. 14 Thoracic ultrasound demonstrating the appearance of A-lines (echogenic horizontal reverberations) and B-lines (hyperechoic, discrete, vertical beams of artifact that generally obliterate A-lines, extend to the bottom of the screen, and move in synchrony with the lung itself)

In normally aerated lung, linear echogenic horizontal reverberations, which are generated by the pleural line itself can be seen extending deep into the lung field repeating at regular intervals. These normal reverberation artifacts are called *A-lines* [23, 24, 37] (Fig. 14). *B-lines* are hyperechoic, discrete, vertical beams of artifact that generally obliterate A-lines, extend to the bottom of the screen, and move in synchrony with the lung itself. B-lines represent increased density in the lung parenchyma and in the right clinical context can be diagnostic of pulmonary edema. Looking in each of the eight scanning regions, a section is designated as *positive* if it has three or more B-lines per lung field at any one point in a respiratory cycle. The presence of two or more *positive* regions, on bilateral hemi-thoraces, is consistent with *diffuse interstitial syndrome (DIS)* [23, 24]. A strictly *quantitative* approach to measuring B-lines also exists, where the exact number of B-lines are counted and correlate with a scoring system of severity [70, 71]. This method is more precise and can be followed over time for more accurate dynamic assessments of interstitial fluid, but is less likely to be useful in the discrete pre-hospital encounter.

DIS is most often due to cardiogenic pulmonary edema, in the setting of volume overload or cardiac dysfunction. However, it is important to note that this is not always the case. Bilateral B-lines and DIS can also be present in acute respiratory distress syndrome (ARDS), pulmonary fibrosis, diffuse parenchymal lung disease, or interstitial/multifocal pneumonia. Additionally, the presence of focal or unilateral B-lines can indicate any of the following: pneumonia, atelectasis, pulmonary contusion, masses, among others [23, 72].

It is also important to keep in mind certain pitfalls when performing lung POCUS. First, be cognizant of the fact that B-lines can soemtimes blur together and coalesce, making it difficult to assess for the *number* of B-lines. However, this is generally associated with significantly increased lung density and severity of edema. Second, *Z-lines* can often appear similar to B-lines. Z-lines are short, vertical, ill-defined artifacts that also arise from the pleural line. They are sometimes referred to *comet tails* and can be mistaken as B-lines. Unlike B-lines, they only extend a few centimeters from the pleural line and are less echogenic and do not obliterate A-lines [23] (Fig. 15). They are normal findings and do not indicate DIS.

POCUS can be very helpful in guiding management by differentiating patients who are not fluid tolerant or responsive as a result of acute decompensated heart

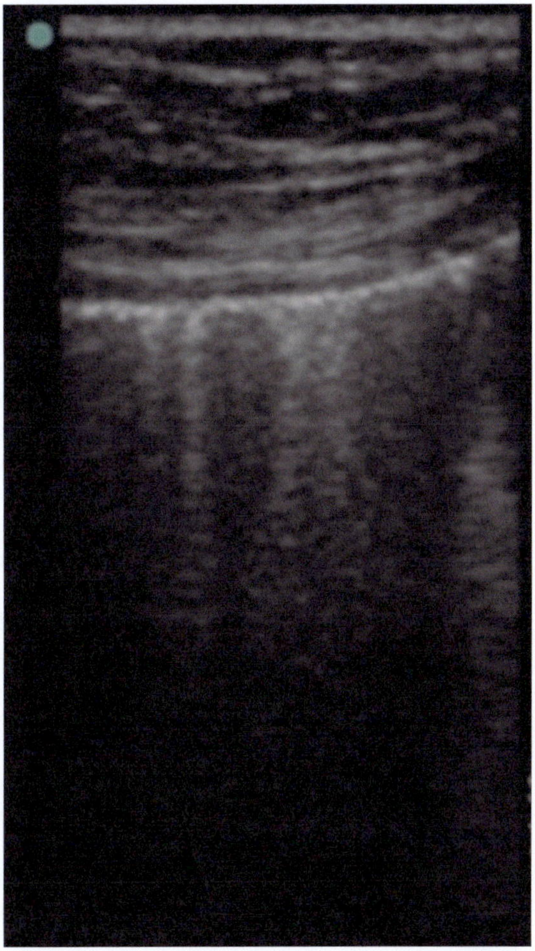

Fig. 15 Superficial Linear ultrasound image demonstrating Z-lines (short, vertical, ill-defined artifacts that also arise from the pleural line). They are sometimes referred to *comet tails* and can be mistaken as B-lines

failure (ADHF). The diagnosis of ADHF can be challenging as traditional diagnostic modalities such as physical exam, plain radiographs, and laboratory testing have variable and limited or mixed utility for the diagnosis. In fact, one study showed that a lung POCUS combined with clinical assessment had a higher diagnostic accuracy than other commonly used diagnostic tools in differentiating ADHF from other causes of acute dyspnea [69, 73]. One study showed that POCUS lead to the diagnostic reclassification of 19% of cases [69]. Another study showed that the combination of LVEF <45%, IVCCI <20%, and presence of DIS is 100% specific for the diagnosis of ADHF, and only takes a few minutes to perform [70].

The information gleaned from the lung POCUS should be combined with the rest of the evaluation as well as the history and physical exam to make determinations regarding the patient's volume status and fluid responsiveness. For example, a patient with no evidence of DIS, in association with a normal or flat IVC and a hyperdynamic heart will likely be fluid tolerant and/or fluid responsive. This patient should get IVF and have a repeat assessment after the initial intervention. Alternatively, a patient with evidence of DIS in conjunction with decreased systolic function and a plethoric (enlarged) IVC is likely going to be neither fluid tolerant, nor fluid responsive, and would likely benefit from vasoactive or inotropic agents and prompt transport to definitive care. Additional blind administration of fluids in this patient would likely only result in further cardiopulmonary compromise and worsening respiratory failure.

FALLS Protocol

The ***F**luid **A**dministration **L**imited by **L**ung **S**onography* (FALLS) protocol is not yet supported by robust clinical trials but can be considered as an additional tool for fluid management. One of the biggest complications of over-resuscitation is respiratory compromise as a result of worsening pulmonary edema [24]. Pulmonary edema generates a thickening of the interlobular septa, which can be easily evaluated with simple lung POCUS, as mentioned in the previous section. The transition from an A-line pattern (normally aerated lung) to a B-line pattern (increased density pattern) can indicate a patient-specific and individualized real-time upper limit of fluid tolerance. One study demonstrated that B-lines appear and vanish rather quickly, making septal thickening an *on-off phenomenon* [24]. Additionally, it is suggested that the appearance of B-lines *precedes* the symptomatic and physiologic manifestations of volume overload.

The FALLS protocol, which is a sequential evaluation for causes of shock and ultrasound-informed fluid resuscitation can be utilized to determine adequate resuscitation. After ruling out obstructive and cardiogenic shock, hypovolemic and distributive shock are remaining. These syndromes generally are treated with IVF resuscitation with or without vasoactive agents. This protocol also advocates for resuscitation until you generate *iatrogenic B-lines*. This is the FALLS end point, and the indicator to withhold further fluid resuscitation [24].

Advanced POCUS Applications for Assessment of Fluid Responsiveness

Not only can POCUS help with the diagnosis of a potential cause of shock, but can also help guide interventions, including IVF resuscitation. As mentioned earlier in the chapter, there are risks associated with fluid administration. Fluids should be considered *medications*. Just as we consider the risks and benefits of administering medications to our patients, similar prudent judgment should be exercised when deciding who would benefit from IVF administration and these interventions should be titrated to the specific needs of the patient.

Traditionally, methods of evaluating fluid responsiveness have involved estimation of central venous pressure (CVP) as a surrogate for right ventricular end-diastolic pressure. This, in combination with the principles of the *Frank-Starling Law*, guided resuscitation and fluid loading. New techniques have been studied and are currently available to assess fluid tolerance and fluid responsiveness more accurately. All of these techniques have some limitations, but they are frequently complementary. However, they should not be examined in isolation, but rather taking into account the entire clinical picture of the patient.

Prior to discussing these more advanced methods, it is important to clarify the difference between *Fluid Tolerance* and *Fluid Responsiveness. Fluid Tolerance* is the patient's ability to receive a fluid challenge without experiencing harm. "Will this harm my patient"? By utilizing the cardiopulmonary assessments described above, one can make a determination if IVF resuscitation is most appropriate for their patient in shock. Alternatively, *Fluid Responsiveness* is meant to determine whether a patient would *benefit* from additional fluid. This question requires more advanced ultrasound techniques that should only be considered in the pre-hospital setting if the provider has advanced training and expects a prolonged transport time that requires reassessment. These advanced techniques aim to answer the question of, "Will my patient have an increase in their stroke volume (SV) and cardiac output (CO), and therefore end-organ perfusion?" More specifically, most studies note that a fluid responsive patient generally has an increase in their stroke volume of approximately 10–15% after receiving a fluid challenge.

Overall, CO monitoring is invasive, expensive, not widely available, and nearly impossible in the pre-hospital setting. Given that determining *Fluid Tolerance* with POCUS in the pre-hospital setting is the less technically demanding approach, it will be the focus of our discussion. Among others, the main adjunctive or supplementary methods evaluate Inferior Vena Cava Indices (IVCCI) and the Passive Leg Raise (PLR) maneuver in conjunction with different ultrasound-guided hemodynamic parameters including the Left Ventricular Outflow Tract (LVOT)-Velocity Time Integral (VTI). There are also advanced techniques that are in early stages of validation such as Corrected Carotid Flow Time (CCFT), and Carotid Blood Flow (CBF) that are beyond the scope of this textbook and will not be discussed.

Passive Leg Raise (PLR)

The most reliable and practical measurement for most patients (with or without mechanical ventilation or arrhythmias) for the estimation of fluid responsiveness is the passive leg-raise (PLR) technique looking at the change in the velocity time integral (VTI) at the left ventricular outflow tract (LVOT) [21]. This was the first validated assessment of fluid responsiveness in *spontaneously* breathing patients.

To perform the PLR, the patient has their stroke volume (SV) measured in a semi-recumbent position, at approximately 45-degrees head of bead elevation. This is accomplished as described in the following section utilizing the product of the VTI and LVOT measurements. After determining the patient's baseline SV, the patient is then laid flat and the legs are raised to 45-degrees and maintained there for approximately 2 minutes as the patient receives an *auto-bolus* during which the intravascular contents of the venous reservoir in their lower extremities return to the central circulation and increase the cardiac preload. The patient then has their SV calculated again. Patients that are fluid responsive sit on the steeper portion of the Frank Starling curve (Fig. 16), where an increase in their preload should cause a resultant increase in SV, and thus, their CO. Certain studies have noted that an increase in the VTI of approximately 12% or greater indicates *fluid-responsiveness* [74].

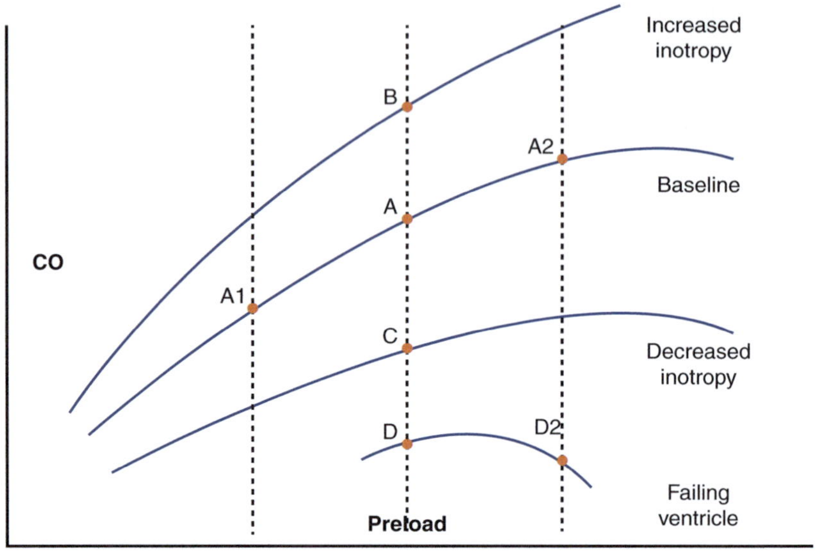

Fig. 16 Starling Curve demonstrating the theoretical relationship between Preload and Cardiac Output (CO)

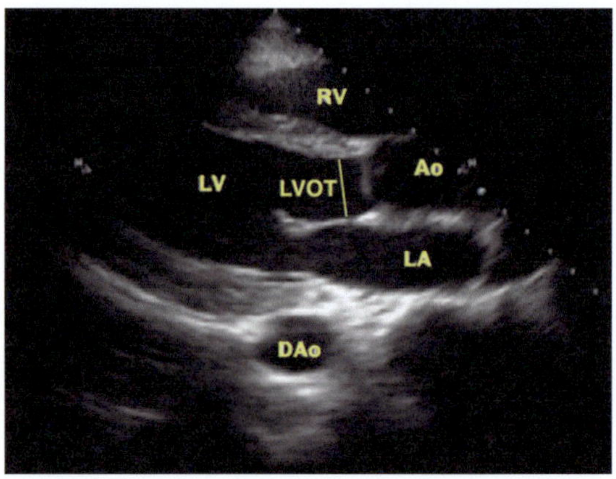

Fig. 17 Parasternal Long Axis Cardiac View demonstrating the location and orientation of the LVOT. LVOT left ventricular outflow track, RV right ventricle, LV left ventricle, LA left atrium, Ao aorta, DAo descending thoracic aorta

Stroke Volume (SV) and the Left Ventricular Outflow Tract (LVOT) - Velocity Time Integral (VTI)

Stroke volume (SV), the amount of blood that is pumped with each cardiac cycle/heartbeat, can be estimated utilizing transthoracic echocardiography (TTE) by calculating the product of the velocity-time integral (VTI) and the left ventricular outflow tract (LVOT) area. The LVOT measurement is generally obtained in the PSL view, (Fig. 17) while the VTI is obtained in the A4C view, with the pulsed wave doppler gate placed at the aortic outflow, in the same place where the LVOT is measured [21, 37, 53, 74] (Fig. 18).

In this equation (Fig. 19), the LVOT is the constant and any resultant changes in the SV are generally a result of the VTI and the patient's fluid responsiveness.

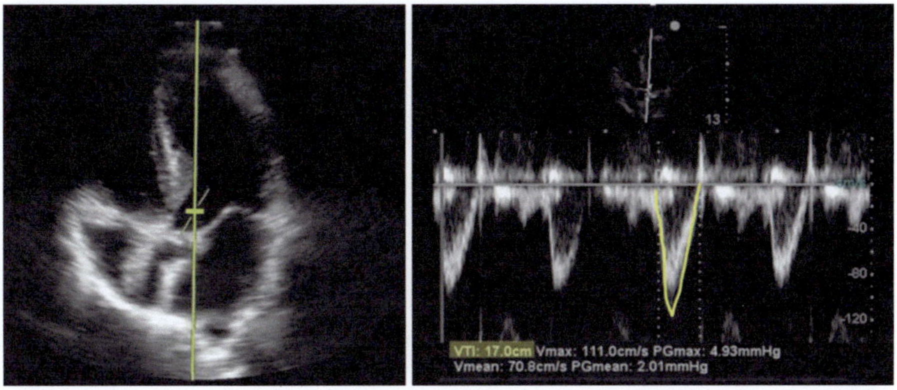

Fig. 18 Left; Apical 4 Chamber Cardiac View demonstrating the orientation and positioning of the pulsed wave doppler gate within the Aortic Outflow Track, at the level of the LVOT. Right; Measurement of the VTI as measured by tracing the pulsed wave doppler gate waveform. LVOT left ventricular outflow track, VTI velocity time integral

$$CO = HR \text{ x } (LVOT \text{ x } VTI)$$

Fig. 19 Equation for cardiac output. CO cardiac output, HR heart rate, LVOT left ventricular outflow track, VTI velocity time integral

Therefore, the VTI measurement has utility in examining the response to fluid loading, drug therapy, or relief of obstructive shock mechanisms [21, 37, 53, 74]. One study demonstrated that an increase in VTI by 12.5% was 77% sensitive and 100% specific for response to a 500 mL fluid bolus [74]. Another study demonstrated that an increase in VTI of 10% after PLR was 97% sensitive and 94% specific for fluid responsiveness [75]. Based on the experience of the authors of one study, the addition of this calculation allows clinicians caring for patients with hypovolemia, hypotension, and shock to rapidly make reliable estimates of cardiac function and track improvements in their CO. Based on their assessment, they recommend an augmented RUSH-VTI protocol, which would combine the ability to not only identify the suspected etiology of shock, but also simutaneously assess for frluid responsiveness, all in 10 minutes or less [21]. This would be beneficial for patients in the prehospital setting or with protracted transport times, where changes in the VTI and thus CO could be monitored throughout the transport process to optimize resuscitation.

Because of the importance of the VTI measurement, any inconsistencies in obtaining this sometimes technically difficult view, can result in potential error. For example, it is important that the angle of insonation of the VTI is consistent and the probe to VTI trajectory is less than 15-degrees to provide an accurate measurement of the true velocity [21, 53]. Additionally, the repeat positioning of the doppler gate within the LVOT may be inconsistent and will affect additional measurements by the same operator, and especially by different operators. If the ultrasound machine requires a manual tracing of the VTI, this creates even more potential variability in the measurement. Also, not all patients are good candidates for this examination. For example, patients with irregular ventricular rhythms (e.g. PVCs, atrial fibrillation) will not give reliable SV values, as the SV will vary depending on diastolic filling time. The routine use of VTI to assess for fluid responsiveness should be approached with caution - advanced training and experience are advised.

Putting It All Together

Integration of Cardiac, IVC, & Lung Ultrasound into Resuscitation of Pre-hospital Patients in Shock

POCUS can provide clinicians with a lot of information but integrating all the components of a comprehensive POCUS exam to make clinical decisions can be challenging, even for experienced providers. The first step in evaluating the patient is to determine the etiology of their undifferentiated shock or hypotension. This can be performed by completing a systematic assessment to rule out a series of potential causes. As described in more detail in chapter "Advanced Diagnostic Topic for Austere Providers: Skeletal Trauma": *Undifferentiated Shock*, utilizing a protocol that is easy to remember, like the *RUSH* protocol, is best. The following mnemonic can be a helpful guide in remembering the components of this exam: **HI-MAP** - **H**eart, **I**VC, **M**orison's (FAST with thoracic views), **A**orta, **P**neumothorax [29].

Once the provider has assessed for possible causes of shock, he or she can focus on the strategy for resuscitation by assessing the patient's potential for fluid tolerance and/or fluid responsiveness. Despite its controversy, evaluation of the IVC can provide useful information to guide the initial IVF resuscitation when used in conjunction with the information obtained from a cardiac and lung POCUS. In general, low IVC diameters and/or high respiratory variation (high IVCCI, >50%) are associated with low CVP states. These patients likely have a distributive or hypovolemic etiology for their shock and are generally fluid *tolerant* and likely need a more robust IVF resuscitation initially prior to vasoactive agents. Provided that they have a normal LVEF and no evidence of pulmonary edema, they can continue to safely receive IVF during their pre-hospital care. Conversely, patients with distended IVCs, generally greater than 2.0–2.5 cm and/or with little to no respirophasic variation (low IVCCI, <50%), are likely to have an elevated CVP and will need further evaluation to assess their fluid tolerance and fluid responsiveness.

Begin by assessing the fluid tolerance of these patients with a POCUS cardiac and lung exam to evaluate the LVEF, IVC distensibility, and presence of pulmonary edema or diffuse interstitial syndrome (DIS). If decreased systolic function and/or pulmonary edema are noted, the patient will likely not be fluid tolerant nor fluid responsive, and further IVF administration will likely cause untoward complications. In fact, these two findings in association with a low IVCCI, are 100% specific for acute decompensated heart failure [70]. These patients would benefit more from interventions that would improve their forward-flow cardiac mechanics, like positive inotropy. If the LVEF is preserved and there is no evidence of pulmonary edema, consider beginning your resuscitation with the appropriate IVF administration. It is prudent to repeat the cardiac, IVC, and lung POCUS after each iterative intervention, especially in the setting of longer transport times in the pre-hospital setting.

For more advanced users or those providing pre-hospital critical care with long transport times, assessment of fluid responsiveness with use of the PLR enables the provider to utilize the patient's own blood volume to deliver an *auto-bolus* of approximately 500 cc. This is a simple, and more importantly, reversible intervention that permits real-time monitoring via changes of non-invasive hemodynamic markers like the LVOT-VTI. These non-invasive hemodynamic markers may help estimate a patient's fluid responsiveness. Based on the most recent evidence, >20% increase of the LVOT-VTI with PLR reliably indicates fluid responsiveness with an increase in the SV and CO of the patient. However, a VTI measurement that changes <10% with PLR indicates that the patient is *unlikely* to be fluid responsive and alternative interventions should be considered, e.g. inotropes or vasopressors.

Depending on the duration of the pre-hospital care, these studies can be repeated as necessary to make ongoing decisions regarding further resuscitative efforts. Frequent re-evaluation of the lungs can help determine the optimal end point to withhold further resuscitation. Utilizing the principles of the *FALLS* protocol, the appearance of B-lines on lung POCUS in the setting of active IVF resuscitation likely indicates the practical limit of fluid tolerance and thus fluid resuscitation. At this point, the provider has probably optimized the patient's location on the Frank-Starling curve, maximizing effective CO, while limiting morbidity and untoward effects of excessive IVF administration (Fig. 20).

This general approach to an *ultrasound-informed* fluid resuscitation in patients with hypotension or shock in the pre-hospital setting has not been validated, nor has it been shown to improve mortality outcomes. In fact, the first randomized controlled trial to compare POCUS to standard care in undifferentiated hypotensive/shock patients failed to show any benefits of survival, CT scanning rates, inotrope use, mortality, or fluid administration [76]. However, this has yet to be studied in the austere and pre-hospital setting.

Future Directions

Artificial Intelligence (AI)

At the time of literature review, there were no studies evaluating the effectiveness of artificial intelligence algorithms to evaluate for LVOT-VTI. However, newer POCUS machines and software packages are being developed with automated features that can help inexperienced healthcare providers evaluate patients with the help of computer software. For example, one study served as the basis for an automated VTI calculator, which would guide the provider and simplify the steps, while reducing variability in obtaining VTI measurements [21]. Other studies that clearly outlined the definition and quantification of B-lines set the foundation for automated learning to count B-lines and map them in accordingly on a virtual lung field map, and track changes over time [23, 24, 71]. Automated IVC software packages also are capable of measuring IVC indices and collapsibility in real time over multiple respiratory cycles to be used in the volume assessment of a patient [54].

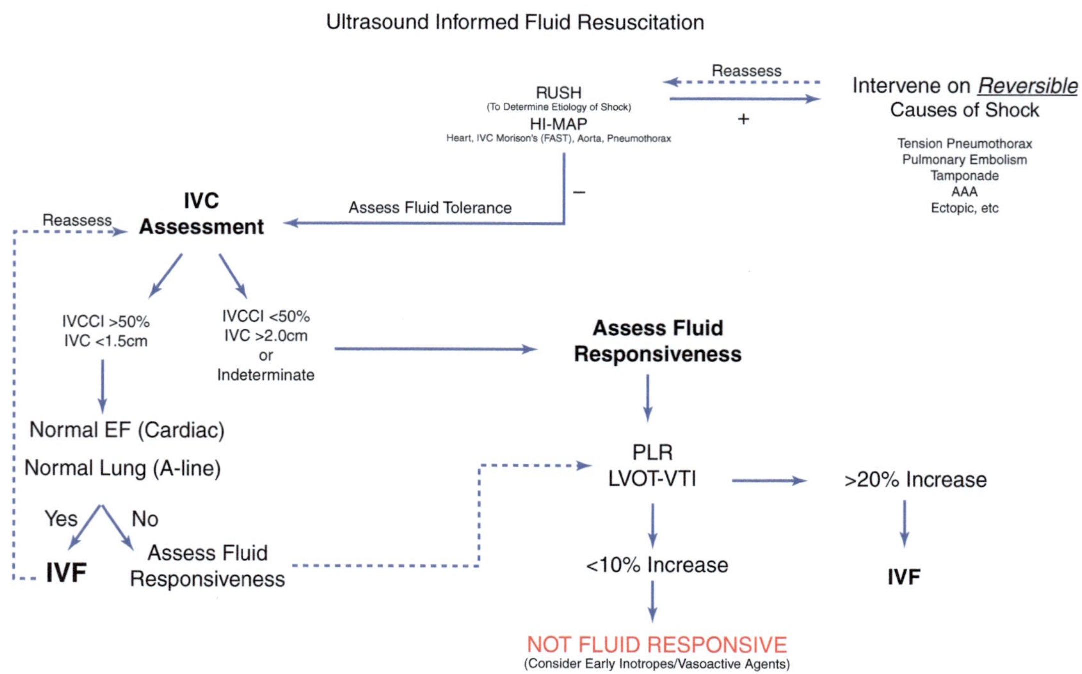

Fig. 20 Algorithm for Ultrasound-Informed Resuscitation. RUSH = Rapid Ultrasound in SHock, AAA abdominal aortic aneurysm, IVC inferior vena cava, IVCCI IVC caval indices, EF ejection fraction, IVF intravenous fluid, PLR passive leg raise, LVOT left ventricular outflow track, VTI velocity time integral

3D IVC Ultrasound

As mentioned in an earlier section, the evaluation of the IVC is prone to inaccuracy due to the lateral displacement of the IVC relative to the probe position that sometimes occurs during inspiration [54, 58]. New innovations are incorporating methods that would be able to help identify, measure, and quantify a collapsibility index automatically with minimal involvement by the provider. Additionally, studies have shown that the geometry of the IVC is complicated and non-cylindrical, and that the movement of this convoluted, pliable, flexible structure can be hard to capture with 2D image acquisition. Studies that have investigated the accuracy of IVC size and collapsibility index obtained by 3D echocardiography for assessing CVP in patients with cardiogenic shock have shown this method to be accurate and reproducible [77].

Carotid Blood Flow and Corrected Carotid Flow Time

Carotid Blood Flow (CBF) and Corrected Carotid Flow Time (CCFT) are newer techniques that can also be added to maneuvers like the Passive Leg Raise as an additional method to help monitor changes in cardiac output and assess fluid responsiveness. These are thought to be more easily accessible and reproducible than the LVOT-VTI measurements given the ease of access to the carotid and more easily attainable views compared to the A4C views that can oftentimes be limited by patient habitus and other anatomic factors. Although still relatively new and seeking large scale validation, these advanced techniques will likely become a component of future ultrasound-informed resuscitative techniques.

Pearls & Pitfalls

Some of these advanced POCUS techniques may not be feasible for pre-hospital providers and require advanced training that may not be realistically attainable or practical for pre-hospital and non-physician providers. A recent critical care consensus statement stated that at least 150 supervised TTE exams are necessary to attain adequate proficiency in these advanced critical care applications [78].

It important to keep in mind the following when performing your POCUS:

- Use a structured approach to determine the cause of shock and hypotension, e.g. RUSH protocol.
- Remember what question you are trying to answer. There is a difference between asking, whether your patient will *tolerate* additional fluid or whether they will *benefit* from additional fluid as manifest by improved stroke volume, cardiac output, and end organ perfusion.
- Understand the limitations of utilizing IVC evaluation for volume status, CVP, and its role in fluid tolerance/responsiveness. CVP is an *inadequate* measure of fluid responsiveness.
- LVOT-VTI is a well validated application, but can be technically challenging, which predisposes it to user error.

- These studies are most accurate in the setting of normal sinus rhythm. Irregular heart rhythms affect the amount of diastolic filling and preload, which impairs resultant cardiac output. In these cases, LVOT-VTI should be measured over multiple beats.
  - Similar changes in preload are associated with respirations.
- Utilize multiple modalities including cardiac echocardiography, thoracic/lung ultrasound, IVCCI, in combination with physical exam and clinical setting to determine the most accurate picture of a patient's fluid tolerance/responsiveness.
  - Advanced providers may additionally utilize PLR and LVOT-VTI.
  - DO NOT USE ANY OF THESE EXAMINATIONS IN ISOLATION.
- The POCUS evaluation is not a discrete data point. Be sure to REPEAT your evaluation throughout the course of the resuscitation to evaluate for changes in the various ultrasonographic indices.

Bibliography

1. Kauvar DS, Lefering R, Wade CE. Impact of hemorrhage on trauma outcome: an overview of epidemiology, clinical presentations, and therapeutic considerations. J Trauma - Inj Infect Crit Care. 2006;60(6 SUPPL):3–11. https://doi.org/10.1097/01.ta.0000199961.02677.19.
2. McGee S, Abernethy WB, Simel DL. Is this patient hypovolemic? J Am Med Assoc. 1999;281(11):1022–9. https://doi.org/10.1001/jama.281.11.1022.
3. Wo CCJ, Shoemaker WC, Appel PL, Bishop MH, Kram HB, Hardin E. Unreliability of blood pressure and heart rate to evaluate cardiac output in emergency resuscitation and critical illness. Crit Care Med. 1993;21(2):218–23. https://doi.org/10.1097/00003246-199302000-00012.
4. Opreanu RC, Arrangoiz R, Stevens P, Morrison CA, Mosher BD, Kepros JP. Hematocrit, systolic blood pressure and heart rate are not accurate predictors for surgery to control hemorrhage in injured patients. Am Surg. 2010;76(3):296–301.
5. King DR, Ogilvie MP, Pereira BMT, et al. Heart rate variability as a triage tool in patients with trauma during prehospital helicopter transport. J Trauma - Inj Infect Crit Care. 2009;67(3):436–40. https://doi.org/10.1097/TA.0b013e3181ad67de.
6. Moore CL, Rose GA, Tayal VS, Sullivan DM, Arrowood JAKJ. Determination of left ventricular function by emergency physician echocardiography of hypotensive patients. Acad Emerg Med. 2002;9(3):186–93.
7. Jones AE, Stiell IG, Nesbitt LP, et al. Nontraumatic out-of-hospital hypotension predicts inhospital mortality. Ann Emerg Med. 2004;43(1):106–13. https://doi.org/10.1016/j.annemergmed.2003.08.008.
8. Durairaj L, Schmidt GA. Fluid therapy in resuscitated sepsis: less is more. Chest. 2008;133(1):252–63. https://doi.org/10.1378/chest.07-1496.
9. Caltabeloti F. Early fluid loading in acute respiratory distress syndrome with septic shock deteriorates lung aeration without impairing arterial oxygenation: a lung ultrasound observational study. Crit Care. 2014;18(R91):1–11. https://doi.org/10.1186/cc13859.
10. Kasotakis G, Sideris A, Yang Y, et al. Aggressive early crystalloid resuscitation adversely affects outcomes in adult blunt trauma patients: an analysis of the Glue Grant database. J Trauma Acute Care Surg. 2013;74(5):1215–22. https://doi.org/10.1097/TA.0b013e3182826e13.
11. Jones AE, Tayal VS, Sullivan DM, Kline JA. Randomized, controlled trial of immediate versus delayed goal-directed ultrasound to identify the cause of nontraumatic hypotension in

emergency department patients. Crit Care Med. 2004;32(8):1703–8. https://doi.org/10.1097/01.CCM.0000133017.34137.82.
12. Rose JS, Bair AE, Mandavia D, Kinser DJ. The UHP ultrasound protocol: a novel ultrasound approach to the empiric evaluation of the undifferentiated hypotensive patient. Am J Emerg Med. 2001;19(4):299–302. https://doi.org/10.1053/ajem.2001.24481.
13. Ferrada P, Anand RJ, Whelan J, et al. Limited transthoracic echocardiogram: so easy any trauma attending can do it. J Trauma - Inj Infect Crit Care. 2011;71(5):1327–31. https://doi.org/10.1097/TA.0b013e3182318574.
14. Ferrada P, Anand RJ, Whelan J, et al. Qualitative assessment of the inferior vena cava: useful tool for the evaluation of fluid status in critically ill patients. Am Surg. 2012;78(4):468–70. http://www.ingentaconnect.com.ezproxy.bu.edu/content/sesc/tas/2012/00000078/00000004/art00039. Accessed 27 Oct 2018.
15. Ferrada P, Evans D, Wolfe L, et al. Findings of a randomized controlled trial using limited transthoracic echocardiogram (LTTE) as a hemodynamic monitoring tool in the trauma bay. J Trauma Acute Care Surg. 2014;76:31–8. https://doi.org/10.1097/TA.0b013e3182a74ad9.
16. Ferrada P, Murthi S, Anand RJ, Bochicchio GV, Scalea T. Transthoracic focused rapid echocardiographic examination: real-time evaluation of fluid status in critically ill trauma patients. J Trauma - Inj Infect Crit Care. 2011;70(1):56–64. https://doi.org/10.1097/TA.0b013e318207e6ee.
17. Gunst M, Ghaemmaghami V, Sperry J, et al. Accuracy of cardiac function and volume status estimates using the bedside echocardiographic assessment in trauma/critical care. J Trauma - Inj Infect Crit Care. 2008;65(3):509–16. https://doi.org/10.1097/TA.0b013e3181825bc5.
18. Atkinson PRT, McAuley DJ, Kendall RJ, et al. Abdominal and Cardiac Evaluation with Sonography in Shock (ACES): an approach by emergency physicians for the use of ultrasound in patients with undifferentiated hypotension. Emerg Med J. 2009;26(2):87–91. https://doi.org/10.1136/emj.2007.056242.
19. O'Dochartaigh D, Douma M. Prehospital ultrasound of the abdomen and thorax changes trauma patient management: a systematic review. Injury. 2015;46(11):2093–102. https://doi.org/10.1016/j.injury.2015.07.007.
20. Taylor J, McLaughlin K, McRae A, Lang E, Anton A. Use of prehospital ultrasound in North America: a survey of emergency medical services medical directors. BMC Emerg Med. 2014;14(1):6. https://doi.org/10.1186/1471-227X-14-6.
21. Blanco P, Aguiar FM, Blaivas M. Rapid ultrasound in shock (RUSH) velocity-time integral: a proposal to expand the RUSH protocol. J Ultrasound Med. 2015;34(9):1691–700. https://doi.org/10.7863/ultra.15.14.08059.
22. Perera P, Mailhot T. The RUSH exam: rapid ultrasound in SHock in the evaluation of th e critically lll. Shock. 2010;28(1):29–56. https://doi.org/10.1016/j.emc.2009.09.010.
23. Lichtenstein D. Lung ultrasound in acute respiratory failure an introduction to the BLUE-protocol. Chest. 2008;134(1):117–25. https://doi.org/10.1378/chest.07-2800, Relevance of Lung Ultrasound in the Diagnosis of Acute Respiratory Failure*: The BLUE Protocol.
24. Lichtenstein DA. BLUE-protocol and FALLS-protocol: two applications of lung ultrasound in the critically ill. Chest. 2015;147(6):1659–70. https://doi.org/10.1378/chest.14-1313.
25. Breitkreutz R, Walcher F, Seeger FH. Focused echocardiographic evaluation in resuscitation management: concept of an advanced life support-conformed algorithm. Crit Care Med. 2007;35(5 Suppl) https://doi.org/10.1097/01.CCM.0000260626.23848.FC.
26. Hypotensive A, Bahner DP. Trinity. J Diagn Med Sonogr. 2002;18(4):193–8.
27. Jensen MB, Sloth E, Larsen KM, Schmidt MB. Transthoracic echocardiography for cardiopulmonary monitoring in intensive care. Eur J Anaesthesiol. 2004;21(9):700–7. https://doi.org/10.1017/S0265021504009068.
28. Lanctôt JF, Valois M, Beaulieu Y. EGLS: Echo-guided life support. Crit Ultrasound J. 2011;3(3):123–9. https://doi.org/10.1007/s13089-011-0083-2.
29. Weingart S. Original RUSH article. https://emcrit.org/rush-exam/original-rush-article/. Published 2008. Accessed 22 Oct 2018.

30. Chin EJ, Chan CH, Mortazavi R, et al. A pilot study examining the viability of a prehospital assessment with ultrasound for emergencies (PAUSE) protocol. J Emerg Med. 2013;44(1):142–9. https://doi.org/10.1016/j.jemermed.2012.02.032.
31. Fitzgibbon JB, Lovallo E, Escajeda J, Radomski MA, Martin-Gill C. Feasibility of out-of-hospital cardiac arrest ultrasound by EMS physicians. Prehospital Emergency Care. https://www.tandfonline.com/doi/full/10.1080/10903127.2018.1518505. Published 17 Oct 2018. Accessed 14 Dec 2018.
32. Kennedy Hall M, Coffey EC, Herbst M, et al. The "5Es" of emergency physician-performed focused cardiac ultrasound: a protocol for rapid identification of effusion, ejection, equality, exit, and entrance. Costantino T, ed. Acad Emerg Med. 2015;22(5):583–93. https://doi.org/10.1111/acem.12652.
33. Tayal VS, Kline JA. Emergency echocardiography to detect pericardial effusion in patients in PEA and near-PEA states. Resuscitation. 2003;59(3):315–8. https://doi.org/10.1016/S0300-9572(03)00245-4.
34. Spodick DH. Acute cardiac tamponade. N Engl J Med. 2003;349:684–90. https://doi.org/10.1056/NEJMra022643.
35. Imazio M, Mayosi BM, Brucato A, Adler Y. Pericardial effusion triage. Int J Cardiol. 2010;145(2):403–4. https://doi.org/10.1016/J.IJCARD.2010.04.031.
36. Armstrong WF, Schilt BF, Helper DJ, Dillon JC, Feigenbaum H. Diastolic collapse of the right ventricle with cardiac tamponade: an echocardiographic study. Circulation. 1982;65(7):1491–6. http://www.ncbi.nlm.nih.gov/pubmed/7074806. Accessed 28 Oct 2018.
37. Noble VE, Nelson B, Sutingco AN. Manual of emergency and critical care ultrasound; 2007. https://doi.org/10.1017/CBO9780511547249.
38. Pérez-Casares A, Cesar S, Brunet-Garcia L, Sanchez-de-Toledo J. Echocardiographic evaluation of pericardial effusion and cardiac tamponade. Front Pediatr. 2017;5:79. https://doi.org/10.3389/fped.2017.00079.
39. Heegaard W, Hildebrandt D, Reardon R, Plummer D, Clinton J, Ho J. Prehospital ultrasound diagnosis of traumatic pericardial effusion. Acad Emerg Med. 2009;16(4):364. https://doi.org/10.1111/j.1553-2712.2009.00379.x.
40. Byhahn C, Bingold TM, Zwissler B, Maier M, Walcher F. Prehospital ultrasound detects pericardial tamponade in a pregnant victim of stabbing assault. Resuscitation. 2008;76(1):146–8. https://doi.org/10.1016/j.resuscitation.2007.07.020.
41. Amico AF, Lichtenberg GS, Reisner SA, Stone CK, Schwartz RG, Meltzer RS. Superiority of visual versus computerized echocardiographic estimation of radionuclide left ventricular ejection fraction. Am Heart J. 1989;118(6):1259–65. http://www.ncbi.nlm.nih.gov/pubmed/2686380. Accessed 28 Oct 2018.
42. Gudmundsson P, Rydberg E, Winter R, Willenheimer R. Visually estimated left ventricular ejection fraction by echocardiography is closely correlated with formal quantitative methods. Int J Cardiol. 2005;101(2):209–12. https://doi.org/10.1016/j.ijcard.2004.03.027.
43. Moore C. Determination of left ventricular function by emergency physician echocardiography of hypotensive patients. Acad Emerg Med. 2002;9(3):186–93.
44. Secko MA, Lazar JM, Salciccioli LA, Stone MB. Can junior emergency physicians use E-point septal separation to accurately estimate left ventricular function in acutely dyspneic patients? Acad Emerg Med. 2011;18(11):1223–6. https://doi.org/10.1111/j.1553-2712.2011.01196.x.
45. Jones AE, Craddock PA, Tayal VS, Kline JA. Diagnostic accuracy of left ventricular function for identifying sepsis among emergency department patients with nontraumatic symptomatic undifferentiated hypotension. Shock. 2006;24(6):513–7. https://doi.org/10.1097/01.shk.0000186931.02852.5f.
46. Nazeyrollas P, Metz D, Jolly D, et al. Use of transthoracic Doppler echocardiography combined with clinical and electrocardiographic data to predict acute pulmonary embolism. Eur Heart J. 1996;17(5):779–86. https://doi.org/10.1093/oxfordjournals.eurheartj.a014946.
47. Torbicki A, Perrier A, Konstantinides S, et al. Guidelines on the diagnosis and management of acute pulmonary embolism. Eur Heart J. 2008;29(18):2276–315. https://doi.org/10.1093/eurheartj/ehn310.

48. Jardin F, Vieillard-Baron A. Ultrasonographic examination of the venae cavae. Appl Physiol Intensive Care Med 2 Physiol Rev Ed. 2012:51–4. https://doi.org/10.1007/978-3-642-28233-1_5.
49. Randazzo MR, Snoey ER, Levitt MA, Binder K. Accuracy of emergency physician assessment of left ventricular ejection fraction and central venous pressure using echocardiography. Acad Emerg Med. 2003;10(9):973–7. https://doi.org/10.1197/S1069-6563(03)00317-8.
50. Tsutsui RS, Borowski A, Tang WHW, Thomas JD, Popović ZB. Precision of echocardiographic estimates of right atrial pressure in patients with acute decompensated heart failure. J Am Soc Echocardiogr. 2014;27(10):1072–8. https://doi.org/10.1016/j.echo.2014.06.002.
51. Kircher BJ, Himelman RB, Schiller NB. Noninvasive estimation of right atrial pressure from the inspiratory collapse of the inferior vena cava. Am J Cardiol. 1990;66(4):493–6. https://doi.org/10.1016/0002-9149(90)90711-9.
52. De Lorenzo RA, Morris MJ, Williams JB, et al. Does a simple bedside sonographic measurement of the inferior vena cava correlate to central venous pressure? J Emerg Med. 2012;42(4):429–36. https://doi.org/10.1016/j.jemermed.2011.05.082.
53. Dawson M, Mallon Mi. Introduction to bedside ultrasound: Volume 1. Emergency Ultrasound Solutions; 2013. https://itunes.apple.com/us/book/introduction-to-bedside-ultrasound-volume-1/id554196012?mt=11.
54. Seif D, Mailhot T, Perera P, Mandavia D. Caval sonography in shock. J Ultrasound Med. 2012;31(12):1885–90. https://doi.org/10.7863/jum.2012.31.12.1885.
55. Wallace DJ, Allison M, Stone MB. Inferior vena cava percentage collapse during respiration is affected by the sampling location: an ultrasound study in healthy volunteers. Acad Emerg Med. 2010;17(1):96–9. https://doi.org/10.1111/j.1553-2712.2009.00627.x.
56. Weekes AJ, Tassone HM, Babcock A, et al. Comparison of serial qualitative and quantitative assessments of caval index and left ventricular systolic function during early fluid resuscitation of hypotensive emergency department patients. Acad Emerg Med. 2011;18(9):912–21. https://doi.org/10.1111/j.1553-2712.2011.01157.x.
57. Yildirimturk O, Tayyareci Y, Erdim R, et al. Assessment of right atrial pressure using echocardiography and correlation with catheterization. J Clin Ultrasound. 2011;39(6):337–43. https://doi.org/10.1002/jcu.20837.
58. Blehar DJ, Resop D, Chin B, Dayno M, Gaspari R. Inferior vena cava displacement during respirophasic ultrasound imaging. Crit Ultrasound J. 2012;4(1):18. https://doi.org/10.1186/2036-7902-4-18.
59. Nagdev AD, Merchant RC, Tirado-Gonzalez A, Sisson CA, Murphy MC. Emergency department bedside ultrasonographic measurement of the caval index for noninvasive determination of low central venous pressure. Ann Emerg Med. 2010;55:290–5. https://doi.org/10.1016/j.annemergmed.2009.04.021.
60. Brennan JM, Blair JE, Goonewardena S, et al. Reappraisal of the use of inferior vena cava for estimating right atrial pressure. J Am Soc Echocardiogr. 2007;20(7):857–61. https://doi.org/10.1016/j.echo.2007.01.005.
61. Lang RM, Badano LP, Mor-Avi V, et al. Recommendations for cardiac chamber quantification by echocardiography in adults: an update from the American society of echocardiography and the European association of cardiovascular imaging. Eur Heart J Cardiovasc Imaging. 2015;16(3):233–71. https://doi.org/10.1093/ehjci/jev014.
62. Feissel M, Michard F, Faller JP, Teboul JL. The respiratory variation in inferior vena cava diameter as a guide to fluid therapy. Intensive Care Med. 2004;30(9):1834–7. https://doi.org/10.1007/s00134-004-2233-5.
63. Barbier C, Loubières Y, Schmit C, et al. Respiratory changes in inferior vena cava diameter are helpful in predicting fluid responsiveness in ventilated septic patients. Intensive Care Med. 2004;30(9):1740–6. https://doi.org/10.1007/s00134-004-2259-8.
64. Yanagawa Y, Sakamoto T, Okada Y. Hypovolemic shock evaluated by sonographic measurement of the inferior vena cava during resuscitation in trauma patients. J Trauma. Background: Inferior vena cava. 2007;63:1245–8. https://doi.org/10.1097/TA.0b013e318068d72b.

65. Marik PE, Baram M, Vahid B. Does central venous pressure predict fluid responsiveness?*: a systematic review of the literature and the tale of seven mares. Chest. 2008;134(1):172–8. https://doi.org/10.1378/chest.07-2331.
66. Marik PE, Cavallazzi R. Does the central venous pressure predict fluid responsiveness? An updated meta-analysis and a plea for some common sense. Crit Care Med. 2013;41(7):1774–81. https://doi.org/10.1097/CCM.0b013e31828a25fd.
67. Corl K, Napoli AM, Gardiner F. Bedside sonographic measurement of the inferior vena cava caval index is a poor predictor of fluid responsiveness in emergency department patients. Emerg Med Australas. 2012;24(5):534–9. https://doi.org/10.1111/j.1742-6723.2012.01596.x.
68. Muller L, Bobbia X, Toumi M, et al. Respiratory variations of inferior vena cava diameter to predict fluid responsiveness in spontaneously breathing patients with acute circulatory failure: need for a cautious use. Crit Care. 2012;16(5):R188. https://doi.org/10.1186/cc11672.
69. Pivetta E, Goffi A, Lupia E, et al. Lung ultrasound-implemented diagnosis of acute decompensated heart failure in the ED: a SIMEU multicenter study. Chest. 2015;148(1):202–10. https://doi.org/10.1378/chest.14-2608.
70. Anderson KL, Jenq KY, Fields JM, Panebianco NL, Dean AJ. Diagnosing heart failure among acutely dyspneic patients with cardiac, inferior vena cava, and lung ultrasonography. Am J Emerg Med. 2013;31(8):1208–14. https://doi.org/10.1016/j.ajem.2013.05.007.
71. Anderson KL, Fields JM, Panebianco NL, Jenq KY, Marin J, Dean AJ. Inter-rater reliability of quantifying pleural B-lines using multiple counting methods. J Ultrasound Med. 2013;32(1):115–20. https://doi.org/10.7863/jum.2013.32.1.115.
72. Volpicelli G, Lamorte A, Tullio M, et al. Point-of-care multiorgan ultrasonography for the evaluation of undifferentiated hypotension in the emergency department. Intensive Care Med. 2013;39(7):1290–8. https://doi.org/10.1007/s00134-013-2919-7.
73. Martindale JL, Wakai A, Collins SP, et al. Diagnosing acute heart failure in the emergency department: a systematic review and meta-analysis. Carpenter C, ed. Acad Emerg Med. 2016;23(3):223–42. https://doi.org/10.1111/acem.12878.
74. Lamia B, Ochagavia A, Monnet X, Chemla D, Richard C, Teboul JL. Echocardiographic prediction of volume responsiveness in critically ill patients with spontaneous breathing activity. Intensive Care Med. 2007;33:1125–32. https://doi.org/10.1097/MCC.0b013e3282fd6e1e.
75. Monnet X, Cipriani F, Camous L, et al. The passive leg raising test to guide fluid removal in critically ill patients. Ann Intensive Care. 2016;6(1):46. https://doi.org/10.1186/s13613-016-0149-1.
76. Atkinson PR, Milne J, Diegelmann L, et al. Does point-of-care ultrasonography improve clinical outcomes in emergency department patients with undifferentiated hypotension? An international randomized controlled trial from the SHoC-ED investigators. Ann Emerg Med. 2018;72(4):478–89. https://doi.org/10.1016/j.annemergmed.2018.04.002.
77. Huguet R, Fard D, D'Humieres T, et al. Three-dimensional inferior vena cava for assessing central venous pressure in patients with cardiogenic shock. J Am Soc Echocardiogr. 2018;31(9):1034–43. https://doi.org/10.1016/j.echo.2018.04.003.
78. Cholley BP. International expert statement on training standards for critical care ultrasonography. Intensive Care Med. 2011;37(7):1077–83. https://doi.org/10.1007/s00134-011-2246-9.

Endotracheal Tube Placement

Matthew Neth and Lori Stolz

Introduction

Endotracheal intubation is a potentially lifesaving procedure performed in the out-of-hospital setting. The goal of the intervention is to optimize oxygenation, ventilation, and aid in airway protection from potential aspiration [1]. When performed successfully, the endotracheal tube (ETT) is placed through the glottic opening and into the trachea, with an appropriate depth in the mid-trachea above the carina.

Like any other intervention or procedure, endotracheal intubation has inherent associated risks, many of which are caused by the failure to recognize a misplaced or dislodged ETT. These complications of airway management can lead to significant morbidity (e.g., pulmonary aspiration, severe hypoxia, anoxic brain injury, esophageal perforation) and possibly even death. Studies report the percentage of unrecognized ETT displacement in the out-of-hospital setting being upward of 25% [2, 3].

In order to limit the potential complications of a misplaced or dislodged ETT, providers should engage multiple methods to confirm appropriate ETT placement. The gold standard is direct visualization of the ETT passing through the vocal cords. When performed with direct laryngoscopy, the effectiveness of this technique is reliant on the skill and experience of the person performing the intubation. The use of video assisted laryngoscopy devices may assist providers in obtaining an improved glottic view, and can allow other members of the care team to help visualize successful ETT passage [3]. Limitations of the direct visualization technique include operator-error, incomplete visualization of the vocal cords, and obstruction of the view by anatomy, blood, emesis or other matter. Direct visualization is

M. Neth (✉)
Department of Emergency Medicine, OHSU, Portland, OR, USA
e-mail: neth@ohsu.edu

L. Stolz
Department of Emergency Medicine, University of Cincinnati, Cincinnati, OH, USA
e-mail: stolzla@ucmail.uc.edu

B. D. Nicholson et al. (eds.), *Manual of Austere and Prehospital Ultrasound*,
https://doi.org/10.1007/978-3-030-64287-7_16

additionally limited due to inability to confirm correct ETT depth in the trachea, and inability to detect ETT dislodgement after the procedure is performed [3]. Auscultation of the bilateral anterolateral chest and over the epigastrium is another commonly used clinical technique to confirm ETT placement. While easy to perform, it should not be used in isolation as this approach has been shown to lead to false positives and negatives, as gastric sounds can be transmitted to the chest wall and normal breath sounds can be transmitted to the epigastrium [4]. Loud noise and an unpredictable environment in the out-of-hospital setting further limits this technique. Other unreliable observation and exam based techniques include condensation within an ETT, as this can be seen with esophageal placement, and equal chest rise with positive pressure ventilation, as this is limited by patients' anatomy and physiologic parameters (e.g., obese body habitus, lung compliance) [5].

The use of specialized devices should be used in conjunction with clinical assessment in order to aid in the confirmation of correct ETT placement. Measuring the patients' oxygenation by pulse oximetry (SpO_2) is commonly used when performing an endotracheal intubation. This technique relies on patient oxygen desaturation to be present in order to detect misplacement or dislodgement of the ETT. As such, recognition of oxygen desaturation is typically a late manifestation of incorrect ETT placement, which can lead to poor patient outcomes.

Measurement of exhaled carbon dioxide has emerged as the gold-standard for confirming ETT placement following intubation and is widely considered the most accurate method available [6, 7]. Measurement can be made with colorimetry, capnometry, and capnography devices which assess either qualitative or quantitative measurements. The colorimetric end-tidal CO_2 ($EtCO_2$) detector is a qualitative capnometric device used for initial confirmation of ETT placement in the out-of-hospital setting [3]. The device changes color when exposed to carbon dioxide and fits inline with an endotracheal tube allowing for quick, simple identification of exhaled carbon dioxide. Waveform capnography involves the measurement of end tidal exhaled CO_2, which is collected non-invasively, displayed quantitatively and in a continuous fashion. Not only can waveform capnography confirm correct ETT placement, but if used continuously, it can be an early indicator for ETT dislodgement [8]. A normal and sustained four-phase waveform capnogram indicates that the ETT is correctly placed through the glottic opening. Waveforms which gradually decline over time (e.g., esophageal intubation), become erratic (e.g., hypopharyngeal placement), or are flat-lines (e.g., esophageal intubation, device failure) generally indicate placement outside of the trachea (assuming normal physiologic parameters). Limitations of waveform $EtCO_2$ capnography include low readings in cases of low pulmonary blood flow (e.g., cardiac arrest, pulmonary embolism), alterations in $EtCO_2$ values with certain medications (e.g., sodium bicarbonate), ventilation changes (e.g., hyperventilation and hypoventilation), device malfunction (e.g., kinked or disconnected tube, secretions in tube), and an inability to detect correct ETT depth [9]. Additionally, carbon dioxide can be transiently detected in the case of esophageal intubation after aggressive bagging or after ingestion of carbonated beverages, thus false positives are possible.

The use of an ultrasound device for the identification of correct ETT placement in the out-of-hospital setting is emerging as a helpful tool for providers as an additional means of confirmation. Ultrasound offers many advantages over the current gold standard detection device (waveform $EtCO_2$ capnography), in that it does not rely on exhaled CO_2 gas (which can be affected by multiple variables) and can be used directly without ventilation. Out-of-hospital ultrasound machines are recently more available, allowing this technology to be utilized as an additional adjunct for the confirmation of ETT placement.

Topic Discussion

The use of ultrasound has several advantages in the out-of-hospital setting in that it is portable, safe (with no radiation exposure), can be rapidly performed, and is not limited by a noisy environment. The device allows for immediate feedback of ETT placement, which can aid clinicians in preventing poor patient outcomes or delays in recognition of tube displacement [3]. Additionally, ultrasound can also allow providers the ability to assess for optimal ETT depth and potential concomitant lung pathology (e.g., pneumothorax, pulmonary edema, pleural effusion) [9].

No standard definition for how to perform an ultrasound examination for ETT confirmation exists. Several methods of assessing for correct ETT placement have been described in the literature. These strategies vary by type of transducer used (e.g., high-frequency linear probe or low-frequency curvilinear probe) and by ultrasound probe placement location (e.g., trachea or chest wall). Two main ultrasound strategies exist: direct and indirect. The direct approach involves assessing the trachea with the ultrasound probe to confirm the ETT presence in the trachea or esophagus. The indirect approach involves assessing bilateral lung sliding and diaphragmatic movement associated with ventilation.

In 2011, Chou et al. described an approach for direct tracheal ultrasound with a technique they termed "tracheal rapid ultrasound exam" (T.R.U.E.) [10] In this technique, a high-frequency, linear ultrasound transducer is placed transversely on the anterior neck, just superior to the suprasternal notch. The trachea is identified by a hyperechoic air-mucosa interface with reverberation artifact posteriorly (comet-tail artifact). (Fig. 1) Endotracheal intubation can be identified if only one air-mucosa interface with comet-tail artifact and posterior shadowing is observed. (Fig. 2) Other nomenclature (the "bullet sign," "snowstorm sign") also describes the same sonographic appearance of an endotracheal tube in the esophagus. If two air-mucosa interfaces with comet-tail artifacts and posterior shadowing are observed (double tract sign or second trachea sign), esophageal intubation is likely identified (Fig. 3) [10, 11]. One downside to this technique is that the esophagus is not positioned in a lateral location to the trachea in all patients. Occasionally, the esophagus will be directly posterior to the trachea, thus obscuring sonographic visualization of an esophageal intubation.

The tracheal ultrasound approach described above, used during the intubation attempt, can be referred to as dynamic. To further assist in ETT identification with

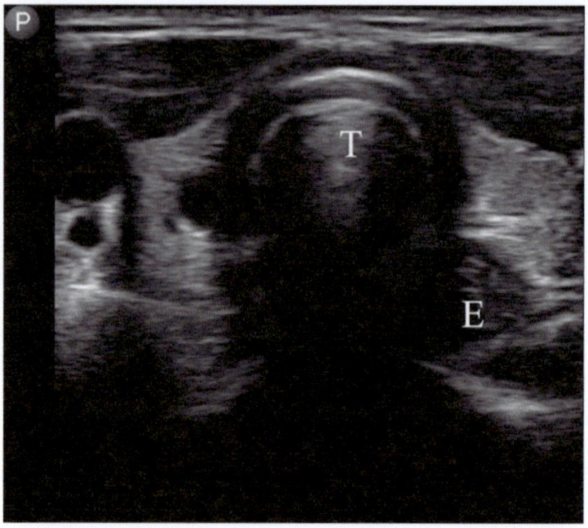

Fig. 1 A transverse plane ultrasound image of the lower anterior neck at the trachea. The trachea is marked with a 'T' and the esophagus is marked with an 'E'

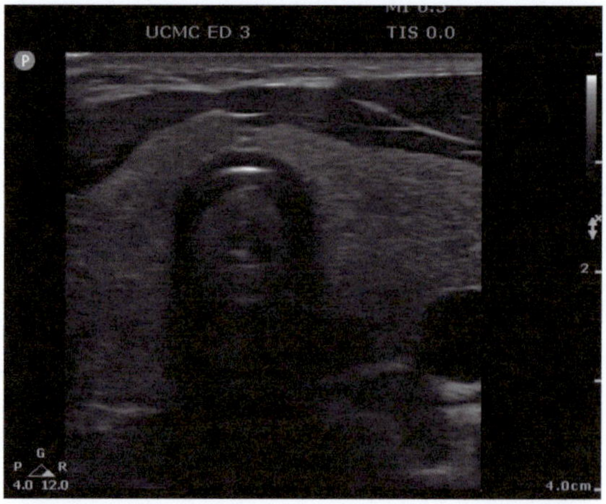

Fig. 2 A transverse plane ultrasound image with an endotracheal tube in proper positioning within the trachea

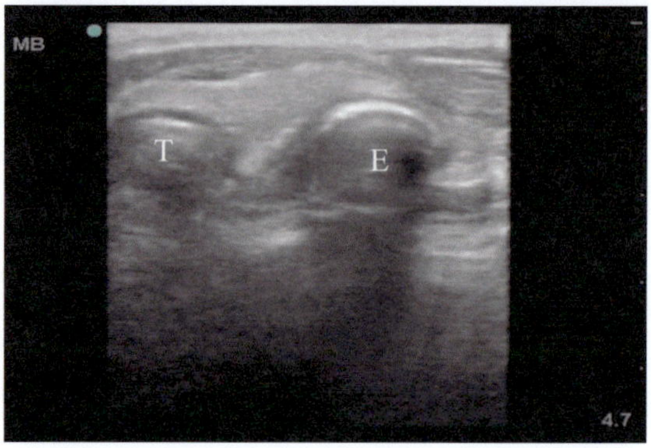

Fig. 3 A transverse plane ultrasound image of an esophageal intubation with the endotracheal tube in the esophagus. The "second trachea" sign can be seen. The trachea is marked with a 'T' and the esophagus (and the endotracheal tube within it) is marked with an 'E'

the direct ultrasound approach, users can perform a static technique. With the static technique, the user places the transducer in a similar location transversely on the anterior neck, just superior to the suprasternal notch before or after intubation. Once the patient is intubated, the person intubating should then gently rotate the ETT side-to-side to create a motion artifact. Endotracheal intubation is confirmed if movement is noted within the trachea. Again, if a double tract sign or second trachea is observed, esophageal intubation is likely [11]. In a 2018 blinded RCT comparing the dynamic versus static approach, no statistically significant difference was identified with either approach in 120 intubations with regards to time to ETT identification, the accuracy of ETT identification, and operator confidence [11]. One advantage of the static technique is that the person performing intubation can also confirm ETT placement with ultrasound; thus, fewer personnel are required to perform the procedure. An additional person to hold the probe and monitor the ultrasound image during intubation is required for the dynamic technique.

Compared to the direct tracheal approach for ETT confirmation, the indirect technique is performed by assessing intercostal (lungs), diaphragm, or subxiphoid (diaphragm) regions. These indirect techniques assess endotracheal intubation by detecting pleural sliding or movement of the diaphragm [10]. In this approach, a transducer is placed on both sides of the chest in the mid-axillary line around the fourth to fifth intercostal space. After intubation, positive pressure ventilation allows for the identification of lung sliding. Bilateral lung sliding during ventilation, in which the parietal and visceral pleura glide over each other, confirms proper endotracheal intubation; whereas, the absence of lung sliding on one side may indicate a contralateral endobronchial intubation (or underlying lung pathology) [12]. If lung sliding is difficult to assess, M-mode on the ultrasound can be helpful. The "sandy beach" sign appears when pleural sliding exists, and the "barcode sign" appears in the absence of pleural sliding (similar to the appearance of a pneumothorax) (Figs. 4 and 5) [13]. Measuring and monitoring diaphragmatic excursion (i.e., diaphragmatic movement) can also assist in confirmation of endotracheal intubation. With this technique, the transducer is placed under the costal margin in the mid-clavicular line. In the presence of positive pressure ventilation, equal bilateral diaphragmatic movement indicates endotracheal intubation, unilateral diaphragmatic movement indicates endobronchial intubation (of the ipsilateral side), and no diaphragmatic movement indicates esophageal intubation [14–16]. Additionally, lung pulse, which is an ultrasonographic sign seen with the indirect approach can assist in detecting endobronchial intubation. This sign is identified by a "pulsation" (i.e., a vertical movement of the pleural line in the absence of lung sliding) synchronous with heart activity. It is seen in cases of complete lung atelectasis, meaning its absence is associated with preserved lung inflation [12, 17].

Unlike the direct approach, the indirect technique requires the application of positive pressure ventilation to the patient, which may be affected by underlying lung pathology (e.g., pneumothorax, pneumonia, or mass) [10]. Additionally, if an esophageal intubation is performed, positive pressure through the ETT can increase the risk of aspiration.

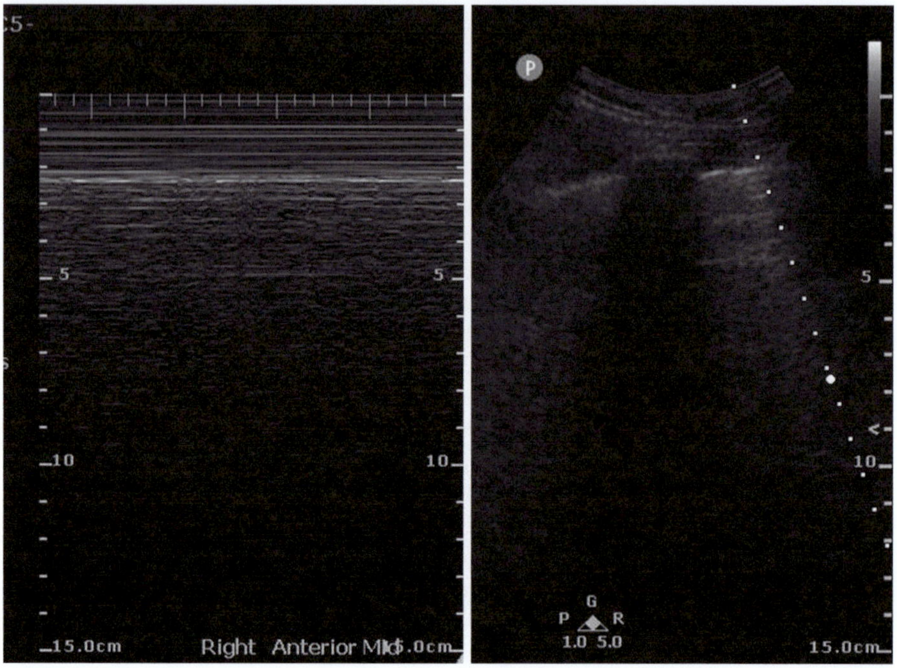

Fig. 4 M-mode of normal lung sliding. In the near field static lines represent the soft tissues. In the far field movement of the lung sliding creates a sandy appearing sonographic signal. This pattern is known as the "sandy beach"

The use of ultrasound for ETT confirmation includes several disadvantages, mainly for the cost of the device, ultrasound gel, cleaning supplies, and storage considerations. Others include time needed to create protocols and train out-of-hospital providers on its use, and time spent developing a quality assurance and quality improvement program. Additionally, as an operator-dependent technique, ultrasound image acquisition can vary significantly between providers regarding quality and speed.

Key Literature Reviewed

Several clinical and cadaveric studies have assessed the use of ultrasound for endotracheal intubation confirmation. These studies have typically been prospective and observational in design, with participants ranging from paramedics to ultrasound trained emergency medicine attending physicians, and settings ranging from cadaver labs to the emergency department. A review of noteworthy recently published studies follows.

The "tracheal rapid ultrasound exam" (T.R.U.E.) approach for ETT confirmation was described by Chou et al. in a 2011 prospective observational study of 112

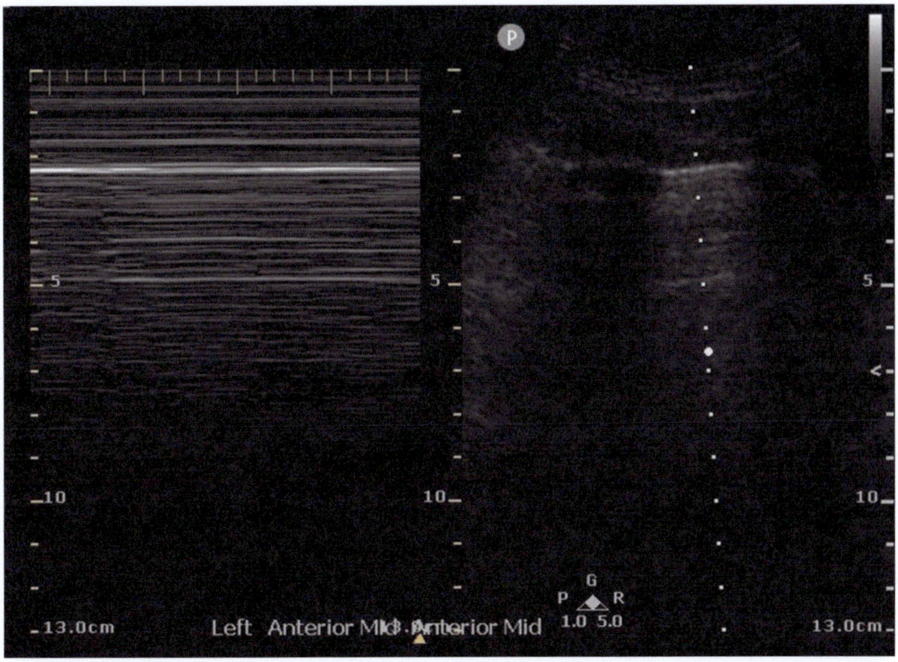

Fig. 5 M-mode of a pneumothorax. Throughout the entire field, static lines show lack of movement and therefore, lack of lung sliding, indicating a pneumothorax. This pattern is known as the "barcode sign"

intubations. The study took place in the emergency department with ultrasonography performed by emergency department residents. The gold standard comparison to ultrasound was waveform $EtCO_2$. The study authors report an overall accuracy of the T.R.U.E. approach as 98.2% with a kappa value of 0.93, indicating a high degree of agreement between the T.R.U.E. approach and waveform capnography. Sensitivity and specificity were reported as 98.9% and 94.1% respectively [10].

Assessment of the indirect ultrasound method for ETT confirmation was evaluated in a 2012 study. Sim, et al. prospectively observed 115 intubations in the emergency department. Intubations were confirmed by emergency department residents with the use of ultrasound assessing for bilateral lung sliding. In this study, chest x-ray was cited as the gold standard control. The authors report an accuracy with this confirmation technique of 88.7%. While methods vary, this technique showed less sensitivity compared to that reported with the T.R.U.E approach discussed above [12].

In the recent years, ultrasound research has begun to assess applications of ultrasound in the out-of-hospital setting and by out-of-hospital participants. In 2015, Zadel et al. prospectively observed 124 intubations in the out-of-hospital setting. Their study compared indirect bilateral lung sliding to auscultation and $EtCO_2$ to confirm appropriate ETT position after urgent endotracheal intubation. The authors report a sensitivity, specificity, positive predicted value, and negative predicted value for ultrasound of 100%. It should be noted that study participants included emergency department physicians with specialized ultrasound training [2].

Lema et al. published a prospective, observational study evaluating paramedics who attempted to determine the position of an ETT on cadavers with use of the ultrasound, with and without manipulation of the ETT. A total of 228 intubations (113 endotracheal and 115 esophageal) were included in the study with direct laryngoscopy confirmation. The authors report improved sensitivity (i.e., esophageal intubation detection) from 52.2% without manipulation to 87.0% with manipulation [18]. This study shows it is feasible for out-of-hospital providers to perform ultrasound for endotracheal intubation confirmation and indicates that manipulation of the ETT may assist in detection of esophageal intubation. Please see Table 1.

Table 1 Ultrasound evaluation of endotracheal intubation [2, 10–12, 18–30]

Author	Year	Intubations	Sonographer (Location)	Ultrasound technique	Sensitivity	Conclusion
Chou	2011	112	EM residents (ED)	T.R.U.E. (Tracheal)	99%	The application of the T.R.U.E. to examine ETT placement during emergency intubation is feasible. Accuracy of 98%
Muslu	2011	150	Anesthesiologist (OR)	Tracheal	100%	US for confirmation of endotracheal intubation is fast and effective
Sim	2012	115	EM residents (ED)	Bilateral lung sliding	92%	The positive predictive value of bilateral lung sliding in confirming proper endotracheal intubation was high at 96%
Adi	2013	107	EM residents (ED)	Tracheal	98%	US can replace waveform capnography in confirming ETT placement in centers without capnography. Accuracy is 98%
Chou	2013	89	EM residents (ED)	Tracheal	100%	Tracheal US in resuscitation management may serve as a powerful adjunct in trained hands

Table 1 (continued)

Author	Year	Intubations	Sonographer (Location)	Ultrasound technique	Sensitivity	Conclusion
Hoffmann	2014	101	EM providers (ED)	Tracheal	100%	US determined ETT locations rapidly with 100% accuracy in the ED
Sun	2014	96	EM residents (ED)	Tracheal	100%	Real-time tracheal US is an accurate method for identifying ETT position during CPR
Abbasi	2015	120	EM residents (ED)	Tracheal (dynamic vs. static)	99%	Acceptable accuracy for prediction of correct ETT placement with the use of dynamic and static US techniques
Chenkin	2015	66	EM residents (Web)	Tracheal	98%	Emergency physicians were able to quickly and accurately interpret ultrasound intubation clips of esophageal and endotracheal intubations. Accuracy of 99.1%
Zadel	2015	124	EM physician (Prehospital)	Lung sliding & Diaphragm excursion	100%	US is an accurate and reliable method for confirming the proper ETT placement in trachea and it is feasible for the out-of-hospital setting
Karacabey	2016	115	EM interns (ED)	Tracheal & Lung sliding	97%	US is a good alternative to $EtCO_2$ for confirming ETT placement
Abhishek	2017	100	Anesthesiologists (OR)	Tracheal	97%	Both capnography and tracheal US examination may be used as primary procedures for the confirmation of ETT placement

(continued)

Table 1 (continued)

Author	Year	Intubations	Sonographer (Location)	Ultrasound technique	Sensitivity	Conclusion
Lahham	2017	72	EM residents (ED)	Tracheal	99%	Tracheal US examination performed by ED resident physicians can be used as an adjunct to help confirm correct ETT placement during intubation
Thomas	2017	100	Sonographer not reported (ED)	Tracheal	98%	US confirmed ETT placement has similar sensitivity and specificity to waveform capnography and is performed more rapidly
Zamani	2017	150	EM residents (ED)	Tracheal	88%	US is a good screening tool in determining endotracheal tube placement
Gottlieb	2018	120	US trained EM physician (Cadaver)	Tracheal (dynamic vs. static)	94%	Both the static and dynamic US approaches were rapid and accurate for confirming ETT location
Lema	2018	228	Paramedic (Cadaver)	Tracheal	87%	Paramedics can accurately identify esophageal intubations with US. ETT manipulation improves identification

Abbreviations: ED emergency department, EM emergency medicine, OR operating room, US ultrasonography

Limitations of Current Knowledge and Opportunities for Future Research

Out-of-Hospital Provider Application

The literature to date seems to agree that ultrasound is a quick procedure, with an acceptable degree of accuracy for the confirmation of endotracheal intubation. As such, it appears to be a valuable adjunct to waveform capnography, especially in situations where $EtCO_2$ is unavailable or unreliable. With the exception of the Zadel et al. study in 2015, most of the studies to date have been performed in the emergency department or operating room and not in the out-of-hospital setting [2]. Additionally, most studies have not assed out-of-hospital providers' (e.g., paramedics) use of the ultrasound device for confirmation of ETT intubation, although the recent study by Lema et al., shows paramedics can accurately identify esophageal intubations with the ultrasound in cadaveric models [18]. As such, a potential opportunity for future research involves studying the clinical performance of the out-of-hospital provider with the application of ultrasound for ETT confirmation.

Another direction for future research would involve defining the optimal length of training programs, learning curves for skill acquisition, and adequate curriculum needed for out-of-hospital provider use of ultrasound for ETT confirmation. Though it should be noted that paramedic ultrasound curriculum for other ultrasound modalities (e.g., focused assessment with sonography in trauma [FAST] and pleural ultrasound) have already been shown to be feasible and time-effective with successful application [31].

Endotracheal Tube Depth

While providers are currently able to indirectly assess for potential endobronchial intubation (through lung and diaphragmatic sliding), ultrasound may also be used to directly measure ETT depth. This can be invaluable in the out-of-hospital setting when traditional measuring techniques like chest x-ray and bronchoscopy are unavailable. This practice is already well accepted in the pediatric population, where ultrasound can measure the optimal ETT to carina depth given the lack of sternal calcification [32]. However, in adults, this measurement is somewhat challenging. Dong et al., recently reported a pilot study which explored how to indirectly measure the ETT depth by measuring the aortic arch depth, upper margin of the ETT cuff depth, and patient height. They derived a formula which can then be used to estimate ETT depth [33]. Although the authors report feasibility with this approach, more prospective clinical data is needed.

Pearls and Pitfalls

- To date, $EtCO_2$ capnography is the current gold standard when confirming ETT positioning and should be performed whenever possible. However, in cases when waveform capnography is not available or is malfunctioning (e.g., in cases of low pulmonary blood flow, ventilation changes, and device malfunction), it is reasonable to use ultrasound for ETT intubation confirmation.
- Ultrasound can be used to complement ETT confirmation along with waveform capnography.

- Providers should not exclusively rely on one method for ETT confirmation and should utilize a multimodal approach. This can include clinical examination (e.g., auscultation, visualization of ETT passage through glottis opening, chest rise) or other monitoring devices (e.g., endtidal capnography, ultrasound and pulse oximetry) [10].
- When performing sonography with a transverse plane image on the trachea, direct visualization of the endotracheal tube passing through the trachea can be observed. The air-mucosal interface can also be appreciated in an endotracheal intubation.
- Esophageal intubations may demonstrate a second air-mucosal interface adjacent to the trachea indicating the endotracheal tube in the esophagus.
- If the esophagus is located immediately posterior to the trachea, the trachea's shadowing may obscure an esophageal intubation (i.e., the double trachea sign may not be present in an esophageal intubation).
- Most of the studies evaluating ultrasound for endotracheal intubation excluded patients with abnormal anatomy or with difficult airway predictors. These would include but are not limited to the following: neck trauma, neck mass, history of neck operation or tracheostomy, cervical spine disease, aspiration risk factors, esophageal disease, age less than 18 years old (unless otherwise specified), or other abnormal anatomic features [19].

References

1. Prekker ME, Kwok H, Shin J, Carlbom D, Grabinsky A, Rea TD. The process of prehospital airway management: challenges and solutions during paramedic endotracheal intubation. Crit Care Med. 2014;42:1372–8.
2. Zadel S, Strnad M, Prosen G, Mekiš D. Point of care ultrasound for orotracheal tube placement assessment in out-of hospital setting. Resuscitation. 2014;2015(87):1–6.
3. Straker T, Urdaneta F. Confirmation of tracheal intubation. In: Hagberg and Benumof's airway management. 4th ed. US: Elsevier; 2018. p. 540–550.e3.
4. Caplan RA, Posner KL, Ward RJ, Cheney FW. Adverse respiratory events in anesthesia: a closed claims analysis. Anesthesiology. 1990;72:828–33.
5. Andersen KH, Hald A. Assessing the position of the tracheal tube. The reliability of different methods. Anaesthesia. 1989;44:984–5.
6. Grmec S. Comparison of three different methods to confirm tracheal tube placement in emergency intubation. Intensive Care Med. 2002;28:701–4.
7. Roberts RJ. Roberts and Hedges' clinical procedures in emergency medicine and acute care. 7th ed. US: Elsevier; 2017.
8. Silvestri S, Ralls GA, Krauss B, et al. The effectiveness of out-of-hospital use of continuous end-tidal carbon dioxide monitoring on the rate of unrecognized misplaced intubation within a regional emergency medical services system. Ann Emerg Med. 2005;45:497–503.
9. Brun P, Bessereau J, Cazes N, Querellou E, Chenaitia H. Lung ultrasound associated to capnography to verify correct endotracheal tube positioning in prehospital. Am J Emerg Med. 2012;30:2080.e5–6.
10. Chou H, Tseng W, Wang C, et al. Tracheal rapid ultrasound exam (T.R.U.E.) for confirming endotracheal tube placement during emergency intubation. Resuscitation. 2011;82:1279–84.

11. Gottlieb M, Nakitende D, Sundaram T, Serici A, Shah S, Bailitz J. Comparison of static versus dynamic ultrasound for the detection of endotracheal intubation. West J Emerg Med. 2018;19:412.
12. Sim S, Lien W, Chou H, et al. Ultrasonographic lung sliding sign in confirming proper endotracheal intubation during emergency intubation. Resuscitation. 2011;2012(83):307–12.
13. Hu W, Xu L, Zhang Q, Wei L, Zhang W. Point-of-care ultrasound versus auscultation in determining the position of double-lumen tube. Medicine. 2018;97:e9311.
14. Kerrey BT, Geis GL, Quinn AM, Hornung RW, Ruddy RM. A prospective comparison of diaphragmatic ultrasound and chest radiography to determine endotracheal tube position in a pediatric emergency department. Pediatrics. 2009;123:e1039–44.
15. Palkar A, Mayo P, Singh K, et al. Serial diaphragm ultrasonography to predict successful discontinuation of mechanical ventilation. Lung. 2018;196:363–8.
16. Piette E, Daoust R, Denault A. Basic concepts in the use of thoracic and lung ultrasound. Curr Opin Anaesthesiol. 2013;26:20–30.
17. Lichtenstein DA, Lascols N, Prin S, Mezière G. The "lung pulse": an early ultrasound sign of complete atelectasis. Intensive Care Med. 2003;29:2187–92.
18. Lema P, O'Brien M, Wilson J, et al. Avoid the goose! Paramedic identification of esophageal intubation by ultrasound. Prehosp Disaster Med. 2018;33:406–10.
19. Muslu B, Sert H, Kaya A, et al. Use of sonography for rapid identification of esophageal and tracheal intubations in adult patients. J Ultrasound Med. 2011;30:671–6.
20. Adi O, Chuan TW, Rishya M. A feasibility study on bedside upper airway ultrasonography compared to waveform capnography for verifying endotracheal tube location after intubation. Crit Ultrasound J. 2013;5:1–11.
21. Chou H, Chong K, Sim S, et al. Real-time tracheal ultrasonography for confirmation of endotracheal tube placement during cardiopulmonary resuscitation. Resuscitation. 2013;84:1708–12.
22. Hoffmann B, Gullett J, Hill H, et al. Bedside ultrasound of the neck confirms endotracheal tube position in emergency intubations. Ultraschall Med. 2014;35:451–8.
23. Sun JT, Sim SS, Chou HC, et al. Ultrasonography for proper endotracheal tube placement confirmation in out-of-hospital cardiac arrest patients: two-center experience. Crit Ultrasound J. 2014;6(suppl 1):A29.
24. Abbasi S, Farsi D, Zare MA, et al. Direct ultrasound methods: a confirmatory technique for proper endotracheal intubation in the emergency department. Eur J Emerg Med. 2015;22:10–6.
25. Chenkin J, McCartney CJL, Jelic T, Romano M, Heslop C, Bandiera G. Defining the learning curve of point-of-care ultrasound for confirming endotracheal tube placement by emergency physicians. Crit Ultrasound J. 2015;7:1–7.
26. Karacabey S, Sanrı E, Gencer EG, Guneysel O. Tracheal ultrasonography and ultrasonographic lung sliding for confirming endotracheal tube placement: speed and reliability. Am J Emerg Med. 2016;34:953–6.
27. Abhishek C, Munta K, Rao SM, Chandrasekhar CN. End-tidal capnography and upper airway ultrasonography in the rapid confirmation of endotracheal tube placement in patients requiring intubation for general anaesthesia. Indian J Anaesth. 2017;61:486.
28. Lahham S, Baydoun J, Bailey J, et al. A prospective evaluation of transverse tracheal sonography during emergent intubation by emergency medicine resident physicians: tracheal sonography during intubation by emergency medicine residents. J Ultrasound Med. 2017;36:2079–85.
29. Thomas VK, Paul C, Rajeev PC, Palatty BU. Reliability of ultrasonography in confirming endotracheal tube placement in an emergency setting. Indian J Crit Care Med: peer-reviewed, official publication of Indian Society of Critical Care Medicine. 2017;21:257–61.
30. Zamani Moghadam H, Sharifi MD, Rajabi H, et al. Screening characteristics of bedside ultrasonography in confirming endotracheal tube placement: a diagnostic accuracy study. Emerg (Tehran). 2017;5:e19.
31. McCallum J, Vu E, Sweet D, Kanji HD. Assessment of paramedic ultrasound curricula: a systematic review. Air Med J. 2015;34:360–8.
32. Jaeel P, Sheth M, Nguyen J. Ultrasonography for endotracheal tube position in infants and children. Eur J Pediatr. 2017;176:293–300.
33. Dong F, Zhu C, Xu H, et al. Measuring endotracheal tube depth by bedside ultrasound in adult patients in an intensive care unit: a pilot study. Ultrasound Med Biol. 2017;43:1163–70.

Intracranial Pressure Evaluation

Jenna M. B. White, Amanda Medoro, and Luke Welle

Optic nerve sheath diameter (ONSD) measurement with ophthalmologic ultrasound is an adjunctive tool used by physicians in the hospital setting to evaluate patients for elevated intracranial pressure (ICP). ONSD measurement is performed using a high-frequency linear transducer applied to the patient's closed eye covered with a clear barrier dressing. The linear probe is oriented with the indicator towards the supine patient's right side and gel is applied over the barrier dressing (Fig. 1).

The optic nerve is identifiable as a hypoechoic structure posterior to the retina. A transverse measurement of the nerve is obtained 3 mm posterior to the retina (Fig. 2). Measurements are obtained on both eyes to ensure accuracy. An ONSD measurement greater than 5 mm correlates with elevated ICP [3, 6, 9] (Fig. 3).

What is the utility of ONSD by emergency medical services (EMS) providers in the prehospital setting? Altered mental status is a common reason for EMS activation. A subset of these patients will have elevated ICP as the cause of their altered mentation. The ability of prehospital providers to detect elevated ICP or the presence of a serious intracranial injury with existing prehospital resources is limited. Current practice strategies focus on obtaining a historical report of trauma to the cranium and identifying external signs of head trauma. In the absence of these factors, prehospital providers report various clinical findings and utilize both the Glasgow Coma Scale (GCS) and the Alert, Responsive to Verbal Stimuli, Responsive to Painful Stimuli, and Unresponsive (AVPU) Scale to convey the depth of coma in a patient [7, 12]. With the increased availability and use of prehospital ultrasound, ONSD measurement can provide EMS with an objective measure to identify elevated ICP in patients with poorly differentiated altered mental status and confirm ICP elevation in traumatic head injury.

With the introduction of any new technology it is necessary to question how such an addition will improve patient care or EMS workflow. Detecting elevated

J. M. B. White (✉) · A. Medoro · L. Welle
Department of Emergency Medicine, University of New Mexico, Albuquerque, NM, USA
e-mail: jmwhite@salud.unm.edu; AMMedoro@salud.unm.edu; LuWelle@salud.unm.edu

B. D. Nicholson et al. (eds.), *Manual of Austere and Prehospital Ultrasound*,
https://doi.org/10.1007/978-3-030-64287-7_17

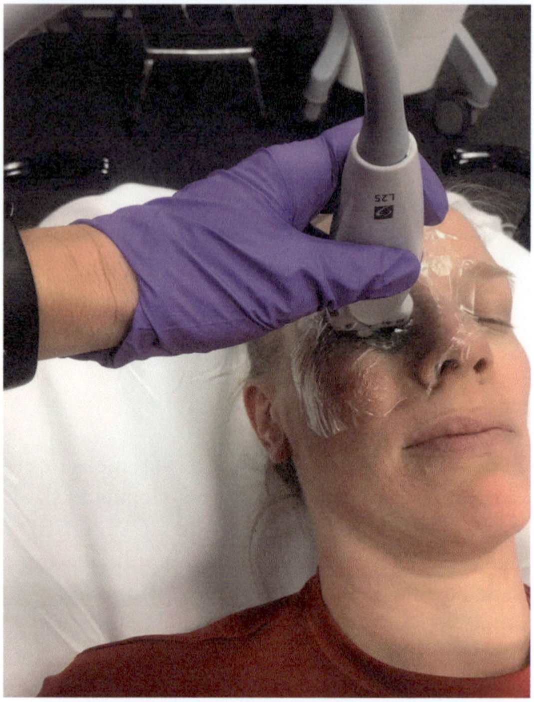

Fig. 1 Patient and transducer positioning for ONSD measurement

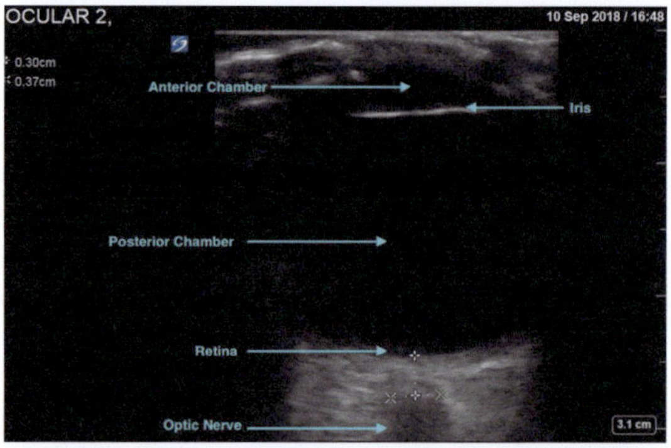

Fig. 2 Normal ophthalmic anatomy and ONSD measurement

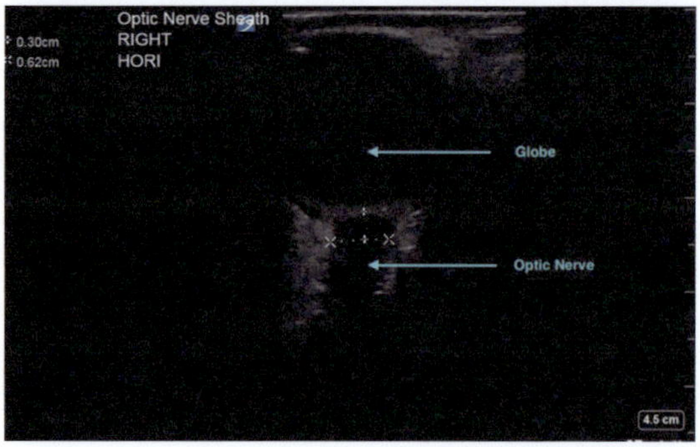

Fig. 3 Abnormal ONSD measurement

ICP in the field has the potential to change prehospital patient management, as has been previously demonstrated with the performance of prehospital FAST exams [13]. An abnormal ONSD measurement in the field may prompt crews to consider transporting the patient to a neurosurgically-equipped receiving facility, to request pre-arrival activation of the trauma team at a destination hospital with a trauma designation, or to request air medical transport from the scene in geographically isolated areas. In extremely austere settings or in clinical environments where computed topography is not possible (such as in polar research stations, high altitude base camps or disaster zones), ONSD measurement may be the only non-invasive diagnostic means of ICP evaluation. Clinical signs of impending herniation coupled with elevated ONSD can additionally lead to earlier administration of an osmotic agent.

While there exists an abundance of research confirming that paramedics and other prehospital non-physician providers can learn ultrasound exams with ease and perform them with a high degree of accuracy and proficiency [1, 11], ONSD measurement has not been studied in this manner. Additionally, most studies that report a high degree of accuracy of ONSD measurement utilize a small cohort of highly trained physicians with extensive ultrasound backgrounds [4]. Among ultrasound fellowship-trained physician sonographers, considerable inter-rater agreement exists [5, 10]. The inter-rater reliability of this exam across ultrasonographers with less training is unknown. Additionally, patients with critical head injuries are likely to have other pressing clinical needs such as airway management, intravenous access, anticonvulsant administration in the case of seizure activity, cardiac monitoring, and ventilatory support, which the EMS provider must balance with the precision skill of ONSD measurement.

The prehospital environment presents a unique set of challenges to obtaining quality ultrasound images. The noise level, varying light conditions, and the need to perform skills while an EMS transport unit is in motion together create a scanning environment that is very different from the emergency department or intensive care unit, where most research assessing the validity of ONSD measurements has been conducted [8]. While one study demonstrated the feasibility of obtaining this exam in the prehospital setting, the sonographers in this study were also physicians with robust ultrasound training backgrounds [2].

Additional challenges to the implementation of an ultrasound-based treatment guideline in the prehospital setting include the time and resources required to train providers and to maintain competency over time. Current accredited paramedic training programs require over 1000 clock hours of training, and the National Registry of Emergency Medical Technicians (NREMT) requires 60 additional hours of continuing education every 2 years for paramedics to maintain membership [14]. Locally, EMS providers at all levels are required to perform skill maintenance, training on protocol updates, and clinical measures. These requirements of practice pose a significant demand on prehospital providers. To further mandate additional training requirements for the maintenance of ultrasound skills may disproportionately strain rural EMS agencies, ironically where the ONSD measurement skill would likely be most impactful.

In summary, the evidence does not yet support broadly incorporating this exam in general EMS provider training, nor in the routine prehospital acquisition of ONSD in the evaluation of patients with altered mental status. In remote settings or areas where neurological diagnostics are not readily accessed, ONSD measurement may support clinical decision-making to sufficiently warrant its use. In these situations, a training protocol should be developed for prehospital providers, and their performance assessed by an experienced sonographer. Further research and investigation on ONSD evaluation in the prehospital setting is necessary prior to broad implementation.

References

1. Brooke M, Walton J, Scutt D, et al. Acquisition and interpretation of focused diagnostic ultrasound images by ultrasound-naïve advanced paramedics: trialing a PHUS education programme. Emerg Med J. 2012;29:322.
2. Houze-Cerfon CH, Bounes V, Guemon J, et al. Quality and feasibility of sonographic measurement of the optic nerve sheath diameter to estimate the risk of raised intracranial pressure after traumatic brain injury in the prehospital setting. Prehosp Emerg Care. 2019;23(2):277–83.
3. Kimberly HH, Shah S, Marrill K, et al. Correlation of optic nerve sheath diameter with direct measurement of intracranial pressure. Acad Emerg Med. 2008;15(2):201.
4. Lochner P, Brio F, Zedde ML, et al. Feasibility and usefulness of ultrasonography in idiopathic intracranial hypertension or secondary intracranial hypertension. BMC Neurol. 2016;16:85.
5. Oberfoell S, Murphy D, French A, et al. Inter-rater reliability of sonographic optic nerve sheath diameter measurements by emergency physicians. J Ultrasound Med. 2017;36:1579.
6. Ohle R, McIsaac S, Woo MY, et al. Sonography of the optic nerve sheath diameter for detection of raised intracranial pressure compared to computed tomography. J Ultrasound Med. 2015;34:1285.
7. Pollack AN. Emergency care and transportation of the sick and injured 10th edition. Burlington; Jones and Bartlett Learning. 2011.
8. Qayyum H, Ramlakhan S. Can ocular ultrasound predict intracranial hypertension? A pilot diagnostic accuracy evaluation in a UK emergency department. Eur J Emerg Med. 2013;20(2)
9. Rajajee V, Vanaman M, Fletcher JJ, et al. Optic nerve ultrasound for the detection of raised intracranial pressure. Neurocrit Care. 2011;15:506.
10. Robba C, Santori G, Czosnyka M, et al. Optic nerve sheath diameter measured sonographically as non-invasive estimator of intracranial pressure: a systematic review and meta-analysis. Intensive Care Med. 2018;44:1284.
11. Rooney KP, Lahham S, Lahham S, et al. Pre-hospital assessment with ultrasound emergencies: implementation in the field. World J Emerg Med. 2016;7(2):117.
12. Teasdale G, Jennett B. Assessment of coma and impaired consciousness: a practical scale. Lancet. 1974;304:81–4.
13. Walcher F, Weinlich M, Conrad G, et al. Prehospital ultrasound imaging improves management of abdominal trauma. Br J Surg. 2006;93:238.
14. National Registry of Emergency Medical Technicians. www.nremt.org. Accessed 27 Nov 2018.

Bladder Volume and Assessment of Hydronephrosis

Alex Kranc and Catalina Gonzalez-Marques

Introduction

The body is constantly utilizing energy and maintaining a delicate balance of electrolytes in a process call homeostasis. This process generates liquid and solid waste products which must be disposed of. The kidney, as the collecting system for liquid in the body, is one of the main organs that helps to filter this liquid waste and preserve this delicate balance of electrolytes. Any malfunction in this process can lead to serious electrolyte abnormalities and build-up of toxins within the body. While there are many causes of intrinsic renal injury, or injuries within the kidney this chapter will focus on post-renal pathology, mainly urinary tract obstruction (UTO) and its sequelae.

Waste products from the blood are filtered through a complex collecting system within the kidney producing urine. This liquid waste then flows through two small tubes composed of smooth muscle, called ureters, and into a large vesicular structure for temporary storage, called the bladder. Waste is finally excreted from the bladder through the urethra in a process called urination. There are a number of pathologic processes that can occur preventing proper excretion of urine, one of which, is urinary tract obstruction. UTO can occur at any time and any place along the urinary tract. It is more common in men, and prevalence increases with age [10–12]. Obstructive processes may be chronic or acute, unilateral or bilateral, partial or complete. UTO has different causes, some of which include benign prostatic hyperplasia (in men), renal stones, medications, tumors, infections, or trauma. Urinary tract injury can occur in up to 10% of trauma patients. Blunt trauma is the cause of 90% of traumatic renal injuries and the most commonly injured area of the

A. Kranc (✉)
Emergency Department, Lexington Medical Center, West Columbia, SC, USA
e-mail: dakranc@lexhealth.org

C. Gonzalez-Marques
Brigham and Women's Department of Emergency Medicine, Boston, MA, USA

B. D. Nicholson et al. (eds.), *Manual of Austere and Prehospital Ultrasound*,
https://doi.org/10.1007/978-3-030-64287-7_18

urinary tract is the kidney [14]. Depending on the location of the obstruction or injury, urine may back up into the bladder, ureters, or kidneys. This may lead to kidney injury, electrolyte abnormalities, urinary tract infections (UTIs), and can cause sepsis. In the hospital and in austere environments, ultrasound is the ideal imaging modality to assess for the sequelae of UTO: hydronephrosis. It should be noted that hydroureter, a back-up of fluid into the ureters, can also be found in UTO. However, this is difficult to detect via ultrasound. For the purposes of this chapter we will define hydroureter as dilation of ureter >4 mm [15]. We define hydronephrosis as the pathologic dilation and swelling of the kidney that occurs due to a failure in the normal flow and drainage of urine from the kidneys to the bladder, often due to blockage (more on this later).

Topic Discussion

Patients with UTO may present with a range of complaints from simple suprapubic pain, to frank altered mental status, hypotension, and sepsis. Other symptoms can include oliguria (decrease in urine output), hematuria (blood in the urine), and flank pain. Pain may be mild or severe, however severe pain may indicate a renal stone, or acute obstruction. As there are two kidneys and ureters, it is possible to have an obstruction but still produce adequate urine. This can be seen in partial or unilateral obstructions. More distal obstructions can lead to acute urinary retention. On physical exam you may observe a palpable bladder in the pelvis and potentially abdominal distension. However, these are late manifestations of UTO. Early identification of UTO allows for timely intervention and treatment, avoiding the deleterious effects of sustained obstruction.

Ultrasound is the preferred imaging modality for diagnosis of UTO in the austere or limited-resource environment due to its portability and high sensitivity in the hands of a trained operator [1, 5, 7]. If the provider suspects obstruction, the positive predictive value of a renal/bladder. Ultrasound is adequate for diagnosis [5, 7]. Ultrasound is >90% sensitive and specific for hydronephrosis [13]. However, false positives can occur as some patients will have chronic mild hydronephrosis. While evaluation of the ureters and kidneys is slightly more technically challenging, evaluation of bladder volume is much more simplistic and straightforward (technique and calculations are shown later in this chapter).

Though very complex, it is easy to think of the kidney as being comprised of two different parts: the cortex which filters blood, and the renal medulla (also known as pyramid or collecting system), which collects and filters urine. The characteristic finding of UTO on ultrasound is dilation of the renal collecting system or ureters. This can occur in one or both kidneys depending on the level and side of obstruction. A system for grading the severity of hydronephrosis exists, however this scale has questionable clinical significance, and would be of minimal use to the austere provider.

If found, care should be taken to identify the exact location of the area of hypoechogenicitiy as renal cysts arising from the cortex are common and may occasionally be mistaken for a dilated collecting system. There also exists a condition (polycystic kidney disease) in which the kidney is comprised of many cysts, which makes evaluation of hydronephrosis extremely difficult.

Procedure

In evaluation of suspected UTO, providers should start with imaging of the bladder. This is done using either the phased array or curvilinear transducer. Prior to initiating the exam the patient should be laid supine. The probe should then be placed on the lower abdomen, midline, just superior to the symphysis pubis, with the indicator facing to the left. The transducer should be angled in all four directions, sweeping through all sides of the bladder. A normal distended bladder should appear as an anechoic structure located midline in the pelvis. It should be triangular shape in the sagittal plane and oval shape in the transaxial plane [13]. The wall of the bladder should appear uniform and 3–4 mm in thickness [13]. If the patient is dehydrated or recently urinated, it may not be possible to identify the bladder. If found, there are several different methods of calculating bladder volume, however we recommend the prolate ellipsoid method. This is simply (length × width × heig ht × 0.52). For simplicity, providers can use 0.5 instead of 0.52. The first image obtained should be the transverse view, and the measurement should be taken at the widest width. For the second and third calculations, the probe should be turned 90° counterclockwise so the indicator is pointing towards the patient's head (the sagittal plane). Once oriented, the bladder length and anterior/posterior width should be measured. A normal bladder can hold 300–400 mL of urine, though higher volumes are possible [8]. While these measurements will estimate bladder volume, interpretation should be based on the clinical picture as there is a reasonable margin of error [4–6] (Figs. 1 and 2).

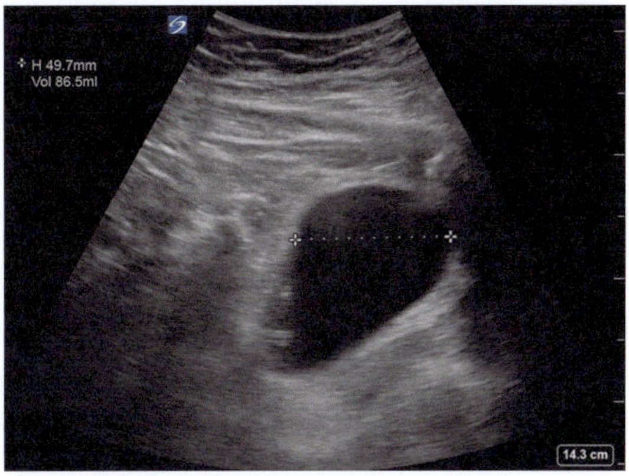

Fig. 1 Bladder volume measurement in transverse: In a transverse plane, measure across the bladder to obtain length (L) and from anterior to posterior to obtain width (W)

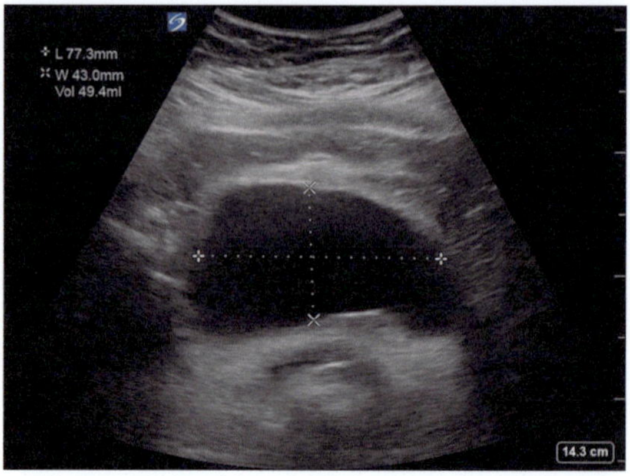

Fig. 2 Bladder volume measurement in sagittal: In sagittal orientation, measure superior to inferior to obtain the height (H) measurement

Renal ultrasound is slightly more technical, however can be easily performed by the austere provider. Indications for this procedure include hematuria, oliguria with bladder distension or blunt abdominal trauma as part of the FAST exam. The kidneys are located on the flanks just below the ribs, slightly towards the back. This exam is also performed while the patient is supine using either the phased array or curvilinear probes. The left and right kidneys are in slightly different locations, and their imaging locations are thus slightly different. On the right, the probe should be placed just below the ribs on the mid-axillary line, angled slightly posterior. Depth should be adjusted to the provider can see just deep to the kidney on the screen. The probe should be fanned through the kidney so the whole organ is imaged from the upper pole of the kidney to the lower pole. The left kidney is slightly more superior and retroperitoneal than the right kidney, and thus the probe should be placed slightly higher than the right side. Again, the probe should be fanned so the entire kidney is imaged. The provider should evaluate the kidneys for distension, free fluid, or stones. Stones will appear as bright, hyperechoic structures with posterior acoustic shadowing. Calculi within the renal pelvis are often of little significance but can mobilize to the ureter potentially causing UTO.

Literature Review

The authors were only able to find one case report of austere bladder ultrasound [9]. In this case a bedside ultrasound was used for a soldier with bladder discomfort and ultimately resulted in transfer to a higher level of care. There are several reports of austere renal ultrasound, however most are case reports which show utility of this imaging modality [2, 3]. There is clearly a need for more research in this area, however we feel the data obtained in a hospital environment would be easily reproduced in the field.

Pearls and Pitfalls

Ultrasound has great utility in the evaluation of UTO and for renal complaints, as described above. The increased portability and durability of this device make it the ideal austere imaging modality and can change patient management and disposition [1]. It can be used effectively to evaluate for UTO, hydronephrosis and bladder volume. While bladder volume can be easily calculated, this measurement can be prone to error depending on the areas measured. Hydronephrosis can also be evaluated easily and diagnosed via ultrasound. This exam is indicated if the provide is suspicious of UTO.

The pitfalls of these procedures are related to care after diagnosis. It is unlikely that a provider will have appropriate medical equipment in the field to help relieve UTO e.g. a foley catheter (though in emergencies suprapubic aspiration may be indicated). Additionally this device may be of no use if the UTO is located proximal to the bladder. If diagnosed, care should be directed at pain relief and expedited transport to a higher level of care.

References

1. Blaivas M, et al. Change in differential diagnosis and patient management with the use of portable ultrasound in a remote setting. Wilderness Environ Med. 2005;16(1):38–41.
2. Cramer JS, Forrest K. Renal Lithiasis: addressing the risks of Austere Desert deployments. Aviat Space Environ Med. 2006;77(6):649–53.
3. Dean AJ, et al. The utility of handheld ultrasound in an austere medical setting in Guatemala after a natural disaster. Am J Disaster Med. 2007;2(5):249–56.
4. Dicuio M., et al. (PDF) Measurements of urinary bladder volume: comparison of five ultrasound calculation methods in volunteers. ResearchGate. https://www.researchgate.net/publication/7834367_Measurements_of_urinary_bladder_volume_Comparison_of_five_ultrasound_calculation_methods_in_volunteers. Accessed 27 Nov 2018.
5. Ellenbogen P, et al. Sensitivity of gray scale ultrasound in detecting urinary tract obstruction. Am J Roentgenol. 1978;130(4):731–3. Crossref,. https://doi.org/10.2214/ajr.130.4.731.
6. Hvarness H, et al. Urinary bladder volume measurements: Comparison of three ultrasound calculation methods. Scand J Urol Nephrol. 2002;36(3):177–81. Taylor and Francis+NEJM. https://doi.org/10.1080/003655902320131839.
7. Kamholtz RG, et al. Obstruction and the minimally dilated renal collecting system: US evaluation. Radiology. 1989;170(1):51–3. *pubs.rsna.org (Atypon)*. https://doi.org/10.1148/radiology.170.1.2642347.
8. Lukacz ES, et al. A healthy bladder: a consensus statement. Int J Clin Pract. 2011;65(10):1026–36. PubMed Central,. https://doi.org/10.1111/j.1742-1241.2011.02763.x.
9. Lunceford N, et al. Utilization of bedside urogenital ultrasound in an austere combat setting: enterovesicular fistula case report. Mil Med. 2013;178(3):e376–9. academic.oup.com,. https://doi.org/10.7205/MILMED-D-12-00320.
10. Meigs JB, et al. Incidence rates and risk factors for acute urinary retention: the health professionals followup study. J Urol. 1999;162(2):376–82. www.jurology.com,. https://doi.org/10.1016/S0022-5347(05)68563-1.

11. Selius BA, Subedi R. Urinary retention in adults: diagnosis and initial management. Am Fam Physician. 2008;77(5):643–50.
12. Urethral Stricture - Care at Mayo Clinic - Mayo Clinic. https://www.mayoclinic.org/diseases-conditions/urethral-stricture/care-at-mayo-clinic/mac-20362386. Accessed 27 Nov 2018.
13. Zagoria RJ, et al. An introduction to radiologic methods. In: Genitourinary imaging: the requisites. 3rd ed: Elsevier; 2016. p. 1–39. *Clinical Key*, https://www-clinicalkey-com.revproxy.brown.edu/#!/content/book/3-s2.0-B9780323057752000015?scrollTo=%23hl0001299.
14. Zagoria RJ, et al. The kidney: diffuse parenchymal abnormalities. In: Genitourinary imaging: the requisites. 3rd ed: Elsevier; 2016. p. 107–45. *Clinical Key*, https://www-clinicalkey-com.revproxy.brown.edu/#!/content/book/3-s2.0-B9780323057752000040?scrollTo=%23hl0001263.
15. Zelenko N, et al. Normal ureter size on unenhanced helical CT. Am J Roentgenol. 2004;182(4):1039–41. ajronline.org (Atypon),. https://doi.org/10.2214/ajr.182.4.1821039.

Part V

Introduction to Procedures

The benefits of ultrasound in procedures include the ability to confirm pathology, such as the case of an abscess prior to attempting an incision and drainage, or directly visualizing the advancement of a needle to perform an injection, such as in the case of nerve blocks, or appropriately avoiding structures. In the hospital setting, ultrasound guidance has become the standard of care for high-risk procedures such as central line placement or peripheral nerve blocks. Out-of-hospital providers performing similar procedures should strongly consider adding ultrasound guidance to their practice.

Vascular Access

Kelly Mayo and Joseph R. Pare

Introduction

Obtaining vascular access is essential in both the pre-hospital and emergency department settings. Up to 150–200 million peripheral intravenous lines (PIVs) are placed every year in the United States [1]. As the prevalence of obesity, drug abuse, and chronic illness increase, so do the number of patients who present with challenges in obtaining IV access. These patients may be critically ill and subjected to repeated attempts at IV placement. It is estimated 8–23% of ED patients meet criteria for difficult venous access (DVA), and may require additional efforts beyond a PIV placed by landmark technique to provide medical care [1]. The use of ultrasound has allowed medical providers to locate and cannulate vessels below the skin that may be too deep for a traditional PIV or are unable to be palpated due to soft tissues. Because of the ability to visualize deeper and possibly larger vessels, ultrasound-guided peripheral venous access has become an important approach with increased success rates compared to landmark technique, higher patient satisfaction, decreased complications, and reduced rates of central-venous catheter placement [2, 3].

This chapter will discuss the anatomy of the applicable venous systems, vessels frequently selected for cannulation, necessary equipment, technique, possible complications, pediatric applications, and options for device selection for venous access in the DVA patient.

K. Mayo (✉) · J. R. Pare
Department of Emergency Medicine, Boston University School of Medicine,
Boston Medical Center, Boston, MA, USA
e-mail: Kelly.Mayo@bmc.org; Joseph.Pare@bmc.org

B. D. Nicholson et al. (eds.), *Manual of Austere and Prehospital Ultrasound*,
https://doi.org/10.1007/978-3-030-64287-7_19

Anatomy

Commonly used veins for ultrasound-guided IVs are in the upper extremity and include the cephalic, basilic and brachial veins. While these are frequently accessed in the antecubital fossa, it is important to consider that this location may restrict mobility of the arm. The cephalic vein, which is located along the entire radial side of the arm, is most accessible from the lateral surface of the upper arm. If accessed, the cephalic vein can be particularly useful in contracted patients and may be more comfortable. The brachial vein runs along with the brachial artery and nerve and often exists as a set of paired veins within the antecubital fossa before they join deeper in the upper arm. Because this is a deeper vein it tends to have a higher rate of infiltration as compared to more superficial veins, but is still an acceptable option [4]. The basilic vein runs along the ulnar aspect of the arm and is typically best accessed only with US-guidance. While useful for temporary peripheral access, the basilic vein is also used for more permanent IV access such as with peripherally inserted central catheters (PICC) lines and midline catheters.

It is feasible and sometimes preferred to obtain access in the more distal upper extremities such as the forearm and hand. This is especially useful in stable patients who are not expected to need imaging studies with IV contrast, which may require access in the antecubital fossa or above. These forearm veins are typically the distal cephalic or the median anti-brachial veins and tend to be more superficial.

In the lower extremity, the great saphenous vein provides an alternative option for peripheral access. This vein passes anterior to the medial malleolus and courses upwards along the medial aspect of the leg. It is widest and most superficial immediately above the medial malleolus and can be more easily visualized in the reverse trendelenburg position [5]. (Fig. 1). The use of leg veins is generally recommended only after the use of alternative upper extremity sites.

It is also possible to access the external and internal jugular veins of the neck with ultrasound guidance. The external jugular vein passes from the angle of the mandible towards the heart, obliquely across the sternocleidomastoid muscle and under the clavicle to meet the subclavian vein. The internal jugular vein passes through the jugular foramen and runs downwards, lateral to the internal carotid artery and then lateral to the common carotid artery before joining the subclavian vein. Cannulating the internal jugular vein peripherally is a fairly new approach, and though there is limited evidence for its use, it is thought to be an alternative option in the DVA patient population [6, 7] (Fig. 2).

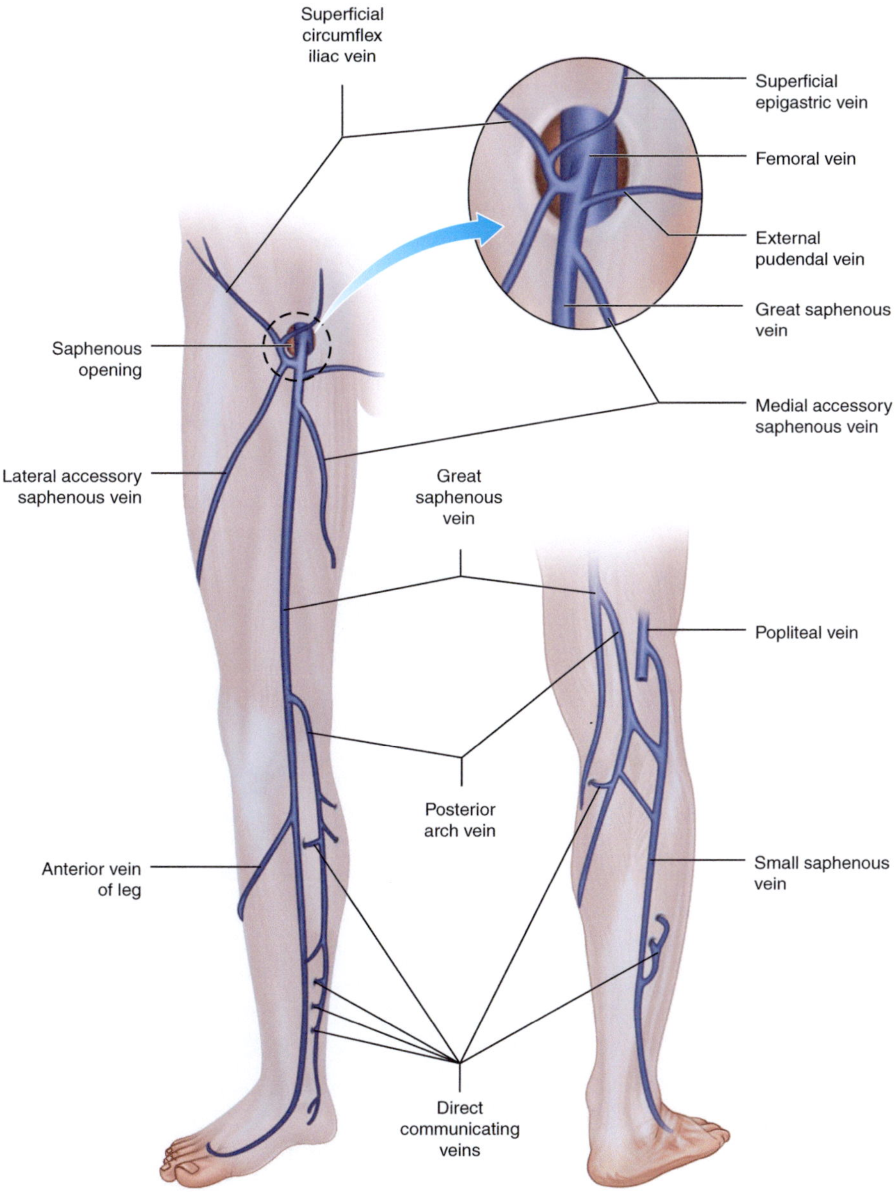

Fig. 1 Diagram of lower extremity venous anatomy

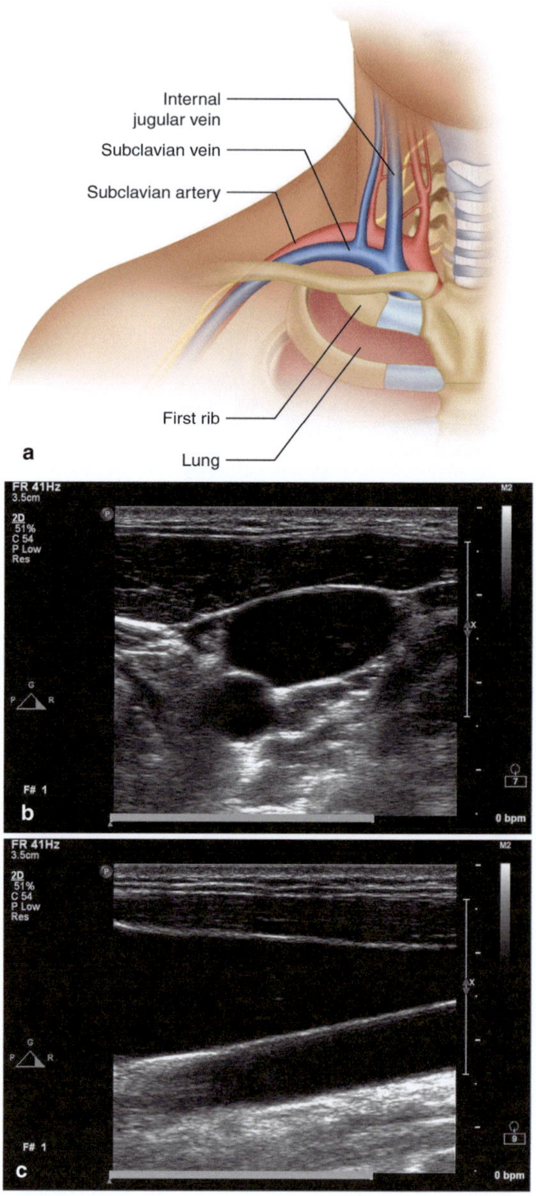

Fig. 2 Illustrates the anatomy of the internal jugular vein and its relationship to the carotid artery and subclavian vein (**a**). Ultrasound imaging of the internal jugular vein (IJV) and carotid artery (CA) is demonstrated in short axis (**b**) and in long axis (**c**)

Procedure

Peripheral access with the ultrasound machine requires a dynamic approach, where the operator identifies and cannulates the vein using real time ultrasound guidance. Described below is a suggested technique for the procedure adapted from previously suggested checklists and descriptions in addition to clinical experience of the authors [8, 9].

1. Recommended supplies:
    - Ultrasound machine
    - Gloves
    - Tegaderm × 2 (one for the probe for cleanliness and one for securing the site)
    - Sterile gel
    - Tourniquet device
    - Skin cleansing agent
    - Device catheter
    - Gauze
    - IV tubing
    - Blood collection materials if drawing blood samples
    - Saline flush
    - Dressing
2. Prep the patient and ultrasound machine:
    - Position arm to fully maximize vein exposure, this may include placing patient in a more supine position or extending the arm on a table (Fig. 3).
    - Place the ultrasound on the side of the desired vein and so the screen can be easily viewed.
    - Use the high frequency linear array probe (7.5–10.0 MHz) under "vascular" mode or other superficial setting, which will provide higher resolution for superficial structures.
    - Though not always necessary, the focus and gain of the machine can be adjusted to increase the resolution and clarity of the blood vessels and surrounding structures.
3. Prepare to scan:
    - Place a tegaderm over the surface of the transducer and apply sterile gel over the tegaderm.
    - Cleanse the patient's skin with approved antiseptic agent.

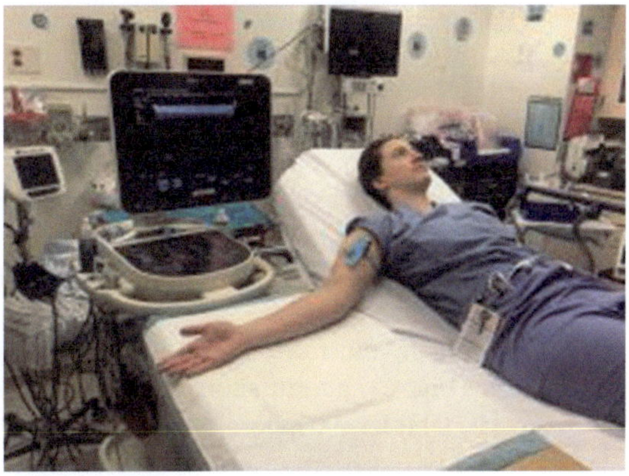

Fig. 3 Patient positioning

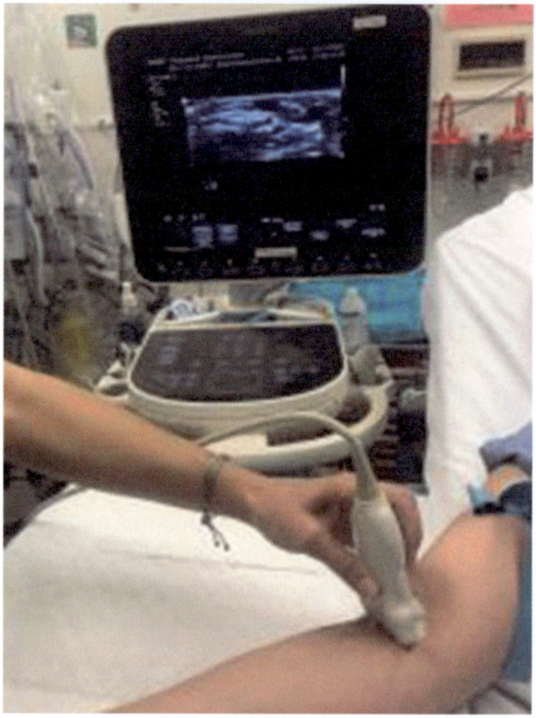

Fig. 4 Probe placement

- Position the tourniquet as close to the axilla as possible.
- Place the transducer in the transverse orientation with the probe marker towards the right of the patient. The patient's right side will now be displayed on the left side of the ultrasound monitor. Therefore, when the transducer is moved right and left, the image on the screen will be in the proper orientation from the operator's point-of-view (Fig. 4).
- Start with the probe in the antecubital fossa. Veins will appear as anechoic circular structures in the transverse (short axis) orientation and as anechoic horizontal structures in the longitudinal (long axis) orientation (Fig. 5a).

4. Choose an appropriate vein:
   - Look for a vein with large diameter and superficial location, and evaluate the vein's location in relation to surrounding arteries and nerves. Make sure to track the chosen vein both proximally and distally along the arm, keeping the vein in the center of the screen the entire time. This will make sure the transducer is entirely perpendicular to the vein. Check if the vein quickly dives deep or if there are branch points along the vein before choosing a suitable access point.
   - Distinguish vein from artery. Start by compressing the vessel with the transducer (Fig. 6); a vein should easily collapse, while an artery will not. As a caveat, smaller peripheral arteries may collapse with pressure, especially in hypotensive patients, and excessive pressure will collapse both vein and

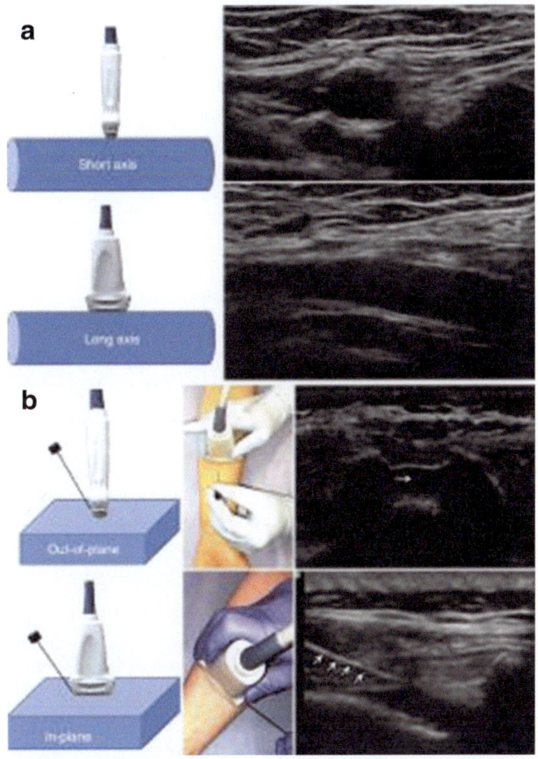

Fig. 5 (**a**) Ultrasound appearance of vein in both short and long axis. (**b**) Needle angle on insertion for both out-of-plane and in-plane approach

artery. If needed, the color-flow Doppler or pulsed-wave Doppler can be utilized to help differentiate between the venous and arterial systems: arteries with have a pulsatile flow while veins will have a more stable, lower amplitude flow. If an artery is accidentally cannulated the catheter and needle should be removed and firm pressure should be held for several minutes. The site should then be inspected for signs of ongoing bleeding or hematoma formation.

- Evaluate for potential venous clot, which can be done by checking the vein for internal echoes and assessing compressibility. A vessel that contains a clot should not be fully compressible and should not be cannulated (Fig. 7).
- Once a suitable vein is selected, an image may be captured for documentation purposes.
- As a rule of thumb, those recommendations for peripheral IV site selection still hold true for using the ultrasound such as not using arms with dialysis fistulas or surgical histories such as mastectomies.

5. Access and cannulate the vein:
   - Place the vein in the center of the screen and adjust the depth so the vein is well visualized; too shallow of a view and it may be difficult to continue to visualize the vein if it begins to dive deeper.

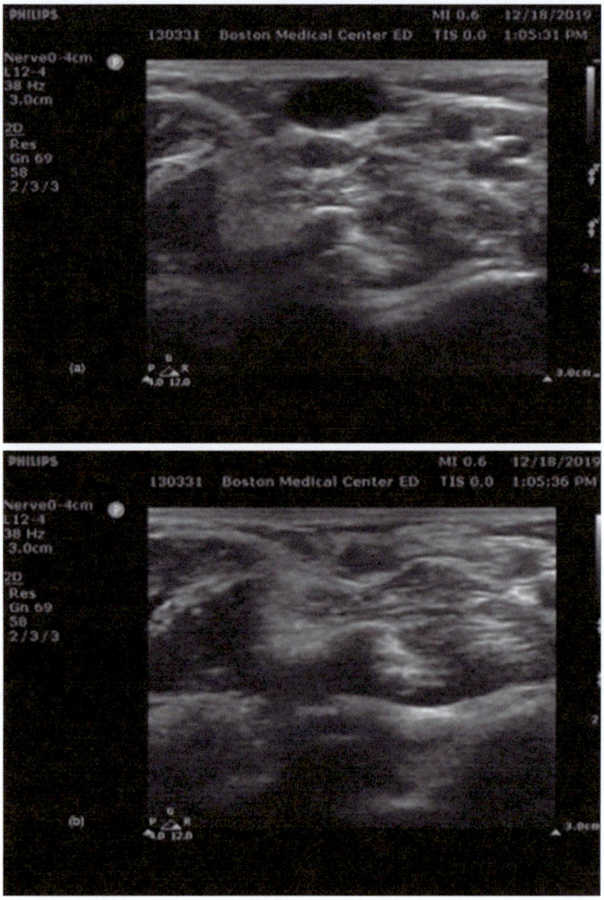

Fig. 6 (**a**) vein in short axis (**b**) vein in short axis after compression

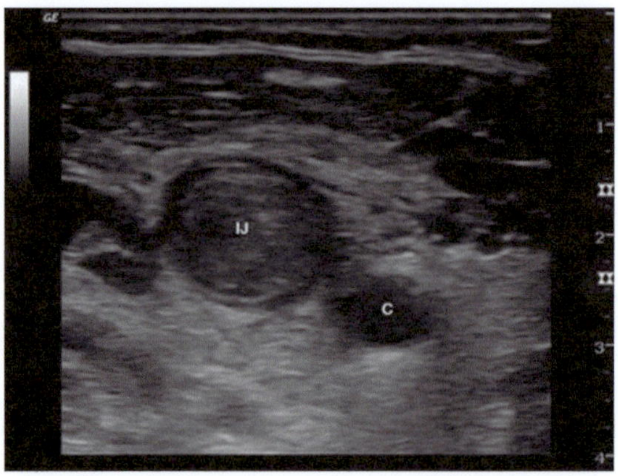

Fig. 7 Venous clot

- Assess the depth of the vein using the markings on the side of the ultrasound monitor. Choose a catheter based on the depth of the chosen vein. Unless the vein is very superficial (e.g. <1 cm from the skin) a longer angiocatheter is a better choice. A standard angiocatheter is typically about 3.2 cm long, while a longer angiocatheter is about 5 cm [10]. We recommend trying to cannulate a vessel less than 1.5 cm in depth if using a 5 cm length angiocatheter as deeper vessels will have higher rates of failure.
- Stabilize probe position by resting your wrist, hand or fingertips on the patient.
- Insert the needle at a 45-degree angle in the center of the probe at the same distance from the probe as the depth of the vein (Fig. 5b). On the screen, the needle will appear as a bright, white, hyperechoic dot (Fig. 8).
- Slowly advance the needle towards the vein while adjusting the transducer more proximally up the arm. Track the needle tip sequentially in 1–2 mm increments, advancing the transducer proximally up the arm while advancing the needle, maintaining visualization of the needle tip throughout. This is known as the "out-of-plane" technique.
- Once the needle tip reaches the vein, the operator can visualize the needle tip "tenting" the vein and then entering the vein so that a "target sign" appears on the screen (Fig. 9) [10]. There may be a popping sensation as this happens. It is possible to see a "target sign" without having "popped" through the vein and there will be no flash of blood in the catheter. If this happens, advance the needle further into the vein while maintaining the "target sign" until a flash of blood is seen. Maintaining the "target sign" throughout helps prevent "back-walling" or breaking through the posterior wall of the vein (Fig. 10). If the needle becomes lost on the screen during the procedure, gently jiggle the needle tip and move the transducer slowly up and down the arm until the bright tip of the needle is relocated. We recommend caution while advancing and moving the needle as it can damage tissues such as nerves and arteries.
- Once a flash of blood is seen, drop the angle of the needle as needed to maintain the "target sign".

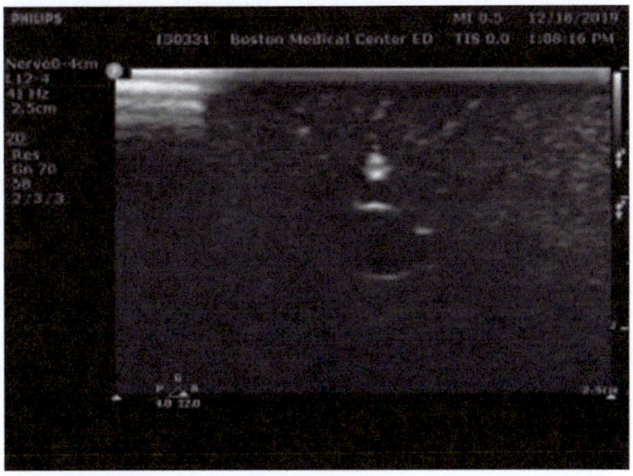

Fig. 8 Needle visualized as hyperechoic dot above vein in out-of-plane technique. (Of note a simulation gel was used instead of human tissue for this image)

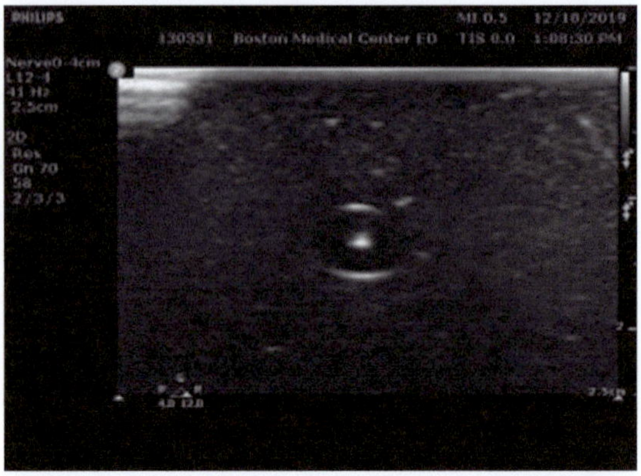

Fig. 9 Target sign. (Of note a simulation gel was used instead of human tissue for this image)

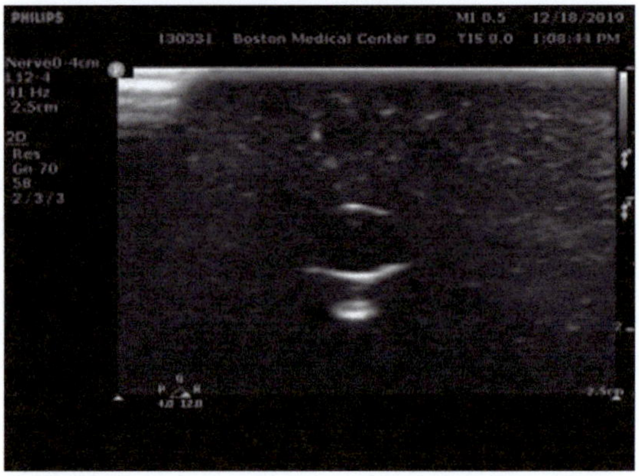

Fig. 10 Needle tip through the back wall of the vein. (Of note a simulation gel was used instead of human tissue for this image)

- Advance the transducer up the arm until the needle tip disappears and then advance the needle another 1–2 mm until the target signs reappears. This is known as the "vanishing target sign", and can be done sequentially until the operator is confident the catheter can be advanced safely. For deeper veins it is a good idea to sequentially advance the needle several times to avoid the needle coming out of the vein when probe pressure is removed.
- The next steps are identical to standard peripheral IV placement, including advancing the plastic catheter off the needle, retracting the needle, attaching IV tubing, and securing the IV. There may be a significant amount of blood return from the angiocatheter after retracting the needle, especially when a larger vein is cannulated. Gauze tactfully placed underneath the angiocatheter prior to retracting the needle may prevent blood from getting on the patient, sheets and other materials. It is also helpful to apply pressure with one hand above the catheter over the vein to slow bleeding. Securing the IV is especially important in ultrasound-guided peripheral lines and should not be overlooked. One may find that the sterile gel will impede adhesive devices and special attention should be paid to clean the skin carefully prior to applying a dressing.

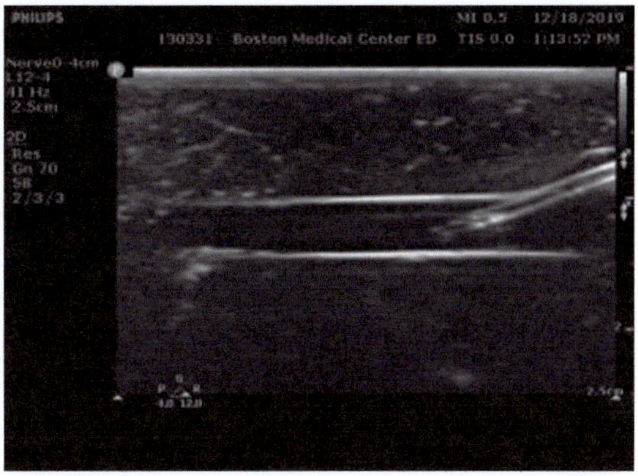

Fig. 11 In-plane image of catheter inserting into the vein. (Of note a simulation gel was used instead of human tissue for this image)

6. Confirm placement:
   - As in standard IV placement, aspiration of blood from the angiocatheter suggests correct location within the vein.
   - Using the ultrasound, one can adjust the transducer to the sagittal or "in-plane" orientation so that the vein is visible going from left to right across the screen. Probe adjustment may be required, however the catheter should be visible within the vessel (Fig. 11).
   - The operator can also place the probe proximal to the catheter location and inject agitated saline into the catheter; if it is in the correct position there will be small hyperechoic dots within the vein on the screen representing micro-bubbles.
7. Finishing touches:
   - Remove the tegaderm from the transducer and clean with an approved solution.
   - Dispose of sharps and clean the work area.
   - If desired, save an image clip of the target vessel or catheter within the vessel in order to bill for or have proof of proper venous placement.

Pearls and Pitfalls

- Two tourniquets may be necessary for more obese patients to promote sufficient venous dilation.
- It is a good idea to clean the entire antecubital fossa and distal upper arm so there will be several options for an access point.
- Some providers prefer the "in-plane" or longitudinal technique for cannulating the vein. In this technique, the entire length of the vein is visualized across the screen and the needle will be seen entering from a top corner of the screen in plane with the transducer and vessel (Fig. 5b). In this view, one should be able to visualize the needle entering the vein without having

to adjust the transducer to track the needle tip. While this may lead to decreased "back-walling" as compared to the "out of plane" technique, it may be more difficult for novice operators as it requires fairly precise alignment of the vein, transducer and needle. An additional option is the "2-axis" technique in which the operator begins with the "out-of-plane" technique until they achieve a "target sign" and then rotates the transducer 90° to the longitudinal view. At this point the operator can adjust the angle of the needle and advance the tip as needed before advancing the catheter. An advantage to this technique is being able to confirm catheter placement.

Limitations

As described in the chapter, obtaining vascular access is extremely important for the DVA population and can be successfully performed using ultrasound guidance. In this section we will review some of the limitations surrounding US-guided peripheral access including complications, pediatric applications, and device selection.

Complications

The most common complications that can arise from US-guided peripheral IVs are damage to surrounding structures including nerves and arteries, in addition to infection and bleeding. One study showed no difference in infection rates between US-guided and landmark-guided PIVs, however it was unclear if there was a significant difference in damage to surrounding structures [11]. US-guided IVs also have a significant potential to fail for various reasons including infiltration, dislodgement, and extravasation. One study found a 100% failure rate when <30% of the catheter resides in the vein, and optimum IV survival occurs when >65% of the catheter resides in the vein [12]. This reinforces the use of the longer angiocatheter for deeper vessels. In extreme cases of infiltration compartment syndrome can ensue, but is rare. Compartment syndrome can result in requiring surgical intervention and possibly limb amputation. Risks for compartment syndrome include age <1 year and barriers to alert providers of complications of IVs such as alerted level of consciousness or impaired sensation [13].

Pediatric Applications

As of now, the utility of ultrasound for peripheral IV access in the pediatric DVA population is unclear. Some studies are similar to adults and show increased success with ultrasound guidance, while some show decreased or not statistically significant difference in success [14, 15]. However, these studies have limitations including small study populations and inclusion of providers who were "early adopters" to ultrasound.

That being said, obtaining access in the DVA pediatric patient is challenging, and ultrasound remains a viable option. As with adults, it is possible to access the upper extremity veins as mentioned above. Additionally, the greater saphenous vein can be a suitable and possibly safe alternative to upper extremity veins, especially in children. If US-guidance is required for access in the stable pediatric patient, there are some steps the provider can take during this procedure to help the patient feel calmer. In addition to helping the child be comfortable with a large machine near them, the provider can warm the gel and use topical anesthetics before attempting the IV. Of course in the critically ill patient, these steps will not be as important.

Device Selection

There are numerous devices available for clinical use for IV access with ultrasound. We have already reviewed standard IV catheters and those with longer catheter length for use with ultrasound. There are also long dwell peripheral IVs, midline catheters, peripherally inserted central catheters (PICCs), and central lines, which may be used with ultrasound. Midline catheters (MC) have started to gain popularity as a potential access device for the DVA population in the emergency department [16]. Midline catheters are longer catheters (typically 8–20 cm) that have either one or two lumens, and may have a Seldinger device for placement. They typically are placed with ultrasound-guidance a few centimeters proximal to the antecubital fossa and should be placed so that the catheter tip rests distal to the axillary vein. In this position, they are not considered to be in the central circulation as are central venous catheters (CVC) and PICC lines. MCs generally are approved for use up to 28 days, while PIVs tend to fail in <48 hrs [16]. MCs do have a comparable rate of bloodstream infection to standard peripherally inserted IVs, and still include risks of infiltration, dislodgement and thrombophlebitis [17]. Benefits of MCs include potential lower complication rates, fewer needle sticks, lower rates of CVC placement and decreased central-line-associated bloodstream infections (CLABSI), all of which may translate to improved care [17]. While a larger randomized-controlled-trial comparing MCs to standard PIVs, CVCs and PICC lines needs to be explored, there appears to be increasing evidence that placement on MCs in the emergency department is a generally safe option for the DVA population and should be further considered. It is noted that a PICC or CVC should be considered for placement if medications that need to be administered centrally is required. For the trauma patient a single large bore central line should be considered so rapid administration of blood or fluids can be provided.

Conclusion

As many patients may have difficult vascular access, understanding and experience with placing ultrasound guided IVs is an important clinical skill. The use of ultrasound to place an IV as described has greatly reduced the need for central venous catheters and improved patient safety. Use of ultrasound in the pre-hospital setting will likely increase as handheld devices are becoming more affordable and available. There are numerous factors that may affect selecting the proper device for vascular access, however we have found use of ultrasound IVs has been of great clinical utility.

References

1. Gottlieb M, Sundaram T, Holladay D, Nakitende D. Ultrasound-guided peripheral intravenous line placement: A narrative review of evidence-based practices. West J Emerg Med. 2017;18(6):1047–54.
2. Shokoohi H, Boniface K, McCarthy M, Khedir Al-tiae T, Sattarian M, Ding R, et al. Ultrasound-guided peripheral intravenous access program is associated with a marked reduction in central venous catheter use in non critically ill emergency department patients. Ann Emerg Med. 2013;61(2):198–203.
3. Fields JM, Piela NE, Au AK, Ku BS. Risk factors associated with difficult venous access in adult ED patients. Am J Emerg Med. 2014;32(10):1179–82.
4. Korley F. Ultrasound for venous access. In: Carmody K, Moore C, Feller-Kopman D, editors. Handbook of critical care & emergency ultrasound. New York: McGraw-Hill; 2011. p. 219–34.
5. Jones T, Stea N, Stolz U, Adhikari S. Ultrasound evaluation of saphenous vein for peripheral intravenous cannulation in adults. J Vasc Access. 2015;16(5):418–21.
6. Butterfield M, Abdelghani R, Mohamad M, Limsuwat C, Kheir F. Using ultrasound-guided peripheral catheterization of the internal jugular vein in patients with difficult venous access. Am J Ther. 2017;24(6):667–9.
7. Zitek T, Busby E, Hudson H, McCourt JD, Baydoun J, Slattery DE. Ultrasound-guided placement of since lumen peripheral intravenous catheters in the internal jugular vein. West J Emerg Med. 2018;19(5):808–12.
8. Jung CF, Breaud AH, Sheng AY, Byrne MW, Muruganandan KM, Dhanani M, et al. Delphi method validation of a procedural performance checklist for insertion of an ultrasound-guided peripheral intravenous catheter. Am J Emerg Med. 2016;34(11):2227–30.
9. Liu SW, Zane RD, Butts C. Peripheral intravenous access. In: Roberts J, Custalow C, Thomsen T, Hedges J, editors. Roberts and Hedges' clinical procedures in emergency medicine. 6th ed. Philadelphia: Elsevier Saunders; 2014. p. 385–96.
10. Elia F, Ferrari G, Molino P, Converso M, De Filippi G, Milan A, Apra F. Standard-length catheters vs long catheters in ultrasound-guided peripheral vein cannulation. Am J Emerg Med. 2012;30(5):712–6.
11. Adhikari S, Blaivas M, Morrison D, Lander L. Comparison of infection rates among ultrasound-guided versus traditionally placed peripheral intravenous lines. J Ultrasound Med. 2010;29(5):741–7.
12. Pandurangadu AV, Tucker J, Brackney AR, Bahl A. Ultrasound-guided intravenous catheter survival impacted by amount of catheter residing in the vein. Emerg Med J. 2018;35(9):550–5.
13. Pare J, Moore CL. Intravenous infiltration resulting in compartment syndrome. J Patient Saf. 2018;14(2):e6–8.
14. Otani T, Morikawa Y, Hayakawa I, Atsumi Y, Tomari K, Tomobe Y, et al. Ultrasound-guided peripheral intravenous access placement for children in the emergency department. Eur J Pediatr. 2018;177(10):1443–9.
15. Doniger SJ, Ishimine P, Fox JC, Kanegaye JT. Randomized controlled trial of ultrasound-guided peripheral intravenous catheter placement versus traditional techniques in difficult-access pediatric patients. Pediatr Emerg Care. 2009;25(3):154–9.
16. Scoppettuolo G, Pittiruti M, Pitoni S, Dolcetti L, Emoli A, Mitidieri A, et al. Ultrasound-guided "short" midline catheters for difficult venous access in the emergency department: a retrospective analysis. Int J Emerg Med. 2016;9(1):3.
17. Adams Z, Little A, Vinsant C, Khandelwal S. The midline catheter: a clinical review. J Emerg Med. 2016;51(3):252–8.

Pericardiocentesis

Stephanie K. Louka

Introduction

Cardiac tamponade is an emergent, life-threatening cause of shock and cardiac arrest. Early recognition is crucial but difficult without ultrasound. Additionally, "blind" performance of pericardiocentesis is associated with increased risk of complications and low success rate in correcting tamponade physiology [1]. Prehospital pericardiocentesis is a temporizing measure until a patient can reach definitive care.

Topic Discussion

Ultrasound for Recognition of Tamponade Physiology

Pericardial effusions are easily identifiable using portable ultrasound. When pericardial effusions are large enough, or occur rapidly, patients are at risk for developing cardiac tamponade. Cardiac tamponade occurs when the pressure from fluid in the pericardial space rises and impedes the ability of the heart to fill and contract effectively. The result is hypotension and shock. The volume of a pericardial effusion does not dictate clinical significance. The presence of physiologic fluid, from 15 mL to 50 mL, can be normal. Patients with large volume pericardial effusions (>500 mL) may not exhibit tamponade physiology if accumulation has been slow [1].

Clinically significant pericardial effusions are best visualized via the parasternal long axis and subxiphoid views. The most sensitive and earliest sign of tamponade physiology is collapse of the right atrium during systole, while the most specific sign is collapse of the right ventricle during diastole [2].

S. K. Louka (✉)
VCU Health, Richmond, VA, USA
e-mail: stephanie.louka@vcuhealth.org

B. D. Nicholson et al. (eds.), *Manual of Austere and Prehospital Ultrasound*,
https://doi.org/10.1007/978-3-030-64287-7_20

Ultrasound for Procedural Guidance

Whenever possible, performance of pericardiocentesis under ultrasound guidance is preferred over blind techniques. When ultrasound is used in-hospital for drainage of significant effusions, procedural success rates near 100% versus blind performance which has shown a risk of life-threatening complications as high as 20.9% [3].

In-hospital, if ultrasonography is available and the clinical situation allows, the recommended anatomic approach for pericardiocentesis is parasternal as it avoids most critical anatomic structures [4]. The subxiphoid approach, while safest in blind performance, is associated with the highest rates of morbidity and mortality [5]. Per ATLS guidelines, blind performance of pericardiocentesis with subxiphoid approach is accepted practice in emergent situations such as cardiac arrest or hemodynamic compromise with high suspicion for cardiac tamponade as cause [6]. The parasternal approach is not mentioned or taught in most prehospital courses. This is unlikely deliberate and more likely a relic of earlier times when portable ultrasound technology was just not available in this environment (Figs. 1 and 2).

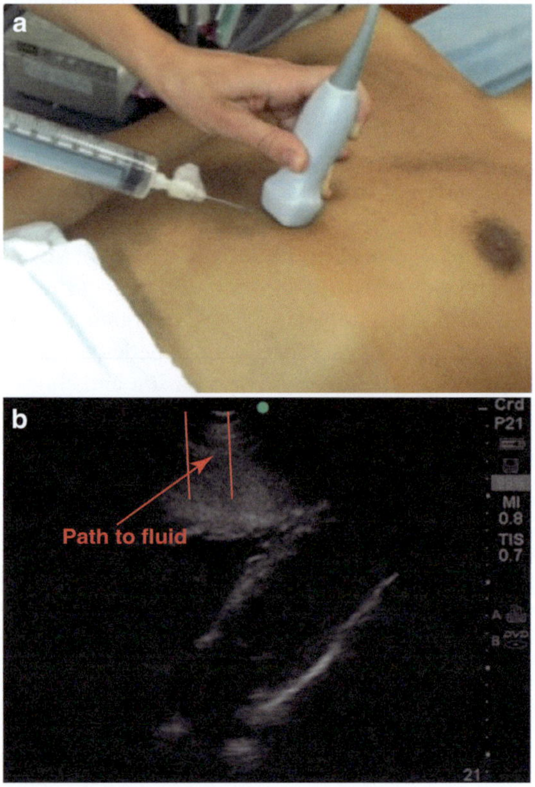

Fig. 1 Subxiphoid approach utilizing dynamic ultrasound guidance

Fig. 2 Apical approach utilizing dynamic ultrasound guidance

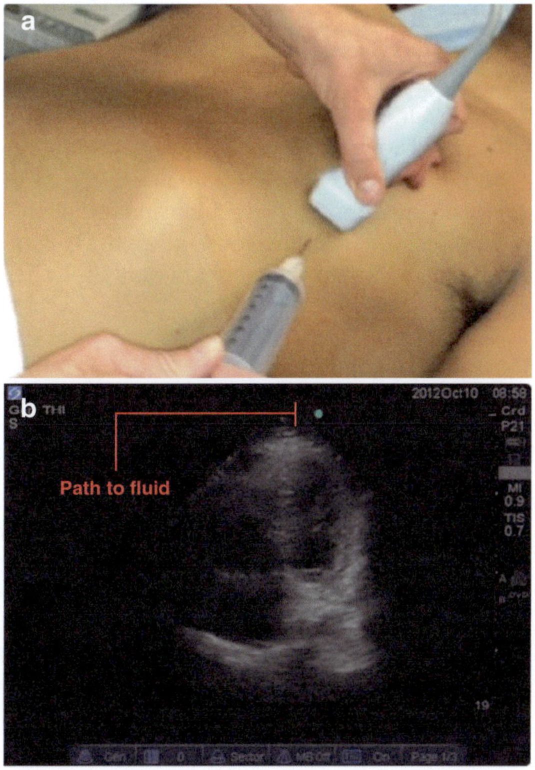

Key Literature Reviewed

There is a notable absence of literature surrounding the performance of pericardiocentesis in the prehospital setting, nevertheless ultrasound-guided pericardiocentesis in the prehospital setting. There are scattered case reports of emergency physician-performed pericardiocentesis, but no case reports of pericardiocentesis by non-physician EMS providers or formal studies with multiple subjects.

In a case report published in 2008, an anesthesia-boarded EMS Physician identified cardiac tamponade via subxiphoid ultrasound in a pregnant stabbing victim in cardiac arrest. Pericardiocentesis was performed on scene in the patient's apartment with immediate return of spontaneous circulation. She made a full neurologic recovery, but the 26 week fetus was lost [7]. In this case from Ireland, the provider performing both the ultrasound and pericardiocentesis was an anesthesia-boarded physician practicing in the prehospital setting where physician-staffed ambulances are common.

Limitations of Current Knowledge and Opportunities for Future Research

There is currently no data supporting the use of the parasternal approach over the subxiphoid approach in the prehospital setting when ultrasound is readily available. Currently the subxiphoid approach is the primary, and in some cases the only, approach taught in standard prehospital trauma and critical care courses. This is an opportunity for study; however, given the lack of familiarity of alternative anatomic approaches, additional training of non-physician EMS providers is needed.

Procedure Performance

Indications

The indication for an emergent, prehospital pericardiocentesis is detection of a clinically significant pericardial effusion with evidence of tamponade physiology (right atrial collapse during systole and/or right ventricular collapse during diastole) on bedside ultrasound. Patients will exhibit hemodynamic instability in the form of shock or cardiac arrest.

The prehospital pericardiocentesis is always for therapeutic purposes. There is no role in the prehospital setting for a diagnostic pericardiocentesis.

Contraindications

There are no absolute contraindications to emergent pericardiocentesis. Relative contraindications include: coagulopathy, presence of cardiac devices (pacemakers, AICD, prosthetic heart valve), previous thoracoabdominal surgery, and poor visualization of effusion and/or cardiac structures on ultrasound [1].

Preparation

1. Equipment
   (a) Required:
       16 or 18 g, 6 in. (15 cm) catheter/needle or longer
       35 mL or 60 mL luer lock syringe
       3-way stopcock
   (b) Optional:
       Ultrasound machine with curvilinear or phased array probe
       Lidocaine 1% solution
       10 cc syringe
       Small caliber injection needle
       Alcohol prep/Chlorhexidine/Betadine or other antiseptic
       Cardiac monitor and leads

2. Patient preparation & positioning
   (a) Supine position
   (b) On cardiac monitor (Lead II displaying)
3. Approach
   (a) Subxiphoid (blind or with ultrasound guidance)
       Needle insertion 1 cm inferior to the xiphoid process and left xiphocostal angle
       30° angle of needle to patient skin
       Ultrasound guidance with curvilinear or phased array probe in subxiphoid orientation
       Advance toward patient's left shoulder
   (b) Parasternal (with ultrasound guidance)
       Needle insertion adjacent to and left of the sternum, fifth intercostal space, above the rib to avoid the inferior vascular bundle
       45–60° angle of needle to patient skin
       Ultrasound guidance with curvilinear or phased array probe. Identify maximal fluid collection and orient probe so this collection is closest to the transducer. Needle and probe in longitudinal orientation with probe indicator pointing toward apex [5].
   (c) Alternative Approaches (not indicated in emergency situations)
       Apical [4]

Procedure

Ultrasound

1. Using either a parasternal long axis or subxiphoid view, verify presence of a pericardial effusion with tamponade physiology.
2. Of these views, select the one that allows best visualization of the pericardial effusion at its deepest (ideally >20 mm of separation between the pericardium and myocardial tissue).
3. Elect for either subxiphoid or parasternal approach for pericardiocentesis based on this information.

Analgesia

1. After locating the landmark for needle insertion, if time allows and patient's condition warrants, insert the medication needle and inject lidocaine into the tissue surrounding the needle insertion site.
2. Local anesthetic may not be required in some circumstances (e.g. cardiac arrest).

Needle Insertion & Aspiration

1. Using a subxiphoid or parasternal approach, insert the aspiration needle into the skin.
2. Pull back on the plunger to aspirate as you advance the needle, checking the syringe for return of blood or other fluids. In cases of traumatic pericardial effusions, blood return is to be expected. In cases of atraumatic pericardial effusions,

aspiration of frank blood may indicate penetration of a vessel or chamber of the heart. If frank blood is noted, conisder leaving the needle in place if additional equipment is available to make a separate drainage attempt as removal of the needle could provide a pathway for escape of blood from the affected chamber into the pericardial sac. If a second set of equipment is not available, retract the needle and reevaluate your approach.

3. Visualize the needle advance through the pericardium and into the pericardial space. At this point, there should be return of pericardial fluid. As soon as fluid return is identified, stop advancing the aspiration needle.
4. Continue to aspirate fluid from the pericardial space into the syringe. If aspiration suddenly becomes difficult, reconfirm presence of fluid still remaining within the pericardial space. If the fluid is absent, proceed to securing catheter as described below. If fluid is still present, adjust the needle by advancing or retracting slightly to change position. In cases of traumatic effusion, consider clotted blood as a likely cause of needle occlusion and adjust needle accordingly, attempting to aspirate any non-clotted blood [1, 4–6]. Aspiration of just a small volume of pericardial fluid (35–50 mL) is often adequate to achieve return of spontaneous circulation (ROSC) or hemodynamic stability [1].
5. Whenever advancing the needle, it is important to monitor the ECG tracing for a "current of injury" pattern (ST-segment elevation) that suggests contact of the needle with the myocardial surface. Additionally, ectopic beats such as premature ventricular contracts (PVCs) also indicate possible myocardial contact [6]. If these ECG changes are noted, the needle should be withdrawn until the baseline ECG tracing returns. If possible, connect a V lead directly to the aspiration needle to best visualize the "current of injury" phenomenon [1].

Securing the Catheter

1. Upon completion of aspiration, remove the needle and syringe, leaving the catheter in place.
2. Attach a 3-way stopcock to the catheter and leave it in the closed position.
3. Suture or tape the catheter in place, and cover with a dry dressing. Do not excessively tape, as the 3-way stopcock must be quickly accessible should the effusion reaccumulate and hemodynamic instability recur.

Repeat Aspiration

1. If after the initial fluid aspiration, the patient experiences a deterioration in hemodynamic stability and return of shock state, consider reaccumulation of the pericardial effusion as cause. Obtain repeat ultrasound views in the parasternal long axis and/or the subxiphoid views.
2. If the effusion has reaccumulated, reattach the syringe to the 3-way stopcock and attempt to aspirate additional fluid [6].

Pericardiocentesis Catheter (Optional)

1. If available prehospital or upon Emergency Department arrival, consider changing out the initial IV catheter with a flexible catheter. Using a Seldinger technique, pass a guidewire through the initial catheter into the pericardial space. This can be done with active ultrasound guidance to ensure correct location of the guidewire.
2. Remove the initial catheter, leaving the guidewire in place.
3. Pass a 14-gauge flexible pericardiocentesis catheter over the guidewire.
4. Attach a 3-way stopcock.
5. Secure in place with sutures (preferred) or other available material [6].

References

1. "Pericardiocentesis." Clinical procedures in emergency medicine, by James R. Roberts and Jerris R. Hedges, Saunders/Elsevier, 2010.
2. Chapter 3: Cardiac ultrasound – pericardial effusion and tamponade. Clinical ultrasound: a pocket manual, by Angela Creditt et al., Springer, 2018, pp. 69–73.
3. Kil UH, Jung HO, Koh YS, Park HJ, Park CS, Kim PJ, Baek SH, Seung KB, Choi KB. Prognosis of large, symptomatic pericardial effusion treated by echo-guided percutaneous pericardiocentesis. Clin Cardiol. 2008;31:531–7.
4. Loukas M, Walters A, Boon JM, Welch TP, Meiring JH, Abrahams PH. Pericardiocentesis: a clinical anatomy review. Clin Anat. 2012;25:872–81.
5. Tsang TS, Freeman WK, Sinak LJ, Seward JB. Echocardiographically guided pericardiocentesis: evolution and state-of-the-art technique. Mayo Clin Proc. 1998;73:647–52.
6. "Skill Station VII: Chest trauma management." Advanced Trauma Life Support: ATLS Student Course Manual, American College of Surgeons. 2012. pp. 120–121.
7. Byhahn C, Bingold T, Zwissler B, Maier M, Walcher F. Prehospital ultrasound detects pericardial tamponade in a pregnant victim of stabbing assault. Resuscitation. 2008;76(1):146–8.

Surgical Cricothyroidotomy

Randy M. Kring, Christopher F. Allison,
and David C. Mackenzie

Introduction

For a medical provider in an austere setting, perhaps no procedure is more vital or anxiety-provoking than the surgical airway. In a cannot-intubate, cannot-ventilate situation—often a consequence of significant facial trauma—the surgical cricothyrotomy is a last resort, life-saving procedure. Fortunately, the equipment required to perform this procedure is minimal. A surgical airway can be successfully obtained with a scalpel, bougie, and 6-0 cuffed endotracheal tube.

Traditionally, the surgical cricothyrotomy has been performed as a landmark-guided procedure, with inspection and palpation providing the only guidance to cannulate the cricothyroid membrane (CTM). Ultrasound can be used to dramatically improve localization of the CTM, especially in patients with difficult anatomy [1–3]. This chapter describes the ultrasound techniques used to identify the CTM, a step-by-step strategy for performing ultrasound-guided surgical cricothyrotomy, and review the literature supporting this strategy for obtaining a surgical airway.

Topic Discussion

General Strategy

There are two general strategies for ultrasound-guided surgical cricothyrotomy which have been described in the literature [4, 5]. In the first strategy, the location of the cricothyroid membrane (CTM) is pre-marked using ultrasound guidance. Pre-marking the CTM has the advantage of allowing the provider to have both hands free to obtain the surgical airway after marking is complete. However, this

R. M. Kring (✉) · C. F. Allison · D. C. Mackenzie
Department of Emergency Medicine, Maine Medical Center, Portland, ME, USA

B. D. Nicholson et al. (eds.), *Manual of Austere and Prehospital Ultrasound*,
https://doi.org/10.1007/978-3-030-64287-7_21

strategy does require advance preparation, and relies on accurate marking for success. In the second strategy, the provider uses real-time point of care ultrasound to identify the CTM while performing the surgical airway. This strategy allows for dynamic evaluation of airway anatomy and more rapid placement of a surgical airway as no pre-marking is required. However, it does require the provider to devote one hand to point-of-care ultrasound use during the procedure. These two strategies are not mutually exclusive, as the provider may choose to mark the location of the cricothyroid membrane as a first step, and use real-time point of care ultrasound to evaluate the airway while performing the surgical airway. We recommend providers be familiar with both strategies, as the strategy ultimately selected will depend on preparation time available and clinical context. Furthermore, we advise providers to recognize that ultrasound should likely not be used in the "crash," failed airway due to need for rapid placement of a surgical airway. In this time-critical context, the traditional landmark-guided technique for surgical cricothyrotomy is likely superior.

Ultrasound Evaluation of the Trachea

As a relatively superficial structure, the trachea is best evaluated by the linear probe (15-6 MHz). If a linear probe is not available, a curvilinear probe (5-2 MHz) will provide an adequate image, but care should be taken to ensure minimum depth is used to optimize image resolution. In patients with minimal subcutaneous fat overlying the trachea, sufficient gel should be used to allow sliding the probe over the elevated cartilaginous rings of the trachea.

The trachea can be evaluated in both a transverse and longitudinal (sagittal) plane. We find that the longitudinal plane provides better visualization of the anatomy and easier identification of the CTM. As is convention, the probe marker should be positioned towards the patient's right for a transverse evaluation of the trachea, and towards the patient's head for a longitudinal evaluation of the trachea.

Prior to placing the ultrasound probe on the patient's neck, the anatomy of the trachea should be palpated. This is best done with the patient's head in as much extension as possible, while still maintaining cervical spine stabilization if necessary. Key anatomic landmarks to palpate (from cephalad to caudad) include the thyroid cartilage, the cricothyroid membrane, the cricoid cartilage, and the tracheal rings (Fig. 1).

The midline of the trachea should then be identified, and the ultrasound probe placed in longitudinal orientation just caudad to the thyroid cartilage (Fig. 2a). The following image will be obtained (Fig. 2b). Note that the cartilage of the thyroid cartilage, cricoid cartilage, and tracheal rings appear as hypoechoic oval structures in cross section. A bright white hyperechoic line seen just deep to these cartilaginous structures identifies the air within the trachea, similar to the pleural lines seen on ultrasound of the chest. If this hyperechoic line is not seen, the ultrasound probe may not be on midline and appropriate adjustment should be made. To localize the

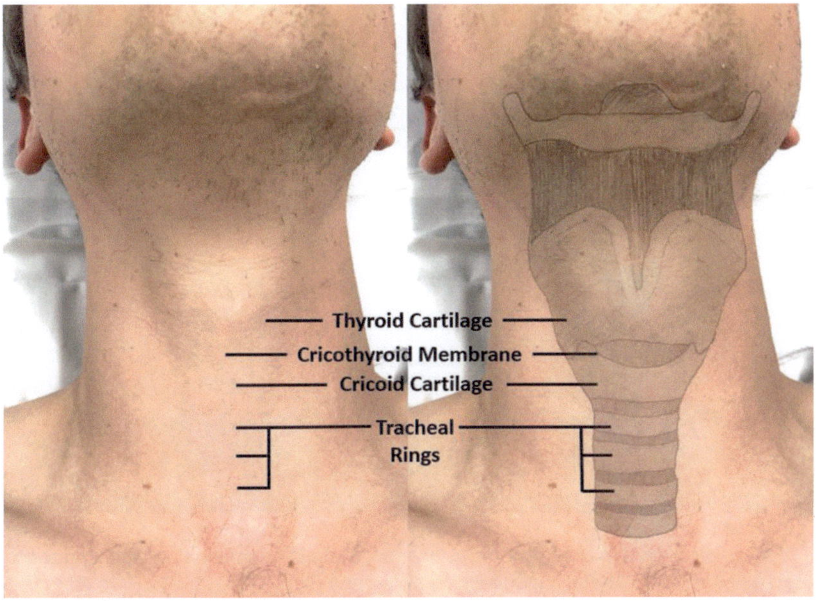

Fig. 1 Palpable anatomic landmarks along the anterior neck to identify in anticipation of a surgical cricothyroidotomy

CTM on ultrasound, the thyroid cartilage and cricoid cartilage must first be identified. In general, the thyroid cartilage will be a very prominent cartilaginous structure. The cricoid cartilage can be most reliably identified by thinking of the tracheal rings as "pearls on a string," with the "pearls" being the hypoechoic cartilage connected by the "string" of the air within the trachea. The cricoid cartilage is a slightly more prominent "pearl" at the cephalad end of this "string of pearls." The CTM will lie directly between the thyroid cartilage and cricoid cartilage.

Site Marking

Once the CTM is identified in longitudinal orientation as above, a skin marker can be used to mark its location on the patient's skin. We recommend lining the arrow of the ultrasound probe up with the CTM in order to maximize marking accuracy (Fig. 3). The ultrasound probe is then rotated into a transverse orientation, and midline is identified based on location of the hyperechoic line representing air within the trachea (Fig. 4a, b). Marking midline will allow accurate localization of the CTM (Fig. 4c). An alternative approach is to slide a hyperechoic needle between the probe and the patient's skin in order to identify the transverse location of the CTM, without need for skin marking (Fig. 5).

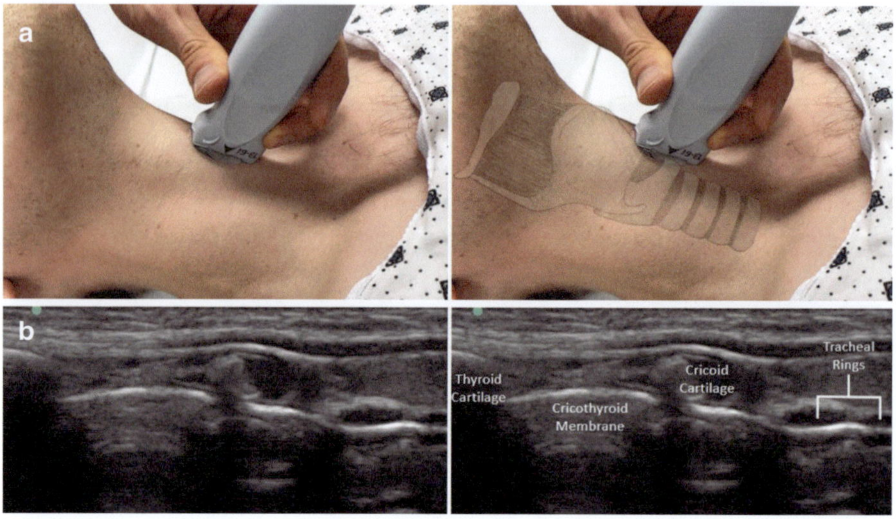

Fig. 2 Proper placement of the linear probe in a longitudinal orientation on the anterior neck (**a**) and appearance of key anatomic landmarks on ultrasound (**b**)

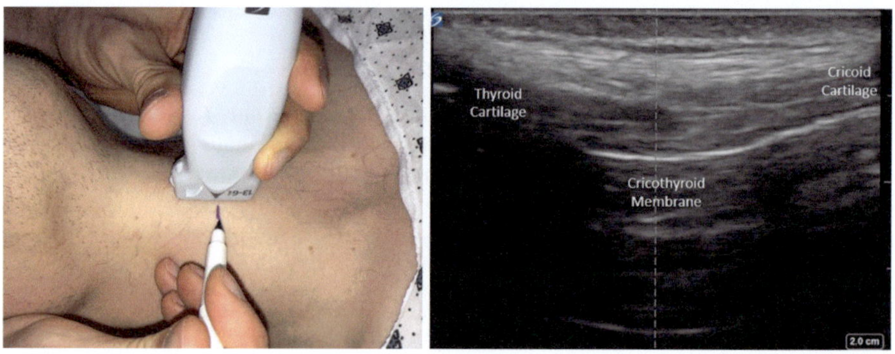

Fig. 3 Marking of the transverse plane of the cricothyroid membrane using the linear ultrasound probe in longitudinal orientation

Performing Surgical Cricothyrotomy

We recommend approaching ultrasound-guided surgical cricothyrotomy from the head of the bed, as this is already the position the provider will be in after a failed attempt at oral intubation. In this position, the ultrasound probe is held in the provider's left hand, with the ultrasound machine at the patient's feet (Fig. 6). If time allows, site marking as discussed above should be performed. However, if time does not allow for site marking, the CTM can be identified real-time in longitudinal orientation.

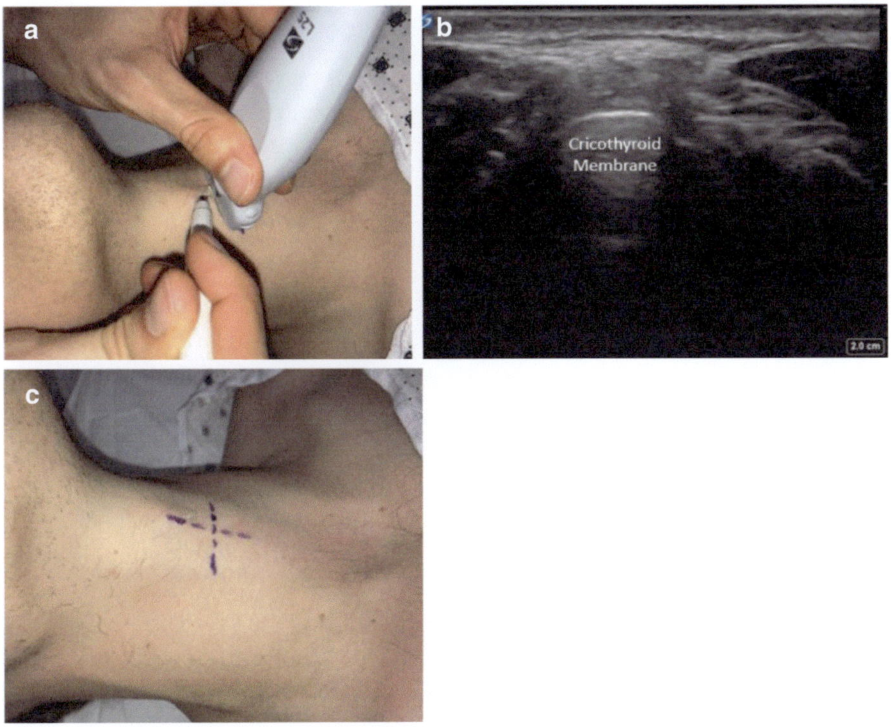

Fig. 4 (**a**) Marking the longitudinal plane of the cricothyroid membrane using the linear ultrasound probe in transverse orientation, with (**b**) the probe centered over the cricothyroid membrane. (**c**) Accurate marking of the transverse and longitudinal plane of the cricothyroid membrane

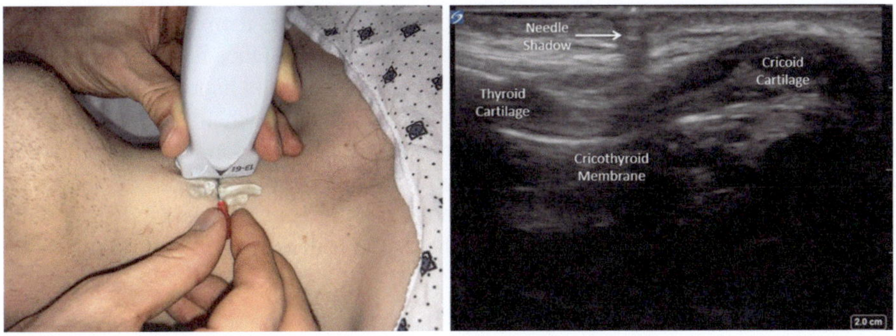

Fig. 5 Blunt fill needle placed between the linear probe in longitudinal orientation and the patient's skin to identify the transverse plane of the cricothyroid membrane

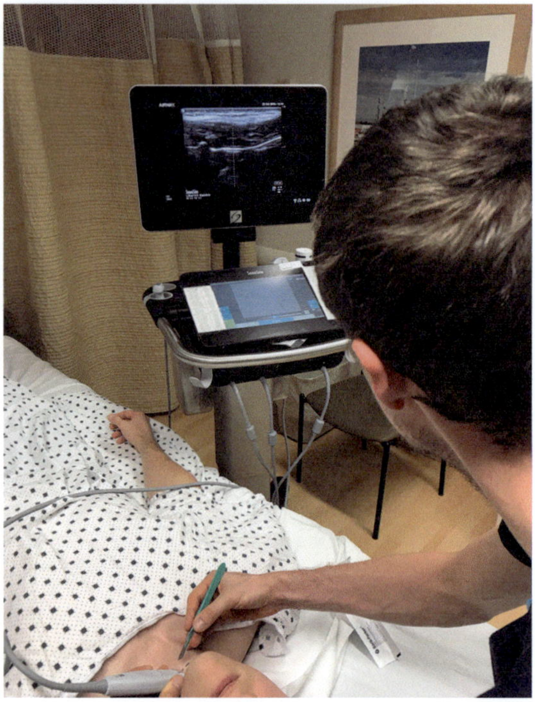

Fig. 6 Ideal placement of the ultrasound machine and linear probe for ultrasound guidance of cricothyroidotomy

Perform a surgical cricothyrotomy as follows. The scalpel, held in the right hand, is inserted into the CTM with a single horizontal stab incision, ensuring depth of the incision exceeds the depth to the CTM as visualized on ultrasound. After this stab incision is made, the scalpel must be kept within the lumen of the trachea. The scalpel is rotated 90 degrees to enlarge the opening in the CTM. The left hand then releases the ultrasound probe and picks up the bougie. The bougie is then passed through the incision into the trachea. The bougie is advanced until resistance is met to ensure the bougie is in the trachea. The scalpel is then removed. The right hand then passes a 6-0 endotracheal tube over the bougie. The endotracheal tube is then advanced into the airway. The cuff is inflated and successful placement of the endotracheal tube into the trachea is confirmed via auscultation and end-tidal CO_2 monitoring if available. The presence of lung sliding visualized bilaterally with thoracic ultrasound also supports that the tube is in the airway. The endotracheal tube is then secured to the skin.

Pearls and Pitfalls

Crucial to successful performance of a surgical cricothyrotomy is to not overthink and delay the procedure when it is indicated. Undoubtedly when you are called on to perform this procedure it will be in a highly stressful situation.

- Recognize potentially difficult oral airways, and be prepared for a surgical airway in these cases. Gather your equipment in advance—scalpel, bougie, 6–0 endotracheal tube, and ultrasound machine with linear transducer.

- If time allows, mark the site for a surgical airway on every anticipated difficult oral airway before initiating attempt at orotracheal intubation.
- If oral airway attempts fail and a surgical airway is required, stay at the head of the bed as you prepare for the procedure. Position the ultrasound machine at the patient's feet. Pick up the linear probe in your left hand. Pick up the scalpel in your right hand.
- Place the patient's head in as much extension as possible, keeping in mind cervical spine stabilization if necessary.
- For ultrasound guidance, obtain a longitudinal visualization of the thyroid cartilage and cricoid cartilage, at the end of the "string of pearls" created by the tracheal rings.
- Be aware that marked soft tissue can shift with patient movement. Confirm the location of the CTM using ultrasound just prior to entering the skin with the scalpel.
- Do not remove the scalpel from the airway until the bougie is in the airway. Do not remove the bougie from the airway until the endotracheal tube is in the airway.
- Recognize that ultrasound should likely <u>not</u> be used in the "crash," failed airway due to need for rapid placement of a surgical airway. In this time-critical context, the traditional landmark-guided technique for surgical cricothyrotomy is likely superior.

Review of the Literature

Early in the investigations of ultrasound guidance for surgical cricothyrotomy, Nicholls et al. demonstrated the feasibility of emergency physicians with minimal training visualizing the cricothyroid membrane in a convenience sample of 50 patients in an emergency department setting. They reported mean time to visualize the cricothyroid membrane as less than 25 seconds [6].

This application was investigated further by Siddiqui et al. in a randomized trial of ultrasound-guided versus palpation-guided cricothyrotomy performed by anesthesiology residents on 52 human cadavers [1]. In this study, there was no significant difference in first-attempt cricothyrotomy success rate in all cadavers; but in the subgroup of cadavers with difficult or impossible to palpate landmarks, proper airway placement had a 5.6 times higher probability ($p = 0.043$) in the ultrasound group. Ultrasound-guidance was significantly slower, with a mean time of insertion of 196 seconds versus 110 seconds in the palpation-guided group. However, injuries to the trachea and larynx were significantly less frequent and less severe in the ultrasound group.

Additional studies have shown the benefit of ultrasound guidance in pre-marking landmarks in patients with abnormal neck anatomy. Okano et al. published a compelling case report of an obese patient with a large neck abscess. This study demonstrated how ultrasound easily identified the cricothyroid membrane when it was impossible to palpate and allowed the team to be prepared if orotracheal intubation failed [2]. A study by Siddiqui et al. of 223 patients with abnormal neck anatomy (history of neck surgery, irradiation, and/or neck mass) randomized patients to identification of cricothyrotomy anticipated entry point by palpation versus bedside ultrasonography. Ultrasound was superior at identifying entry point within 5 mm of that defined by CT, with a rate of 81% (92/114) vs. 8% (9/109) for palpation [3]. Note that cricothyrotomy was not performed on the patients in these studies.

There are concerns that landmarks identified and marked on the skin prior to failed intubation will no longer be accurate following the neck manipulation performed during intubation attempts. Mallin et al. reduced this concern in a study comparing ultrasound-guided landmarks drawn with invisible ink before simulated failed intubation and ultrasound-guided landmarks drawn afterward; the average difference in sagittal and axial planes was about 1 mm [7]. This suggests that it is reasonable to mark the neck with ultrasound-obtained landmarks before an anticipated difficult airway for which cricothyrotomy may be needed as a rescue maneuver.

Limitations of Current Literature

Current literature supports the notion that ultrasound facilitates accurate identification of cricothyrotomy landmarks in patients with factors that limit easy palpation of the cricothyroid membrane. However, this has not been prospectively studied in patients requiring urgent cricothyrotomy, and thus we lack data to assess if ultrasound improves outcomes such as success rate and time to endotracheal intubation. Given the rarity of cricothyrotomy, it will be difficult to produce a study with sufficient power to show improved clinical outcomes. This remains an opportunity for research. When time permits and landmarks cannot be easily palpated, ultrasonographic identification of the cricothyroid membrane is a reasonable step that will likely facilitate emergent cricothyrotomy.

References

1. Siddiqui N, Arzola C, Friedman Z, Guerina L, You-Ten KE. Ultrasound improves cricothyrotomy success in cadavers with poorly defined neck anatomy: a randomized control trial. Anesthesiology. 2015;11:1033–41.
2. Okano H, Kohji U, Watanabe K, et al. Ultrasound-guided identification of the cricothyroid membrane in a patient with a difficult airway: a case report. BMC Emerg Med. 2018;18:5.
3. Siddiqui N, Yu E, Boulis S, You-Ten KE. Ultrasound is superior to palpation in identifying the cricothyroid membrane in subjects with poorly defined neck landmarks. Anesthesiology. 2018;129:1132.
4. Curtis K, Ahern M, Dawson M, Mallin M. Ultrasound-guided, Bougie-assisted cricothyroidotomy: a description of a novel technique in cadaveric models. Acad Emerg Med. 2012;19:876–9.
5. Kristensen MS, Teoh WH, Rudolph SS. Ultrasonographic identification of the cricothyroid membrane: best evidence, techniques, and clinical impact. Br J Anaesth. 2016;117(S1):i39–48.
6. Nicholls SE, Sweeney TW, Ferre RM, Strout TD. Bedside sonography by emergency physicians for the rapid identification of landmarks relevant to cricothyrotomy. Am J Emerg Med. 2008;26(8):852–6.
7. Mallin M, Curtis K, Dawson M, Ockerse P, Ahern M. Accuracy of ultrasound-guided marking of the cricothyroid membrane before simulated failed intubation. Am J Emerg Med. 2014;32(1):61–3.

Advanced Procedure Topic for Austere Providers: Thoracentesis

Amir Louka

Introduction

Unlike most procedures, accessing the pleural space is performed both routinely and emergently, for both diagnostic and therapeutic purposes. In general, the aim of the procedure is to remove fluid or air from the pleural space, between the lung and chest wall. Traditionally, confirmation of both pneumothorax and pleural effusion has been via chest radiography, either CT or x-ray, and practitioners have relied on physical exam to determine landmarks at the time of the procedure. Chest ultrasound, however, lends itself well to all aspects of the procedure. Ultrasound may be used for the diagnosis of chest pathology including pleural effusion and pneumothorax, administration of local anesthesia, identification of landmarks and procedural guidance. By incorporating ultrasound, chest drain placement can be done quickly, safely and effectively.

Discussion

Thoracentesis

Thoracentesis refers to the act of placing a needle through the chest wall, into the pleural space for the purpose of removing air or fluid. In stable patients, this may be done to relieve symptoms of dyspnea and/or to collect a fluid sample for laboratory analysis. There are many causes for fluid to collect in the pleural space including malignancy, infection, intrathoracic bleeding and edema, or any combination of these. For cases in which the diagnosis is unclear or a single therapy is expected to

A. Louka (✉)
Department of Emergency Medicine, VCU Medical Center/VCU Health, Richmond, VA, USA
e-mail: amir.louka@vcuhealth.org

B. D. Nicholson et al. (eds.), *Manual of Austere and Prehospital Ultrasound*,
https://doi.org/10.1007/978-3-030-64287-7_22

be sufficient or temporizing, thoracentesis provides a less invasive means of drainage than thoracostomy and can be done without leaving a catheter in place, if desired.

Extra-pulmonary air, on the other hand, often collects due to damage to the lung, bronchus, trachea or esophagus, allowing air to escape into the pleural space. This may be spontaneous or due to trauma, blunt or penetrating. Alternatively, trauma to the chest wall may occur, allowing air to be drawn in from outside of the chest. In either case, rapid diagnosis and treatment are needed to prevent the development of tension pneumothorax, a potentially life-threatening condition in which extra-pulmonary air exerts pressure on the heart, preventing diastolic filling and leading to hemodynamic collapse.

In stable but symptomatic patients, serial drainage or the placement of a drainage catheter may be required to facilitate removal of accumulating fluid or air. A variety of catheter-over-needle products are available to facilitate the placement of a temporary drain.

Diagnosis

Ultrasound can be used to detect both pneumothorax and pleural effusion. This is primarily accomplished by determining the presence of "lung-slide," the sonographic image of lung tissue passing back and forth across the parietal pleura as the patient breaths. Unlike other parts of the body, ultrasound cannot provide a clear image of normal lung tissue due to the presence of air. Nevertheless, a sonographer can clearly visualize the pleura as a thin, bright, hyperechoic line extending horizontally across the screen. Just above the pleural line, ribs are visible in cross section as ovoid echogenic objects with posterior shadowing. Together, when an ultrasound probe is placed on the chest wall, these structures create an image of a "shimmering" pleural line, sometimes referred to as resembling "ants on a string."

The presence of sliding lung requires contact between the parietal and visceral pleura. Separation of the two by air, such as would be found in a patient with pneumothorax, causes the pleural line to appear static, with no back and forth quality. Because extra-pulmonary air raises, this is most commonly found at the most elevated portion of the chest, anterior in a supine patient and apical in an upright patient. As the ultrasound probe is moved around the chest, lung slide may become visible, delineating the border of the pneumothorax. The interface between the sliding and non-sliding lung is termed a "lung point." The absence of lung slide confirms the diagnosis of pneumothorax, while the presence of lung points may aid in determining the size of the collection.

Similarly, a pleural effusion is identified by a lack of sliding lung. However, pleural fluid is more likely to be dependent, collecting first in the posterior thorax, just above the diaphragm. Unlike extra-pulmonary air, ultrasound waves easily penetrate pleural fluid and provide an image of dark, hypoechoic fluid below the bright pleural line or above the similarly echogenic diaphram. Collapsed lung tissue may be visible deep to the collection as an echogenic, irregular shape moving freely within the fluid (Fig. 1).

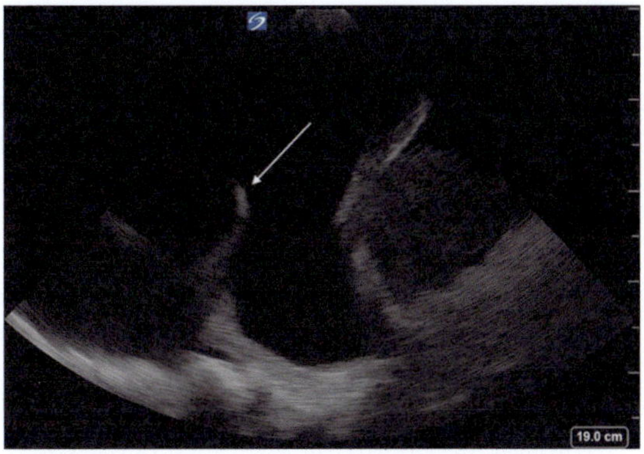

Fig. 1 Floating lung: With large pleural effusions, the lung will appear to be floating in the fluid, creating what looks like a flag flapping in the wind (flag sign)

Landmarks

Thoracentesis is usually performed in the posterior, mid-scapular line in patients able to sit upright or in the mid-axillary line on supine patients. Ultrasound is employed primarily to determine the level at which to insert the needle, with utmost care being taken to avoid insertion below the diaphragm. In contrast to physical exam which relies on imprecise techniques such as percussion and tactile fremitus, ultrasound is a painless, harmless and highly accurate means of "seeing" the targeted air or fluid collection (see section "Diagnosis").

Once the level for insertion is determined, the ribs are identified deep to the skin and subcutaneous tissue. The neurovascular bundle should be noted, most commonly along the inferior border of each rib. The intercostal nerve is visualized as a small bundle of echogenic fibers in close proximity to the hypoechoic vascular structures. Deep to the ribs, the pleural line is identified as described above.

Contraindications

There are no absolute contraindications to thoracentesis or the use of ultrasound, but there a number of relative contraindications. Primarily, overlying skin infection at the planned procedure site increases the risk of developing further infection including empyema. Additionally, a collection too small to allow for safe passage of the needle into the pleural space adds to the risk of iatrogenic lung trauma and pneumothorax. A distance greater than 1 cm between lung and chest wall is generally considered sufficient for safe drainage under ultrasound guidance. Traditionally, bleeding risk due to elevated INR or low platelets (<50,000), has been considered a contraindication. However, more recent case series have not shown this to result in a significantly increased risk of bleeding or morbidity [1].

Equipment

In the absence of a commercially available kit specific to the thoracentesis procedure, the following equipment may be assembled:

- Sterile gloves, gown and drapes
- Marking pen
- Skin sterilizing liquid such as chlorhexidine or povidone-iodine solution
- Local anesthetic such as 1–2% lidocaine, with or without epinephrine
- Needles including 21 to 25-gauge for skin/subcutaneous anesthetic and 18-gauge for drainage or over-the-needle catheter of sufficient diameter (note: wide range available depending on presumed density and viscosity of fluid to be drained)
- Drainage tubing, stopcock and collection bags or vacuum bottles
- Syringes for both infiltrating anesthetic and advancing the drainage needle (10–20 cc)
- Ultrasound machine with sterile gel, high-frequency probe and sterile probe cover

Technique

Landmarks are identified as above using a high-frequency ultrasound probe with the patient in either the upright or supine position. When the targeted collection is identified and confirmed to be of sufficient size to be amenable to percutaneous drainage, the planned access site is marked ensuring it is well above the diaphragm. Due to the potential for diaphragmatic movement during the procedure, insertion below the ninth rib is generally avoided. The marked site and surrounding skin are sterilized using chlorhexidine or povidone-iodine solution. Sterile drapes should now be applied and sterile technique followed by the provider, including the use of a sterile probe cover and ultrasound gel.

Local anesthetic is applied to the skin and subcutaneous tissue at the marked site. Using ultrasound, the neurovascular bundle is again identified below the nearest rib, and additional anesthetic can be provided directly to the intercostal nerve using in-plane technique. This can be repeated at the ribs above and below the access site for more complete regional anesthesia if planning to use a larger bore drainage catheter.

Generally, dynamic guidance is not needed for insertion of the drainage needle, but it can be used if landmarks are difficult to palpate or distorted by trauma, for example. Attached to a 10–20 cc syringe, the needle is inserted perpendicular to the skin at the marked site, maintaining negative pressure on the syringe as the needle is advanced through the skin, subcutaneous tissue, over the nearest rib and through the pleura. Entry into the collection is noted by the sudden release of negative pressure on the syringe. At this time, the catheter can be advanced over the needle and drainage tubing attached or a sample collection syringe attached, fluid aspirated and the needle withdrawn.

Key Literature Reviewed

A paucity of literature exists regarding ultrasound guided austere or prehospital thoracentesis. However, a growing fund of knowledge describes the limitations of prehospital thoracentesis for tension pneumothorax, more commonly referred to as needle-decompression. Multiple studies have aimed to determine the efficacy of traditional blind insertion of a 5 cm needle at the second intercostal space in the mid-clavicular line, most notably the work of Inaba et al. using both radiographic measurements and cadavers to confirm differences in tissue depth in the anterior vs lateral approaches, concluding up to 57% of anteriorly placed needles may be insufficient to access the pleural space, let alone drain a pneumothorax [2, 3]. Even when done correctly, blindly placed catheters have a high propensity to fail due to kinking, obstruction, and dislodgement – over 50% in one study [4]. Others, such as Ferrie et al., have shown blind placement to be limited by an inability of even highly trained providers to reliably identify landmarks for needle placement [5]. Perhaps most tellingly, in 2003 Diacon et al. showed 15% of proposed thoracentesis puncture sites identified by physicians using physical exam alone to be inaccurate when confirmed via ultrasound, and in 17% no puncture site could be identified at all using physical exam alone [6]. The inclusion of ultrasound has been shown to improve efficacy and safety, with risk of pneumothorax reduced in one study by 19%, with no added risk to the patient or provider and minimal added time to the procedure [7–9].

Limitations and Opportunities for Future Research

The overwhelming majority of data regarding the safety and efficacy of ultrasound guided thoracentesis is based on in-hospital treatment, specifically highly resourced hospitals. There is growing recognition of the ability of ultrasound to bring advanced care to under-resourced facilities and even austere environments. It remains to be seen how the use of ultrasound will affect care, particularly of trauma patients requiring emergent intervention, in prehospital and limited-resource settings. As cost continues to decrease and availability increases, the capability to diagnose and manage significant thoracic pathology will provide new options for clinical care in these unique and challenging environments.

Pearls and Pitfalls

- Ultrasound should be deployed early for reliable diagnosis of potentially life-threatening intrathoracic pathology such as pneumothorax.
- Traditional physical exam and blind insertion are unreliable and should be avoided when possible.
- Landmark identification using ultrasound provides added safety and improved efficacy of chest drain placement.

- Static lung tissue (ex: right-mainstem bronchial intubation or adhesive disease) appears identical to pneumothorax on ultrasound and should be considered prior to needle insertion.
- Sterile technique should be followed whenever possible to avoid introducing infection to the pleural space.

References

1. Patel MD, Joshi SD. Abnormal preprocedural international normalized ratio and platelet counts are not associated with increased bleeding complications after ultrasound-guided thoracentesis. AJR Am J Roentgenol. 2011;197:W164.
2. Inaba K, et al. Optimal positioning for emergent needle thoracostomy: a cadaver-based study. J Trauma. 2011;71(1):099–103.
3. Inaba K, et al. Radiologic evaluation of alternative sites for needle decompression of tension pneumothorax. Arch Surg. 2012;147(9):813–8.
4. Martin M, Satterly S, Inaba K, Blair K. Does needle thoracostomy provide adequate and effective decompression of tension pneumothorax? J Trauma Acute Care Surg. 2012;73(6):1,412–7.
5. Ferrie EP, Collum N, McGovern S. The right place in the right space? Awareness of site for needle thoracocentesis. Emerg Med J. 2005;22(11):788–9.
6. Diacon AH, Brutsche MH, Solèr M. Accuracy of pleural puncture sites: a prospective comparison of clinical examination with ultrasound. Chest. 2003;123:436.
7. Daniels CE, Ryu JH. Improving the safety of thoracentesis. Curr Opin Pulm Med. 2011;17:232.
8. Mercaldi CJ, Lanes SF. Ultrasound guidance decreases complications and improves the cost of care among patients undergoing thoracentesis and paracentesis. Chest. 2013;143:532.
9. Salamonsen M, Ellis S, Paul E, et al. Thoracic ultrasound demonstrates variable location of the intercostal artery. Respiration. 2012;83:323.

Advanced Procedure Topic for Austere Providers: Upper Extremity Nerve Blocks

Jacob Wayman and David Evans

Introduction

Nerve blocks of the upper extremity can provide rapid analgesia in the setting of acute pain, helping facilitate procedures and interventions in the field. When performed properly, many of these blocks have a low rate of complications when completed under ultrasound guidance [4]. This chapter will provide an overview of relevant anatomy and instructions for the most common upper extremity nerve blocks performed under ultrasound guidance [1], as well as a review of the relevant literature.

Common Blocks

Interscalene Blocks

Effectively blocks C5-C7 nerve roots and superficial cervical plexus providing analgesia for the shoulder and upper arm. The block will not provide analgesia for the hand, especially the ulnar aspect.

With your patient supine and facing away from the side of the block place the probe on the lateral aspect of the patient's neck at the level of the cricoid cartilage then insert your needle in plane from lateral to medial (Fig. 1) towards the nerve roots between the scalene muscles at the level of C6 (Fig. 2). Infiltrate with 20–30 mL of anesthetic.

J. Wayman · D. Evans (✉)
Department of Emergency Medicine, Virginia Commonwealth University, Richmond, VA, USA
e-mail: david.evans@vcuhealth.org

B. D. Nicholson et al. (eds.), *Manual of Austere and Prehospital Ultrasound*,
https://doi.org/10.1007/978-3-030-64287-7_23

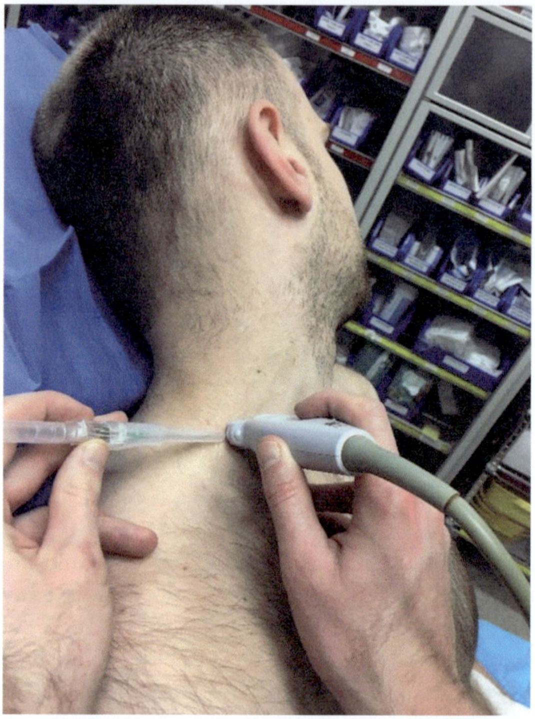

Fig. 1 Interscalene block approach

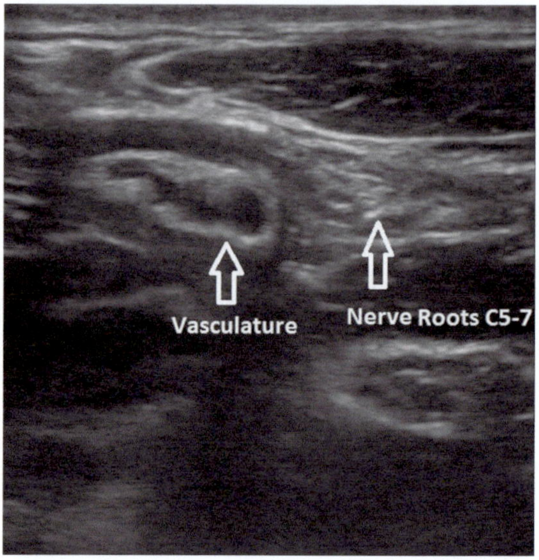

Fig. 2 Interscalene nerve roots and nearby vasculature

Interscalene blocks can be complicated by accidently blocking the phrenic nerve. This could potentially limit a patient's respiratory capacity. Other reported complications include horner syndrome from an accidental block of the sympathetic trunk, and voice changes from block of the recurrent laryngeal nerve.

Supraclavicular Block

Blocks sensation to the humerus, elbow, forearm and hand.

With your patient supine, head turned toward the contralateral side (Fig. 3). Using a high-frequency probe, scan the supraclavicular area to identify a short-axis view of the subclavian artery (Fig. 4). You should be able to see the first rib under the vessel. Superolateral to the artery you should see a collection of hypoechoic structures (trunks and divisions of the brachial plexus. Using an in-plane technique in a lateral to medial direction, insert a 5-cm block needle toward the "corner pocket," formed by the intersection between the subclavian artery and the first rib. Infiltrate the area with 20–40 mL of local anesthetic.

Infraclavicular

Blocks sensation to the humerus, elbow, forearm and hand.

With your patient positioned supine, arm is flexed so that the forearm and hand can rest comfortably on the torso. Place your high-frequency ultrasound probe in the infraclavicular fossa, medial to the coracoid process, to obtain a short-axis view of the axillary vessels. Identify the axillary artery and vein which can be found under the pectoralis major and minor muscles. Using an in-plane technique in a cephalad to caudad direction, a long, 10 cm, block needle is advanced until the tip lies just dorsal to the artery. Infiltrate the skin, subcutaneous tissues, and pectoralis muscles with 30–40 mL of local anesthetic. Usually, a pop can be felt just before the needle assumes the correct position.

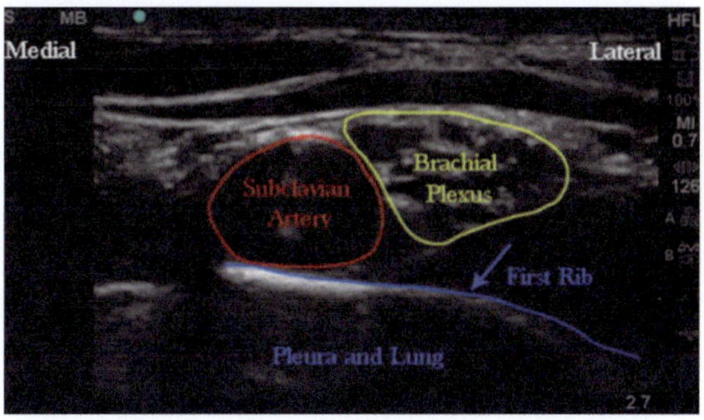

Fig. 3 Supraclavicular block approach

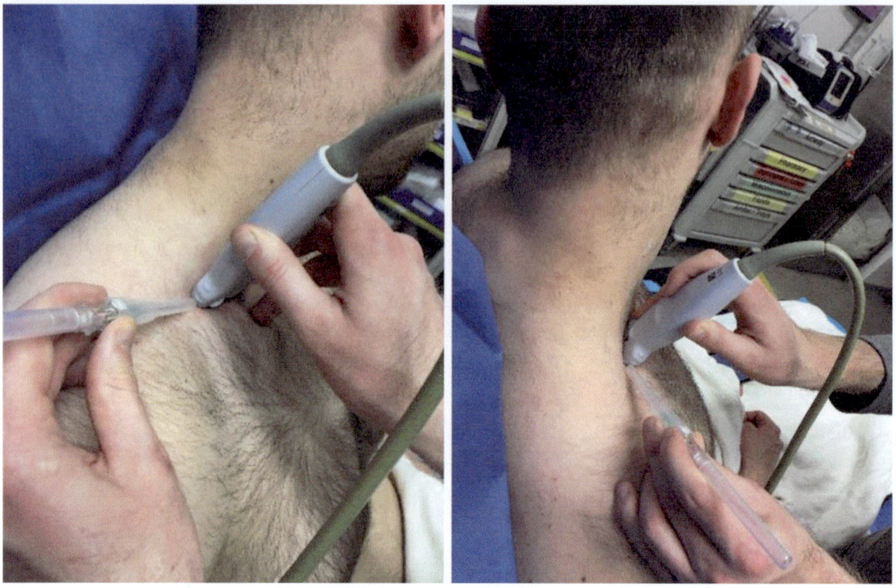

Fig. 4 Brachial plexus and adjacent subclavian artery

Axillary Block

Blocks sensation to the elbow, forearm and hand.

With your patients shoulder abducted and the elbow flexed (Fig. 5), scan the axilla with a high-frequency linear ultrasound probe to identify a short-axis view of the axillary artery and the musculocutaneous nerve, a hyperechoic structure which can be found anterior and lateral to the artery in the belly of the coracobrachialis muscles, or in a plane between the coracobrachialis and biceps muscles.

Using an in-plane technique, direct a 5-cm block needle toward the musculocutaneous nerve, infiltrate the surrounding tissue with 5 mL of local anesthetic. Then, redirected toward each of the three remaining nerves surrounding the axillary artery (Fig. 6)and repeat the infiltration process. Using 1–5 mL per nerve.

An alternative technique, in the event of difficulty with access or identification of the nerve branches, is to hydrodissect the circumference of the axillary artery which should suffice to effect the targeted nerves typically in the range of 30 mL.

Median Nerve Block

Blocks the radial aspect of the palm.

With your patient supine, arm extended, place the probe proximal to the elbow and insert the needle from medial to lateral in plane with the probe to the nerve

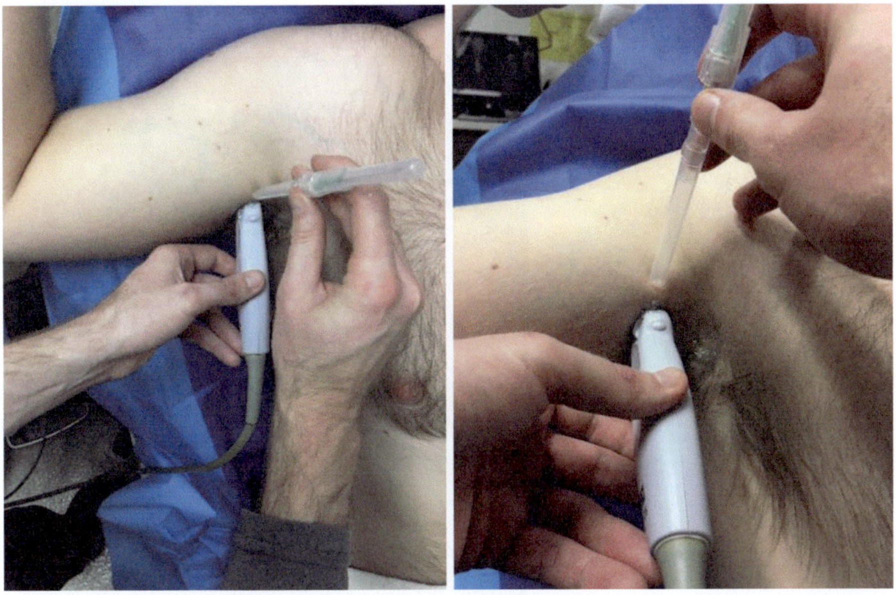

Fig. 5 Axillary artery approach

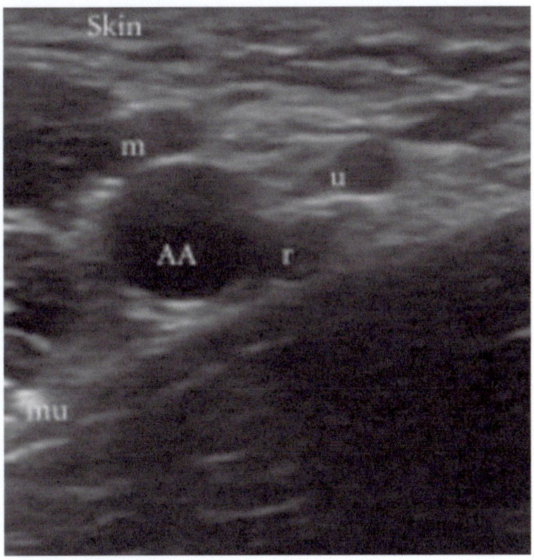

Fig. 6 Axillary artery (AA) and surrounding median (m), radial (r) and ulnar (u) arteries

found coursing medial to the brachial artery. (5 mL) Alternatively the block can be performed in distal third of the forearm with the probe placed on the volar aspect of the arm (Fig. 8). The distal approach will limit the effects of the block on the muscles of the forearm.

Fig. 7 Median Nerve

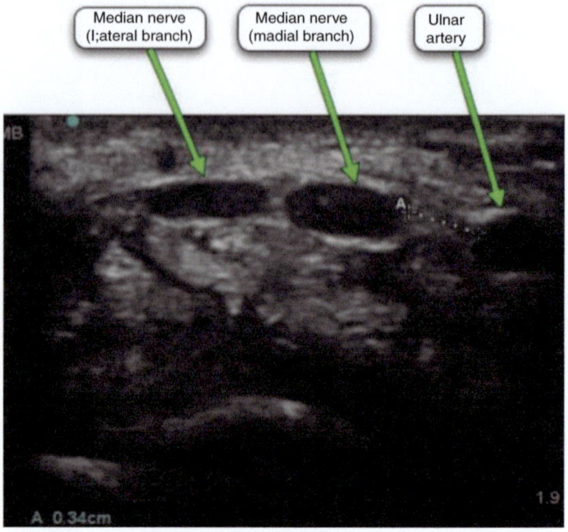

Fig. 8 Forearm median nerve block approach

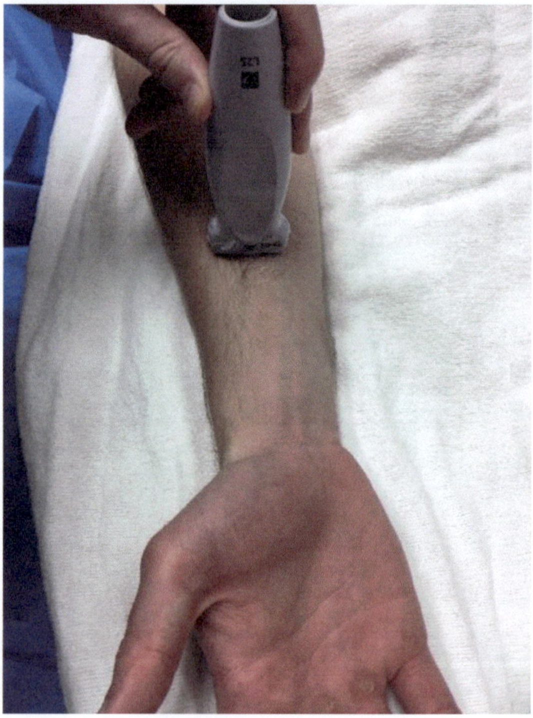

Radial Nerve Block

Blocks the dorsal aspect of the forearm and the majority of the dorsal aspect of the first through fourth digits.

With your patient supine, arm extended, place the probe over the lateral aspect of lateral epicondyle (Fig. 10) and insert your needle from medial to lateral in plane with the probe to the nerve found between the brachioradialis and brachialis muscles (Fig. 9). Infiltrate the area with 5 ml of local anesthetic.

Ulnar Nerve Block

Blocks the medial aspect of the hand.

With your patient supine, arm rotated outward in extension (Fig. 12), place the probe on the ventromedial aspect of the proximal forearm, several centimeters distal to the medial epicondyle and insert the needle in plane from medial to lateral towards the nerve found between the flexor digitorum superficialis and profundus (Fig. 11).

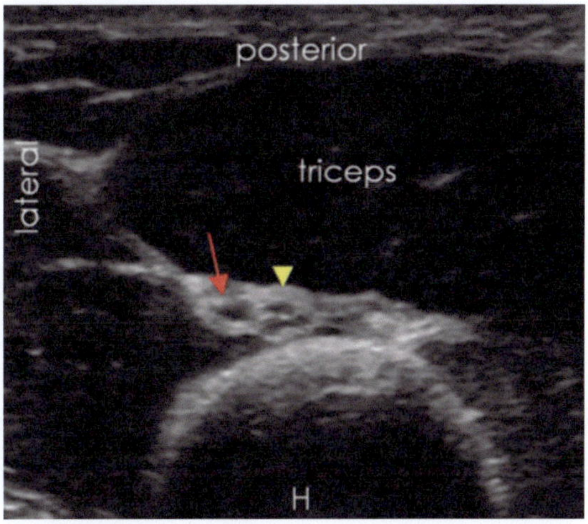

Fig. 9 Radial nerve

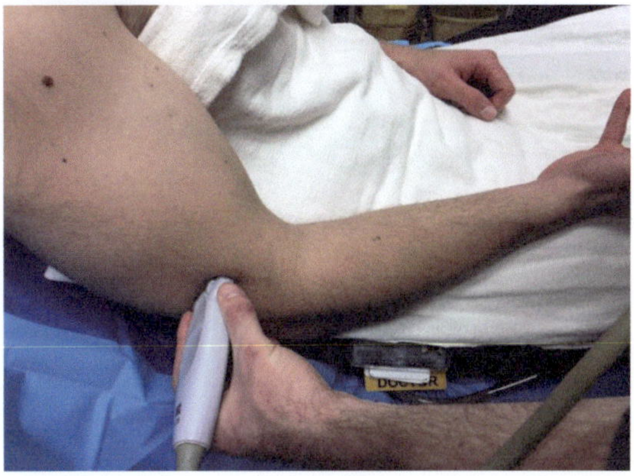

Fig. 10 Radial nerve block approach

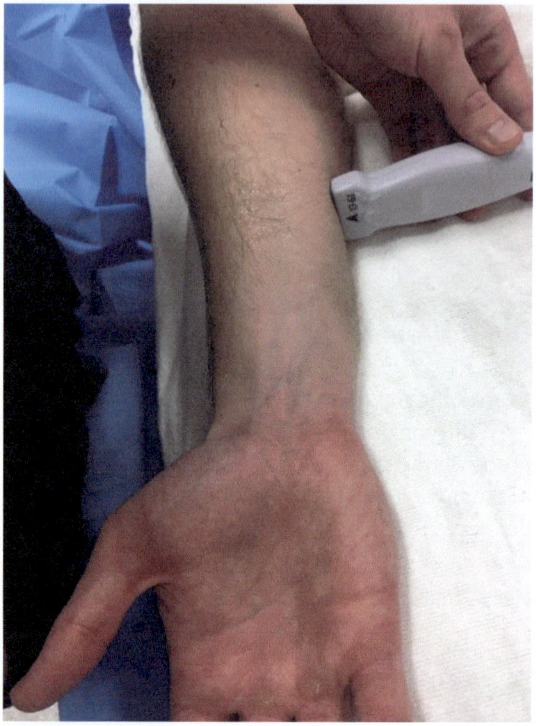

Fig. 11 Ulnar nerve and ulnar artery

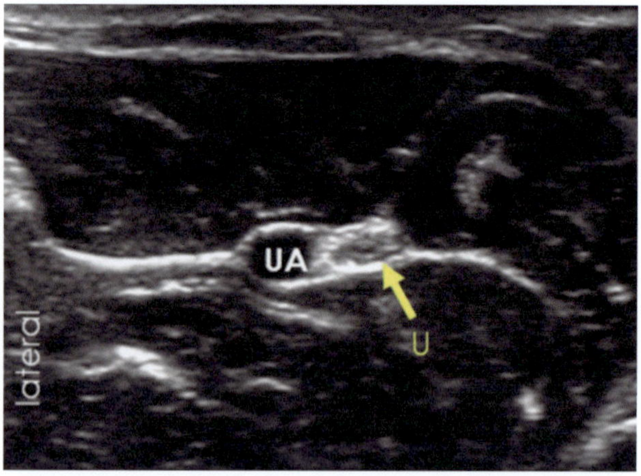

Fig. 12 Ulnar nerve block approach

Key Literature Reviewed

PUBMED was searched (between November and December of 2018) using the following terms: upper extremity nerve block, ultrasound guided upper extremity nerve block, and ultrasound guided upper extremity peripheral nerve block. Review articles and expert panel recommendations were included and form the basis for the procedural recommendations in the Topic Discussion section, they have been listed in the works cited. RCT studies dealing with specific issues regarding relative efficacy of the blocks, complications, and alternative techniques have been included in the pearls and pitfalls section of the chapter.

Limitations of Current Knowledge and Opportunities for Future Research

Although there is a growing body of evidence surrounding the use of peripheral nerve blocks and specifically the use of US guidance in facilitating these blocks, the vast majority of the studies come from the Anesthesia literature and operating room settings. These controlled environments and expert operators with additional resources and limit the generalizability of many of their findings and likely underestimate the rate of failure or complications in a less controlled setting; current data notwithstanding, there is a growing body of literature for the use peripheral nerve blocks in the prehospital and out of hospital environment, most notably for femoral nerve and fascia iliaca in the setting of femoral fractures [2, 3, 5].

As the prevalence of prehospital ultrasound increases there is tremendous opportunity for new studies to demonstrate the efficacy and reproducibility of all the established upper extremity blocks listed in this chapter in the prehospital setting. The military is on the leading edge of this movement as peripheral nerve blocks are moving closer to the front lines of battle [5].

Pearls and Pitfalls

All patients receiving regional anesthesia should receive a detailed neurovascular exam. Providers performing the block should note the pulses, strength, sensation, and pain in the affected limb.

Prior to considering a nerve block, patients need to be evaluated for compartment syndrome. Any patient that receives a block should be monitored appropriately for the development of compartment syndrome as long as the block is in effect. Compartment syndrome is primary a clinical diagnosis, characterized classically as pain out of proportion to exam, pallor, paresthesia, paralysis, and pulselessness. Pain out of proportion with passive stretching of the fingers is an early sign of possible compartment pressure and should warrant emergent testing of compartment pressures. As pain will be lessened by the block, compartments should be felt for changes and any unusually firm or pale tissue should be checked formally with an intracompartmental pressure measurement device.

When choosing a local anesthetic there are a variety of options with different half-lives and side effect profiles. Lidocaine without epinephrine offers a relatively low side effect profile, is commonly available, and has a rapid onset making it often the local anesthetic of choice for peripheral blocks. Dosing of lidocaine should not exceed 4.5 mg/kg per dose with doses spaced at least 2 hours.

Generally speaking, more proximal blocks are used to anaesthetize more proximal areas of the upper extremity as well as to block larger regions with minimal numbers of injections and the lowest volume possible of local anesthetic. More distal blocks will tend to be more limited to the affected area, often require smaller volumes of local anesthetic, and are further removed from the more important central structures that cause the more serious complications associated with the proximal blocks [6].

An area of active research is the relative risks and benefits of the infraclavicular vs supraclavicular approach to brachial plexus blocks. While some studies have suggested the supraclavicular approach may be faster in some populations [8], the infraclavicular approach was actually completed more rapidly in at least one study [7] and consistently associated with fewer side effects than the supraclavicular approach [7, 8].

The axillary brachial plexus block, carries significantly less risk than more proximal blocks. An effective axillary block provide anesthesia of the four main branches of plexus: the median, ulnar, musculocutaneous, and radial nerves. Use of perineural infiltration allows for minimal quantities of local anesthetic and more rapid time to effective block [8]. However, in the prehospital setting a perivascular approach would likely be more practical considering relative ease in identifying the axillary artery relative to the surrounding peripheral nerves as well as the fewer number of needle sticks required and infiltrate the anesthetic [8].

Median ulnar and radial nerve blocks can be achieved either at the levels described above in the chapter or more distally for injuries that are isolated to the hand. Regardless of the site of injection, care should be taken to avoid vascular structures and providers should keep a high index of suspicion for potential compartment syndrome.

References

1. Barrington MJ, Watts SA, Gledhill SR, Thomas RD, Said SA, Snyder GL, Tay VS, Jamrozik K. Preliminary results of the Australasian regional anaesthesia collaboration. Reg Anesth Pain Med. 2009;34:534–41.
2. Kwofie K, Shastri U, Vandepitte C. Standard approaches for upper extremity nerve blocks with an emphasis on outpatient surgery. Curr Opin Anaesthesiol. 2013;26:501–8.
3. Jing L, Xinchao Y. Nerve blocks for initial pain management of femoral fractures in children. Orthop Nurs. 2014;33:235.
4. Black KJ, Murphy NG, Thompson K, Bevan CA, Howard JJ. Nerve blocks for initial pain management of femoral fractures in children. Cochrane Database Syst Rev. 2012; https://doi.org/10.1002/14651858.cd009587.
5. Gelfand HJ, Kent ML, Buckenmaier CC. Management of acute pain of the war wounded during short and long-distance transport and "Casevac". Tech Orthop. 2017;32:263–9.
6. Sehmbi H, Shah U, Madjdpour C, Chin K. Ultrasound guided distal peripheral nerve block of the upper limb: a technical review. J Anaesthesiol Clin Pharmacol. 2015;31:296.
7. Matsuda H, Oka Y, Takatsu S, Katsube R, Yoshida R, Oyama T, Takeda Y, Miyazaki M. Ultrasound-guided block of selective branches of the brachial plexus for vascular access surgery in the forearm: a preliminary report. J Vasc Access. 2016;17:284–90.
8. María BDJ, Banús E, Egea MN, Serrano S, Perelló M, Mabrok M. Ultrasound-guided supraclavicular vs infraclavicular brachial plexus blocks in children. Pediatr Anesth. 2008;18:838–84.

Advanced Procedure Topic for Austere Providers: Lower Extremity Nerve Blocks

Fredrik Granholm

Lower Extremity Nerve Blocks

Introduction

Lower limb nerve blocks may be extremely useful in an austere or combat environment and there has been a rapid development in this area the last 10 years. Mainly because of the development of smaller and better ultrasound machines but also because of the experiences from current international conflicts and the prolonged field care concept. Nerve blocks can be useful as pain control after trauma, as an adjunct to sedation or general anesthesia, or to facilitate surgical interventions on their own.

The use of ultrasound has led to improved success and made it easier to perform these interventions even for people with limited training in regional anesthesia. Just a decade ago most techniques relied on blind techniques and nerve stimulators. Nowadays the modality of ultrasound guided nerve blocks is within the scope of practice for most healthcare providers in an austere and combat setting.

However, it is important to point out that nerve blocks are not without serious risks and it is paramount that anyone performing these interventions has the proper training and a sound knowledge of the underlying theory and anatomy. Preferably the training on these skills have been done in a less stressful environment.

Even with optimal ultrasound technique, and safest possible local anesthetics used, the risk of systemic toxicity is not eliminated. Therefore, relevant monitoring must be used all times and the maximum safe doses must not be exceeded.

The use of nerve blocks of the lower limb will reduce the need for systemic opioids or other potent analgesics/sedatives like Ketamine. This may reduce complications like over sedation, respiratory depression and nausea/vomiting. Good pain

F. Granholm (✉)
Department of Emergency and Ambulance, Sundsvall County Hospital, Sundsvall, Sweden
e-mail: fredrik.granholm@rvn.se

B. D. Nicholson et al. (eds.), *Manual of Austere and Prehospital Ultrasound*,
https://doi.org/10.1007/978-3-030-64287-7_24

control may also facilitate evacuation and transportation of a trauma victim in the austere environment. It has also been shown that regional anesthesia may reduce the stress response to trauma and that with good pain control PTSD can be limited.

Even single shot nerve blocks can provide fairly long periods of pain relief depending on which local anesthetic being used and on the use of adjunct medications like Clonidine.

Most basic blocks of the lower limb are relatively easy to perform with ultrasound but they require good knowledge of the anatomy of the leg. Both for choosing the correct block and for localization of the nerve. The anatomy of the leg, from the femoral crease and down to the foot, should be very familiar. Including the distribution of cutaneous nerves. (Bild).

To maximize nerve block success it is often good to have an assistant who can inject the local anesthetics while the operator advances and places the needle close to the nerve. Often the assistant holds a syringe with local anesthetics connected to a suitable needle using plastic tubing.

With all nerve block procedures it is paramount to clean the area where the needle is injected and to follow local guidelines regarding preventive measures for infection (Figs. 1, 2, and 3).

Local Anesthetics in Lower Extremity Nerve Blocks

Usually long acting agents are preferred in an austere setting (ropivacaine, bupivacaine, levo-bupivacaine) and they may provide pain relief for 4–10 h but this may vary. However, in a resource limited setting flexibility is important, so short acting drugs like lidocaine should be familiar to the individual performing the block. Even when using ultrasound, and getting close to the nerve, one should be prepared to use a relatively large dose of local anesthetics to maximise the duration of the block.

Clonidine is an an alpha agonist that may be used as an adjuvant to local anesthetics.

1 mg/kg can be added to the local anesthetics and this has been shown to prolong the duration of the block by several hours. However, the use increases the risk of hypotensive episodes and sedation so there must be continuous monitoring of vital signs. And the risks must be weighted against the gains.

Nerve Anatomy of the Lower Extremity: A Primer

The nerve supply to the lower limb is derived from the lumbar plexus (L1-L4) through the femoral, obturator, and lateral cutaneous nerve of the thigh. The remainder is largely supplied by the sciatic nerve (L4/5-S1/3).

The nerve supply of the lower limb distal to the knee is provided by the sciatic nerve (L4-S3) with the exception of the medial cutaneous aspect of the calf. This is supplied by the saphenous nerve (L3-L4), which is derived from the femoral nerve

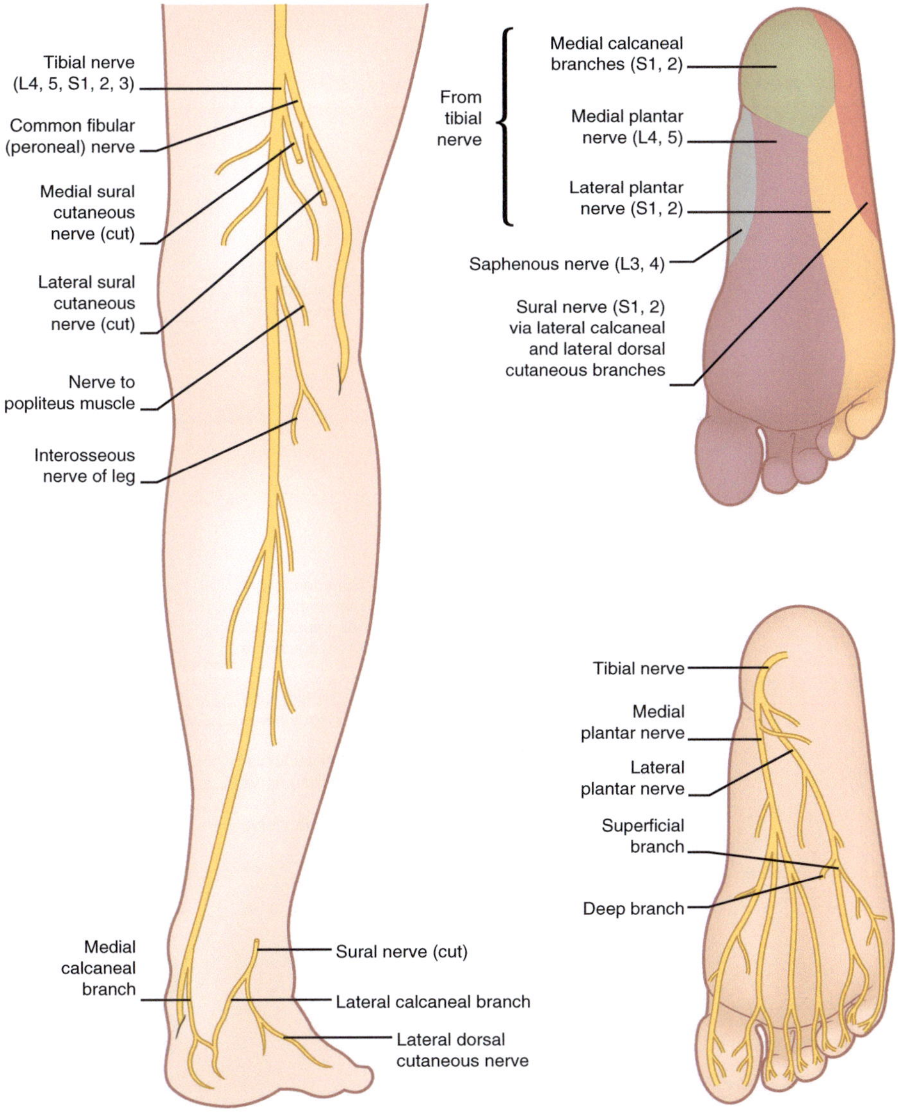

Fig. 1 Posterior and plantar sensory nerve distributions and innervations of the sole

(L2-L4). For this reason, most simple operations on the foot can be performed using sciatic block alone.

The sciatic nerve branches into the tibial and the common peroneal nerves near the apex of the popliteal fossa, about 5–10 cm proximal to the posterior knee skin crease. The tibial nerve divides into the medial and lateral plantar nerves distal to the medial malleolus and supplies sensation to the sole and foot. Both the tibial and

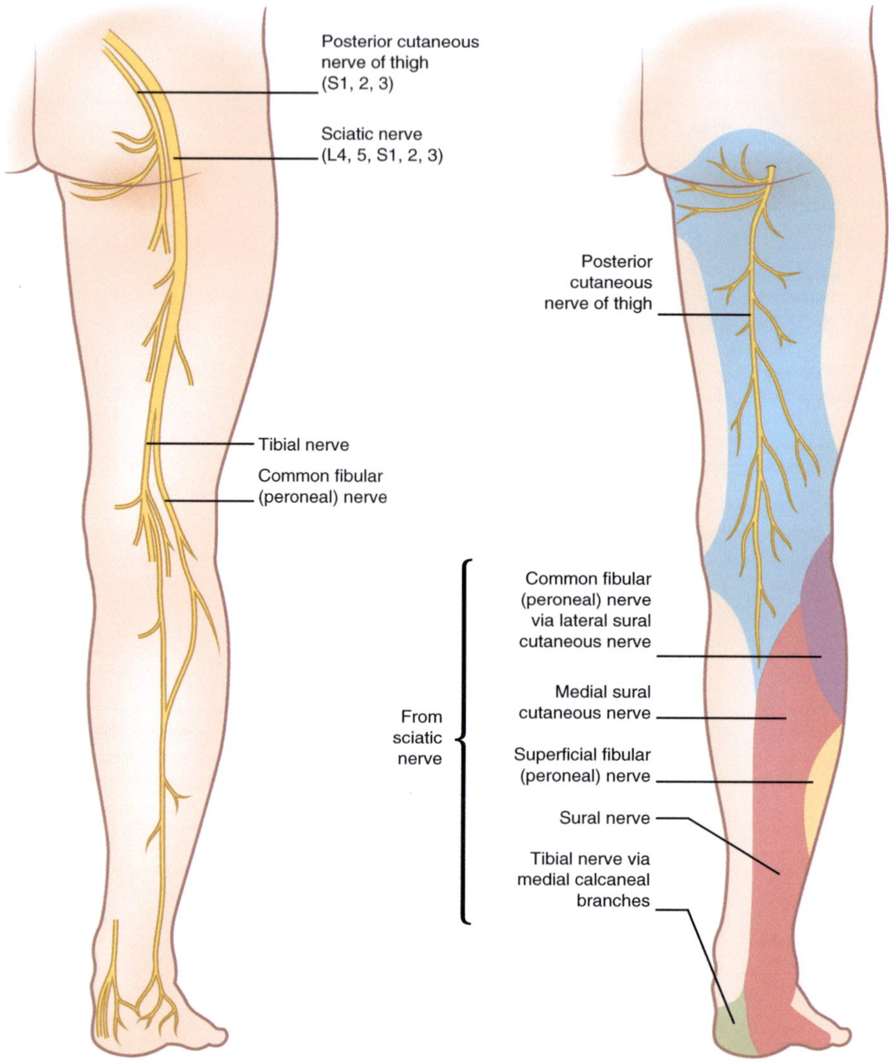

Fig. 2 Posterior leg sensory nerve distribution and innervations of heel

common peroneal nerves provide sensory fibres to the sural nerve, which supplies sensation to the lateral aspect of the calf and foot.

Femoral Nerve Block

Indication and Background

The femoral nerve block, in the austere environment, is very good for analgesia of the hip, femoral fractures and minor surgical procedures on the front of the thigh

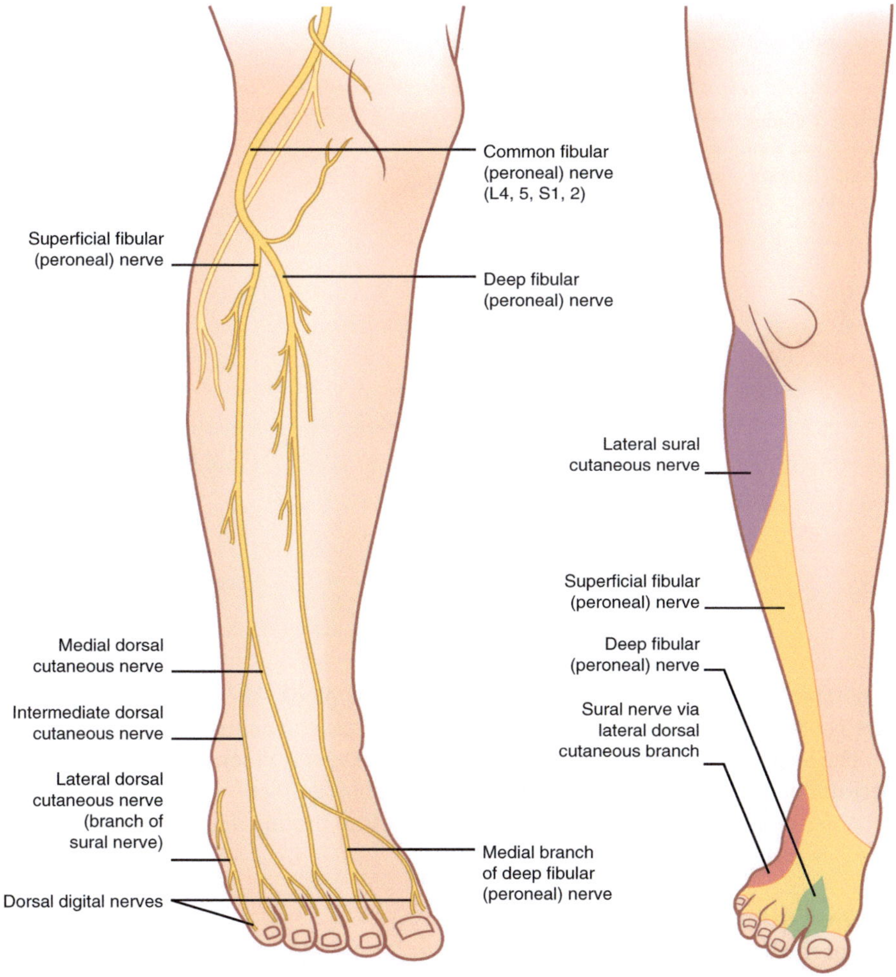

Fig. 3 Anterior leg sensory nerve distribution and innervations

down to the knee. However, it may only cover part of the knee joint since it is also innervated by the obturator and sciatic nerve.

Anatomy

The femoral nerve is the largest terminal branch of the lumbar plexus (L2-L4). The nerve travels caudally into the thigh under the inguinal ligament and between the iliacus and psoas muscles. It is located under the fascia iliaca which usually can be felt as a structure with some resistance when advancing the needle (Fig. 4)

Superficial to the femoral nerve are skin, subcutaneous tissue, fascia lata and fascia iliaca. Medially to the nerve is the femoral artery and the femoral vein. It is

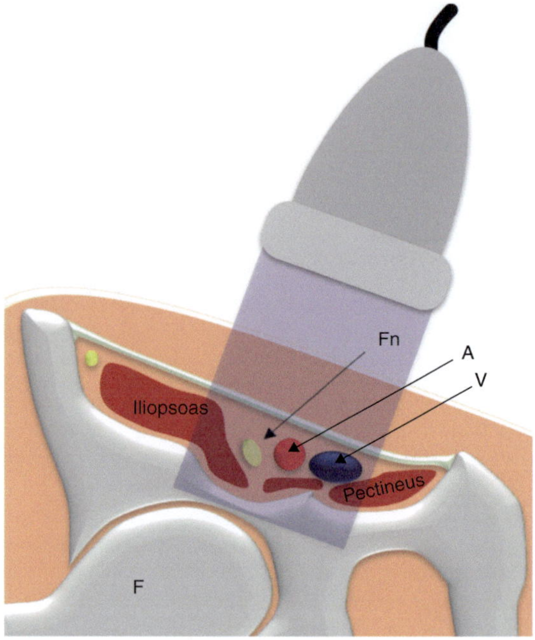

Fig. 4 A trans-sectional view of the thigh showing the adductor canal. IP biceps muscle, P brachialis muscle, F femur, Fn with black arrow femoral nerve close to femoral artery and vein

paramount to avoid vessel damage performing this block. However, a vessel puncture is often quickly identified and the vessels are easy to compress.

The anatomic location of the femoral nerve makes this block one of the easiest to perform because the landmarks are usually simply identified.

A nerve block is usually performed just below the inguinal crease where the nerve is relatively superficial.

Probe/Equipment

Linear transducer. 70–100 mm needle

Technique

This block typically is performed with the patient in the supine position, with the bed or table flattened to maximize operator access to the inguinal area.

If possible, it is optimal to have the leg abducted and slightly externally rotated. If needed the patient may be given some analgesics to facilitate optimal positioning.

Place the ultrasound machine opposite to the person performing the block, optimizing a view across the bed. If a handheld ultrasound machine is used an assistant may help by holding the machine in the line of sight of the operator.

It is often good to start with palpating the femoral pulse as a useful landmark. However, this is not mandatory since the artery should be readily visualized by placing a linear probe (5–12 Mhz) on the inguinal crease with the probe marker to the operator's right. If the artery is not seen use slow movements laterally or medially to localize the artery and the vein. It is important to identify the fascia iliaca, the artery, the vein and the nerve. If the ultrasound machine has doppler this may be used to identify vessels. Also make sure that you visualize any other smaller vessels as well in the proximity of the nerve. To differentiate between artery and vein look for pulsations, which indicate arterial flow, and try to compress the vessel. Veins are more easy to compress than arteries.

The nerve usually has a slightly triangular or oval shaped hyperechoic appearance. Even though it is fairly large it can be difficult to see, so a good starting point is to look for the femoral artery and the fascia iliaca to localize the nerve. When you see the artery and the fascia iliaca, move the probe slightly lateral and slowly fan up and down. Sometimes it may also help rotating the probe a bit (Fig. 5).

The block is most often performed in a lateral to medial, in-plane technique. After a small wheal of local anesthetics, the skin is entered on the lateral side of the probe using a long needle (>70 mm) with a 30 degree angle. The needle tip should always be seen during the procedure and the aim is to place it lateral to, or just below the inferior border of the nerve. If you cannot see the tip of the needle the stop and try to tilt, rotate or angulate the probe.

To facilitate the visualization of the needle tip hydrodissection can also be used, where very small volumes of saline or local anesthetics is injected to facilitate the view of the tip. The fluid will appear black on the screen as it is injected.

A needle passage through the fascia iliaca is often felt as a resistance or a small "pop".

When the needle tip is in place aspiration is performed to check for intravascular placement. A small volume (1–2 ml) should first be injected to make sure that the needle is below the fascia iliaca and that the fluid is spreading around the nerve. In an optimal nerve placement the nerve will be surrounded, and sometimes lifted, by the local anesthetics. Thereafter, 30 ml of local anesthetics is injected and the rationale for this high volume is to both increase the duration of the block as well as to increase the spread towards the lateral femoral cutaneous nerve. Of course the volume must be correlated to the maximum dose of the specific local anesthetic given. The appearance of local anesthetic above the nerve only may indicate deposition above the fascia iliaca and result in inadequate analgesia. In that case the needle should be re-directed.

Remember that it should always be easy to inject and if the patient experiences pain on injection the needle tip may be intraneural. It should then be removed and another attempt may done.

Popliteal Sciatic Nerve Block

Indication and Background

Blocking the sciatic nerve in the popliteal fossa is very useful for surgery and pain control in the lower leg, foot and ankle.

Combined with a sapenhous nerve block it will give full analgesia for the foot and ankle.

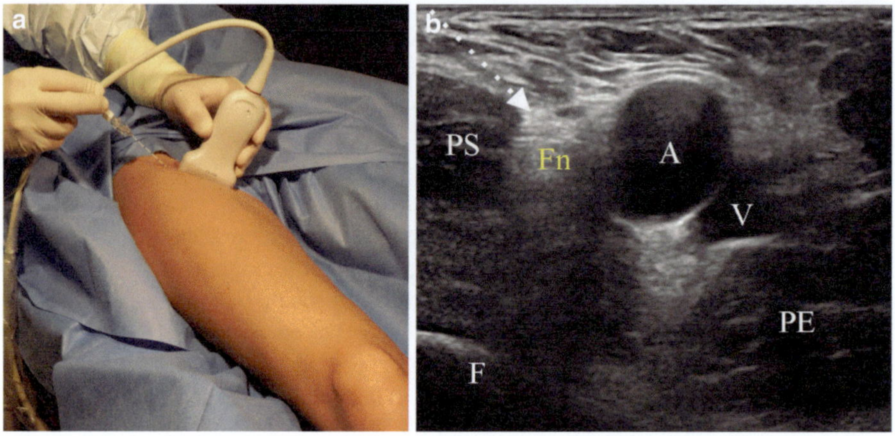

Fig. 5 (**a**) Patient position and needle entry point. (**b**) Sonoanatomy of the inguinal area. Fn femoral nerve, PS iliopsoas muscle, PE pectineus muscle, A femoral artery, V femoral vein, F femur

Fig. 6 Schema of popliteal fossa anatomy BF Biceps femoris muscle, *ST* Semitendinosus muscle, *SM* semimembranosus muscle, *LG* Gastrocnemius lateral head, *MG* Gastrocnemius medial head

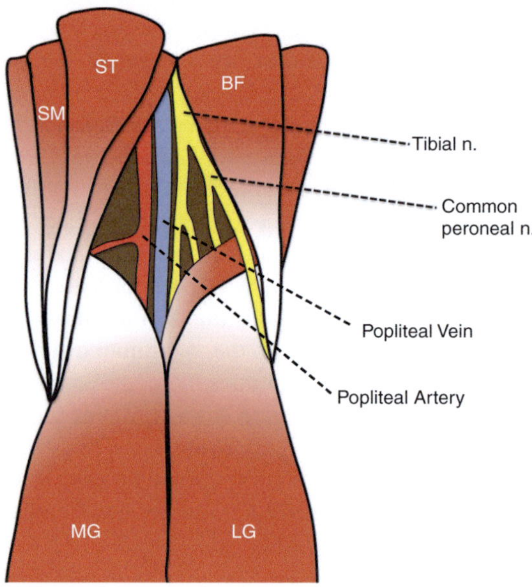

Anatomy

The nerve supply of the lower limb distal to the knee is provided by the sciatic nerve, with the exception of the medial aspect of the calf and the medial part of the foot. This is supplied by the saphenous nerve which is derived from the femoral nerve. The sciatic nerve branches into the tibial and the common peroneal nerves near the apex of the popliteal fossa, about 5–10 cm proximal to the knee crease (Fig. 6).

Probe/Equipment

Linear transducer. 100 mm needle

Technique

This block is performed with the patient in the prone or supine position.

The supine lateral approach has some advantages in the austere environment. For example, a trauma patient can stay supine and does not have to be turned to the side or lay prone. In the lateral approach the patient should rest the foot on pillows or flexing the knee while an assistant stabilizes the foot and ankle. There should be enough space under the knee to place and move the probe.

If needed the patient may be given some analgesics to facilitate optimal position.

Even if ultrasound is used it is good practice to study the anatomy of the patient and to palpate the relevant structures. One should palpate the popliteal crease and measure a distance of ca 10 cm cephalad in the groove between the vastus lateralis and biceps femoris muscles of the thigh.

Beginning with a high frequency linear probe in the transverse position at the popliteal crease, the popliteal artery is identified, aided with color Doppler when necessary. The popliteal artery is your main landmark for this block. The depth of the artery is usually 3–4 cm. The popliteal vein follows the artery at it is positioned just superficial or posterior to it. Compress the vessels to differentiate between artery and vein.

The tibial nerve is positioned superficial and lateral to the vein and is seen as a hyperechoic, oval or round structure. Usually, tilting the transducer caudally can improve the view of the nerve. If possible, the patient can flex the ankle to make the sciatic nerve branches move. Sliding the transducer slightly proximal or distal may improve the quality of the image and make it easier to visualize it from the background tissue (Fig. 7).

Once you have found the tibial nerve lateral to the artery slide the probe proximally until it is visualized together with the peroneal nerves as they are coming together to form the sciatic nerve. This junction usually is 5–10 cm from the popliteal crease.

When the correct injection site has been identified start with injecting a small wheal of local anesthetics, the skin is then entered on the lateral side of the probe using a long needle (>70 mm?)

The needle is inserted lateral to the probe allowing visualization of the tip in an in-plane view. If you cannot see the needle then do not advance. Optimize the view by slowly fanning with the probe. When the needle is in direct contact with the nerve 1–2 mL of local anesthetic is injected to confirm the proper injection site. Such injection should result in a distribution of local anesthetic within the nerve sheath.

If the needle placement is correct, 30–40 ml of local anesthetic is then injected. The nerve should be completely embedded in a donut shape. If the circumferential spread is incomplete, withdraw, redirect and inject at any missed areas.

Remember that it should always be easy to inject and if the patient experiences pain on injection the needle tip may be intraneural. It should then be removed and another attempt may done.

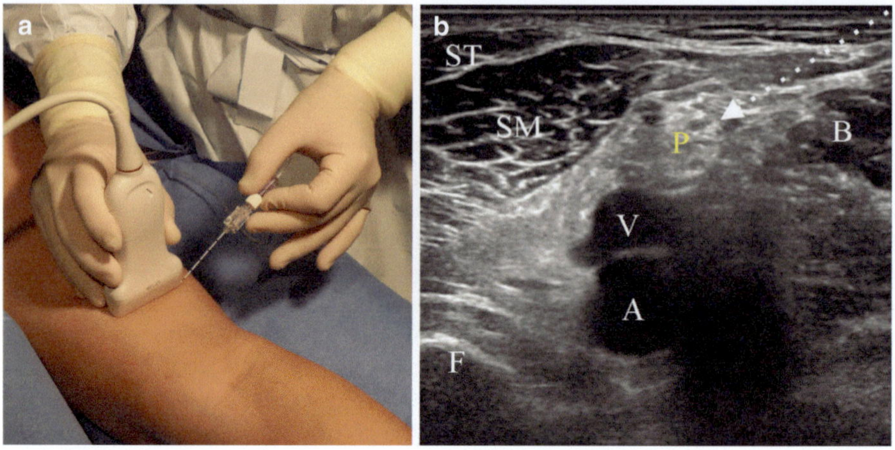

Fig. 7 (**a**) Patient position and needle entry point. (**b**) Sonoanatomy in a transverse section of popliteal region showing popliteal nerve, vein, and artery. F femur, ST semitendonosus muscle, SM semimembranosus muscle. Long white arrow needle direction and target point

Ankle Block

Indication and Background

Analgesia and surgery of the distal foot and toes.

Ankle blocks are fairly easy to perform and can be used both for anaesthesia during surgery as well as for pain control. This may be advantageous in the austere setting with limited resources.

This block may be performed as a 100% ultrasound guided block but this may be challenging for most people who do not have a lot of experience with the technique. It is our recommendation to use the ultrasound to locate vessels in the proximity of the nerves. And use these easily identified structures to maximize block success and to avoid vessel damage and intravascular injection of local anesthetics.

The ankle block is one of the more uncomfortable block procedures for patients.

This is because several needle insertions has to be done through the sensitive skin of the foot and ankle. The multiple subcutaneous injections thereafter are also painful. It is therefore prudent to provide suitable analgesics and/or sedation before the procedure.

Anatomy

Five peripheral nerves supply the foot: the tibial nerve, the deep peroneal nerve, the superficial peroneal nerve, the sural nerve and the saphenous nerve. All cross the ankle and are derived from the sciatic nerve except for the saphenous nerve which is derived from the femoral nerve. The tibial and deep peroneal nerves supply deep structures of the foot and must be blocked beneath the deep fascia of the ankle. The remaining nerves supply sensory innervation to the skin and can be blocked superficially.

Tibial Nerve

This nerve is located posterior to the posterior tibial artery at the level of the medial malleolus (Fig. 8).

Deep Peroneal Nerve

This nerve runs lateral to the dorsalis pedis artery at the level of the foot.

Superficial Peroneal Nerve

This nerve is located between the peroneus brevis muscle and the intermuscular septum in the distal half of the leg in the lateral compartment.

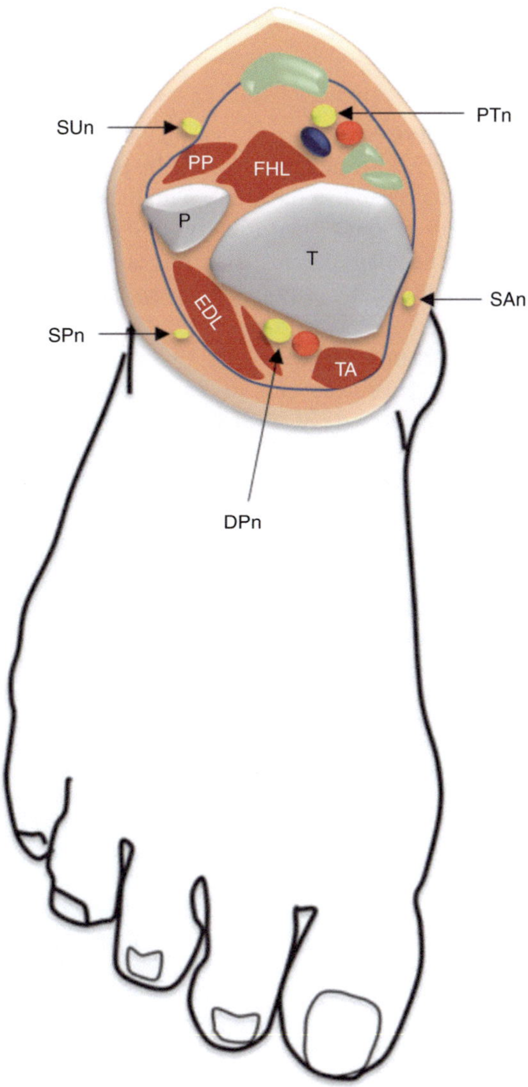

Fig. 8 Schema of ankle nerves anatomy PTn posterior tibial nerve, SAn saphenous nerve, DPn deep peroneal nerve, SPn superficial peroneal nerve, SUn surak nerve. T tibia, P Fibula, EDL extensor digitorum longus muscle, TA tibial anterior muscle, FHL flexor hallucis longus, PP peroneus muscles

Saphenous Nerve

In the lower third of the leg the saphenous nerve runs posterior to the medial aspect of the tibia.

Sural Nerve

Is an extension of the tibial nerve entering the foot between the Achilles tendon and lateral malleolus.

Probe/Equipment

Linear transducer.

Technique

Tibial Nerve

This nerve is located posterior to the posterior tibial artery at the level of the medial malleolus. Visualize the artery with the ultrasound and insert the needle posterior to the artery. If you have difficulty try using the doppler. The needle will usually contact the medial malleolus, after this occurs, slightly withdraw the needle. Inject 5 ml of local anesthetic after negative aspiration for blood (Fig. 9).

Deep Peroneal Nerve

This nerve runs lateral to the dorsalis pedis artery at the level of the foot. Visualize the artery with the ultrasound and insert the needle lateral to the artery. If you have difficulty use doppler. If bone is contacted, withdraw the

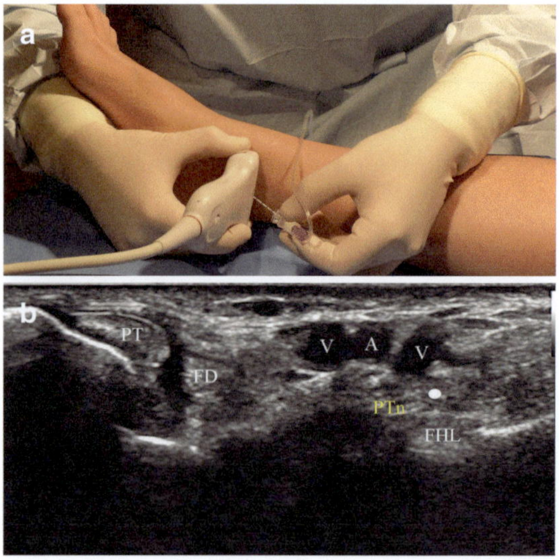

Fig. 9 (**a**) Patient position and needle entry point. (**b**) Sonoanatomy of the tibial nerve at the ankle. PTn posterior tibial nerve, A tibial artery, V tibial vein, FHL flexor hallucis longus, White dot needle target point

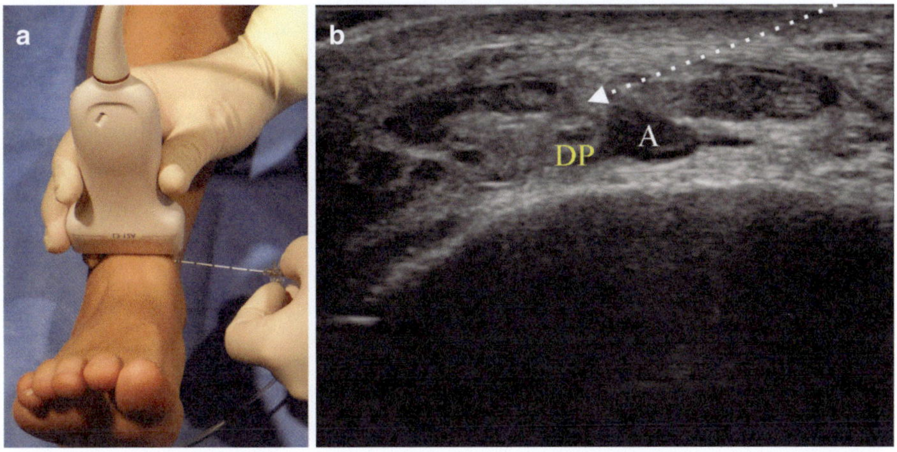

Fig. 10 (**a**) Patient position and needle entry point. (**b**) Sonoanatomy. DP deep peroneal nerve, A anterior tibial artery, Long white arrow needle direction and target point

needle slightly before injecting 5 ml local anesthetics after negative aspiration for blood (Fig. 10).

Superficial Peroneal Nerve

Inject a subcutaneous wheal of local anesthetics (LA) from the anterior border of the tibia to the lateral malleolus. Inject 5 ml after negative aspiration for blood (Fig. 11).

Saphenous Nerve

Inject a subcutaneous wheal of local anesthetics (5 ml), directing it posteriorly from the tibial ridge to the medial malleolus (Fig. 12).

Sural Nerve

Insert the needle between the Achilles tendon and lateral malleolus. Let the needle come in contact with the bone of the lateral malleolus. Withdraw slightly and subcutaneously infiltrate 5 ml of LA (Fig. 13).

Hematoma Block

Indication

The use of ultrasound in orthopedic injuries can be very helpful in the austere environment. Often plain x-ray is not readily available but the ultrasound can often answer the question if there is an interruption in the cortex of the bone as a sign of a fracture. In selected fractures this modality has been used for quite some time (forearm, ribs, sternum) while the ultrasound evaluation of ankle fractures are more

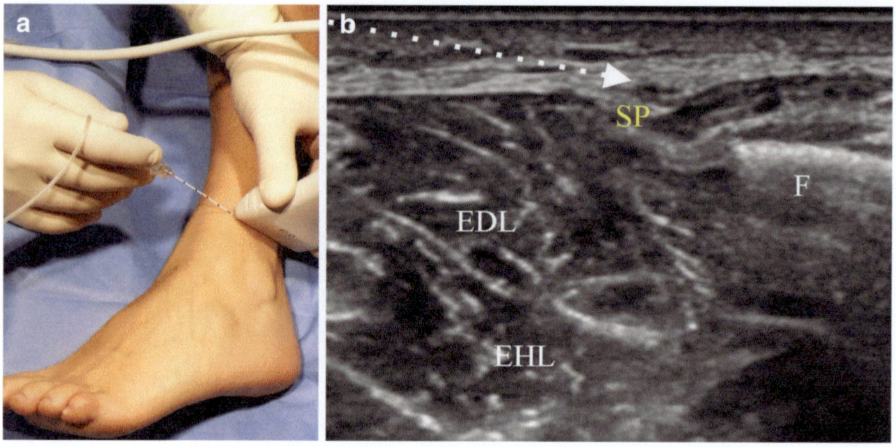

Fig. 11 (**a**) Patient position and needle entry point. (**b**) Sonoanatomy. SP superficial peroneal nerve, F fibula, EDL extensor digitorum longus muscle, EHL Extensor hallucis longus. Long white arrow needle direction and target point

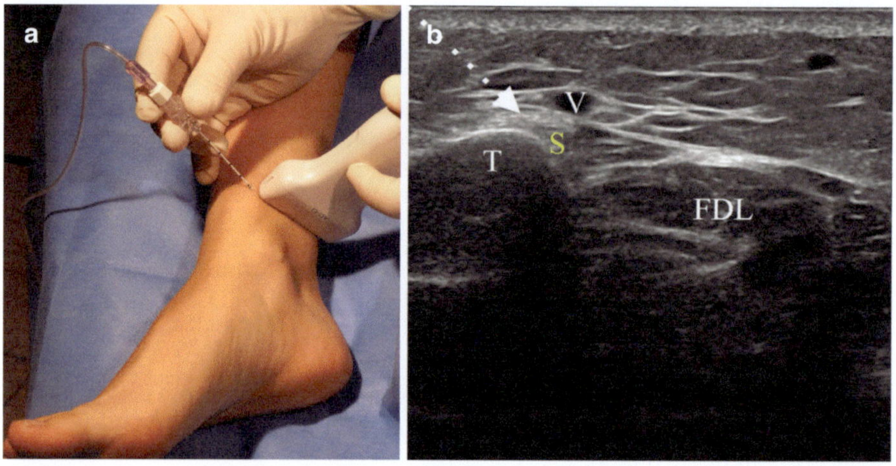

Fig. 12 (**a**) Patient position and needle entry point. (**b**) Sonoanatomy. S saphenous nerve, V saphenous vein, T tibia, FDL flexor digitorum longus. Long white arrow needle direction and target point

new. The radial fracture hematoma block is often used for closed reduction of the fracture.

If an interruption in the cortex is found using ultrasound it is relatively easy to perform a hematoma block.

The hematoma block is a technique to inject a local anesthetic into the hematoma and preferably between the fractured bone fragments.

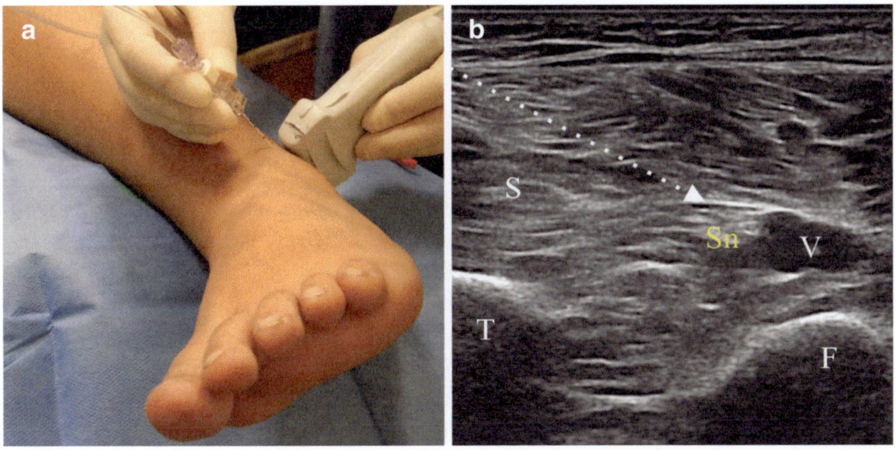

Fig. 13 (**a**) Patient position and needle entry point. (**b**) Sonoanatomy. Sn sural nerve, V small saphenous vein, F fibula, T tibia. Long white arrow needle direction and target point

Literature shows that these hematoma blocks provide good analgesia with low risk of systemic effects and infections. They reduce the need for opioids, ketamine or other potent analgesics that may have negative side effects.

Since there may be a larger risk for systemic effect than in regular nerve blocks the recommendation is to use local anesthetics with a lower risk for cardiac side effects. Like Lidocaine instead of Bupivacaine.

A hematoma block should not be performed in an open fracture.

Anatomy

Bone is readily seen as a white line with distal shadows. This is due to the very high echogenicity of the bone reflecting the ultrasound beam.

Probe/Equipment

Linear transducer

Technique

When using an ultrasound in the assessment of fractures it is vital to have a good knowledge of what bone and soft tissue look like. Bone is reflecting the beams and appear very bright.

Start scanning proximal to the point of suspected fracture and notice what the intact bony cortex looks like. Then slide the probe slowly more distally towards the injury in a longitudinal plane. The fracture will appear as a disruption of the white cortex line.

Insert the needle from in an in-line approach with direct visualization of the needle tip. The aim of the tip is to place it between the bony fragments. Local anesthetics is then injected. For ex. 10–15 ml of 1% Lidocaine. Pain reduction is often seen within 3–5 minutes.

Key Literature Reviewed

Hadzic A, et al. Hadzic's peripheral nerve blocks and anatomy for ultrasound-guided regional anaesthesia. 2nd edn. New York: McGraw Hill Medical; 2017

Salinas FV. Evidence basis for ultrasound guidance for lower-extremity peripheral nerve block. Reg Anesth Pain Med. 2016;41:261–74

Gharahbaghian L, et al. Point-of-care ultrasound in austere environments: a complete review of its utilization, pitfalls, and technique for common applications in austere settings. Emerg Med Clin North Am. 2017;35(2):409–41.

Fleming I, Egeler C. Regional anaesthesia for trauma: an update. Contin Educ Anaesth Crit Care Pain. 2014;14:136–41.

Choi JJ, Lin E, Gadsen J. Regional anesthesia for trauma outside the operating theatre. Curr Opin Anestesiol. 2013, 26:495–500

Gadsden J, Warlick A. Regional anesthesia for the trauma patient: improving patient outcomes. Local Reg Anesth. 2015;8:45–55

Pamplin J, Fischer AD, Hampton K, et al. Analgesia and sedation management during prolonged field care (CPG ID:61). Joint Trauma System Clinical Practice Guideline 01 Apr 2017

Al-Haddad MF, Coventry DM. Major nerve blocks of the lower limb. BJA CEPD Rev. 2003;3(4):102–5

Kopka A, Serpell MG. Distal nerve blocks of the lower limb. Continu Educ Anaesth Crit Care Pain. 2005;5(5):166–70

Marhofer T, Chan VWS. Ultrasound-guided regional anesthesia: current concepts and future trends. Anesth Analges. 2007;104(5):1265–9

Antonakakis JG, Scalzo DC, Jorgenson AS, et al. Ultrasound does not improve the success rate of a deep peroneal nerve block at the ankle. Reg Anesth Pain Med 2010;35:217–21.

Crystal C, et al. Ultrasound guided hematoma block: a novel use of ultrasound in the traumatized patient. J Trauma. 2007;62:532–3.

Komorowski M, Fleming S, Mawkin M, Hinkelbein J. Anaesthesia in austere environments: literature review and considerations for future space exploration missions. NPJ Microgravity. 2018;4:5.

Limitations of Current Knowledge and Opportunities for Future Research

There is currently only limited research on the long term effects and outcomes after prehospital nerve blocks. Further studies are required to give more information about the impact on PTSD and chronic post traumatic pain. There is also limited knowledge regarding the training needed to perform these interventions in an austere setting and the current success rates.

Pearls and Pitfalls

- Optimization of the patient positioning, and the ultrasound machine, is often key to success.
- Use the internet resources that are available to learn the ultrasound anatomy of a block.
- Train needle/eye coordination using ultrasound phantoms. These can be homemade and there are plenty of resources on the internet.
- Always aspirate before injecting to avoid fatal systemic effects.
- Always visualize the needle tip. Otherwise stop and move the probe to see the tip.

Part VI

Training

Initial Training, Credentialing, and Quality Assurance/Quality Improvement Processes

Harinder S. Dhindsa, Michael J. Vitto, and Benjamin D. Nicholson

Introduction

The use of point of care ultrasound or emergency ultrasound (EUS) has grown tremendously over the past decade in the out of hospital environment. The ability to improve diagnostic ability and serve as a tool to facilitate therapeutic intervention is continuing to rapidly evolve. Unlike emergency medicine physicians and other physicians who typically receive formal training in ultrasound during residency or through formal courses that are often required for credentialing, there is a relative paucity of training opportunities and a lack of standardization with respect to curriculum and training standards for nonphysician prehospital providers. Numerous articles have demonstrated that nonphysician providers can be trained in accurate image acquisition and interpretation in various settings and exam types (refs). However, there are no widely accepted standards with respect to curriculum or quality oversight. That said, there is a growing interest to develop such standards in order to provide high quality training, oversight, and ultimately care delivery to patients.

In the US, clinical care including scope of practice provided by emergency medical services are regulated primarily at the state level of government. In the majority of states, EMS providers typically work under the direction or supervision of a physician medical director as a delegated provider. In some states, EMS providers are licensed to practice independently. On the other hand, in many of the European countries, the issue of delegated practice is a non-issue as many EMS agencies are

H. S. Dhindsa · M. J. Vitto · B. D. Nicholson (✉)
Department of Emergency Medicine, Virginia Commonwealth University School of Medicine, Richmond, VA, USA
e-mail: Benjamin.nicholson@vcuhealth.org

B. D. Nicholson et al. (eds.), *Manual of Austere and Prehospital Ultrasound*,
https://doi.org/10.1007/978-3-030-64287-7_25

staffed by physicians who are independently licensed. In situations where EMS personnel are practicing under the supervision of a physician, it is important that training, the achievement of competence, oversight, and quality assurance standards are clearly outlined and followed. The risk of not having training standards and quality assurance is that clinical decisions and interventions may reach a patient by well meaning providers who have not been properly trained in image acquisition and interpretation.

Initial Training Program Goals and Requirements

In order to establish and maintain provider competency, each program or agency should establish an initial training program. The program's goals should align with the agency or unit's goals for the use of ultrasound, including scope of practice, ability to adequately train to achieve competencies, and maintain ongoing quality assurance (QA) and quality improvement (QI) in the targeted areas.

Although there are a number of studies evaluating initial training for EUS as well as performance in the field, there are no uniform standards with respect to ideal curriculum and training for prehospital providers.

Initial training should follow a step-wise or graduated approach to ensure adequate skills prior to image acquisition and interpretation that impacts clinical decisions. Our recommendation is that any process includes the following components: formal didactics program; standardized patient or simulator hands on practice under direct supervision; image acquisition with 100% quality assurance review on live patients but the trainee should not use these training images for their medical decision making and should work within their standard operating procedures; a final exam to demonstrate that the trainee can obtain images of sufficient quality to interpret and an interpretation exam using an image bank of both normal and pathologic images.

The formal didactics program should introduce equipment, image acquisition, image file management, and the process for submitting for QA/QI. Providers must demonstrate comfort with equipment operation and image optimization. Proper sanitization, and care of the equipment should also be covered.

Additional training should introduce specific scans consistent with the scope of the agency's mission. Many programs focus on the FAST or eFAST as the initial study. This offers several benefits. First, there already exists a large body of literature evaluating its utility and it has been incorporated into trauma certification courses as part of the initial patient survey. Second, trauma is a common patient type encountered in the prehospital environment offering providers frequent contact with this group. Third, the FAST depends on understanding probe movement to maximize image quality and helps providers develop this key skill as novices. Finally, it involves less subjectivity compared to interpreting volume status, left ventricle ejection fraction, or cardiac activity in cardiac arrest. Providers are therefore able to better focus on fundamental aspects of image acquisition while they are novices.

Ultrasound simulators should be available as a learning adjunct. These are most frequently employed when providers are developing procedural skills such as IV access. Many of these procedure based phantoms can be built inexpensively with household products. Prior to performing any procedure on a patient, providers should demonstrate proficiency on a simulator.

For non-procedure based ultrasound imaging, training should incorporate standardized patient scanning under direct observation. In many programs, this should be included with the initial didactic training and represent the core knowledge prior to scanning patients in the clinical environment under direct observation. Self scanning on team members could be used when standardized ultrasound models are not available or cost prohibitive.

As part of this graduated approach, providers should then scan on their own with quality review for technique and accuracy. A reasonable benchmark including standardized patient imaging is approximately 25 scans that undergo 100% quality review and are determined to be of sufficient quality for image interpretation. This should be repeated for any new studies, though the number of initial scans may vary based on the application.

Finally, a summary examination should be required that assesses both image acquisition and image interpretation. Similar to other medical training, this should be in the form of an Objective Structured Clinical Examination (OSCE) for the study in question. Assurance of image interpretation knowledge should be assessed through a formal examination involving both normal and pathologic ultrasound images. Images of insufficient quality for interpretation should also be reviewed to encourage the novice ultrasonographer to hold definitive interpretation when the images are not of sufficient quality.

Credentialing

Each agency or department should determine what the requirements for credentialing should be for their providers. Ideally, credentialing standards should help to establish the minimum number of initial scans of sufficient quality for interpretation that must be obtained to achieve reasonably consistent image acquisition and the requirements for confirmation of image interpretation abilities. It is important to note that these two aspects of ultrasonography are separate and there may be times when providers only need to be able to obtain images such as when teleultrasound is implemented.

Quality Assurance/Quality Improvement Process

Systems must be in place to ensure continuous quality image acquisition and appropriate interpretation. This often falls to the senior leadership of the organization or the medical director; however, we encourage this process to involve the providers credentialed to perform ultrasound as this increases the number of studies they review and interpret. It also offers an opportunity for any feedback to reach a larger number of providers (both the providers acquiring images and the ones providing feedback). Good QA/QI processes not only assure high quality of care at the patient level, they also can reveal areas of opportunities for improvement both at the system as well as the provider level.

Conclusion

Instituting an ultrasound program in the out of hospital environment must include a plan for initial training, a credentialing process that is equitable, and a QA/QI process that ensures a safe and efficacious ultrasound program.

Key Literature

1. Becker T, Martin-Gill, Callaway, Guyette, Schott. 398 Emergency Medical Services and Bilateral Lung Ultrasound in Emergency (EMS BLUE) Study. Ann Emerg Med. 2017;70.4: S156. Web.
2. Cone DC. Ultrasound Applications in EMS. Emergency Medical Services. Chichester: Wiley; 2015. p. 483–88. Web.
3. Garrone M. Prehospital ultrasound as the evolution of the Franco-German model of prehospital EMS. Crit Ultrasound J. 2011;3.3:141–47. Web.
4. Fitzgibbon JB, Lovallo E, Escajeda J, Radomski MA, Martin-Gill C. Feasibility of out-of-hospital cardiac arrest ultrasound by EMS physicians. Prehospital Emerg Care. 2019;23.3:297–303. Web.
5. Nelson B, Sanghvi P. Out of hospital point of care ultrasound: current use models and future directions. Eur J Trauma Emerg Surg. 2016;42.2:139–50. Web.
6. Press GM, Miller SK, Hassan IA, Blankenship R, Del Junco D, Camp E, Holcomb JB. Evaluation of a training curriculum for prehospital trauma ultrasound. J Emerg Med. 2013;45.6: 856–64. Web.
7. Russell TC, Crawford PF. Ultrasound in the austere environment: a review of the history, indications, and specifications. Mil Med. 2013;178.1: 21–8. Web
8. Jones SB. Ultrasonography in a forward-deployed military hospital. Mil Med. 2005;170.2: 99–102. Web.

Care of Equipment

Douglas C. George and Jenna M. B. White

As ultrasound technology becomes more accessible in the form of handheld devices and as the price of devices also falls, its utility in the prehospital setting has become more apparent. Handheld devices and transducers that connect to users' existing smartphones or tablets seem practically purpose-built for the prehospital environment. Despite their portability and ease of use, ultrasound devices are medical diagnostic equipment that must meet the same industry standards. Additionally, ultrasound devices utilized in the prehospital environment are subject to environmental stresses that devices which always remain indoors may not be [1-3]. Their small size and portability makes handheld ultrasound devices subject to potential damage, loss, or theft. Prehospital providers utilizing ultrasound must be keenly aware of these equipment considerations.

Device Care and Protection

Unlike a hospital which has access to a clinical engineering department that can be relied upon to inspect, repair, and maintain equipment, most prehospital care agencies maintain their own equipment, or contract with equipment vendors to provide routine maintenance and updates. At the time of purchase of an ultrasound device, the purchaser should understand fully what types of maintenance and repair are included in the purchase package. It should be noted whether warranty covers specific threats unique to the prehospital environment. Purchasers should be aware of the length of the warranty, and be informed regarding at what point a device will no

D. C. George (✉)
Division of Emergency Medicine, University of Vermont Medical Center, Burlington, VT, USA
e-mail: douglas.george@uvmhealth.org

J. M. B. White
Department of Emergency Medicine, University of New Mexico, Albuquerque, NM, USA

B. D. Nicholson et al. (eds.), *Manual of Austere and Prehospital Ultrasound*,
https://doi.org/10.1007/978-3-030-64287-7_26

longer be serviced. What tests does the manufacturer recommend to ensure that image integrity is preserved over time, and that the device continues to display images with high resolution and sharp contrast?

Numerous multidisciplinary groups have issued professional recommendations on how ultrasound transducers should be cleaned and disinfected. Low-level disinfection is suitable for most prehospital point-of-care ultrasound application (surface ultrasounds performed on closed skin). A soap and water cleanse or the use of a quaternary ammonia spray or wipes is recommended. Device manufacturers will provide lists of approved brands of solutions suitable for use with their product. Prepackaged disinfecting wipes are convenient, but it should be noted that these may desiccate if stored for a period of time in high heat, low humidity conditions. Disposable barrier devices such as sterile ultrasound probe covers, clean gloves, transparent film dressings (***tegaderms – copyright name***) or condoms could be utilized to minimize contamination and facilitate efficient cleanup, yet these add to operational costs and direct probe disinfection is still recommended after use [4].

As with adding any device to the field or in the hospital regular device maintenance and daily quality checks may be necessary. Establishing a routine and even a checklist will assist in keeping a device in-service and increase the ultrasound's lifespan. Examples of checklist topics include: sufficient battery life/power supply, ensuring that the probes are clean and cleaning supplies are restocked, checking for software updates, adequate amount of non-expired gel and inspecting for any damage to the probe or cables/connections.

Protecting ultrasound equipment is an important consideration. Storage of prehospital ultrasound devices will vary greatly depending on the planned use of the device, the environmental threats anticipated and the configuration of the ultrasound components. Hard-lined cases with internal customizable foam offer a great deal of protection from falls and environmental elements yet they are usually large and add substantial weight. While larger bulky cases are reasonable for storage on a vehicle or aircraft, their size and weight can hinder responders from bringing ultrasound devices to the scene or on prolonged field responses [5]. Storage devices that piggyback onto or are built into "first-in bags" are more likely to make it to the patient bedside yet could subject the device and transducer to structural damage and environmental exposure. Adjunct supplies for ultrasound use (disinfection supplies, procedural equipment, non-sterile and sterile gel) should ideally be co-stored with the ultrasound device to ensure availability and utilization by prehospital personnel.

Storage considerations should be specific to the type of ultrasound device and transducers chosen and most manufactures can provide storage and device protection recommendations. The prehospital setting has become an ideal opportunity to examine the use of application-based platforms (tablets, smartphones, laptops) given their multi-functional capabilities, light-weight, small size and long battery life. Popular application-based devices offer innumerable options when considering device protection, such as fall and water proofing. Many of the cases utilize military standardization for protective ratings/classification. In the future ultrasound software and the appropriate connectivity (cabled vs wireless) may also be integrated into cardiac monitors which will require attached storage of transducers and possibly cables.

While commercially available cases have many advantages, only a select few cases may provide additional support for sensitive cable connections that are frequently at risk for structural damage. Reinforcing cords at the point of connection to the probe/device and purchasing cable protectors may require more initial investment but can mitigate long term replacement costs by increasing cord life and preventing cord/connection damage [6]. During selection of ultrasound and probe devices prehospital providers should critically identify the vulnerabilities of each device individually. For example, exchangeable probes which can detach from connecting cables at their base, can be efficient and more functional in the prehospital setting due to their smaller size, yet this convenience comes with increased susceptibility to damage as compare to probes with permanently attached cords. While traditional systems only have one connection interface, these systems have two connection interfaces. The benefits and pitfalls of each unique ultrasound setup need to be evaluated in order to appropriately safeguard this valuable and expensive resource.

Devices that are anticipated to be used primarily during transport could be mounted into an ambulance, which protects the device from nearly all potential hazards. However, permanently affixing the device in this manner may decrease the device's functionality if it cannot be brought out of the vehicle to a scene.

Environmental Operating Conditions: Challenges Posed by the Prehospital Setting

The prehospital setting poses environmental hazards that could damage an ultrasound device, markedly degrade image quality, or cause the device to temporarily malfunction. Manufacturers provide information regarding the optimal temperature and humidity ranges for both storage and operating conditions for their device. Providers utilizing the ultrasound device and gel should be aware of these temperature and humidity parameters and avoid using the device when conditions are clearly outside of these ranges. Bright sunlight, while unlikely to acutely damage ultrasound equipment in short exposure intervals, can significantly impair one's ability to visualize ultrasound images on a screen [7, 8].

Resourcing adequate power supply and planning for sustained field usage is a vital component of prehospital ultrasound systems. EMS agencies must decide whether to power the device directly, or to charge it for portable, cord-free use. Internationally, considerations regarding the available power grid as well as the type of plug adaptors are essential to ensuring continuity of care. In general, the manufacturer will supply information regarding battery life and recharging time for portable devices. The type of batteries utilized by the ultrasound system may also change the management and planning for a prehospital ultrasound program. While lead acid batteries are less expensive, they tend to function poorly in cold environments. In addition, lead acid batteries tend to be less power efficient (ie. weigh more and carry less usable energy) than the more expensive Lithium based batteries. While one may favor lithium batteries, deployable agencies that utilize commercial airliners may have difficulty in traveling with Lithium based devices [5]. In situations where a power supply may be inconsistent or non-existent, programs may investigate off-grid recharging solutions such as solar-based, hydro-based and wind-based charging or even human-powered generators ("hand cranks"). While easily overlooked, battery selection and power sources must be thoroughly considered when implementing prehospital ultrasound systems [5, 9, 10].

Variability and limitations in patient access can be an unforeseen difference between hospital based and prehospital ultrasonography. Patient's in the field are frequently in less than ideal locations and body positions for ultrasound use. In addition, modern day stretchers do not allow for easy patient access to the retroperitoneal spaces which can limit fast exams. Some ambulance and aircraft configurations may not allow for 360 degrees of patient access and this may limit space between the patient and vehicular interior frame. Larger and longer ultrasound probes can provide excellent images or allow a single transducer to function across multiple frequencies [11], yet these larger devices may be difficult to utilize in the presence of limit space and physical obstructions such as those encountered in the less spacious prehospital setting (i.e. consider trying to perform a FAST exam in a confined space or even with specific interior ambulance configurations. Given some of these limitations the physical size of the probes selected for prehospital use should be carefully trialed in their anticipated operational setting.

The use of ultrasound for procedures in the field requires additional logistically planning and management. In the hospital setting, procedural equipment is located in systematic fashion with accessibility based on the critical nature of the procedure. Ideally, equipment for critical procedures would be available at the point of patient contact. This patient-centered concept has been the basis for "jump bags" and "first-in bags" in the field. Equipment for ultrasound-based procedures, especially interventions to address life-threats, need to be readily accessible. These procedural instruments should be co-located or attached to the ultrasound device to ensure immediate availability to prehospital personnel. For example, if within the scope of practice of the prehospital clinician, one should consider storing supplies for emergent ultrasound guided pericardiocentesis with the ultrasound device. Additionally, storing intravenous access supplies and specialized angiocatheters with the ultrasound device for ultrasound guided peripheral access care can improve prehospital care efficiency. While not realistic for all procedures, prehospital providers can improve delivery of care via logistical pre-planning and equipment staging.

While once a distant consideration, the implementation of transesophageal ultrasound in the field is no longer a thing of the future. For those programs and individuals considering implementing the use of transesophageal echocardiogram in the field one must select between disposable and re-usable probes. The current selection of portable TEEs is limited in comparison to hospital/ facility based devices. Cleaning re-usable probes will require close coordination with a sterile-processing department, likely within the hospital system, as well as consulting manufacture recommendations. In addition, given their invasive nature, these probes are temperature sensitive by design and only operate within certain temperature ranges which may limit their functionality in austere settings. Field deployment of these expensive devices usually requires large, heavy protective cases, which is another current limitation. Continued research and evolving technology are needed to determine the future utility and functionality of TEE in the field especially given the logistical considerations in mobilizing this device.

Connectivity and Maintaining Application-Based Platforms

Smartphone and tablet-based ultrasound platforms often require internet connectivity, which may be lacking in many prehospital settings. For this reason, it is important to keep application-based platforms up-to-date whenever connection to the internet is possible. Most of these devices will require at least intermittent internet access in order to download updates; if this is not performed at routine intervals, the platform may not function when desired.

Protecting Patient Information

Several handheld ultrasound devices now permit users to upload images to a cloud-based format, or to save images to a DICOM system for review or storage. Tablet or smartphone-based devices allow images to be shared through email or file sharing. The ease with which images can be shared can potentially violate patient confidentiality. Whenever possible and appropriate, the de-identification of images will protect patient privacy and prevent protected health information (PHI) from being inadvertently shared. A secure cloud-based platform is another storage option, but its degree of encryption must be compliant with requirements set forth by the HIPPA Security Rule. Other technical safeguards to protect patient information must be utilized whenever feasible. In the future, with potential integration of ultrasound software into cardiac monitors, the data and images will require similar protection as electrocardiograms and vital sign data.

References

1. Brooks AJ, Price V, Simms M. FAST on operational military deployment. Emerg Med J. 2005;22:263–5.
2. Nelson BP, Melnick ER, Li J. Portable ultrasound for remote environments, part I: feasibility of field deployment. J Emerg Med. 2011;40(2):190–7.
3. Shah SP, Epino H, Bukhman G, Umulisa I, Dushimiyimana JMV, Reichman A, Noble VE. Impact of the introduction of ultrasound services in a limited resource setting: rural Rwanda 2008. BMC Int Health Hum Rights. 2009;9(1):4.
4. Tayal, VS, Blaivas, M, Foster, TR. Ultrasound program management: a comprehensive resource for administrating point-of-care, emergency, and clinical ultrasound. Cham: Springer, 2018. Chapter 15 Ultrasound Safety and Infection Control https://doi.org/10.1007/978-3-319-63143-1

5. In Auerbach, P. S., In Cushing, T. A., & In Harris, N. S. (2017). Auerbach's wilderness medicine. Volume 2 Ch 109 Ultrasound in the Wilderness
6. Tayal, VS, Blaivas, M, Foster, TR. Ultrasound program management: a comprehensive resource for administrating point-of-care, emergency, and clinical ultrasound. Cham: Springer, 2018. Chapter 13 Ultrasound Safety and Infection Control. https://doi.org/10.1007/978-3-319-63143-1
7. Amaral CB, Ralston DC, Becker TK. Prehospital point-of-care ultrasound: A transformative technology. SAGE Open Medicine. January 2020; https://doi.org/10.1177/2050312120932706.
8. Carlo Andre Canepa and N. Stuart Harris.High Altitude Medicine & Biology.Jun 2019.103-111.https://doi.org/10.1089/ham.2018.0121
9. Gallien J, Sullivan A. Use of Solar Power Production for Point-of-Care Ultrasound: A Comparative Analysis. Prehospital and Disaster Medicine. 2019;34:s96–7. https://doi.org/10.1017/S1049023X19001997
10. Fagenholz PJ, Murray AF, Noble VE, et al. Ultrasound for high altitude research. Ultrasound Med Biol. 2012;38(1):1–12.
11. Liu J, Xu J, Forsberg F, et al. CMUT/CMOS-based Butterfly iQ—a portable personal sonoscope. Adv Ultrasound Diagn Ther. 2019;3:115–8.

Index

B. D. Nicholson et al. (eds.), *Manual of Austere and Prehospital Ultrasound*,
https://doi.org/10.1007/978-3-030-64287-7

MIX
Papier aus verantwortungsvollen Quellen
Paper from responsible sources
FSC® C105338

If you have any concerns about our products,
you can contact us on
ProductSafety@springernature.com

In case Publisher is established outside the EU,
the EU authorized representative is:
Springer Nature Customer Service Center GmbH
Europaplatz 3, 69115 Heidelberg, Germany

Printed by Libri Plureos GmbH
in Hamburg, Germany

Springer Series on Cultural Computing

More information about this series at http://www.springer.com/series/10481

Vasileios Mezaris · Claudia Niederée
Robert H. Logie
Editors

Personal Multimedia Preservation

Remembering or Forgetting Images and Video

Springer

Editors
Vasileios Mezaris
Centre for Research and Technology Hellas
Thermi, Thessaloniki
Greece

Robert H. Logie
University of Edinburgh
Edinburgh
UK

Claudia Niederée
University of Hannover
Hannover
Germany

ISSN 2195-9056 ISSN 2195-9064 (electronic)
Springer Series on Cultural Computing
ISBN 978-3-030-08793-7 ISBN 978-3-319-73465-1 (eBook)
https://doi.org/10.1007/978-3-319-73465-1

Printed on acid-free paper

This Springer imprint is published by Springer Nature
The registered company is Springer International Publishing AG
The registered company address is: Gewerbestrasse 11, 6330 Cham, Switzerland

Preface

The ease of creating digital content, especially photos and videos in nearly all life situations, has created an explosion in the amount of personal digital content that is continuously generated. Although declining storage device prices as well as cloud and social media services provide short-term solutions for keeping this content, over the years what we once stored is subject to a random form of digital forgetting, or is just not revisited, because the mere numbers make this a tedious task, not to mention the impact of changing life situations.

In this book, we advocate a novel forgetful approach to dealing with personal multimedia content on the long run, which is inspired by the effectiveness of human forgetting as a mechanism for helping us humans to stay focused on the important things. We present the different theoretical foundations, technologies, as well as applications and results of studies that help the reader understand the problems and challenges associated with personal digital preservation, and the solutions that can be developed in response to these challenges.

The book is organized into three main parts. Part I presents the necessary Interdisciplinary Foundations, Part II covers Multimedia Preservation Theory, and Part III discusses Multimedia Preservation in Practice.

Part I: Interdisciplinary Foundations

The first question that is often raised when discussing the topic of digital preservation is whether this is something that is really necessary or important to the average individual. Chapter 1, "Multimedia preservation: why bother?," attempts to answer this very question, by explaining that just storing the content today does not mean that this content will remain accessible and meaningful in the long run. Based on the understanding of this fact, Chap. 1 proceeds to motivating a more intelligent and selective approach to personal multimedia preservation. This approach introduces and combines three key building blocks: (a) "managed forgetting," for focusing on important and useful content inspired by human forgetting and remembering; (b) "contextualized remembering," for dealing with evolution and keeping content meaningful over time; and (c) "synergetic preservation," for bridging the gap between active information use and long-term information management.

While Chap. 1 highlights problems and challenges associated with digital preservation, we need to acknowledge that the preservation of information, in general, is not a topic that first appeared in the digital age. To the contrary, it is something that was first dealt with as part of evolution: humans have evolved to be very efficient at preservation of what it is necessary to preserve, and forgetting trivial or irrelevant details when they are no longer needed. In order to allow us to draw inspiration from nature, Chap. 2 looks at remembering and forgetting in human memory. It discusses how the human superpowers of managed preservation and forgetting are achieved, and how a conceptual understanding of human memory function could be used to inspire the design of digital managed preservation and forgetting. Chapter 2 argues that human-inspired digital forgetting is key for achieving a truly synergetic relationship between human and digital memory, and uses a study for exploring and contrasting human management of photographic collections with managed preservation and forgetting of the same photo collection by an example digital system. Altogether, Chap. 2 highlights how understanding the human cognitive function can help us to inspire more useful digital storage systems.

Having discussed how human memory works, Chap. 3 takes us to the opposite side, discussing how computers can understand the digital multimedia content. While for humans understanding what, e.g., a photo depicts is something that comes naturally by just looking at the photo, it is not the same for computers: to them, in the absence of specialized understanding methods, a photo is nothing more than a huge array of bits. Thus, Chap. 3 discusses methods and algorithms that endow computers with capabilities to understand digital content, based on the premise that understanding the digital content is important for subsequently supporting intelligent preservation decisions. The methods discussed in this chapter include (a) photo/video annotation, which refers to the problem of assigning one or more semantic concepts to photos or video fragments; (b) photo/video quality assessment, which refers to the automatic prediction of the aesthetic value of a photo or a video; (c) near-duplicate detection, which aims to identify groups of very similar items in large media collections; and (d) event-based photo clustering and summarization, which concern the selection of the most characteristic photos of a photo collection so as to create a storyline that conveys the gist of this collection.

Part II: Multimedia Preservation Theory

Chapter 4 goes into more depth regarding the intelligent and selective approach to personal multimedia preservation that was sketched in Chap. 1, taking advantage of the insights provided in Chaps. 2 and 3. Specifically, Chap. 4 focuses on a core ingredient of managed forgetting: the assessment of the importance of information items. It introduces two key notions for describing this importance: "Memory Buoyancy," which, in the short-term, considers how information sinks away from the user, and "Preservation Value," which attempts to estimate the future importance of a digital resource in the long run. Chapter 4 then proceeds with outlining methods for Preservation Value computation for different exemplary settings. It also discusses managed forgetting beyond assessing the importance of information items, that is, methods that can be used to implement managed forgetting on top of the values for information importance. This includes methods such as information hiding, forgetful search, summarization and aggregation, as well as deletion.

Making informed assessments of the importance of information items and decisions about their preservation is a big first step, but even this does not ensure that the preserved information will remain understandable and relevant in the long run. For this, Chap. 5 looks into contextualization methods. Fully understanding digital objects often requires knowing the wider context: for example, a family photo is practically useless if you do not know who are the people portrayed. This becomes even more important when considering the long-term preservation of documents, as not only is human memory fallible, but over long periods the people accessing the documents will change. Chapter 5 discusses methods for preserving the context associated with a digital item, and for assessing how this context evolves over time. It looks in detail at the relevant challenges and describes the development of a conceptual framework in which context information can be collected, preserved, evolved, and used to access and interpret documents. A number of techniques are presented showing real examples of context in action that fit within the framework, and applying to both text documents and image collections.

Chapter 6 takes the discussion of the Preserve-or-Forget (PoF) approach introduced in this book to the system level. It proposes a reference model—the PoF Reference Model which incorporates the techniques discussed in previous chapters for Preservation Value assessment, contextualization, etc., while at the same time paying special attention to the functionality which bridges between an Information Management System and a Digital Preservation System (DPS). The design of the PoF Reference Model was driven by the identification of five required characteristics: it has to be integrative, value-driven, brain-inspired, forgetful, and evolution-aware. The proposed PoF Reference Model consists of three layers; Chap. 6 goes on to discuss the main functional entities and the representative workflows of each of them, relating them to existing standards and practices in digital preservation. It also presents an architecture and an exemplary implementation for a system based on the PoF Reference Model.

Part III: Multimedia Preservation in Practice

Based on the foundations and methods presented in the two previous parts of this book, Chap. 7 presents the integration of preservation functionalities in a Personal Information Management (PIM) application. In this application, the "semantification" of the user's resources paves the way for more effective functionalities for automated preservation, forgetting, and remembering embedded in the daily activities of a user. The chapter also details a pilot based on this application, looking in depth into user activities such as photo organization, and the generation of diaries to remember past events. It investigates how forgetting functionalities can be embedded in applications and describes how different variants for forgetting are used in the pilot. Chapter 7 concludes with a discussion of experience of using the pilot in daily work.

Chapter 8 continues with investigating the application of the methods presented earlier in this book to the daily activities of users. In the first part of this chapter, a user study on a photo selection task is presented. Participants are asked to select subsets of the most important pictures from their own collections. Because evaluating the importance of photos to their owners is a complex process, which is often driven by personal attachment, memories behind the content, and personal tastes that are difficult to capture automatically, this study allows us to better understand the selection process. Then, based also on the findings of this study, the second part of this chapter presents methods for automatically selecting important photos from personal collections. Photo importance is modeled according to what photos users perceive as important and would have selected, and an expectation-oriented method for photo selection is presented, where information at both photo- and collection-level is considered to predict the importance of photos.

Thessaloniki, Greece
October 2017

Vasileios Mezaris
Claudia Niederée
Robert H. Logie

Acknowledgements

Most of the work reported throughout this book was supported by the EC's Seventh Framework Programme for Research, under contract FP7-600826 "ForgetIT: Concise Preservation by combining Managed Forgetting and Contextualized Remembering", 2013–2016.

Contents

Contributors

Walter Allasia EURIX Srl, Torino, Italy

Konstantinos Apostolidis Information Technologies Institute (ITI), Centre for Research and Technology Hellas (CERTH), Thermi, Thessaloniki, Greece

Andrea Ceroni L3S Research Center, Leibniz Universität Hannover, Hanover, Germany

Francesco Gallo EURIX Srl, Torino, Italy

Mark A. Greenwood The University of Sheffield, Sheffield, UK

Christian Jilek German Research Center for AI (DFKI), Kaiserslautern, Germany

Nattiya Kanhabua NTENT Inc., Barcelona, Spain

Robert H. Logie University of Edinburgh, Edinburgh, Scotland, UK

Foteini Markatopoulou Information Technologies Institute (ITI), Centre for Research and Technology Hellas (CERTH), Thermi-Thessaloniki, Greece; Queen Mary University of London, London, UK

Heiko Maus German Research Center for AI (DFKI), Kaiserslautern, Germany

Vasileios Mezaris Information Technologies Institute (ITI), Centre for Research and Technology Hellas (CERTH), Thermi, Thessaloniki, Greece

Kaweh Djafari Naini L3S Research Center, Hannover, Germany

Claudia Niederée L3S Research Center, Hannover, Germany

Elaine Niven University of Dundee, Dundee, UK

Ioannis Patras Queen Mary University of London, London, UK

Sven Schwarz German Research Center for AI (DFKI), Kaiserslautern, Germany

Nam Khanh Tran L3S Research Center, Leibniz Universität Hannover, Hannover, Germany

Tuan Tran L3S Research Center, Hannover, Germany

Christos Tzelepis Information Technologies Institute (ITI), Centre for Research and Technology Hellas (CERTH), Thermi-Thessaloniki, Greece; Queen Mary University of London, London, UK

Maria Wolters University of Edinburgh, Edinburgh, Scotland, UK

Part I
Interdisciplinary Foundations

Chapter 1
Multimedia Preservation: Why Bother?

Claudia Niederée, Vasileios Mezaris, Heiko Maus and Robert H. Logie

Abstract Multimedia content and especially personal multimedia content is created in abundance today. Short- to mid-term storage of this content is typically no problem due to decreased storage prices and the availability of storage services. However, for the long-term perspective, i.e., preservation, adequate technologies and best practices for keeping the content accessible and meaningful are still missing. Instead, the breakdown of devices and changes in technologies lead to some form of random survival and random forgetting for digital content. In this chapter, we motivate a more intelligent and selective approach to personal multimedia preservation. This approach introduces and combines three key building blocks: (a) "managed forgetting" for focusing on important and useful content inspired by human forgetting and remembering; (b) "contextualized remembering" for dealing with evolution and keeping content meaningful over time; and (c) "synergetic preservation" for bridging the gap between active information use and long-term information management.

C. Niederée
L3S Research Center, Hannover, Germany
e-mail: niederee@L3S.de

V. Mezaris (✉)
Information Technologies Institute (ITI)/Centre for Research and Technology Hellas (CERTH), 6th Km. Charilaou-Thermi Road, 57001 Thermi-Thessaloniki, Greece
e-mail: bmezaris@iti.gr

H. Maus
German Research Center for AI (DFKI), Kaiserslautern, Germany
e-mail: heiko.maus@dfki.de

R. H. Logie
University of Edinburgh, Edinburgh, Scotland, UK
e-mail: rlogie@ed.ac.uk

V. Mezaris et al. (eds.), *Personal Multimedia Preservation*, Springer Series on Cultural Computing, https://doi.org/10.1007/978-3-319-73465-1_1

1.1 Abundant Creation and Random Survival

With the advent of digital photography, taking photos and videos is nearly effortless and requires few resources, and the widespread use of smartphones with continuously improving camera features and storage capacities has accelerated this trend. A further trigger for growing multimedia content creation is social media with its multifaceted opportunities and incentives for content creation and sharing. In addition, nowadays, taking photos and videos is tolerated nearly everywhere. Hundreds of photos are easily taken by an individual participating in public events, such as concerts, as well as in private events such as a holiday trip. Furthermore, photos and videos are also very often taken of more mundane aspects of life, such as food or in support of everyday activities such as shopping, further increasing the amount of personal multimedia content to be dealt with. Thus, personal multimedia content is created in abundance and with a tendency for further growth.

This raises the question of what happens to all of this personal multimedia content, which has to be considered in the short-term, mid-term, and the long-term perspective. With the decreasing price of storage media, it is not really a problem to store all of this content; either in traditional digital storage devices such as hard disks or also on the cloud, since storage is offered as a service by several cloud storage providers. This situation fosters the adoption of a keep-it-all strategy for the short- to mid-term perspective, where the majority of content created is kept "somewhere" (more or less systematically organized).

However for the mid- to long-term perspective, just storing all of this content often ends up as a kind of "dark archive" of photo, video, and other content collections, which are rarely accessed (and enjoyed) again. The mere size of the collections makes going through them as well as sorting or annotating them a tedious task.

Furthermore, for the long-term perspective, there is the risk of losing personal content by a random form of "digital forgetting" [191]: Over decades, storage devices such as hard disks may break down, and employed storage media become subject to decay, loss, and accidental destruction or even theft. Moreover, even cloud storage is vulnerable if the companies providing the service go out of business. Furthermore, with the development and adoption of new technologies, existing formats and storage media quickly become obsolete. These developments make random parts of personal collections inaccessible. Just consider, for instance, how difficult it would be today to access photos stored years ago in .mos format in a floppy disk, or that even accessing photos stored much more recently in a DVD is not that straightforward any more, given that your new ultrabook laptop does not cater for reading this type of external media. This leads to a random form of survival for personal multimedia content. This weakness of digital content of being seemingly easy to keep but also easy to "lose" has raised discussions about "digital dark ages" already in the late 90s [51, 212]. It is possible to read a 200-year-old book, or look at 100-year-old printed photos, but in a hundred years from now, will the technology exist to read the file and media formats being used today? And, even if pure format readability is ensured by timely transformation to more up-to-date formats and copying in contemporary storage media, more investment is still required for ensuring long-term interpretability of content. Over the years, we might simply forget what or whom a photo shows or why it was taken.

What is actually missing are best practices and supporting technologies for dealing with personal multimedia content in the long run. Both the risk of dark archives and of digital forgetting highlight the need to select, supported by automated methods, the most important content and to invest some effort into keeping them enjoyable and accessible not only over a lifetime but possibly also for future generations.

1.2 State of Affairs in Personal Preservation

"Digital Preservation"—i.e., secure long-term storage of content, considering time frames of decades and longer—is a systematic approach for avoiding random digital forgetting. It embraces tools, technologies, as well as organizational aspects.

However, while preservation of digital content is now well established in memory institutions, such as national libraries and archives, it is still in its infancy in most other organizations, and even more so for personal content. There are several obstacles for the wider adoption of preservation technology in organizational and personal information management: There is a considerable gap between active information use and preservation activities. Active information use refers to dealing with information objects for everyday private or professional activities, typically supported by some information management environment, such as a content management system in an organization or a desktop environment in the context of personal information management. In addition, especially in personal information management, there is typically little awareness for preservation. Although the need for personal preservation has been recognized in theory (e.g., [271]), this has not yet propagated to more practical settings and solutions. As a consequence, readiness for investing considerable resources in terms of time and money for preservation is low. Finally, establishing effective preservation and concise and usable archives still requires a lot of manual work for selecting content that is relevant for preservation and for keeping the archives accessible and meaningful long term, thus entailing expenses much larger than just the storage costs. This is further aggravated by the fact that no benefits are seen for moving from more or less systematic backup to systematic preservation.

A personal information space consists of a substantial number of information objects connected to the person's life such as wedding videos, travel pictures, or graduation keepsakes. It requires serious dedication and cognitive effort to organize all these data and keep them accessible as time passes. Moreover, these digital artifacts often represent past moments but are not associated with a physical memento. Therefore, they form valuable resources for the user and future generations. If the material is lost or corrupted due to improper conservation, it will be useless and memories might be lost. Most users still use backups as their main form of preservation. John et al. in [186] surveyed 2600 academics and members of the digital public about their preservation strategies. 60% of the respondents relied on backups. If data were lost, which happened to 30% of the participants, the most common reason for the loss (70% of all cases) was inability to find the files again.

Furthermore, many people follow the keep-it-all strategy. Marshall [271] points out five main reasons: (a) assessing value of resources in advance is difficult, (b) keep-it-all is currently the best practice, (c) deletion and (d) sorting out resources are cognitively demanding exercises, and (e) archived information resources play an important role as memory prosthesis.

There are preservation guidelines aimed at the general public that show how to go beyond backups. For example, the Library of Congress raises awareness of personal archiving solutions on their website and provides practical information [232, 234]. The recommended steps[1] are as follows:

1. Identify what you want to save.
2. Decide what is most important to you.
3. Organize the content (descriptive file names and folders).
4. Save copies in different places.
5. Manage your archive (including migration plans).

These recommendations are very helpful but leave all steps to the user, i.e., what to save, how to organize, where to store (hard disk and online storage), and when to migrate. This puts a high burden on the user: various decisions need to be made and it requires discipline in, e.g., maintaining and updating the archive.

This cognitive up-front effort is one of the reasons why the cloud storage offered by DropBox, Microsoft OneDrive, or Google Drive is not a preservation system in itself, but only a tool in a larger preservation strategy. Started as syncing, file sharing, and backup solutions, those services offer structuring methods such as file folders or (keyword-) tags, but do not comply with preservation best practices such as the Open Archival Information System (OAIS) standard [68]. Other services, such as Amazon Cloud, comply with OAIS, but do not support users before ingesting data into the store. Either way, users are left on their own for large parts of the preservation process. An overview of the preservation functionality of major cloud services can be found in [331].

Another issue is preserving social media content. While service providers carefully store users' data for in-depth analysis, they often do not provide any support for dedicated archiving and preservation. Even when archivists are called in at a later stage, preservation is not optimal, since it is not part of the business model [308]. As shown, for example, in the survey reported in [189], users often post information in social media, which might be worth preserving in a personal archive such as information about lifestyle and data about travel, festivities/parties, and funny events. Many services have emerged around curating social media content in a form that is easily accessible, and would lend itself well to further preservation. At the most basic level, Twitter allows users to download a compressed file that includes all of their tweets, which can then be viewed in a browser. The Storify service allows users to curate

[1]There are some specializations depending on the media, e.g., video or social media.

conversations on Twitter—tweets that are replies to each other are collated into a single web page and can be annotated further [81].

Having a look at services like Flickr where people collect and share digital moments, or services such as Twitter that focus more on real-time short messaging, long-term preservation is not the first thing which comes into one's mind. Nevertheless, Twitter also treats concerns on archiving: they introduced a service to download a zip archive of the user's tweets. Furthermore, Google and Facebook have introduced formal ways of handling an account in case a user is deceased, such as handing it over to a dedicated contact person with full or partial access [57].

1.3 Preserve or Forget: Managed Forgetting and Digital Preservation

To ease the adoption of more robust and beneficial preservation practices for personal multimedia content, we propose the introduction of a radically more adoptable and sustainable approach, the "Preserve-or-Forget" approach to intelligent preservation management, which combines three novel concepts:

- Inspired by the role of forgetting in the human brain, we envision a concept of **managed forgetting** for systematically dealing with information that progressively ceases in importance and finally becomes obsolete, as well as for redundant information. This concept is expected to help in preservation decisions and to create direct benefits for active information use. At first glance, forgetting seems to contradict the idea of preservation: Preservation is about keeping things, not about throwing them away. However, if no special actions are taken for long-term preservation, we already face a rather random digital forgetting in the digital world today. As discussed above, this is triggered, for example, by changing hardware, hard disk crashes, technology evolution, and changes in life circumstances. We aim to replace such random forgetting processes with managed forgetting, where users are optimally supported in their explicit decisions about what to keep, and how what is kept to be organized and preserved. In particular, we envision an idea of gradual forgetting, where complete digital forgetting is just the extreme, and a wide range of different forgetting actions such as summarizing are foreseen. This draws on the principles of a highly efficient process of forgetting in the human brain for information that is trivial, redundant, or only required on a single occasion for a short time.
- For bridging the chasm that still separates active information use from content preservation activities, we envision the concept of **synergetic preservation**, which couples information management and preservation management, making the intelligent preservation integral to the content life cycle in information management. This clearly supports easier adoption, and by enabling a rich information flow from the information context to the preservation context more intelligent and informed preservation decisions, e.g., for preservation selection and contextualization.

- To bring preserved information back into active use in a meaningful way, even if a long time has passed since their transition into the archive, we envision the concept of **contextualized remembering**, again inspired by processes in the human brain. The idea here is to already equip resources with rich context information when packaging them for preservation (thus preparing them for long-term interpretation) and to gradually evolve this context information, reflecting the evolution in terminology, semantics, and interpretation context, thus reaching a semantic level of preservation.

The vision of our Preserve-or-Forget approach is a transition from pure archives to managing and preserving concise knowledge ecosystems, coupling information management and preservation. Realizing such an ecosystem requires a concise, diversity-aware, and evolution-aware preservation approach which includes a careful selection of what to preserve taking into account coverage, diversity, importance and overlap/redundancy of information, the explicit contextualization of preserved resources into self-contained objects to ensure long-term interpretability, as well as adequately dealing with evolution and with information becoming obsolete.

In this book, we discuss the conceptual foundations, architectural aspects, as well as effective methods for implementing the Preserve-or-Forget approach. Many of the discussed methods and technologies have been developed in the European project ForgetIT, in which the editors and authors of this book were involved.

Chapter 2
Preserving and Forgetting in the Human Brain

Robert H. Logie, Maria Wolters and Elaine Niven

Abstract Humans have evolved to be very efficient at managed preservation of what is necessary to preserve. Humans are also extremely efficient at forgetting trivial or irrelevant details when they are no longer needed. Indeed, managed preservation and forgetting could be viewed as a set of human 'superpowers' achieved through use of a lifetime of accumulated knowledge, highly effective contextualisation, aggregation, organisation, summarisation and reconstruction of key features of experiences. But humans are poor at preservation of large amounts of detail. Typically, memories are partially reconstructed during the retrieval process, and this reconstruction process can sometimes lead to false memories. Many of these strengths and limitations of human memory are well understood by human memory researchers, although important questions and uncertainties remain. In complete contrast, digital systems excel in preserving large amounts of detail, and are getting better at contextualisation. But they remain rather poor at systematic forgetting of irrelevant detail. Often, digital forgetting occurs by accident through disk crashes, incompatible upgrades of software and hardware, lost or stolen storage devices. Even if the data are still present and safely stored, insufficient indexing and poor information retrieval may result in those data effectively being forgotten. This chapter will provide a detailed overview of the state of the science of human memory, based on empirical studies and conceptual modelling. It will discuss how the human superpowers of managed preservation and forgetting are achieved, and show how a conceptual understanding of human memory function could be used to inspire the design of digital managed preservation and forgetting. It will argue that human-inspired digital forgetting is key for achieving a truly synergetic relationship between human and digital memory, and explore how such a synergetic relationship can address aspects of the paradox that massive investment in technology has not necessarily led to the expected increase in

R. H. Logie (✉) · M. Wolters
University of Edinburgh, Edinburgh, Scotland, UK
e-mail: rlogie@ed.ac.uk

M. Wolters
e-mail: maria.wolters@ed.ac.uk

E. Niven
University of Dundee, Dundee, UK
e-mail: e.niven@dundee.ac.uk

V. Mezaris et al. (eds.), *Personal Multimedia Preservation*, Springer Series on Cultural Computing, https://doi.org/10.1007/978-3-319-73465-1_2

productivity (IT/productivity paradox). Next, we will describe an in-depth study of personal, digital photograph collections that were contributed by volunteer research participants. This study explored human management of photographic collections and contrasted it with managed preservation and forgetting of the same photo collection by an example digital system that incorporates automated conceptualisation and forgetting. The chapter will conclude with a summary of how understanding human cognitive function can help to inspire more useful digital storage systems that offer reliable and usable tools to complement and support human memory rather than attempt to replace it.

2.1 Human Memory and Forgetting

2.1.1 What Is Human Memory?

Human memory takes many forms and serves a wide range of purposes that are essential for humans to function in everyday personal and working life. Among the lay public, it is most widely associated with preservation and retrieval of information about public and personal events. However, scientific study takes a much broader view of human memory to include the acquisition, preservation and retrieval of knowledge and skills (semantic memory and procedural memory), events and experiences across a person's lifetime (episodic memory), and remembering to carry out intended actions (prospective memory). It also applies to the temporary storage and moment-to-moment updating of information required for a focus on the current task, an ability known as 'working memory'. Finally, it applies to a range of control functions that can suppress or inhibit information that is irrelevant or redundant and that can detect or recognise whether information has been encountered previously or is linked with previously preserved information.

2.1.2 Research Methods for Human Memory

Each individual has different experiences and different memories of those experiences, as well as different knowledge and skills accumulated over their lifetime. Also, people vary in the efficiency with which they can learn and retrieve new knowledge, and encode, forget, preserve or retrieve details of events that they have experienced. However, the study of human memory is based on the assumption that the general principles that govern human memory organisation and function are the same across all healthy human adults, and are the result of the effect of evolution on the human brain. So, there are common principles across all humans for learning, forgetting, encoding, preserving, retrieval and so on. Many of these principles also apply to many animals. An analogy would be that the principles governing the function of other aspects of physiology, such as the heart, the liver, the kidneys, the lungs, the immune system or the endocrine system, are the same across all healthy human adults, even if these systems differ in their efficiency between individuals. On this principle, if we are collecting objective memory performance data, we need only study the principles of functioning of human memory in a single healthy adult and these principles should generalise to all healthy human memory.

However, experimental data are inevitably noisy and an individual who is studied might have some underlying anomaly such as subtle undetected brain damage, or be simply uncooperative. Therefore, in practice, multiple healthy participants are recruited and allocated randomly to different experimental groups for the purposes of comparison. Using this approach, the numbers in each group need not be large, although there is usually a matching in the age range and educational level to mitigate the variability from differences in memory efficiency. Data are then averaged and analysed statistically across participants within each group to reduce the impact of possible idiosyncrasies of any one participant. In contrast to studies that involve subjective opinions, self-report or survey data, in experimental studies of this kind, there is less emphasis on sampling from cross sections of the population. Therefore, most research on human memory involves designing and running experiments with human volunteers who are presented with material and are subsequently tested on their memory for that material.

Experiments are designed according to theoretical, conceptual models of how a specific aspect of human memory might function, and conclusions are drawn from detailed analyses of the pattern of memory errors that result from different experimental manipulations or different kinds of material. Some of the experiments involve assessing the processes and accuracy of retrieval of real-life events, whereas others involve relatively artificial materials. There is also a large amount of research of this kind with volunteers who have suffered specific forms of brain damage, and these studies can reveal some of the characteristics of healthy human memory as well as the nature of memory impairments from which the patients suffer. Other experiments involve exploring the patterns of brain activation while human volunteers are completing memory tasks. The development of the theoretical, conceptual models is driven by the patterns of results from these experiments, and converging evidence across studies.

2.1.3 General Principles of Human Memory

The research approach described in the previous section has generated a large volume of evidence for some general principles of memory function. Most human memory researchers agree about these principles (for an overview see [27]), but there are ongoing debates about the details of the conceptual models of memory and the interpretation of patterns of results. As a result, there is currently no universally accepted conceptual model of human memory. An example of one conceptual model of human memory is illustrated in Fig. 2.1. Some of the details of this model have

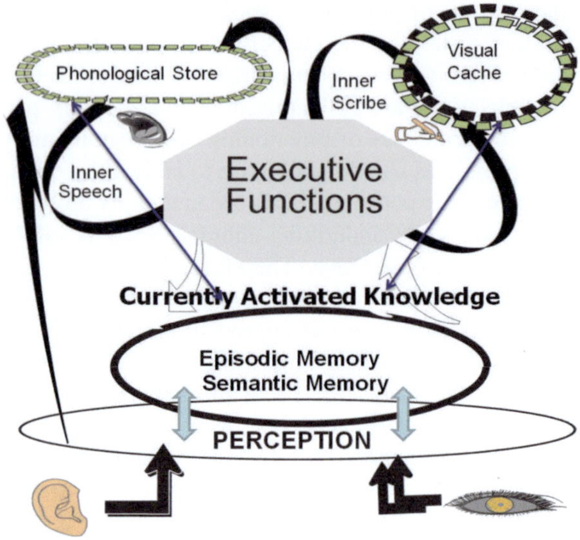

Fig. 2.1 A Conceptual Model of Human Memory

been developed by the first author of this chapter (e.g. [251–253]), based on a simpler model originally proposed in [29]. However, it has characteristics that are similar to other contemporary conceptual models.

In summary, this conceptual model indicates that information from auditory, visual and other forms of perception (e.g. tactile) activates stored knowledge accumulated over a lifetime regarding knowledge about the world and about the self ('semantic memory') and preserved information about individual events ('episodic memory') related to the perceived stimuli. Some of the activated knowledge is held on a temporary basis in a collection of interacting, domain-specific temporary memory systems or components of working memory, and processed by a range of executive functions. For example, combinations of meaning, shape and sound may be held together as Currently Activated Knowledge. Details of recently perceived stimuli that have been seen or heard may be held as sound-based codes in the phonological store component or as visually based codes in the Visual Cache component. Both types of code decay within around 2 s, but the inner speech component can allow the sound-based codes to be held for longer by mentally repeating the sounds. The Inner Scribe component holds and can mentally rehearse sequences of movements and can allow visual codes to be held longer by mentally rehearsing the codes held in the Visual Cache.

It should be noted that the theoretical, conceptual models of human memory such as the one shown in Fig. 2.1 are used as frameworks to generate hypotheses and to guide the design of memory experiments. They are not formal computational models that have clearly defined characteristics for each component, or that describe precisely what information flows along the arrows between components. There are some formal computational models of specific functions of human memory (for example of the phonological store and inner speech shown in Fig. 2.1), and these are used to run simulations of the behavioural data patterns obtained from memory experiments with human volunteers. However, these formal models are beyond the scope of the current chapter. Figure 2.1 is included here to set a context for the reader who is unfamiliar with the approaches and style of research summarised later in this chapter.

2.1.4 Semantic and Episodic Memory

A key distinction is between semantic and episodic memory. Semantic memory includes knowledge acquired through life experience (e.g. language, facts about the world, people and the self) and learned skills, sometimes referred to as procedural memory (e.g. swimming, riding a bicycle, mathematics). Episodic memory refers to memory for specific experiences of events that took place at a particular place and at a particular time (e.g. a particular holiday, meeting, lecture or social event or what you had for dinner yesterday). In [394], the authors introduced the concept of episodic memory as a system that underlies the 'what-when-where' specifics of an event, and as such is distinct from factual knowledge in semantic memory [391]).

Forgetting from episodic memory is rapid and substantial. Forgetting from semantic memory is much less rapid and information is well preserved over long periods or never lost. Semantic memory is thought to develop across the lifetime by extracting features that are common across similar events, and building what are known as schema for specific types of events, a concept first proposed by Bartlett [34]. Details of the occasion on which the information was first encountered are forgotten.

For example, a restaurant schema includes tables, menus, food, conversation, waiting staff and paying a bill, but we probably cannot recall when we first learned these features of restaurants. In the same way, we know that the capital of France is Paris, but are unlikely to remember when that fact was first encountered. This means that the schema sets the general context for each restaurant visit, and provides a 'framework' on which to build the memory for key details of specific visits to restaurants. The features that are common to each restaurant visit need not be stored on every occasion. The same is true of any common experience, such as a working day, a visit to a swimming pool, a train or aeroplane journey. The framework or context can then be used to aid retrieval of information about specific events. When recalling a restaurant visit, we can assume that there was a menu, food, a table, a bill, etc., and so only have to store and retrieve the key information such as who else was at the table, and what was important about the conversation or about the food. In summary, human memory tends to preserve generic information that is repeated across similar experiences and events without 'tagging' that information with a time and place. Human memory tends to forget details that are unique to individual experiences or events, except when the unique features of a particular event are particularly important for the individual.

A further role for a schema or context is in the understanding or interpretation of presented information or events. Take, for example, the following paragraph.

> The procedure is actually quite simple. First, you arrange the items into different groups. Of course, one pile might be sufficient depending on how much there is to do. If you have to go somewhere else due to lack of facilities, that is the next step; otherwise, you are pretty well set. It is important not to overdo things. That is, it is better to do too few things at once than too many. In the short run, this may not seem important but complications can easily arise. A mistake can be expensive as well. After the procedure is completed, one arranges the material into different groups again. They then can be put into their appropriate places. Eventually, they will be used once more and the whole cycle will then have to be repeated [52, 134-5].

This passage is difficult to understand and also is difficult to remember because there is no context. Most of the material from the passage will already have been forgotten as you are reading this sentence. However, after the context for the passage is given as 'washing clothes', then the interpretation of the text is trivial and memory for the sequence of procedures can be generated from existing knowledge in the schema without having to remember the exact wording. The use of the schema can be repeated every time this kind of activity is required, and precise details of each occasion do not have to be preserved in memory, unless, for example, an error on one occasion is to be avoided on future occasions, or a small change to the procedure results in a benefit that should be remembered for future repetition.

However, even when a context is available, substantial forgetting of detail occurs within minutes. For example, although the general meaning of the washing clothes paragraph could be regenerated, the precise wording is unlikely to be remembered accurately. Likewise, within a few seconds of reading the text of the current paragraph, any reader will have forgotten the exact wording used but will remember the meaning of the text. For readers who are not already familiar with the topic of how human memory functions (i.e. have no accurate or detailed existing schema or context), many of the detailed facts presented in this chapter will be forgotten within an hour after it has been read, unless this material is relearned before this forgetting occurs (e.g. [195]).

Therefore, a great deal of information concerning an event is never stored in memory. Because there is a large number of schemata and a large amount of information accumulated in semantic memory over the lifetime of each individual, the human memory system can select what information is necessary to set the context for the current environment or information presented, and can inhibit or ignore information that is irrelevant or can be assumed from the context. This aspect of human memory is a major strength in that it avoids the distraction of information that is irrelevant or redundant for the current task, and avoids the storage of large amounts of irrelevant or redundant information, making it very efficient for storing and retrieving key details about an event, or retrieving key facts and skills that are required for the current task.

2.1.5 Forgetting from Episodic and Semantic Memory

The process of forgetting from semantic or episodic human memory typically refers to the inability to retrieve information that has previously been stored, and this is often

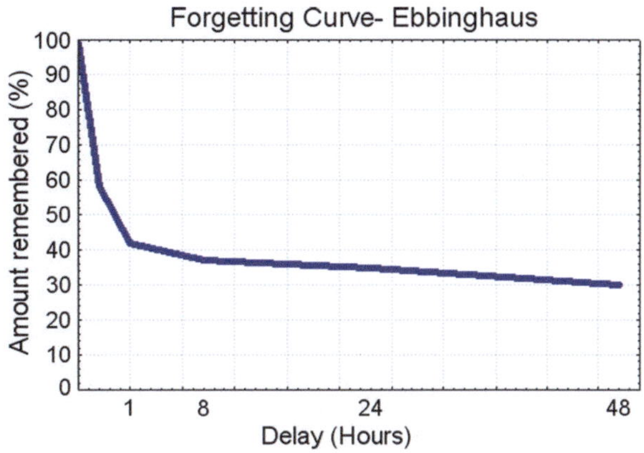

Fig. 2.2 Human forgetting over time

viewed as an unwelcome limitation. However, detailed analysis shows forgetting to be more complex, and to be a benefit to humans most of the time. As should be clear from the previous section, a substantial amount of detail is never encoded in memory. It is equally well established that of the details that are encoded, a substantial amount is forgotten within a short time after the initial experience. This prevents the memory system from being filled with information for which there is no clear context, or that is largely irrelevant, or which is required only on a temporary basis, and preservation is not normally required. Consequently, only information that is important for understanding and functioning in the world tends to be preserved.

The forgetting of information that lacks context was first subject to systematic study by the German researcher Ebbinghaus [122] who experimented with learning and remembering ‘nonsense material’, specifically three-letter syllables (e.g. BAZ FUB YOX DAX LEQ VUM . . .) for which he had no established schema. Therefore, this kind of material was selected to assess ‘pure’ episodic memory without the support of semantic memory. In his experiments, he would spend several minutes trying to learn sequences of these nonsense syllables, and then tested his memory by attempting to relearn the material at different time periods after the initial learning. Typical results from his experiments are shown in Fig. 2.2. It is clear from the figure that most of the forgetting had occurred within one hour of the learning, but the small amount of material that was retained after one hour was retained for at least 48 h.

Although the work of Ebbinghaus was important for understanding memory and forgetting, it was unclear as to why the material was being forgotten. The research was criticised because of the reliance on memory for nonsense material and because only one individual was tested, namely Ebbinghaus himself. It is rare that adult humans are required to remember material for which they have no schema or context, and as mentioned above, most experimental studies of memory involve an investigation of the aggregate results from groups of individuals. The issue of what might be the main causes of forgetting has been the subject of scientific debate ever since the time of Ebbinghaus, with the major possibilities being decay of the material over time, or other material causing interference with the memory representation.

In the case of decay, information is lost over time through gradual deletion from memory of material that is rarely or never accessed and retrieved. In the case of interference, the forgetting may arise from an inability to retrieve key details of an event because of interference from previously stored details about similar events ('proactive interference'—e.g. [398], or because of interference from stored details of similar subsequent events ('retroactive interference', e.g. [287]. More recent studies have demonstrated interference-based forgetting of a first language when trying to learn a second language [177]), an example of retroactive interference: learning of the new language interferes with memory for the previously learned language. Other studies have shown that parking a car in different spaces in the same car park multiple times (e.g. at work or near a retail centre) can make it difficult to remember where the car was parked today [97]. This is a common experience and often suggests to people that their car has been stolen until they realise that they are looking in the space that they used for their car yesterday or last week. This is an example of proactive interference: multiple similar previous experiences interfere with the ability to remember details of the most recent instance of this experience.

The Ebbinghaus forgetting function applies beyond the forgetting of context-less material. It also applies to the forgetting of material that can be supported by context from semantic memory. Take, for example, the results from a study published 100 years after the Ebbinghaus studies. McKenna and Glendon [288] tested memory in people who had undertaken and successfully completed a first aid course. At intervals varying from 3 to 36 months, they were tested on their memory for their ability to diagnose the health problem associated with particular symptoms, their resuscitation technique and performance as well as on a total score for the knowledge they had retained from the course. Despite spending several days on the first aid course, and passing the test at the end of the course, within 3 months they had forgotten 70% of their knowledge about diagnosis, and after 6 months they had forgotten 60% of even their best preserved ability, namely their technique for cardiopulmonary resuscitation (CPR). However, over the following 30 months, the rate of forgetting was very much slower than it was during the first 6 months. In the case of Ebbinghaus, learning took place over a few minutes with no schema or context, and forgetting was over periods of minutes and hours. In the McKenna and Glendon study, learning took place over several days and involved information and skills within the schema or context of first aid care. In this latter case, the forgetting was over periods of months rather than hours. So, context as well as amount of initial learning greatly slows down the speed of forgetting. However, the shapes of the forgetting functions were remarkably similar, even if over different time periods. Equivalent results were found in [31] for English native speakers remembering Spanish learned at school over delays of up to 50 years, and retention of information learned at University up to 30 years later [88]. In both studies, there was substantial forgetting within the first few years after leaving the formal learning environment, but then a much slower rate of forgetting thereafter.

These well-established studies show that when memory is supported by context or schema, then the material can be retained for periods of months or years, but even with this support, most of the forgetting of details still occurs within a relatively

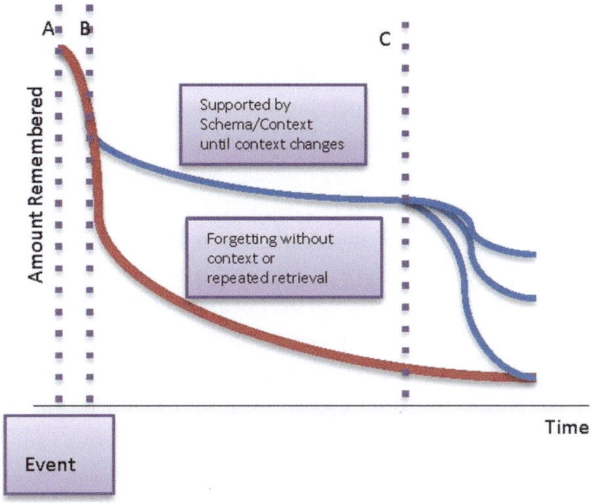

Fig. 2.3 Forgetting with context support versus forgetting without context support

short period and the material that remains after that initial period is forgotten much more slowly. If never ‘relearned’ from time to time, all of the information may be forgotten. For example, the people in the study in [31] who used Spanish in their daily lives after leaving school retained their knowledge of Spanish very much more successfully than those who had few subsequent opportunities to practice using the Spanish they had learned. The same was true of the material learned at university in the study in [88]. The difference in forgetting supported by context and without such support is illustrated in Fig. 2.3.

A further everyday example of the support from context (also illustrated in Fig. 2.3) is remembering the number of a hotel room for the period of staying in the hotel, or remembering a flight number. The context of being in a particular hotel is supported by the repeated requirement to retrieve the room number when asking for the key, going into breakfast, or returning to the room, but after leaving the hotel there is no requirement to retrieve the room number and so it is forgotten. The same is true for the flight number which need only be retrieved while at the airport but is not retrieved again after the travelling is complete, and so is forgotten. Paper and electronic aids are of course extremely useful in these circumstances, and are used widely to avoid the need to retain this kind of information in memory even on a temporary basis.

Context and schema work well in supporting memory most of the time, but because much of memory retrieval involves reconstruction of details based on schema rather than actual memory for details, the reconstruction process can result in major errors and false memories that the individual is convinced are genuine. For example, a witness to a crime or accident can have a false memory for details of the people present or of the incident. These false memories can arise because people assume ‘what must have happened’ based on their schema for such events rather than what actually happened. False memories also arise because of subsequent experiences (retroactive interference) and can result in accusing an innocent bystander of being the criminal, or recognising a face as vaguely familiar and falsely remembering them as the person who had committed the crime. For example, a psychology researcher who is also qualified as a legal practitioner, Donald Thomson was involved in the case of a witness identifying their attacker as someone (Thomson himself) who was appearing on a live television programme that the witness was watching at the time of the attack. Thomson was arrested by the police but rapidly was able to prove that he was somewhere else at the time of the incident. The witness had falsely remembered the face of someone on the television programme (Thomson) as the face of the person who committed the crime (see discussion in [27, p. 344]).

False memories also arise because of the phrasing of questions to the witness: a question such as ‘how fast was the car travelling when it smashed into the wall?’ will generate higher estimates of speed than the question ‘how fast was the car travelling when it hit the wall?’, even although exactly the same incident was witnessed in each case. The memory for the speed estimate is changed by the use of the phrase ‘smashed into’, when questioning the witness [248]. There are hundreds of documented cases of innocent people being arrested and convicted of crimes on the basis of mistaken eyewitness identification, but for whom subsequent DNA or other evidence has proved their innocence. In many cases, their innocence was established after many years in prison, or in some cases after imposition of the death penalty. Despite this, the legal system in many countries relies heavily on the testimony of eyewitnesses and many members of the legal profession, including judges, seem unaware of the fallibility of human memory for events (for reviews of eyewitness research see [241]). So, while one of the strengths of human memory is in the use of schemas to allow memory reconstruction and avoid overloading with redundant or irrelevant information, this process can also generate errors with serious consequences. Some of these errors could be avoided with the use of external devices that can record events as they occur to support accuracy in subsequent recall, as in the case of the eyewitness.

2.1.6 Forgetting Intentions

A further key everyday aspect of memory is the forming of intentions to carry out an activity at some point in the future, and then remembering to do so. This ability is often referred to as prospective memory, in contrast to episodic memory which is retrospective. Failures of prospective memory can result in embarrassment or irritation when forgetting to meet a friend or mistakenly using shaving cream on the toothbrush instead of toothpaste. However, failures of prospective memory also can result in serious consequences, for example if a flight is missed, medicine is not taken, forgetting to put on a parachute when skydiving, or failing to close the entrance ramp of a car ferry when leaving the harbour. These are just few examples of numerous real incidents that also include major aeroplane and train crashes, and major industrial accidents, and they have been known for some time to have resulted from this kind of human memory error [336].

Ironically, many such errors arise from highly practiced activities that have been performed many hundreds if not thousands of times previously, and so are performed somewhat automatically. A novel distraction or preoccupation with a worry such as an upcoming exam, an important interview, a sudden technical failure in equipment or the breakdown in a relationship, can remove the very small amount of attention required to ensure that these highly practiced activities are performed successfully, resulting in an error that is sometimes referred to as 'absent mindedness'. This could result in absent-mindedly starting to drive on the route to work on a Saturday evening instead of to the theatre. It could also result in an experienced pilot switching off the starboard engine on an aeroplane instead of the port engine that is on fire. The underlying type of memory error is the same, but the consequences are dramatically different.

Absent-minded errors occur over periods of a few seconds or minutes when a novel or threatening scenario displaces an intended action in current memory (known as working memory). Prospective memory failures also occur over longer periods of time when it is impractical to 'keep the intention in mind' or in working memory, and other activities or thoughts intervene. For example, setting off to walk to work with the intention of posting a letter during the 40-min journey can result in arriving at work without the letter being posted, unless posting the letter is the only thought kept active while walking. A cue or reminder such as passing a post box can reduce the chance of a prospective memory failure, but remembering to keep an appointment or the date of a wedding anniversary would not be monitored continuously over periods of days, weeks or years. In the absence of external aids such as a calendar or a reminder on a smart phone, it has been argued that some of the intentions are activated automatically from time to time, thereby acting as internal memory cues (e.g. [283, 285]). However, if there are too many intentions formed then errors are extremely likely without some form of external paper or electronic aid. It is also likely that an intention will be remembered at the correct time (e.g. to catch a flight), but that details required to carry out that intention (e.g. the exact flight time or flight number) might require some external memory aid. An external device that could monitor actions required in specific contexts would also reduce the likelihood of memory errors, for example, by preventing departure of a sky diver from the aeroplane at 3000 m unless the parachute is in place correctly.

2.1.7 Temporary Memory and Working Memory

Equally crucial for everyday functioning is the human ability to retain information on a temporary basis to allow completion of a current task or to function in a novel environment. This ability is often referred to as working memory (e.g. [28, 98]). Here, information is held for only a few seconds and continually updated, so forgetting of details is almost immediate. For example, in order to understand the text you are reading now, it is important to remember the text that you have just read, and the most recently read text is continually being updated as you progress through the document. Likewise, successful driving on the motorway requires rapid and regular updating of memory for the position of nearby traffic and this is continually updated with rapidly changing traffic patterns. In neither example is there normally any requirement to retain precise details such as the exact wording and font of the text read 10 min ago, or the precise position, model and colour of the car that was overtaking 15 min ago. Those details are important at the time, but not subsequently, and so are held for just a few seconds and then are forgotten as the contents of working memory are updated.

Working memory is used for almost every activity while humans are awake; mental arithmetic, navigating around unfamiliar environments, keeping track of current intentions and the flow of a conversation, making a meal, creative thinking, or keying a telephone number. It is thought to have capacity for around 3 or 4 items at any one time (e.g. [98]), but items can be grouped together so as to have 3 or 4 groups or chunks of information. However, its capacity can also be shown to be larger when using rehearsal or when storing different types of information. So there is capacity for holding 7 plus or minus 2 random numbers if the numbers are mentally rehearsed [297], and 7 random numbers can be retained at the same time as a random visual matrix pattern [80]. Without rehearsal, items in working memory are readily replaced by new material on a second-to-second basis.

2.2 When Human Forgetting Is Minimised

Sometimes, people remember new information and events well, to the extent that they can recall highly complex details for a long time. There are three major factors that have been shown to be associated with minimal forgetting:

- Expertise
- Relearning
- Vivid Memories

These are explained in more detail below.

2.2.1 *Effects of Specific Expertise on Memory*

Expertise in the present context refers to the accumulation of specialist and advanced knowledge in a particular domain, typically as a result of many hundreds or thousands of hours of learning and practice in that domain. The expert has very detailed schema that can support memory for details of past events related to the area of expertise. For example, expert chess players can readily remember the positions of pieces from multiple chess game positions [113], soccer fans can remember multiple scores from matches played between teams with which they are familiar [303]. Even residential burglars show superior memory for details of houses that are related to their area of activity [250]).

The expertise can also be very specific. For example, in [130] Ericsson trained an individual (Falloon) to be able to repeat back random sequences of up to 80 digits. The individual had significant expertise in athletics and learned to group parts of the sequences as numbers related to his area of expertise. For example, the sequence 354 would be encoded as 3 min 54 s or a record time for running a mile. By creating multiple combinations of numbers and making these meaningful in the context of athletics, his expertise allowed memory for number sequences that greatly exceeded the typical maximum random sequence length of 7 plus or minus 2 digits that most adults are capable of recalling [297]).

However, the expertise did not confer any general enhancement of memory for material outside the areas of expertise: Chess experts are not better than chess novices when remembering the position of pieces shown at random positions on the board, rather than from a real chess game, soccer experts are no better than those lacking an interest in the game when trying to recall random sets of scores rather than scores from real games, burglars can remember if a house had a burglar alarm but not the colour of the curtains in the window, and Steve Falloon could not remember any more than 7 random letters or words. In summary, the more accumulated knowledge that a person has about a topic, the easier it is for him/her to remember details related to that knowledge whether that be information technology, cognitive psychology, journalism or stamp collecting.

2.2.2 *Effects of Relearning*

Relearning material effectively starts the process of transferring details about a specific event (episodic memory) into knowledge and expertise about the topic of that material (semantic memory). If the relearning occurs very soon after the initial encounter with the material, and before most of the forgetting has occurred, this slows down the rate of forgetting. This then allows a longer time before relearning is required, and this expanding spacing of learning has been shown to be effective in dramatically reducing the rate and amount of forgetting that occurs [218]). An example is illustrated in Fig. 2.4. More recently, in [195], the authors have shown that attempting to retrieve information from memory (self-test) is even more effective than rereading or being represented with the same material.

2.2.3 *Vivid Memories*

Vivid memories are associated with events that are of major personal importance, such as one's own wedding, start of a new job, birth of one's child or of major public importance such political assassinations and resignations, natural disasters, major

Fig. 2.4 Relearning slows forgetting

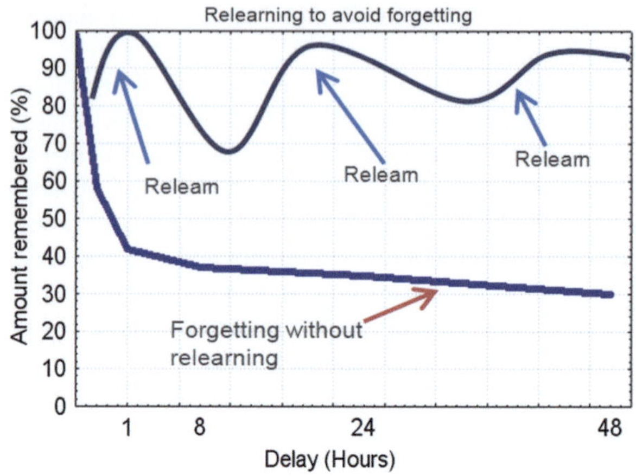

accidents, important sporting events or major human achievements. In these cases, people report having remarkably vivid memories that include many details that are normally forgotten. The best known report was of people remembering where they were, who they were with, what they were doing and what the weather was like at the time that they heard, in 1963, that the US President John F Kennedy had been assassinated, or that Martin Luther King had been assassinated several years later. These memories were reported as remaining vivid more than 10 years after the original event (e.g. [55]. Similar long-term preservation of vivid memories has been recorded for the first moon landing in 1969, the surprise resignation of the British Prime Minister Margaret Thatcher in 1990 [87], and the attack on the World Trade Centre in 2001 [326]. However, even in the case of public events, memories were more vivid for events that were of personal interest. The resignation of Margaret Thatcher was recalled most vividly among UK citizens who had an interest in politics, and the death of the UK Princess Diana in 1997 was more vividly recalled by UK than Italian citizens, although the 2001 attack on the World Trade Centre was remembered equally well in the UK and Italy [215]. The claimed vividness and detail associated with these event-based memories appeared to suggest that these kinds of memories included a great deal more detail and were much more accurate and consistent over time than are memories for other kinds of events (for a review see [258]), including details specifically about place, informant, activity, own affect and aftermath [198].

Several researchers have concluded that these vivid memories arise because there is considerable media coverage at the time, for some time afterwards and on anniversaries of each event. Major public events are also the main topic of conversation for people at the time and for several days, if not weeks afterwards. In sum, the memories for the events are recalled and rehearsed many times over when discussing with friends and through media coverage, making it very likely that those memories will be preserved. The same is true of personal memories of events that are important for the individual. One's own wedding will be a topic of conversation and mental activity for many months in advance and for months and years after the event. So, repeatedly recalling events leads to long-term preservation in memory.

It is worth noting that although many people experience these vivid memories, many of the details that they recall are incorrect, and are not consistent over time, even although people are convinced of their accuracy. A number of researchers have argued that the main difference between vivid memories and memories for other events is that people are much more confident about their recall of the former rather than there being an actual difference in the amount of accurate detail remembered (e.g. [102, 103, 378]). For example, many people in the United States confidently report a vivid memory of watching the television broadcast of the first plane to hit the World Trade Centre on 11 September, 2001, but that event was not recorded or televised. Only the aftermath of the crash and the video recording of the second plane crashing into the building were available. This major error was not only true of many US citizens [326], but also of the US President George W Bush [155]. Similar recall errors have been found for other vivid memories of major public events.

So, vivid memories are subject to the same process of reconstruction as are other memories. These kinds of memories were originally referred to as 'flashbulb memories', suggesting that they involve preservation in memory of considerably more detail than is the case for most memories of events. However, the finding that these memories are often not accurate has led to more widespread use of the term 'vivid memories' to reflect the personal experience of individuals rather than the accuracy of the preserved memory (although not all researchers agree, see [105]). That is, they follow the same general principles of remembering and forgetting of episodic memory, but may be subject to considerably more rehearsal, are experienced as more vivid, often have more emotional content and are recalled with greater confidence than other memories. Moreover, they are just as error prone and therefore do not appear to be subject to any different forms of processing or memory preservation compared with other memories [103].

2.3 Autobiographical or Personal Memory

2.3.1 Definitions of Autobiographical Episodic and Semantic Memory

One major focus for this book is the preservation of personal information, and thus far we have mainly referred to this kind of information primarily in order to illustrate how a conceptual understanding of human memory has been developed using results from controlled, experimental studies of memories for experienced events. However, there is also a research literature involving both experimental research and theoretical development of conceptual frameworks regarding how personal memories, and memories about the self are stored and accessed. Personal memories can be understood broadly within the same set of memory systems described earlier, with episodic memory being the host for memories of personal events, semantic memory being the host for general information about oneself, and working memory for holding in mind information regarding current activities.

However, when referring to personal memory, the term autobiographical memory is often used instead of episodic memory to emphasise that the research is focused on memory for real-life everyday personal experiences, as distinct from episodic memory for numbers, letters, word lists or visual patterns that are used when studying this form of memory in controlled laboratory experiments. Tulving [392] extended the concept of episodic memory to include: a sense of subjective time (that we mentally revisit/travel back in time), autonoetic awareness (that we are aware of our memory experience as different to our experience of the immediate environment) and a sense of self (specifically, a sense of self that can exist in subjective time). He has also argued [391, 392] that memory measures of a task completed in a laboratory should not be considered autobiographical because they are focused on 'what' (remembering content) rather than an integration of 'what-when-where' information. Moreover, the specific reference to an autobiographical episodic memory (e.g. [91, 260]) refers to a memory with personal relevance. Such an approach again requires that the memory preserves 'specific spatio-temporal context', though it may be from the recent or distant past, and acknowledges that event-specific recall will draw upon and be influenced by more general knowledge about the world and general knowledge about the self (history, different life periods, name, etc.) from autobiographical semantic memory.

A distinction between autobiographical episodic memory and autobiographical semantic memory was demonstrated in [393]. They described an individual, who, following brain damage showed a severe impairment of memory for autobiographical events while having intact semantic memory about family and personal history, occupation, residence and car owned. More recently, Renault et al. [337] argued for a further distinction between personal semantics (consisting of knowledge about oneself, self-identity and one's experiences) and general semantic knowledge (facts about the world).

Conway and Pleydell-Pearce [91] proposed a 'Self-Memory System' as a conceptual model of autobiographical memory. This relates development over the lifetime of autobiographical memory knowledge to event-specific knowledge (after [415]), through reciprocal connections with a working self. The working self refers to current short-term goals that are embedded within a hierarchy of longer term (including lifelong) goals, which are in turn framed and constrained by self-image and autobiographical knowledge. In [392], the author argued that information represented in episodic memory is the product of sensory information passing along a serial processing chain through perceptual representation and semantic representation systems, which may or may not result in an episodic representation. In contrast, Williams, Conway and Baddeley maintain that episodic representations 'originate in working memory, where they derive from mental models of online experience' [417, p. 40]. Such episodic representations are given conceptual context by stored autobiographical knowledge, through automatic access to stored knowledge and through operations of the working self, such as inhibiting information that is not relevant to the current goal, that competes with the current goal or that is unrelated to one's own representation of self.

In [89], the authors have argued further that autobiographical knowledge can also be represented as an hierarchical, nested structure comprising a semantic memory of the self in which episodic memories can become integrated with representations of 'general life events' (repeated events with common structure, property or theme), which are themselves further represented within 'lifetime periods' (such as 'when I worked at a specific institution', 'when I was mother to a young child') which are further represented as life stories, contributing to self-images and ultimately a 'conceptual self'. Short-term goals that an individual sets can become part of an autobiographical record of specific memories integrated with an immediate context, or with general life events or a lifetime history. Conway's concept of a Self-Memory System [85, 86, 91] allows for creation of a 'personal history' and ability to access memories in varied ways, for different reasons, throughout changing personal contexts and personal circumstances, while still maintaining an overarching sense of self throughout the lifetime.

Episodic memories for events that are experienced but that have limited personal relevance may or may not become integrated with autobiographical memories. Whether they are integrated partly depends upon the richness and detail of conceptual context available at encoding, and upon subsequent retrieval (among other influences, see [89]). As Conway emphasises, 'the function of episodic memories is to keep a record of progress with short-term goals and access to most episodic memories is lost soon after their formation' [86, p. 2305], consistent with the broader characteristics of memory identified by Ebbinghaus in 1885. Additionally, Conway [86] has noted that within episodic memory, not all components of a memory are equally accessible and has suggested that goal structure at the time of the experience determines the activation, and subsequent accessibility, of features within a memory (for retrieval within that memory context). If episodic memories are to be voluntarily recalled, they must be further integrated into autobiographical knowledge to enable generative retrieval—an often strategic and iterative process of cue elaboration; if this integration is lacking, episodic memories may be brought into awareness only through direct cueing. This latter (involuntary) process would require an unlikely encountered specificity of cue to directly access elements of an episodic memory [89]). A similar concept was proposed by Tulving [391, 392], who suggested the principle of encoding specificity, namely that details encoded and set in a particular context at the time of an event will act as effective cues for prompting later recall of details of the event. For example, if the reader is given the cue 'washing clothes', that can act as a cue to retrieve the passage of text given in Sect. 2.1.4 because that context was used to encode the information in memory. The cue word 'expensive' is a much less effective cue for retrieving that same passage, because it was most likely not used as part of the context or schema for encoding, even though the word appeared in that text. If we consider the notion that each individual has a 'schema of the self', then this schema can set the context for experiences and be used to help retrieve whatever was preserved in memory from those experiences.

As implied in the above model of Conway and colleagues [85, 86, 89, 91]), recalling an autobiographical memory requires an interplay and interaction of episodic information and semantic elements of an individual's personal history. As noted in Sect. 2.1.5, recall of a memory is always a reconstruction from those details of an event that have been encoded within the context of a schema that is used to make assumptions about details that have been forgotten. It is not a veridical record of the event. Cabeza and St Jacques [58] list the most influential factors in determining the episodic versus semantic composition of an event during the reconstruction process at recall: age of memories, event frequency, rehearsal and age of participants. As may be expected, in the real-world context of a person's life history, these factors do not operate in isolation, rather they interact.

2.3.2 Methodologies for the Study of Autobiographical Memory

The systematic study of autobiographical memory is complicated by the large number of factors that have to be considered, and the lack of experimental control over spontaneous or even planned events that occur in everyday life. Individuals also differ in the extent to which they retain details, even of the same event, and which details are retained. Finally, rarely is there a full objective record of an event that can be used to assess the accuracy of the individual's memory for that event. This last feature is particularly problematic given the reconstructive nature of memory.

An early approach to the study of autobiographical memory involved participants keeping a diary or log of events. After delays of days, weeks, months or years, one detail from a recorded event can be used as a cue for participants to recall other details of those events. The original record can be used to check for recall accuracy (e.g. [242]). A related approach has been to prompt participants at random intervals (e.g. via a pager [53]) to record details of the most recent events in their daily life, and again use these records as sources to cue specific events for later recall and for checking accuracy. However, these methods suffer from two major limitations. First, the fact that participants choose the events and the details of those events, and take some time to record them, acts as a form of mental rehearsal of the events that would make it more likely that those events will be recalled when tested at a later date. Second, given the difficulties of running studies over more than a few weeks or months, the method does not allow testing of memory for events from the more distant past. The study in [242] took place over 6 years, but that involved a single participant (Linton herself) and few research projects have the resources for this length of study, or for the numbers of participants that would be required for a comprehensive study.

When there has been no specific documented record of an event, other sources such as family and friends can be used to check recall accuracy, but they too will be subject to memory recall errors. If it was a public event then there may be publicly available documentation, video or audio records to verify memory accuracy. This method has been used very successfully to demonstrate errors in recall of major public events, such as errors in the recall by President George W Bush of the tragic events of 11 September, 2001 [155]. Therefore, many researchers have focused their investigations on memory for, or surrounding public events as described above. The studies of memory for public events indicated that the importance of an event for the individual, or their emotional response to an event is a major factor in the level of detail that can be recalled. Kopple et al. [207] found that after delays of around 4 months following a major public event, the ratings of 'emotional intensity' and 'personal importance' regarding the events were the best predictors of the level of consistency in their recall of the event. However, the fact that an event resulted in an emotional response or was of personal importance would also lead to the individual repeatedly thinking about or talking about the event, thereby having repeated recalls and rehearsal of the event before the formal test of their memory within the study. The extent of media coverage of the event may also be important in driving this form of repeated recall.

A further approach has been to simulate natural autobiographical events by staging them within a controlled experimental setting. This has the advantage that the same or very similar events can be experienced by a large number of participants, thereby removing the confounding factor that some events are more memorable than others or include different amounts of detail (e.g. [343]). Such experiences and associated memory will not be 'pure' or free from the influence of a participant's personal, autobiographical knowledge. For example, certain elements of a constructed experience may resonate strongly with some participants more than others because of their individual past experiences. However, if a sufficiently large number of participants are included then averaging the results across participants can help mitigate the influence of these individual influences on recall. Moreover, constructed situations allow researchers to manipulate components of experiences, enabling generalisable insight into the features of interest in any given experiment such as delay until recall, nature of the event, number of times recall is repeated, effects of different memory cues and so on.

Difficulties inherent in trying to characterise, measure, quantify and understand the information that remains available and accessible from an experienced event still persist even when many of the external characteristics of the experience are under the control of an experimenter. Williams, Conway and Baddeley [417] made an attempt to address some of these factors by tackling the question of event boundaries in memory: when does an event begin and end, and does this change over time? The approach builds on the work of Zacks and colleagues (e.g. [213, 430, 431]), regarding boundaries of events when looking at and perceiving the world, and conceptual features (for example, hierarchically nested goals, which can determine fine or coarser grained events). In the context of Conway's general framework (e.g. [85, 86]), episodic memory is considered a record, or the product of, carrying out short-term goals in the service of increasingly greater overarching goals; while moment-to-moment goals are necessarily dynamic and short-lived, goals further up the hierarchy are more stable and enduring.

Williams, Conway and Baddeley [417] asked participants to freely recall their morning commute on the day of testing, to identify how they would segment this into 'discrete memories' and then to recall the same commute one week later. After analysing the memory elements that began and ended a segment, the authors determined that actions were more likely (but not exclusively) to characterise a beginning, with a fact (more likely but not exclusively) ending the segment. Other features changed with time of recall. This so-called 'action-fact' structure to the memories was replicated for three memories from a more remote time of a recent holiday, and was taken as support of memories defined around goal structure, with actions indicating an initiation of the current short-term goal. Notably, the authors observed that despite the general pattern of facts ending a segment, the properties with which a segment could end were more variable than those with which they would start, and this indicated that goals may be terminated in various ways.

Hohman, Peynircioğlu and Beason-Held [169] tested event memory for events from different time points in the lives of individual participants. They found that college age and middle age adults were more likely to be flexible in their attribution of event boundaries with increasing time—that is, once a memory was recalled and probed for further information, the more time that had passed since the event, the more likely the adults were to accept information outside of the original boundaries for the event as belonging to the original event (therefore moving event boundaries). Overall, older adults were more likely than college age adults to move event boundaries, indicating an age-related component to event structure. Such results are important in demonstrating that not only does the nature of creation of event boundaries at encoding determine how we should approach our memories for events, but so too does the nature of event boundaries at retrieval/reconstruction.

Using a method originally devised in [144], in which participants are asked to provide memories in response to cue words (for example, think of a memory for an event related to the word 'river' or the word 'holiday'), and in [100], the authors demonstrated that fewer memories are produced from early life years. Participants are less likely to recall memories from the first 5 years of their childhood and more likely to recall detailed memories from the more recent past. Moreover, older autobiographical memories contain less detail and are more abstract than those from the more recent past [58, 328].

An exception to the pattern of memory recall frequency is a reminiscence bump found in participants over 40 years of age who produce many memories from their early adulthood (age 18–30 years old; [140]). It has been suggested that such a period may contain life 'firsts' and meaningful, life-defining events (such as jobs, children and marriage; [41]), which serve as anchors in our memory and a basis upon which our life story (or narrative) is built. Glück and Bluck [149] observed a reminiscence bump only for positive (not negative or neutral) memories, in which participants indicated they had perceived themselves as having had control of their lives. This is consistent with the idea that individuals create a positive and defining life story for themselves (see also [86]). A bias towards recall of positive life events is especially present in older adults [272]).

Detailed memory for events throughout the lifespan requires a complex interplay of a number of aspects of the memory system (see [86]) in addition to decline in the integrity of the brain with age. Levine and colleagues [227] reviewed the history of research showing negative effects of age on recall of episodic memories. They demonstrated that older adults provide answers with fewer episodic details and more semantic content than do younger adults, even when probes for episodic detail are provided. St Jacques and Levine [373] demonstrated further that this age-related pattern of fewer episodic details provided by older than younger adults holds true for emotional memories, even when positive emotional memories elicit more episodic details than neutral memories.

As noted in [343], memory for personal events is subject to the same general principles as other types of memory—such as proactive and retroactive interference mentioned earlier. As people age, so the number of similar experiences increases, therefore the effects of interference among memories of those experiences also increase. Meeting thousands of people over one's lifetime, many of whom have similar first names, builds up a lifetime of proactive interference. This makes it increasingly difficult with age to remember the name of someone just met for the first time. It also builds up retroactive interference, making it increasingly difficult to remember the name of someone met a few years ago because of experiencing the names of all of the people met subsequently. This problem with names applies to memory for details of many similar events that have been experienced over a lifetime, making it more likely that there will be increasing reliance on reconstruction from more generic and less specific semantic knowledge, with schema supporting recall [58]. Reconstruction takes place even for events which appear to be unique in many aspects and which the individual believes that they retain in a detailed, episodic format.

2.3.3 Photograph Use and Event Memory

The use of personal photographs offers an illustration of the relationship between the conceptual understanding of human memory and use of digital or physical preservation of information. Their use for research has been widespread in both controlled laboratory settings and in everyday settings. For example, in a laboratory-based experiment, Koutstaal et al. [208] investigated the effect of viewing photographs on people's memory for events. Participants watched a video of action taking place and their memory for the content of this video was tested. Subsequent to watching the video, but prior to testing, participants were shown photographs that included elements from parts of the video, or presented with verbal descriptions of these elements. Koutsaal et al. found older and younger adults remembered more from the parts of the video that had been viewed in the photographs or verbally reviewed than they did sections that had not been reviewed. Such an increase in memory performance following photograph viewing after witnessing events was also replicated by Schacter and colleagues [354].

Despite evidence that reviewing photographs is supportive and beneficial to memory [208, 354, 374], further evidence suggests that photo use may not be without negative consequences. For example, following presentation of photographs that contained images indicating items which were either present or absent in a previously viewed video, older adult participants cued on these latter items were also more likely to attribute them to having been present in the video [354]. More recently, St Jacques and Schacter [374] asked participants to complete a tour of a museum, wearing a camera which automatically took pictures during the tour. They were then presented with photographs which were either strong cues (photographs from a natural perspective) or weak cues (photographs from an unusual perspective) to memory for aspects of the tour. The authors then presented photos of entirely novel items, or other items from the tour, and asked participants whether the items had been a part of their visit. Strong cues produced a higher level of accuracy than weak cues in detecting photographs that depicted items from the tour, but also produced an increase in erroneous selection of photographs of objects that had not been seen on the tour. This reinforces the general conclusion discussed earlier that memories are reconstructed and subject to change. The study also highlights how photographs can influence the reconstruction process.

Koutsaal and colleagues (e.g. [209]) cautioned against possible effects of selective rehearsal when seemingly viewing photographs to help memory. Such effects were demonstrated when participants were asked to view photographs that pertained to elements of a series of activities in which they had been involved in the laboratory; tasks that were carried out but were not then reviewed were more poorly recalled than both reviewed activities and performance of a control group who carried out the same tasks with no subsequent review (a baseline condition). That is, selectively reviewing certain elements of associated activities (or sub-events) led to a reduction in memory recall for activities not studied.

Results reported in [163] have also been used to advocate a need for further understanding of how the act of taking photographs interacts with our natural memory abilities. Participants in this experiment were instructed, throughout an art museum tour, to visit a list of objects and to either only look at them or to look at them and photograph them, with the relevant action for each object dictated by the experimenter. Subsequently, the number of objects, and amount of detail, remembered between these two conditions was compared. In a second experiment, an additional condition was introduced where participants were instructed to zoom in to specific sections of objects to be photographed. When required to perform the zoomed-in photography task, participants' memory (recognition of objects or for detail) was comparable to the observation only (no photography) condition. This was true for the original specific part of the object that was photographed as well as for other parts of items that were not included in the photograph. In contrast, in both experiments, memory was poorer for objects that participants had been instructed to photograph (without zooming). While participants were told in initial instructions that they would be asked about the appearance of the objects of art, Henkel suggested that results indicated a reliance on outsourced memory storage that has negative effects for our own memory. Specifically, that taking a photo could serve as a cue to 'dismiss and forget'. The cognitive effort and attention expended on a zooming task appears to counteract this effect. However, as acknowledged by Henkel, this apparent detriment to memory may not extend to situations in which people exert a choice over taking a photograph, or where the photograph is driven by interest. She suggested that further work is needed to disentangle the factors that may contribute to memory in a real-life situation.

2.4 Remembering and Forgetting in IT Systems

This section discusses methods and technologies in IT which are related to human remembering and forgetting. Our approach is to consider IT systems that are designed to complement (not to replace) the processes of human remembering and forgetting.

The advent of Big Data and the development of ever more effective storage technologies may suggest that forgetting need not occur in digital systems, because there is sufficient storage capacity to keep everything. However, forgetting mechanisms are still necessary, be it to ensure privacy [48, 187, 402], to remove or correct errors (e.g. [279]), or to ensure that the information which was selected for preservation can be retrieved and processed effectively without being swamped by stored irrelevant detail that need not have been preserved. These forms of 'managed digital forgetting' contrast sharply with unintentional digital forgetting that occurs when storage media and file formats become outdated and inaccessible, or when storage media are lost or damaged.

2.4.1 Inferences from Data

When making new inferences from existing data, we always face the problem of noise, i.e. data that look like they might be useful or applicable to the problem, but are not. Some of this noise could arise from information that is available but is trivial or irrelevant, and failure to exclude such information could result in misleading or completely incorrect inferences. This is the kind of information that human memory does not ever encode, because, as discussed in Sect. 2.1.4, initial selection of information to preserve, even on a temporary basis, is driven by context. Use of context derived from prior inferences about the kind of information being stored can help decisions about what data can be excluded from processing or preserving.

A second source of noise is the recording of redundant or repeated information as separate sets of data records. Again, from Sect. 2.1.4, in the case of human memory, each repetition is not recorded separately, but repetitions accumulate by strengthening the representations in memory for features that overlap between repetitions, and using this accumulation to set a context when the same, or similar information is repeated in the future.

A third source of noise can arise from inconsistencies. These could perhaps be seen as an irritation, but may be highly informative. Take for example the task of deriving common features of the class of birds. Most birds can fly, but ostriches and penguins cannot. If we assume that all birds can fly, we have a contradiction. One approach would be to ignore the inconsistency by forgetting the information that causes it, so that the criteria for being a bird no longer includes the ability to fly. Numerous techniques have been proposed for identifying and eliminating variables that lead to such inconsistencies, and for reasoning with inconsistent data [126, 219].

In a system with managed digital forgetting, we can say that internally consistent information should be given a high priority for long-term preservation, or has a high preservation value. However, if we consider that the functioning of human memory categorisation can be based on a match with the majority of criteria rather than an exact match with all criteria, this allows for exceptions. A human memory schema for a bird would contain the key criteria that are true of all birds (e.g. a warm blooded animal that lays eggs, has feathers, and modification of the forelimbs to form wings) plus the extremely useful information that most, but not all members of this category can fly. A similar problem emerges when we consider instance-based learning algorithms, where new examples are classified by retrieving similar items from a database and inferring the class of the new item from the class of these similar items. One approach for items that are irregular and that lead to misclassification is to eliminate them from the database, that is to forget [54].

However, using irregular items to refine the criteria in the database could lead to much greater accuracy in categorisation, so penguins and ostriches would still be categorised correctly, and the information about the majority of the category members is not lost. So too in natural language processing, where irregular spellings and word forms abound, particularly in English, it is important to remember these irregular forms [107]. Having a computational taxonomy learn from instances of exceptions, through a process of taxonomic revision can further enhance effectiveness (e.g. [7, 8, 216, 370]). Therefore, inconsistencies should refine the context rather than be forgotten.

2.4.2 User Models and Companions

IT systems that are personalised to particular users often rely on detailed user models, which consist of general information about the user, such as gender and age, but which can also cover the history of interactions between system and user. Other information about the user such as the languages they speak and at what level of proficiency, or other particular skills and experience that they have might also be useful. Displaying a human-like memory for information about the user is key to appearing intelligent and responsive [236, 338], and so may maximise utility. This complements the notion of a schema for the self, discussed in Sect. 2.3. User models are often fully or partially inferred from data about the user's behaviour, and some longitudinal models can take account of changes in user preferences over time. These data can come from sources of information outside the actual application, such as linked social media accounts, or web browsing history, as documented by cookies.

When it comes to maintaining a human–IT interaction history, not everything should be stored. For example, Vargas et al. [402] make a case for ensuring that privacy and confidentiality are preserved. Barua et al. [35] propose to give users a degree of control over the information that is preserved and the information that is forgotten, which is key to addressing privacy issues. For example, the system might store information about 'work-related self' such as periods when the individual had particular sets of responsibilities or was at a particular stage in career. There could also be storage of work-related relationships with colleagues to support communication and networking. The representations of these relationships could be dynamic, with their prominence or Memory Buoyancy driven by the frequency and recency of interactions. The user would make a personal choice about whether equivalent information about personal relationships and life periods would be included.

Agents that can simulate an autobiographical memory are often designed to recall significant experiences in great detail, equivalent to episodic specific knowledge, and compress everyday routines into scripts that simulate schema within semantic memory [166]. Robot companions should be able to remember both their own experiences and those of the people over whom they watch. These experiences should be easy to retrieve [238], with constraints on the level of detail set by the context at the time of retrieval.

The implementation of such digital memories is based on computational models of the neurobiology of memory, such as Adaptive Resonance Theory [64]. Memories are stored in a network. Accessing a particular item of knowledge or experience activates related memories through a spreading activation framework that simulates relevant interactions between groups of neurons in the brain. In actual robot companion systems, this autobiographical component is integrated into a memory model that covers a store for incoming perceptual information through sensors, working memory and long-term memory [165]. Throughout these systems, in particular when dealing with the details of sensory input, forgetting is key to keeping memory requirements in check [375]. Forgetting can be implemented as removal of transient traces of incoming information, through decay with the passage of time [237], and through generalisation [403]. Forgetting could also be implemented as developing a schema for common features of repeated events, removing the requirement to store the repeated details of those events.

2.4.3 Reminder Systems and Decision Support

The classic example for technology that supports human memory is reminder systems, designed to support prospective memory by giving people cues that help them remember to do things (c.f. Sect. 2.1.6). They can also cover warnings or alerts, and can support complex decision-making. For example, computerised prescription order entry systems routinely warn prescribers about potentially problematic drug/drug interactions (e.g. [344]).

Most of the extensive work on reminder and decision support systems focuses on safety critical work places, such as aviation or medicine (e.g. [125, 332]), while others have addressed solutions for the home (e.g. [286]). Both reminders and key information to support decisions need to be intelligible and acceptable. Being intelligible means that people can perceive the reminder or other information and understand the message. Acceptability means that people are willing to attend to the reminder or to use the information when they make decisions, and that the information is relevant for the user. People often dismiss or disregard reminders because they have received too many irrelevant reminders in the past or because the reminder irritates them. This is 'alert fatigue', and it is one of the main reasons why reminder or alert systems fail, as Thimbleby [381] has discussed. Similar problems arise when professional healthcare staff are provided with information about patients in their care that is in too complex a format or is simply not relevant to their specific healthcare role (e.g. [249, 400]).

2.4.4 Augmented Memory for Personal Information

Another way in which technology can support human memory is by storing personal information so it can be recalled later. Here, we briefly review the literature on a particular type of personal data that we discussed in Sect. 2.3.2, namely, digital photos.

In [206], the authors studied what people do with their photos after these have been taken. They term these activities 'photo work' and they encompass reviewing, downloading, organising, filing and editing. In [10], the authors investigated photo work on camera phones and found a similar rich set of activities related to managing and manipulating photos. Kirk, Sellen, Rother and Wood [206] suggested that as part of photo work, people tend to browse rather than search photos. Browsing is a less goal-directed activity with room for serendipity and following new associations. Interfaces for browsing use a range of different design metaphors that are inspired by ways in which users arrange and search through information, such as a timeline [159], locations, [257] or a choice of contexts including data from friends [399]. At the time of writing, in 2017, Google and Apple organise their users' photos by location and time. Google automatically detects trips and invites users to revisit highlights of a day, while Apple highlights common locations in the photo timeline.

When it comes to preserving photos for later browsing, a key problem is preserving not just the photo itself, but also its meaning. People often forget details such as where or why a photo was taken or the names of people depicted. Such information is particularly difficult to recover if the person who decided to preserve the photo can no longer remember the event or has died. Many automatic analysis techniques have been developed for extracting content information from photos, such as automatic detection of people and faces, or automatic grouping of photos into events [94].

The techniques developed within the ForgetIT project are summarised in Chap. 3. Here, we focus on solutions that are inspired by the way people interact with photos. For example, Frohlich and Fennell [142] suggest several ways of embedding digital photos in a rich context that will preserve information about their meaning, such as linking them to other physical memorabilia or augmenting them with audio narrations. For more information about how this issue was approached within ForgetIT, see Chap. 7.

An important aspect of photo context is the reason why a photo was taken. In a 2004 study of early camera phones [205], Kindberg and colleagues found that people took photos for both affective and functional reasons, and that photos could be either for oneself or for sharing with others. Affective reasons included documenting a shared experience, communicating with absent friends or family, and individual reflection and reminiscence. Photos taken for functional reasons contained information to support a task that was either personal or was shared with others, who might or might not be at the same location. Annotating photos with detailed tags that can then be stored as metadata would be ideal for retrieval and contextualisation, but it is a very burdensome activity that requires well-designed user interfaces to keep users engaged and motivated [194]).

Another form of annotating photos are interactions, where people share reactions, comments, and information. Platforms such as Flickr or Facebook offer this facility routinely, but largely for typed interactions. For example, Vennelakanti et al. [404] proposed a system, Pixene, that can capture conversations about photos and record when each photo had been mentioned during a conversation. Cosley et al. [96] describe a system called Pensieve, which uses social media content as memory cues. The Pensieve sends users random snippets of the social media content that they have generated over the years, with the aim to encourage users to reminisce and reflect on past experiences. Facebook now has similar functionality, 'On This Day' memories, that retrieve a post from past years and display it again in the user's timeline, with the option of sharing it again.

2.4.5 *Digital Heirlooms*

Researchers in the field of digital heritage and personal digital archives have investigated how people use both physical and digital objects as mementos of the past. Van den Hoven and Eggen [172] set out design principles for augmented memory systems inspired by autobiographical memory research. They recommended that augmented digital memories should rely heavily on memory cues that allow people to reconstruct memories. The memories held may not need to be related to specific episodes, they could also refer to lifetime periods or general life events as outlined in [89], where specific information has been forgotten. Digital memory systems should also consider different reasons for retrieving autobiographical memories, be it to support one's identity, to inform decision-making or to share experiences with others.

From the user interface design point of view, augmented digital memory systems should be capable of integrating 'souvenirs', that is, auditory, visual or tactile materials that are particularly good at evoking memories in users. As Kaye et al. [199] have shown, when it comes to personal archives, the physical and the digital can be impossible to separate. Indeed, as Petrelli, van den Hoven and Whittaker [324] found, when asked to construct a time capsule of their life, people preferred a few well chosen, but barely annotated physical objects to a richly annotated large set of digital recordings. Barthel and colleagues [33] report a solution for integrating physical objects into digital networks that relies on a tagging system. Objects are labelled using two-dimensional QR codes or RFID tags that link stories to objects. Compared to physical objects, digital mementos may be seen as less valuable, they are accessed less frequently, because sharing them can be cumbersome, and they are mostly limited to photos and videos [325].

Banks, Kirk and Sellen [32] reanalysed both their own data and other published studies to determine themes around the interaction with digital mementos. Four main themes emerged: how the mementos relate to people, how the mementos connect to memory, qualities of the objects serving as memento and the kind of record that a memento represents. The 'people' theme revolves around access. Are the mementos for oneself, to be shared with others, or can they be made public? This is an important distinction [240]. Were they constructed specifically to be preserved for future generations? What are others expected to do with these mementos?

Mementos can be a record of many different things. They can be intended to capture a place, such as the house of a deceased relative before it was sold or to document a timeline, such as sets of school photos through the years, or a lifelog. They can also encompass material from different modalities, such as the smell of a favourite cologne or the sound of a voice singing. Objects that serve as mementos may also have specific qualities. They may show signs of wear and tear, they may have been crafted exquisitely well, or they may have been handmade with more love than skill. The main connection to memory is through narrative. Mementos serve as cues to specific episodic knowledge in autobiographical memory that can be retrieved and recounted, and they are also linked to such knowledge about the people who used to own that item. As digital means of communication become widespread, it may be tempting to assume that there will be fewer physical mementos, and that people's practices of remembering will focus more on the digital. However, this needs to be empirically tested.

2.4.6 Reminiscence Therapy

Reminiscence therapy uses artefacts related to people's past to stimulate memories. It is particularly popular for people with dementia, as memories that are important for the individual and that will have been retrieved many times during their lifetime are usually less vulnerable to the disease. This arises because each retrieval can strengthen the memory trace, even if memory for some of the details changes with each retrieval. Reminiscence therapy can take place both in person and remotely through teleconferencing [214].

Kalnikaite and Whittaker [190] designed a reminiscence system called Memory-Lane that is based around pictures of mementos. Users can write or record stories about these mementos and store them in a home, save them in a photo frame (for people), or assign them to places on a map. One of the most sophisticated reminiscence systems is CIRCA [153]. The CIRCA system is designed to evoke memories in older users and to stimulate verbal or non-verbal communication about the material that is presented. Materials include songs, video, pictures, animation, text and Virtual Reality reproductions of environments such as a 1930s pub. They cover life experiences and events that were common to the older generation. The interface also uses metaphors that are familiar to older users. For example, songs can be played on a virtual record player, or they can come from an old radio.

An alternative to systems that are built around specific mementos of the past are systems that are built on ongoing lifelogging. The most popular example is SenseCam, developed by Microsoft. SenseCam is a camera worn on a lanyard around the neck that automatically takes photos at set intervals. SenseCam can be paused for up to 7 min, taken off or turned towards the user, if there is a need for more privacy [202]. A variety of published case studies, such as [167], have shown that SenseCam can help people with memory impairments recall what has happened to them. Through reviewing SenseCam images, these patients were able to recall the events associated with those images far better and more vividly. For people without memory impairments, SenseCam does not appear to be more efficient in stimulating recall of episodes than other techniques, such as social reminiscing [359]). However, Sellen and colleagues [360] found that SenseCam helped healthy users activate background knowledge about other things that happened on the same day that the SenseCam images were taken.

2.5 A Sample Experimental Study on Personal Digital Photograph Use

Thus far, this chapter has focused on discussing the current understanding of human memory and forgetting, along with a description of the research methodologies that are used and the scientific evidence that has led to our current understanding. There are many remaining unanswered questions about the details of how human memory is organised and functions, and these questions are major drivers for a large international scientific effort and a large volume of published research (for a review see [27]). We have also discussed some of the research that has been carried out on use of digital memory systems and their relationship with human memory. The current book is focused on personal multimedia preservation, and so in the final main section of this chapter, we describe an experimental study that drew on the understanding and research methodologies of human memory to investigate the relationship between human memory and one of the most ubiquitous forms of personal multimedia, namely digital photographs. These offer an ideal example use case for ForgetIT in that every individual with a camera on their smart phone stores very large numbers of photographs simply because the camera function is extremely easy to use, the smart phone is nearly always readily available, and for most devices there is capacity for many hundreds if not thousands of photographs.

This clearly illustrates the major challenge of how to organise the very large volumes of photographs that accumulate, and how to ensure that photographs that the individual might want to preserve are stored securely long term and that they can easily be retrieved. Some automatic sorting can occur, for example by date and time when the photograph was taken, and for some devices, photographs can be uploaded automatically to cloud services.

As discussed in Chap. 1, the problem of increasing volumes of photographs remains. It is very easy to look at printed photographs that were taken over a hundred years ago and kept in a family album. However, it is very challenging to look at photographs that might have been stored on a floppy disk 20 years ago. Complete collections of photographs could have been lost when switching to a new phone, a new operating system, a new computer, new software that cannot read older file formats, or if the digital device is lost or stolen. Selecting from the many thousands of digital photographs, a subset that an individual feels that they would want to preserve would allow for low-cost long-term storage solutions. Indeed the popularity of printed 'photobook' services suggests that many individuals may still see printing on paper as a reliable method for preserving a small selection of important photographs.

With the above context in mind, our study focused on asking people to take digital photographs of buildings, people and street theatre events during a major international arts festival. After a range of delays from one hour through one week and one month and one year, they were asked to decide which photographs they would like to keep and which they would be happy to delete. They were also asked what they could remember of the events that they photographed. Here, we will briefly summarise the methodological approach, the study and the results. Full reports of the study are available in [1, 2, 418, 419].

2.5.1 An Experimental Study on Personal Digital Photograph Use

In order to design a system that will be adopted by potential users, it is crucial to identify how such potential users currently use digital storage for personal information, and how that use impacts on their biological memory for the original source information, such as an experienced event. In this section, we report on an experimental study in which objective data were collected for this use case scenario. The study took place during the annual Edinburgh Fringe Arts Festival, a large street fair (musicians, acrobats, street theatre, stand-up comedy) that takes place in the

Table 2.1 Demographic details of participant groups

Group	1	2	3	4
Number of participants	20	18	18	18
Age (years)	31.65 ± 5.52 (19–68)	38.61 ± 20.41 (19–71)	33.94 ± 17.54 (20–72)	35.17 ± 15.02 (19–59)
Males	3	8	5	10

centre of Edinburgh, UK over 4 weeks in August each year. In this study, participants spent an hour at the street fair and were tasked with taking snapshots every 3 min to document this experience. Through using the Edinburgh Festival Fringe as a setting for studies centred around photograph use to support memory for an event, we were able to take advantage of a great deal of activity happening in a fairly well-defined area: approximately 400 m along one street. This provided a substantial amount of potential information that participants might want to remember, and also provided a rich opportunity and variety of contexts with which to link their photographs upon subsequent reviewing. More specifically, this enabled investigation of a series of research questions about photograph use when experiencing and mentally revisiting an event.

Here, we focus on how we investigated participant engagement with photographs of the events that they experienced during the one hour visit to the street fair: which photographs they chose to keep, and their methods for organising photographs into meaningful groups. These elements were investigated for changes over time.

For testing, participants were split into four pseudorandomly selected groups. This involved random allocation of people to groups, but this was constrained by dates upon which participants were able to commit to returning for a second test session. Table 2.1 shows the demographic details for each group. Immediately after their hour of festival experience finished (hereafter referred to as Time 1), all participants returned to be interviewed: they orally recalled their experiences in as much detail as possible. In order to assess changes in the preservation value of each photograph, these participants returned to the laboratory a second time (hereafter referred to as Time 2) after one day (Group 1), or after one week (Group 2), or after one month (Group 3), and were again asked recall their experiences and decide which photographs they would like to keep and which they would like to delete. This allowed us to investigate changes over time (from Time 1 to Time 2). Participants in Group 4 were not asked to review their photographs or to make any keep/delete decisions immediately after taking the photographs, but were asked to return after one month to do so. For illustration purposes in this chapter, we will present a summary of the photograph keep/delete decisions over time. An analysis of the keep/delete decision results is available in [418], while a full report of the analysis of the oral recall is available in [1].

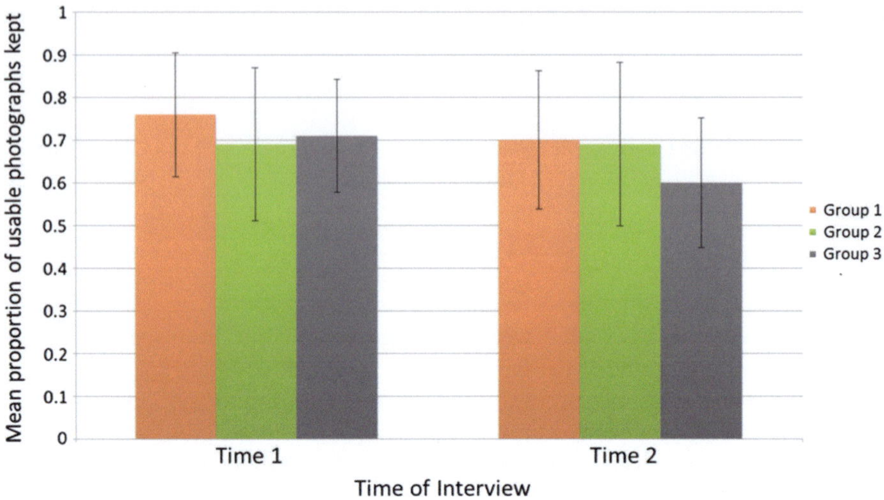

Fig. 2.5 Proportion of photos that participants choose to keep at Time 1 and Time 2, broken down by group (1-one day, 2-one week, 3-one month). Standard error bars are shown

2.5.1.1 Photograph Data

Participants took a mean of 19 photographs (range 12–20) during the one hour set for doing so. The results for Groups 1, 2 and 3 are illustrated in Fig. 2.5. At Time 1, on average, 28% of photographs were selected for deletion (median: 26%, range 0–58%, SD 15%). At Time 2 (a day, week, or month later), these participants deleted on average 33% of their photographs (median: 30%, range: 0–70%, SD 17%). This average difference between Time 1 and Time 2 corresponds to one photograph and is statistically significant ($t(55) = 3.3352$, $p < 0.001$, 95% CI for median).

When further probing the keep or delete decisions, it was observed that seven participants (13%) decided to keep exactly the same photographs when interviewed at both Time 1 and Time 2, while seven other participants (13%) chose to delete four or more photographs at Time 2 that they had previously chosen to keep at Time 1. Overall, 32 participants (59%) did not choose to keep any photographs at Time 2 that they had selected to delete at Time 1, while 37% decided to keep one–three additional photographs at Time 2 compared to Time 1, and two outliers added seven and nine photographs at Time 2 compared to those they had opted to keep at Time 1. Of note, the percentage of photographs chosen for deletion at Time 2 did not differ significantly between the different groups of participants, indicating that whether the retest occurred a day, a week, or a month later made no difference to the keep/delete decisions. That is, there was a similar pattern of results for all three groups.

Participants in Group 4 (that is, those who first saw and interacted with their photographs a month after the initial experience) deleted on average 33% of their photographs (median: 31%, range: 0%-78%, SD 19%) at Time 2. This number is comparable to that observed in Groups 1–3 at Time 2, indicating that viewing photographs immediately after an experience does not produce a strong influence on deletion decisions made one month later.

In order to better understand the decision process of participants, following their keep/delete decisions participants were probed with further questions. Of those photographs that they opted to keep, participants were asked for five, randomly chosen pictures to provide an explanation for why they wanted to keep that particular photograph. Likewise, among the photographs that were chosen for deletion, each participant was asked for the motivation behind each of their decisions. Six categories of reasons for keeping photographs were derived from all provided explanations. Likewise, six reasons for deletion were derived. Results are summarised in Table 2.2. This method enabled participants to provide more than one reason (category) per explanation or per photograph, for example, 'Enjoyed their music'. Not a good photo composition but it is a reminder of the 'atmosphere' (see also Chap. 8).

The reasons that people provided as motivation behind keep and delete decisions for their small photograph collection from one hour of experiences were in part highly predictable, while in part also very subjective. Therefore, it appears that criteria that mimic or simulate these judgments could potentially be computed (semi-)automatically for some photographs. However, for photographs associated with highly subjective value judgments, any automated digital system would be required to include a learning algorithm for the preferences of a given user. This would most likely require substantial user input, in order to either support or simulate user decision-making.

Figure 2.6 shows the percentage of deletion explanations containing a justification/reason per category, collapsed across participants in Groups 1–3. For example, from all of the Time 1 deletion decisions for these groups, 39.5% referenced poor photo quality/aesthetics. Additionally, 42% mentioned that they evoked a negative reaction. Across Time 1 and Time 2 (collapsed across groups), it is evident that there are slight but not drastic changes. The largest differences emerged in 'aesthetic' and 'random' deletion reasons; specifically, participants' aesthetic judgments appeared to feature more in decision-making at Time 2 than they did at Time 1, whereas they were less likely to suggest 'random' for deletion at Time 2, than they were at Time 1.

It is important to note that our participants' decisions to keep or delete photographs were often explicitly made in relation to other photos, for example, '(I have) Another one that's better' or 'Was walking out of frame; have other better shots of her'. Moreover, this factor is also evident when looking more closely at descriptions that did not explicitly state a reason for deletion that could be identified as surplus, for example, the description 'Not a good angle, things included are okay but e.g., too much of chairs would rather reshoot' does not preclude the possibility that this non-optimal photograph would be kept if other photographs of the event did not exist. That is, sometimes a non-optimal photograph is better than no photograph. Therefore, these data suggest that to best support keep/delete decisions, interfaces for digital storage should make it easy for users to browse sets of related pictures. Related pictures may refer to, among other properties: pictures taken at a certain time, of a certain location, of particular buildings or event pictures that represent visually

Table 2.2 Definitions and relevant examples for each category of reason produced by thematic analysis of participants keep and delete decision explanations

Decision	Category of reason	Definition of category	Example quote[a]
Keep	Typical	Photo as something typical of Festival/Edinburgh/Scotland etc.	'Shows Scotland'
	Aesthetics	The composition, quality or staging (or aesthetics otherwise) of the photograph.	'Came out well'
	Reaction	Something the person found funny/ interesting/scary, etc.	'It shocked me the way his eyes are painted different and unusual'
	Sharing	Would be used to tell stories about the person's experience of street fair.	'The man whose mask kept falling off! ...would tell people the story when showing them the photo'
	Subject matter	Specific act, item or view etc.	'It's a Storm Trooper!'
	Personal	Personal relevance to person, their life, or time at street fair.	'Start of Journey. Not successful photo, but start of journey'
Delete	Aesthetics	Bad quality (such as, blurry, fingers blocking view)	'It's fuzzy'
	Surplus	Content was already covered (better) in another picture	'I've already got a picture of them'
	Random	Pictures were just taken because the task alarm went off, indicating a picture should be taken	'buzzer shot'
	No shows	Photograph did not capture content participant had intended to photograph	'Wanted a picture of the street but here (there is a) bus and no view'
	Untypical	Photograph included intended subject matter, but on viewing did not represent the city/country/festival	'The photo could also be Christmas, not necessarily Fringe'
	Reaction	Photograph evoked negative feelings or connections, or were uninteresting	'Didn't like act'

[a]Note that example quotes may demonstrate more than the example category they are listed alongside

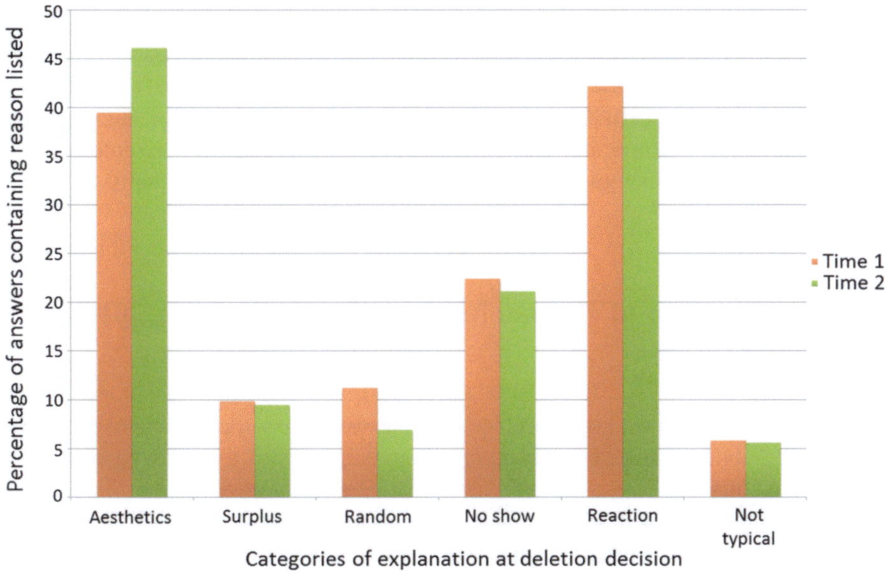

Fig. 2.6 Percentage of different explanations for delete decisions, observed at Time 1 (day of testing) and Time 2 (day, week, month later), collapsed across Groups 1-3

similar views, despite originating in different places. It is important to offer users flexibility in the views they can define.

Finally, a sample of the photographs from the study was processed by an automated system (see Chap. 3) that incorporates feature detection and automated suggestions for deletion of, for example, duplicates, or poor quality photographs. We then compared the results from the automated system with the human decisions for these same photographs. There was a reasonable match between categorisation by humans who took the photographs, and the automated categorisation, although there were some errors (e.g. detecting trees when no trees were depicted). The automated system generated a selection of photographs for preservation and for deletion that were similar to the human selection, but selected some photographs for deletion that the human participant had chosen to keep because, for example, it was the only photograph of an event that they had enjoyed, or it reminded them of a previous experience. These discrepancies between the automated and human categorisations and selection emphasise the need for semi-automated systems, with the digital technologies generating suggestions but with the humans having the final decision. While automatic image annotation and managed preservation and forgetting can support the process, flexible tagging facilities are also required.

These results also indicate that strict binary keep/delete judgments might not be realistic for managed preservation and forgetting with digital storage of photographs. Instead, participants appeared to use three categories, ‘definitely keep’, ‘potentially keep’ and ‘definitely delete’. Photos that should definitely be kept are also far more likely to be chosen as landmarks. This is reminiscent of the way in which Google creates stories from sets of photos, where highlights of a photo collection associated with a certain time and location are assembled into a slide show. If this finding is confirmed in more formal studies, it suggests innovative ways for eliciting data on personal preservation preferences, such as editing automatically assembled slide shows, or creating scrap books that combine photos with videos, comments and other documents.

2.6 Key Features of Human Memory for Designing Digital Preservation

Human memory is a complex, multifaceted collection of interacting and overlapping systems that continues to be the subject of an abundance of psychological studies. Discoveries are made daily, and therefore our understanding of memory is flexible, and will change as new evidence accumulates. Nevertheless, there are central and discernible features of memory upon which many researchers agree. On the basis of the literature reviewed above, and the example small study of engagement with photographs as reminders of an event, it is recommended that the following key features of human memory are considered when designing digital preservation tools:

1. Human memory is often considered to be 'episodic', referring to details about specific events, or 'semantic', referring to knowledge accumulated over the lifetime. Within semantic memory are domains of knowledge or schema that group key features that are repeatedly experienced in specific scenarios. There are schema that are similar across people, such as for a restaurant, the office, the home, the swimming pool, a holiday and so on. Each individual also has a schema of the 'self', including knowledge of life periods, name, date of birth, relationships, etc.
2. Preservation of information about specific events in human memory is heavily influenced by contextualising the information about those events within schema. Recall from memory involves reconstruction of details of events based on schema, rather than retrieval of a veridical record.
3. The level of detail for preservation in human memory is determined by what is required to set the context and to preserve the key features of an event. This means that many details of an event will not be stored. For example, the fact that a particular restaurant was visited on holiday and who else was at the meal may be preserved in memory, but the precise colours and design of the walls and floor coverings, the food eaten and layout of the food on the plate will not be stored in memory or will be forgotten rapidly, unless these were key features of the experience.
4. Forgetting of details of events is extremely rapid and substantial, with most details of any given event forgotten within minutes or hours. The amount forgotten and the rate of forgetting is largely determined by the length of time spent on experiencing the event or actively attempting to preserve in memory details of that event, and

the links with a context or existing schema. Most of the information that remains after the initial period of forgetting is preserved in memory long term.

5. Some details of an event are required only on a temporary basis in order to complete a particular task, and are unlikely ever to be required again in the future. These kinds of details may therefore be retained for only a few seconds, or in some cases for less than a second, and not preserved. Examples could be the positions, colours and models of cars seen briefly while travelling on a motorway, or retaining a telephone number only long enough to successfully press the keys in the correct order on the telephone.
6. Some details are required for periods of hours or days but are forgotten completely after they serve no purpose and are therefore not repeatedly recalled or supported by a different context. Examples here might be a flight number after a particular journey is complete, or the number of the room occupied in a hotel after returning home or moving to a different hotel.
7. Memories for events can be changed as a result of interference from other experiences or information, such as viewing photographs subsequent to the event, or as a result of the process of reconstructing memories from schema or context. This can result in 'false memories' or 'memory illusions' with the individual being unaware of the error and convinced of the accuracy of their retrieval.
8. Memories for major public or personal events that are experienced as being vivid and highly detailed are preserved in memory largely because of rehearsal and multiple retrievals of those details at the time of the event and subsequently. Many of the details that are personally experienced as vivid may be false recollections as a result of many memories being reconstructions and rationalisations based on schema and context.
9. Design of digital storage systems for personal use should:

   - incorporate, but not necessarily duplicate, elements of categorisation, contextualisation, and summarisation analogous to those found in human memory.
   - incorporate algorithms to estimate preservation value of information as a driver for (a) storing all details, (b) storing summaries with options for reconstruction of details (c) selecting to delete.
   - incorporate algorithms to assess what information may be needed for a current task, but can be summarised or deleted after the task is complete or after some specified period.
   - incorporate succession protocols to ensure that information with high, long-term preservation value continues to be available indefinitely with changing software and operating systems, digital hardware and changing file formats and storage media.
   - incorporate sufficient redundancy to ensure preservation following failure of hardware, storage media, software or corporate and organisational failure of storage services.
   - incorporate the fundamental principle that digital storage should complement and support human memory, not attempt to replace it.

Chapter 3
Multimedia Processing Essentials

Konstantinos Apostolidis, Foteini Markatopoulou, Christos Tzelepis, Vasileios Mezaris and Ioannis Patras

Abstract As multimedia applications have become part of our life, preservation and long-term access to the multimedia elements that are continuously produced is a major consideration, both for many organizations that generate or collect and need to maintain digital content, and for individuals. In this chapter, we focus primarily on the following multimedia analysis and organization techniques that provide the basis for multimedia preservation: (a) photo/video annotation, which refers to the problem of assigning one or more semantic concepts to photos or video fragments, (b) photo/video quality assessment, which refers to the automatic prediction of a photo's or video's aesthetic value, (c) near-duplicate detection, which aims to identify groups of very similar items in large media collections, and (d) event-based photo clustering and summarization, which concern the selection of the most characteristic photos of a photo collection so as to create a storyline that conveys the gist of this collection.

3.1 Introduction

Either for organizational or personal use, the amount of media items produced every day is huge. In the case of organizations, taking into account the information located in their web sites, and in the documents and media produced and used internally, we

---

K. Apostolidis · F. Markatopoulou · C. Tzelepis · V. Mezaris (✉)
Information Technologies Institute (ITI)/Centre for Research
and Technology Hellas (CERTH), 6th Km. Charilaou-Thermi Road,
57001 Thermi-Thessaloniki, Greece
e-mail: bmezaris@iti.gr

K. Apostolidis
e-mail: kapost@iti.gr

F. Markatopoulou
e-mail: markatopoulou@iti.gr

C. Tzelepis
e-mail: tzelepis@iti.gr

F. Markatopoulou · C. Tzelepis · I. Patras
Queen Mary University of London, Mile end Campus, London E1 4NS, UK
e-mail: i.patras@qmul.ac.uk

V. Mezaris et al. (eds.), *Personal Multimedia Preservation*, Springer Series
on Cultural Computing, https://doi.org/10.1007/978-3-319-73465-1_3

realize that the amount of data that is created continuously grows at an increasing pace. Similarly, for individuals, digital cameras, mobile phone cameras, webcams, etc. are frequently used, giving them the opportunity to capture events important for them, like weddings, birthday parties, a trip, as well as everyday situations like a coffee break with friends, a walk to the beach, etc. These constitute a considerable volume of data, nevertheless, not all of them are important and should be preserved along time. Many documents become outdated at some point, and often photos exist that are just duplicates or of poor quality. In order to support human-memory-inspired approaches for organizing, retrieving, processing, and finally preserving these media items efficiently and effectively, multimedia content analysis and condensation methods are essential for evaluating the preservation value of each photo or video. Such methods should be able to answer questions such as:

- What does a photo "*A*" show? What are the high-level concepts describing it? Which items in a photo/video collection depict the same concepts as photo "*A*"?
- What is the aesthetic value of a photo/video? How can we assess this in an automatic way (without the need for user interaction)? Which items in a photo/video collection are characterized by poor aesthetic quality?
- Are there any items in a photo/video collection that are very similar (or nearly identical) to photo "*A*"? And, more generally, are there any items in a photo/video collection that are very similar (or nearly identical) with each other?
- How to present a large photo collection concerning an event to the user in a compact way?

In this chapter, we present multimedia processing techniques that will help a Preserve-or-Forget system (PoF, see Chap. 6) answer such questions, and/or give clues about which items can be "forgotten" and which should be "preserved" as input to in a preservation value estimation method (see Chap. 4).

We focus primarily on the following multimedia analysis and organization tasks: (a) photo/video annotation, (b) photo/video quality assessment, (c) near-duplicate detection, and (d) event-based photo clustering and summarization. Photo/video annotation refers to the problem of assigning one or more semantic concepts to photos or video fragments. We focus on deep learning techniques that have shown excellent results during the last years. We show how to take advantage of state-of-the-art pretrained deep convolutional neural networks (DCNNs) in smaller collections by fine-tuning their parameters, and we also present a method that improves the photo/video annotation accuracy by performing multi-task learning in combination with DCNN-based features. Photo/video aesthetic quality assessment refers to the automatic prediction of the aesthetic value of a photo/video. To this end, we investigate comprehensive image- and motion-based features, as well as a sophisticated learning method that takes the input features' uncertainty into consideration. Near-duplicate detection and retrieval aim to identify very similar media items in large collections. We present various approaches for near-duplicate detection and retrieval based on the use of different types of features extracted from photos. On top of all the presented approaches, we propose a graph-based analysis of a photo/video collection to support both near-duplicate detection and near-duplicate retrieval scenarios. Event-based photo clustering and summarization consist in segmenting an event-centered photo collection to groups, each depicting a distinct part of the event. This is an essential preprocessing step for being able to summarize an event-centered photo collection by selecting the most characteristic photos of each subevent, thus creating a storyline that conveys the gist of the collection. For all of the above techniques, we review the state of the art, propose an own approach, and perform extensive experiments and comparisons.

3.2 Photo and Video Annotation

Photo/video annotation, aka concept detection, refers to the task of assigning semantic labels to photos or video fragments (e.g., shots) based on a predefined list of labels [369]. Photos/videos are commonly annotated with concept labels (aka keywords or tags) that refer to objects (e.g., "car" and "chair"), activities (e.g., "running" and "dancing"), scenes (e.g., "hills" and "beach"), etc. Automatically understanding the content of photos/videos is a challenging and intensively investigated problem. Typically, a two-step label detection procedure for photo annotation is followed: (a) Extraction of features; referring to interest point detection, local feature extraction and feature encoding, or DCNN-based (deep convolutional neural network) features. (b) Classification; referring to the process of building classifiers that learn the associations between the extracted features and semantic labels. A similar process can be followed for video annotation. In this case, video sequences are first segmented into one or more video fragments; one or more keyframes are selected for each fragment, and these keyframes can subsequently be treated as still images.

In this section, we discuss how deep learning can be applied to photo/video annotation, focusing mainly on the optimal training of DCNNs on small-sized datasets using transfer learning, and on how improved concept detection accuracy can be achieved by employing multitask learning (MTL) techniques in combination with DCNN-based features. A recent trend in video annotation is to learn features directly from the raw keyframe pixels using DCNNs. A DCNN consists of several layers that are placed sequentially the one after the other. Three main types of layers can be distinguished: convolutional, pooling, and fully-connected. In a typical architecture, the most-bottom layers are convolutional layers, after each convolution layer, there may be a pooling layer, and finally, after several convolutional and pooling layers one or more fully-connected layers follow. A fully-connected layer takes all neurons in the previous layer and connects it to every single neuron it has. Fully-connected layers can be visualized as d-dimensional vectors. Essentially, the convolutional layers are providing a meaningful, low-dimensional, and somewhat invariant feature space, and the fully-connected layer is learning a (possibly nonlinear) function in that space. DCNN training requires the learning of millions of parameters, which means that a small-sized training set could easily over-fit the DCNN on the training data. Transferring a pretrained network in a new dataset by fine-tuning its parameters is a common strategy that can take advantage of the bottom generic layers and adjust the top layers to the target dataset and the new target concepts [74, 147, 428]. Most DCNN-based approaches use the pretrained or fine-tuned DCNN as a standalone classifier, i.e., they perform the final class label prediction directly, using for example, a softmax layer [210, 363]. Other approaches use the DCNN as a feature generator, i.e., they train classifiers with features extracted from one or more layers of the DCNN [266]. Specifically, for each target concept one supervised learning classifier (e.g., SVM) is trained to solve a binary classification problem (i.e, decide on the presence or absence of the concept) [369]. Independently, training concept detectors (i.e., using SVMs) is a single-task learning (STL) process, where each task involves recognizing one concept. STL ignores the fact that groups of concepts can be related. Some recent methods use MTL in order to build many concept detectors together at the same time, which can improve concept detection accuracy. In the remainder of this section, we survey the literature on DCNN transfer learning and MTL for video/photo annotation (Sect. 3.2.1), and then we present in more detail:

- Three fine-tuning strategies that can be used for transferring a pretrained DCNN to a new target domain (Sect. 3.2.2.1).
- A lifelong MTL algorithm for photo/video concept detection (Sect. 3.2.2.2).

3.2.1 Related Work

Concept detection is a multi-label classification problem (one photo/keyframe may be annotated with more than one semantic concepts), that can be treated as multiple independent binary classification problems, where for each concept a model can be learned to distinguish photos/keyframes that the concept appears in from those that the concept does not appear in. Given feature-based photo/keyframe representations and the ground-truth annotations for each photo/keyframe (i.e., the concepts that are present), any supervised machine learning algorithm that solves classification problems can be used in order to learn the relations between the low-level photo/keyframe representations and the high-level semantic concepts. The most commonly used machine learning algorithms are support vector machines (SVM) and logistic regression (LR). Chi-square kernels, that were originally considered to be optimal for use in SVMs [182, 433] are now often replaced by Histogram Intersection kernels [261] or even Linear SVMs. Other machine learning algorithms have also been used, such as Random Forest and Lazy style algorithms (e.g., *k*nn); however, achieving lower performance or presenting higher computational complexity. A recent trend in video annotation is to learn features directly from the raw keyframe pixels using DCNNs. DCNNs consist of many layers of feature extractors, which makes them have a more sophisticated structure than simply using a single hand-crafted representation or combinations of a few such. DCNNs can be used either as feature generators, as described in the beginning of this section, or as standalone classifiers, i.e., unlabeled keyframes are forward propagated by a DCNN that performs the final class label prediction directly, using typically a softmax or a hinge loss layer [210, 363].

The small number of labeled training examples is a common problem, especially in video datasets, making it difficult to train a deep network from scratch without overfitting its parameters on the training set [368]. For this reason, it is common to use transfer learning, i.e., to take a network that has been trained on a large-scale source dataset (e.g., ImageNet [345]) and fine-tune its parameters for the target dataset. Fine-tuning is a process where the weights of a pretrained DCNN are used as the starting point for a new target training set and they are modified in order to adapt the pretrained DCNN to the new target dataset. Different DCNN-based transfer learning approaches have been successfully applied in many datasets. The most straightforward approach replaces the classification layer of a pretrained DCNN with a new output layer that corresponds to the categories that should be learned with respect to the target dataset, [74, 147, 428]. Generalizing this approach, the weights of the first K network layers can remain frozen, i.e., they are copied from the pretrained DCNN and kept unchanged, and the rest of the layers (be it just the last one or more than one) are learned from scratch [60, 316]. Alternatively, the copies of the first K layers could be allowed to adapt to the target dataset with a low learning rate. For example, [428] investigates which layers of Alexnet [210] are generic, i.e., can be directly transferred to a target domain, and which layers are dataset-specific. Furthermore, experiments in [428] show that fine-tuning the transferred layers of a network work better than freezing them. Other studies extend the pretrained network by one or more fully-connected layers, which seems to improve the above transfer learning strategies [60, 316, 329, 368]. In Sect. 3.2.2.1 we present the most commonly used fine-tuning strategies and we compare them in order to find the most suitable one for photo/video annotation.

Given a pretrained or a fine-tuned DCNN, more elaborate methods that promote the sharing of information between concepts, such as multitask learning (MTL) methods instead of STL ones (e.g., training SVM classifiers on DCNN-based features), have been proposed in order to improve concept detection accuracy. Specifically, a pretrained or fine-tuned DCNN is applied on a ground-truth annotated video/image dataset in order to extract DCNN-based features; then, a MTL classifier can be trained on these features in order to learn task models for all of the concepts together at the same time by exploiting the relations across the different concept models. Many MTL methods have been proposed that exploit task relatedness towards improving the overall concept detection accuracy. The main difference of MTL methods is the way they define task relatedness. Some methods identify shared features between different tasks and use regularization to model task relatedness [20, 305, 313]. Other methods identify a shared subspace over the task parameters [21, 112, 132]. The methods above make the strong assumption that all tasks are related; some newer methods consider the fact that some tasks may be unrelated. For example, the clustered MTL algorithm (CMTL) [438] uses a clustering approach to assign to the same cluster parameters of tasks that lie nearby in terms of their L_2 distance. Adaptive MTL (AMTL) [376] decomposes the task parameters into a low-rank structure that captures task relations, and a group-sparse structure that detects outlier tasks.

The GO-MTL algorithm [211] uses a dictionary-based method that allows two tasks from different groups to overlap by having one or more basis in common. In general, MTL methods have high-computational cost, because the shared representation of all tasks is learned at once. Online or lifelong MTL, in contrast, can learn consecutive tasks that arrive in a sequence. The ELLA algorithm [121] is the online version of GO-MTL [211], presenting similar performance but being three orders of magnitude faster in training. In Sect. 3.2.2.2 we show how ELLA can be used as the starting point for devising an online MTL algorithm suitable for image/video concept detection.

3.2.2 Method

3.2.2.1 DCNN-Based Features and Fine-Tuning Strategies

Let D_{so} denote a pretrained DCNN, trained on T_{so} categories using a source dataset, and D_{ta} denote the target DCNN, fine-tuned on T_{ta} categories of a different target dataset. In this section, we present three fine-tuning strategies (Fig. 3.1) that can be used for the problem of visual annotation, in order to effectively fine-tune DCNNs D_{so} that were trained on a large visual dataset for a new target video/image dataset. These three fine-tuning strategies are as follows:

- FT1-def: Default fine-tuning strategy: This is the typical strategy that modifies the last fully-connected layer of D_{so} to produce the desired number of outputs T_{ta}, by replacing the last fully-connected layer with a new T_{ta}-dimensional classification fully-connected layer.
- FT2-re: Re-initialization strategy: In this scenario, similar to FT1-def, the last fully-connected layer is replaced by a new T_{ta}-dimensional classification layer. The weights of the last N layers, preceding the classification layer, are also reinitialized (i.e., reset and learned from scratch).
- FT3-ex: Extension strategy: Similar to the previous two strategies, the last fully-connected layer is replaced by a new T_{ta}-dimensional classification fully-connected layer. Subsequently, the network is extended with E fully-connected layers of size L that are placed on the bottom of the modified classification layer. These additional layers are initialized and trained from scratch during fine-tuning, at the same rate as the modified classification layer. One example of a modified network, after the insertion of one extension layer for two popular DCNN architectures, is presented in Fig. 3.2. Regarding the GoogLeNet architecture in this figure, which has two additional auxiliary classifiers, an extension layer is also inserted in each of them.

Each fine-tuned network D_{ta} can be used in two different ways to annotate new test keyframes/images with semantic concepts: (a) Direct classification: Each test keyframe/image is forward propagated by D_{ta} and the network's output is used as the final class distribution assigned to the keyframe/image. (b) D_{ta} is used as feature generator: The training set is forward propagated by the network and the features

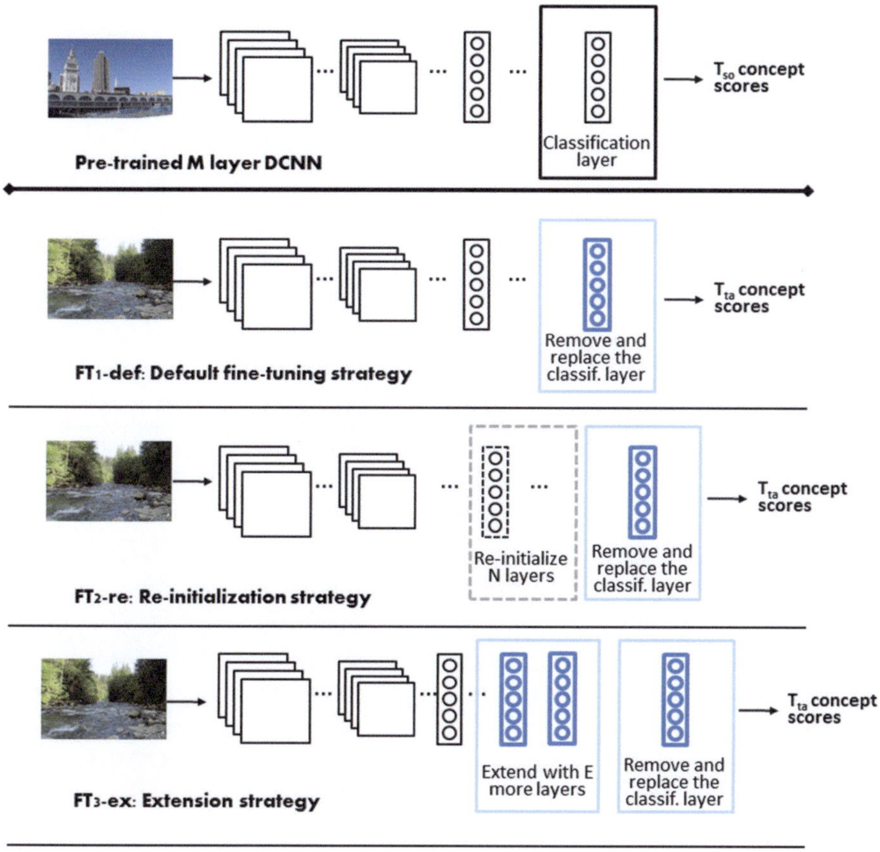

Fig. 3.1 Fine-tuning strategies outline

extracted from one or more layers of D_{ta} are used as feature vectors to subsequently train one supervised classifier (e.g., Logistic Regression) per concept. Then, each test keyframe/image is first described by the DCNN-based features and subsequently, these features serve as input to the trained classifiers.

3.2.2.2 ELLA with Label Constraints: ELLA_LC

In this section, we present a MTL method that uses a trained DCNN (i.e., pretrained or fine-tuned from a source DCNN using any of the three fine-tuning strategies presented in Sect. 3.2.2.1) as a feature generator in order to learn concept detectors. Starting by formulating our problem, a video concept detection system needs to learn a number of supervised learning tasks, one for each target concept. Each task t is associated with one concept detector (task model) $C^{(t)} : \mathbb{R}^d \mapsto \{\pm 1\}$, and the training set available

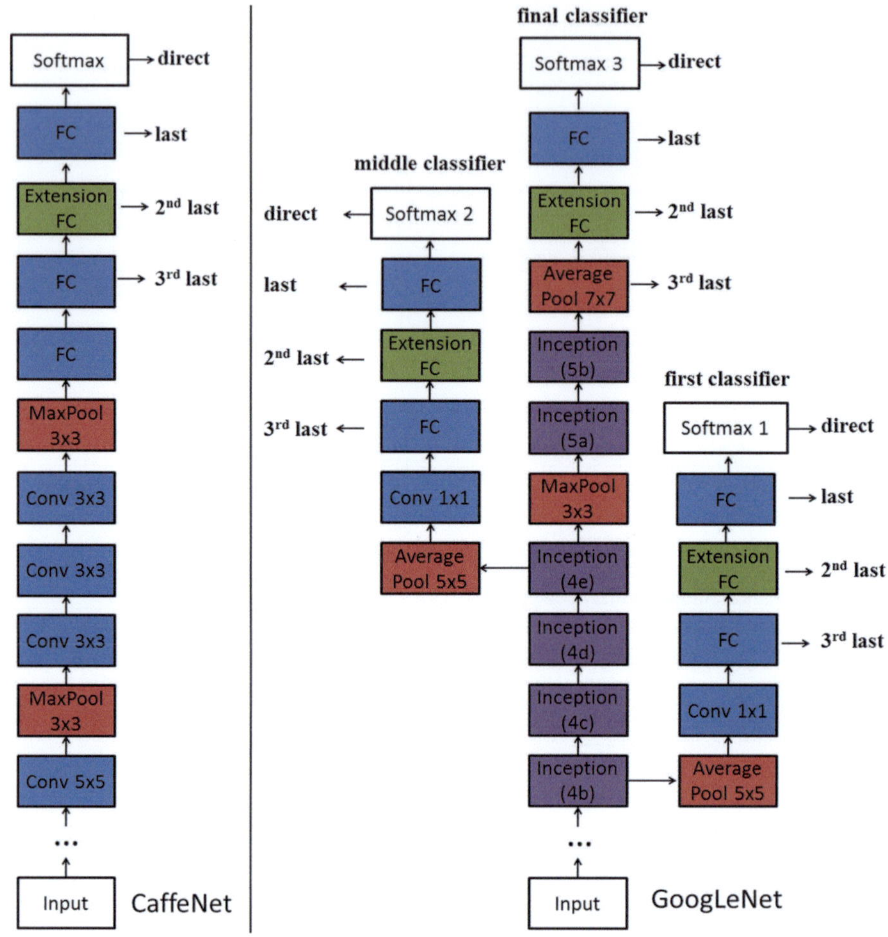

Fig. 3.2 A simplified illustration of the CaffeNet [210] (left) and GoogLeNet [377] (right) architectures used after insertion of one extension layer. Each of the inception layers of GoogLeNet consists of six convolution layers and one pooling layer. The figure also presents the direct output of each network and the output of the last three layers that were used as features w.r.t. the FT3-ex strategy. Similarly, the corresponding layers were used for the FT1-def and FT2-re strategies

for this concept $(\mathbf{x}_i^{(t)}, y_i^{(t)})_{i=1}^{n_t}$, where $\mathbf{x}_i^{(t)} \in \mathbb{R}^d$, a feature vector extracted for the ith keyframe and $y_i^{(t)} \in \{\pm 1\}$ the ground-truth annotation for the ith keyframe and the tth task/concept. A concept detector can be defined as $C^{(t)}(\mathbf{x}^{(t)}) = C(\mathbf{x}^{(t)}; \mathbf{w}^{(t)})$, where $\mathbf{w}^{(t)} \in \mathbb{R}^d$ is the task parameter vector. A concept detection system should be easily extended with new tasks even if the total number of tasks/concepts $T_{\max}$ is not available from the start. Furthermore, task parameters of related concepts may share similar knowledge, but also concept correlations obtained by the ground-truth annotation may provide another source of information regarding the relations between tasks. Considering all the above, in [267] we introduced the ELLA_LC algorithm (Efficient Lifelong Learning Algorithm with Label Constraint), which is presented in the rest of this section.

ELLA_LC is an extension of the ELLA algorithm proposed by Eaton and Ruvolo [121]. Specifically, we add a new label-based constraint on ELLA's model in order to incorporate statistical information of pairwise correlations between concepts that we can acquire from the ground-truth annotation. ELLA_LC uses a knowledge shared basis $\mathbf{L} \in \mathbb{R}^{d \times k}$ for all task models, where the columns of $\mathbf{L}$ correspond to the parameter vectors of k latent tasks. We model the parameter vector $\mathbf{w}^{(t)}$ of observed task t as $\mathbf{w}^{(t)} = \mathbf{L}\mathbf{s}^{(t)}$, where $\mathbf{s}^{(t)} \in \mathbb{R}^k$ is a task-specific weight vector that contains the coefficients of the linear combination. Each linear combination is assumed to be sparse in $\mathbf{L}$; in this way, we assume that there exist a small number of latent basis tasks and the task parameter vector of every observed task $\mathbf{w}^{(t)}$ is a linear combination of them. The overlap in the sparsity patterns of any two tasks controls the amount of sharing between them. ELLA_LC builds a concept detection system that (a) updates the shared basis $\mathbf{L}$ when a new concept arrives without building all the previous task models from scratch; and (b) incorporates the label correlations of the new concept with all of the previously learned concepts in order to improve the learning of the task-specific weight vector regarding the new concept and the shared basis $\mathbf{L}$. The above problem can be formulated by the following objective function:

$$\min_{(\mathbf{L},\mathbf{s}^{(t)})} \frac{1}{T}\sum_{t=1}^{T}\Bigg\{\frac{1}{n_t}\sum_{i=1}^{n_t}\mathscr{L}\left(C(\mathbf{x}_i^{(t)};\mathbf{L}\mathbf{s}^{(t)}),y_i^{(t)}\right)+\mu\left\|\mathbf{s}^{(t)}\right\|_1 \tag{3.1}$$

$$+\beta\left(\sum_{\substack{t'=1\\t'\neq t}}^{T}\frac{1}{T\text{-}1}|r_{t,t'}|\left\|\mathbf{L}(\mathbf{s}^{(t)}-\operatorname{sign}(r_{t,t'})\mathbf{s}^{(t')})\right\|^2\right)\Bigg\}+\lambda\left\|\mathbf{L}\right\|_F^2,$$

where $\mathscr{L}$ refers to the loss function that is used for learning the task-specific parameter vector $\mathbf{w}^{(t)}$; and $\mathbf{w}^{(t)}$ is obtained by building a classifier only using the training data available for task t: $\min_{(\mathbf{w}^{(t)})} \frac{1}{n_t}\sum_{i=1}^{n_t}\mathscr{L}\left(C(\mathbf{x}_i^{(t)};\mathbf{w}^{(t)},y_i^{(t)})\right)$. T is the number of tasks that have been learned so far. $r_{t,t'}$ is the ϕ-correlation coefficient between the concepts learned in tasks t and t', calculated from the ground-truth annotation of the training set.

This is similar to the objective function of ELLA [121] with the addition of the extra term: $|r_{t,t'}|\left\|\mathbf{L}(\mathbf{s}^{(t)}-\operatorname{sign}(r_{t,t'})\mathbf{s}^{(t')})\right\|^2$ that incorporates the label correlations. Specifically, we aim to model highly correlated concepts (positive or negative). We assume that if two concepts are positively correlated, then the underlying task parameters should be similar; on the other hand, if two concepts are negatively correlated, then the task parameters should be opposite. The similarity measure suitable to capture both positive and negative correlations that was selected in this study is the ϕ-correlation coefficient. To model this assumption, we use the above constraint in the objective function of Eq. (3.1). The larger the correlation between two concepts

Algorithm 1 ELLA_LC(k,d,λ,μ,β)

while existMoreTrainingData() **do**
  $T \leftarrow T{+}1, t = T$
  1. $(\mathbf{w}^{(t)}, \mathbf{H}^{(t)}) \leftarrow$ base_learner$(\mathbf{X}^{(t)}_{\text{new}}, \mathbf{y}^{(t)}_{\text{new}})$
  2. $\mathbf{s}^{(t)} \leftarrow$ Eq. (3.3)
  3. $\mathbf{A} \leftarrow \mathbf{A} + \Bigg((\mathbf{s}^{(t)}\mathbf{s}^{(t)\top}) \otimes \mathbf{H}^{(t)}$
  $+\beta\Big(\sum_{\substack{t'=1\\ t'\neq t}}^{T} \frac{1}{T-1} |r_{t,t'}| [\boldsymbol{\phi}_{t,t'}\boldsymbol{\phi}_{t,t'}^{\top} \otimes \mathbf{I}] \Big)\Bigg)$
  4. $\mathbf{b} \leftarrow \mathbf{b} + \text{vec}(\mathbf{s}^{(t)\top} \otimes (\mathbf{w}^{(t)\top}\mathbf{H}^{(t)}))$
  5. $\mathbf{L} \leftarrow \text{mat}((\frac{1}{T}\mathbf{A} + \lambda\mathbf{I})^{-1}\frac{1}{T}\mathbf{b})$
end while

(positive or negative), the higher the imposed constraint. On the other hand, if two concepts are not correlated, using the above function will not impose any constraint. This constraint is applicable to linear classifiers, where positive correlated concepts are forced to return similar responses, while negative correlated concepts are forced to return opposite responses.

Equation (3.1) is not jointly convex in $\mathbf{L}$ and $\mathbf{s}^{(t)}$, so ELLA [121] approximates them using two simplifications that we also follow here: (a) to eliminate the explicit dependence on all previous training data through the inner summation, we approximate Eq. (3.1) using the second-order Taylor expansion of

$$\frac{1}{n_t}\sum_{i=1}^{n_t} \mathscr{L}\left(C\left(\mathbf{x}_i^{(t)}; \mathbf{w}^{(t)}\right), y_i^{(t)}\right)$$

around $\mathbf{w}^{(t)}$. (b) We compute each $\mathbf{s}^{(t)}$ only when training data for task t are available and do not update it when new tasks arrive. These give the following objective function that approximates Eq. (3.1):

$$\min_{(\mathbf{L},\mathbf{s}^{(t)})} \frac{1}{T}\sum_{t=1}^{T}\Bigg\{ \left\|\mathbf{w}^{(t)} - \mathbf{L}\mathbf{s}^{(t)}\right\|^2_{\mathbf{H}^{(t)}} + \mu\left\|\mathbf{s}^{(t)}\right\|_1 + \beta\left(\sum_{\substack{t'=1\\ t'\neq t}}^{T}\frac{1}{T-1}|r_{t,t'}|\left\|\mathbf{L}(\mathbf{s}^{(t)} - \text{sign}(r_{t,t'})\mathbf{s}^{(t')})\right\|^2\right)\Bigg\} + \lambda\left\|\mathbf{L}\right\|^2_F, \tag{3.2}$$

where $\mathbf{H}^{(t)}$ is the Hessian of the loss function $\mathscr{L}$ evaluated on $\mathbf{w}^{(t)}$. To optimize this objective function, consequently to update our model, we perform three steps: (a) we compute the ϕ-correlation coefficient of the concept learned in task t with all the previously learned concepts; (b) we compute the task-specific weight vector $\mathbf{s}^{(t)}$ and (c) we update the shared basis $\mathbf{L}$. Below we describe each of these steps in more details.

To compute $\mathbf{s}^{(t)}$ we solve Eq. (3.2) for $\mathbf{s}^{(t)}$, when the task t arrives (i.e., $t = T$):

$$\min_{\mathbf{s}^{(t)}} \left\{ \left\| \mathbf{w}^{(t)} - \mathbf{L}\mathbf{s}^{(t)} \right\|_{\mathbf{H}^{(t)}}^2 + \mu \left\| \mathbf{s}^{(t)} \right\|_1 + \beta \left(\sum_{\substack{t'=1 \\ t' \neq t}}^{t} \frac{1}{t-1} |r_{t,t'}| \left\| \mathbf{L}(\mathbf{s}^{(t)} - \text{sign}(r_{t,t'})\mathbf{s}^{(t')}) \right\|^2 \right) \right\} \tag{3.3}$$

By expanding the above we arrive at the following problem that can be solved using quadratic programming:

$$\min_{\mathbf{s}^{(t)}} \left\{ \mathbf{s}^{(t)^\top} \left[\mathbf{L}^\top \mathbf{H}^{(t)} \mathbf{L} + \beta \left(\sum_{\substack{t'=1 \\ t' \neq t}}^{t} \frac{1}{t-1} |r_{t,t'}| \mathbf{L}^\top \mathbf{L} \right) \right] \mathbf{s}^{(t)} -2 \left[\mathbf{w}^{(t)^\top} \mathbf{H}^{(t)} \mathbf{L} + \frac{\beta}{2} \left(\sum_{\substack{t'=1 \\ t' \neq t}}^{t} \frac{1}{t-1} r_{t,t'} \mathbf{s}^{(t')^\top} \mathbf{L}^\top \mathbf{L} \right) - \frac{\mu}{2} \mathbf{I} \right] \mathbf{s}^{(t)} \right\} \tag{3.4}$$

where $\mathbf{I}$ denotes the identity matrix of order $k \times d$. Similarly, to update $\mathbf{L}$, we solve Eq. (3.2) for $\mathbf{L}$, which equals to:

$$\min_{\mathbf{L}} \frac{1}{T} \sum_{t=1}^{T} \left\{ \left\| \mathbf{w}^{(t)} - \mathbf{L}\mathbf{s}^{(t)} \right\|_H^2 + \beta \left(\sum_{\substack{t'=1 \\ t' \neq t}}^{T} \frac{1}{T-1} |r_{t,t'}| \left\| \mathbf{L}\boldsymbol{\phi}_{t,t'} \right\|^2 \right) \right\} + \lambda \left\| \mathbf{L} \right\|_F^2 , \tag{3.5}$$

where $\boldsymbol{\phi}_{t,t'} = \mathbf{s}^{(t)} - \text{sign}(r_{t,t'})\mathbf{s}^{(t')}$. Then, we null the gradient of Eq. (3.5) and solve for $\mathbf{L}$. This gives a column-wise vectorization of $\mathbf{L}$ as $\mathbf{A}^{-1}\mathbf{b}$ where:

$$\mathbf{A} = \frac{1}{T} \sum_{t=1}^{T} \left\{ (\mathbf{s}^{(t)} \mathbf{s}^{(t)^\top}) \otimes \mathbf{H}^{(t)} + \beta \left(\sum_{\substack{t'=1 \\ t' \neq t}}^{T} \frac{1}{T-1} |r_{t,t'}| [\boldsymbol{\phi}_{t,t'} \boldsymbol{\phi}_{t,t'}^\top \otimes \mathbf{I}] \right) \right\} + \lambda \mathbf{I}, \text{ and} \tag{3.6}$$

$$\mathbf{b} = \frac{1}{T} \sum_{t=1}^{T} vec(\mathbf{s}^{(t)^\top} \otimes (\mathbf{w}^{(t)^\top} \mathbf{H}^{(t)}))$$

where $\otimes$ is the Kronecker product symbol.

Algorithm 1 summarizes the steps that ELLA_LC performs for updating the above parameters and learning consecutive tasks. In each iteration, ELLA_LC receives training data $(\mathbf{X}_{new}^{(t)}, \mathbf{y}_{new}^{(t)})$ for a task t. If this is the first time that task t appears, then ELLA_LC computes the model parameters $\mathbf{w}^{(t)}$ and Hessian $\mathbf{H}^{(t)}$ from only this training data for task t using a base learner (Algorithm 1: Step 1). This step depends on the base learning algorithm; Eaton and Ruvolo [121] provide details for learning linear and logistic regression models using ELLA. In [267] we also show how the hinge loss can be used instead. We compute the ϕ-correlation coefficient of the concept learned in task t with all the previously learned concepts. Subsequently, the correlation information and the shared basis $\mathbf{L}$ are used to compute the task-specific weight vector $\mathbf{s}^{(t)}$ (Algorithm 1: Step 2). Finally, ELLA_LC updates the basis $\mathbf{L}$ to incorporate new knowledge via an incremental update that considers Eq. (3.6) (Algorithm 1: Steps 3–5). If additional training data for a previously learned task is provided, the algorithm can be extended, similarly to [121], in order to concatenate the new data with the past data and then update the vector $\mathbf{s}^{(t)}$ and the shared basis $\mathbf{L}$.

3.2.3 Experimental Study

3.2.3.1 Dataset and Experimental Setup

The TRECVID SIN task 2013 [6] dataset and the PASCAL VOC-2012 [131] dataset were utilized to train and evaluate the concept detection methods presented in the previous sections. The TRECVID SIN dataset consists of low-resolution videos, segmented into video shots; each shot is represented by one keyframe. The dataset is divided into a training and a test set (approx. 600 and 200 h, respectively). The training set is partially annotated with 346 semantic concepts. The test set is evaluated on 38 concepts, i.e., a subset of the 346 concepts. The PASCAL VOC-2012 [131] dataset consists of photos annotated with one object class label of the 20 available object classes. PASCAL VOC-2012 is divided into training, validation, and test sets (consisting of 5717, 5823, and 10991 photos, respectively). We used the training set to train the compared methods, and evaluated them on the validation set. We did not use the original test set because ground-truth annotations are not publicly available for it at the time of writing this chapter. The photo/video indexing problem was examined; that is, given a concept, we measure how well the top retrieved photos/video shots for this concept truly relate to it. Figure 3.3 shows (a) an example regarding the concept-based image annotation problem, i.e., a photo is automatically annotated with the concepts that are depicted in it; (b) an example regarding the concept-based image retrieval problem, i.e., the top photos that are retrieved for concept “river”.

A first set of experiments was developed in order to compare the three fine-tuning strategies presented in Sect. 3.2.2.1. Specifically, in all cases, we replaced the classification fully-connected (FC) layer of the utilized pretrained network, with

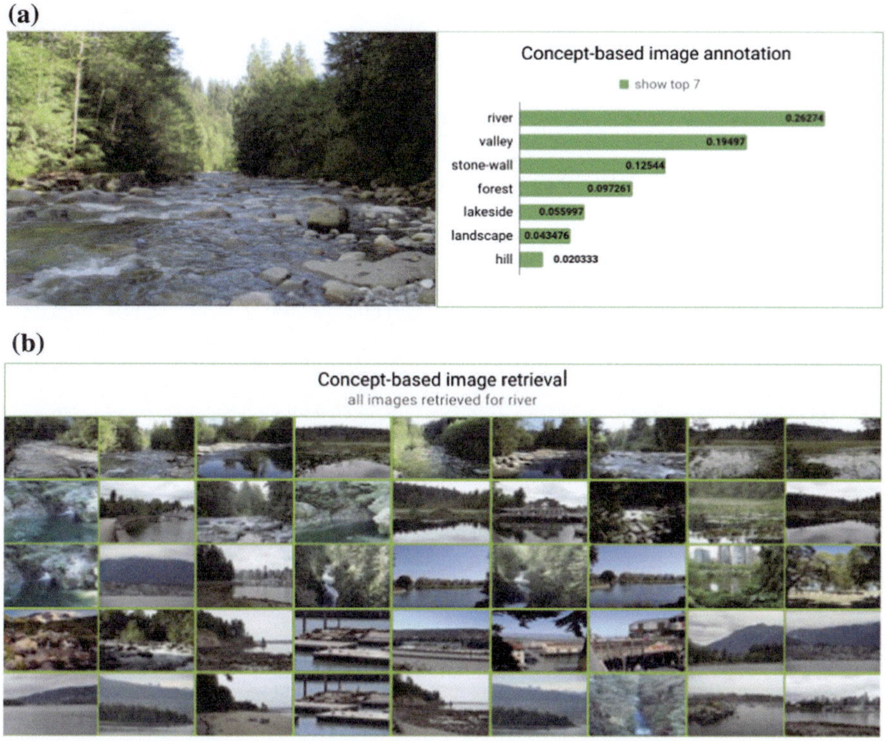

Fig. 3.3 Example of **a** the concept-based image annotation and **b** the concept-based image retrieval problem

a 345-dimensional FC classification layer for the 345 concepts of the TRECVID SIN dataset, or with a 20-dimensional classification layer for the 20 object categories of the PASCAL VOC-2012 dataset. We examined two values for parameter N of the FT2-re strategy; we refer to each configuration as FT2-re1 (for $N = 1$) and FT2-re2 (for $N = 2$). The FT3-ex strategy was examined for two settings of network extensions $E \in \{1, 2\}$: i.e., extending the network by one or two FC layers, respectively, followed by ReLU (Rectified Linear Units) and Dropout layers. Seven values where examined for the size of each extension layer: $L \in \{64, 128, 256, 512, 1024, 2048, 4096\}$. We refer to these configurations as FT3-exE-L. The new layers' learning rate and momentum was set to 0.01 and $5e^{-4}$, whereas the mini-batch size was restricted to 128 (based on the capabilities of the employed PC and GPU).

A second set of experiments was developed to evaluate the MTL approach presented in Sect. 3.2.2.2. We instantiated ELLA_LC with two base classifiers: LR and LSVM. We performed comparisons with the following methods: (a) STL using (i) LR, (ii) LSVM, and (iii) kernel SVM with radial kernel (KSVM); (b) The label powerset (LP) multi-label learning algorithm, that has been used in [268] to model the label relations; (c) AMTL [376], and (d) CMTL [438], two batch MTL methods,

Table 3.1 MXinfAP (%) for GoogLeNet-5k-345-SIN. The best result per column is underlined. The globally best result is bold and underlined

conf/layer	Final classifier					Middle classifier		First classifier	
	Direct (a)	Last (b)	2nd last (c)	3rd last (d)	Fused (e)	Direct (f)	Fused (g)	Direct (h)	Fused (i)
FT1-def	22.45	29.60	<u>29.80</u>	–	30.58	23.08	29.41	<u>21.25</u>	26.00
FT2-re1	20.88	28.44	28.43	–	29.58	22.51	28.55	20.37	25.16
FT2-re2	19.08	27.21	27.17	–	28.02	21.73	28.44	20.07	25.74
FT3-ex1-64	25.48	28.86	26.86	29.22	29.62	23.30	28.37	20.20	24.47
FT3-ex1-128	<u>25.52</u>	29.75	28.66	29.57	30.60	<u>23.98</u>	28.82	20.87	25.38
FT3-ex1-256	24.79	30.16	28.99	<u>30.26</u>	31.11	23.62	29.56	21.06	26.32
FT3-ex1-512	24.28	30.86	29.26	29.68	31.47	23.54	29.86	20.71	26.32
FT3-ex1-1024	24.03	31.02	28.78	29.35	31.55	23.43	29.90	20.53	26.57
FT3-ex1-2048	23.37	31.02	27.24	29.37	31.02	23.29	<u>29.94</u>	20.56	<u>26.61</u>
FT3-ex1-4096	23.07	30.91	28.98	29.61	<u>**31.57**</u>	22.85	29.64	20.82	26.26
FT3-ex2-64	16.44	17.51	19.62	19.95	20.09	11.43	15.12	10.65	13.33
FT3-ex2-128	23.87	26.19	26.73	26.05	27.02	18.70	23.64	14.87	19.95
FT3-ex2-256	24.46	28.94	28.69	28.68	29.57	22.68	26.98	18.75	23.10
FT3-ex2-512	23.95	29.44	29.07	28.94	30.14	22.72	28.22	20.20	24.79
FT3-ex2-1024	23.41	30.03	28.80	29.54	30.63	22.79	29.10	19.74	25.68
FT3-ex2-2048	23.38	30.74	28.98	28.21	30.61	22.29	29.34	19.57	26.23
FT3-ex2-4096	23.07	<u>31.21</u>	28.94	27.98	30.93	22.11	29.40	19.64	26.11

(e) ELLA [121], an online MTL approach. We selected all the parameter values for these methods based on the training data alone. The value of k was set to 38, regularization parameters λ and μ in Eq. (3.1) were kept fixed at e^{-10} and e^{-3}, respectively, for all the online MTL methods, in all experiments. These parameters are expected to depend on the dimensionality of the feature space and the number of examples, and according to preliminary experiments seem to work well for the employed features. The parameter value of β for ELLA_LC was selected from the set $\{e^{-2}, e^{-1}, 1, e^{1}, e^{2}\}$. The ordering of the tasks was fixed and the same for all the online MTL algorithms, and each task was presented sequentially. AMTL and CMTL learned each new task from a single batch of data that contained all training instances of that task.

Table 3.2 MAP % for GoogleNet-5k-VOC. The best result per column is underlined. The globally best result per subtable is bold and underlined

conf/layer	Final classifier					Middle classifier		First classifier	
	Direct (a)	Last (b)	2nd last (c)	3rd last (d)	Fused (e)	Direct (f)	Fused (g)	Direct (h)	Fused (i)
FT1-def	82.39	86.75	86.74	–	88.01	81.10	84.25	78.96	79.06
FT2-re1	80.50	85.21	86.91	–	87.44	79.58	82.76	77.78	77.23
FT2-re2	77.73	78.81	83.13	–	83.11	75.28	77.34	71.99	69.65
FT3-ex1-64	79.74	82.86	86.41	86.26	86.92	76.36	82.72	72.32	77.51
FT3-ex1-128	80.47	85.50	88.26	86.56	88.12	78.57	84.12	74.01	78.76
FT3-ex1-256	81.43	85.81	88.33	86.73	**88.36**	79.31	84.48	75.29	79.12
FT3-ex1-512	81.65	85.91	87.84	86.90	88.33	79.99	84.76	76.25	79.69
FT3-ex1-1024	82.30	86.48	87.01	86.89	88.20	80.68	84.56	77.32	79.32
FT3-ex1-2048	82.51	86.93	86.80	86.96	88.23	81.15	84.51	77.97	79.62
FT3-ex1-4096	82.39	87.20	86.37	87.05	88.13	81.52	84.45	78.43	79.65
FT3-ex2-64	43.85	45.11	53.99	51.67	52.81	39.10	47.22	32.42	38.72
FT3-ex2-128	75.89	70.96	82.85	83.34	82.51	63.27	72.34	54.45	63.64
FT3-ex2-256	78.94	80.30	86.44	86.43	86.01	69.19	77.67	65.31	72.75
FT3-ex2-512	80.47	82.83	87.56	87.00	87.38	75.17	81.44	66.50	74.38
FT3-ex2-1024	81.47	84.54	86.81	86.53	87.58	76.99	82.85	71.09	76.74
FT3-ex2-2048	82.11	85.49	86.90	86.28	87.76	78.15	83.24	73.55	77.69
FT3-ex2-4096	80.50	83.83	85.82	84.71	86.64	77.49	81.79	74.66	78.21

3.2.3.2 Experimental Results

Tables 3.1 and 3.2 present the results of the three fine-tuning strategies of Sect. 3.2.2.1 for the TRECVID SIN and PASCAL VOC dataset, respectively. For each dataset, we fine-tuned the GoogLeNet-5k, which refers to a DCNN that we trained according to the 22-layer GoogLeNet architecture on the ImageNet "fall 2011" dataset for 5055 categories. Specifically, GoogLeNet-5k was fine-tuned on the 345 TRECVID SIN concepts (i.e., all the available TRECVID SIN concepts, except for one which was discarded because only five positive samples are provided for it). We refer to it as GoogLeNet-5k-345-SIN. In addition, GoogLeNet-5k was fine-tuned on the positive examples of the PASCAL VOC-2012 training set. This network is labeled as GoogLeNet-5k-VOC. For the TRECVID SIN dataset, we analyze our results in terms of mean extended inferred average precision (MXinfAP) [427], which is an approximation of the mean average precision (MAP) suitable for the partial ground-truth that accompanies the TRECVID dataset [6]. Table 3.1 presents the MXinfAP of the GoogLeNet-5k-345-SIN and Table 3.2 presents the results in terms of a MAP of the GoogLeNet-5k-VOC.

For each pair of utilized network and fine-tuning strategy we evaluate: First, the direct output of the network (Tables 3.1 and 3.2: col. (a)). Second, logistic regression (LR) classifiers trained on DCNN-based features. Specifically, the output of each of the three last layers of each fine-tuned network was used as a feature to train one LR model per concept (Tables 3.1 and 3.2: col. (b)–(d)). Furthermore, we present results for the late-fused output (arithmetic mean) of the LR classifiers built using the last three layers (Tables 3.1 and 3.2: col. (e)). Evaluations are also reported for the two auxiliary classifiers (Tables 3.1 and 3.2: col. (f)–(i)). The details of the two GoogLeNet architectures and the extracted features are also illustrated in Fig. 3.2. Based on the results reported in the aforementioned tables, we reach the following conclusions:

- For both datasets, the FT3-ex strategy almost always outperforms the other two fine-tuning strategies (FT1-def, FT2-re) for specific (L, E) values.
- With respect to the direct output, FT3-ex1-64 and FT3-ex1-128 constitute the top-two methods for the TRECVID SIN dataset. On the other hand, FT3-ex1-2048 and FT3-ex1-4096 are the top-two methods for the PASCAL VOC-2012 dataset. That is, the FT3-ex strategy with one extension layer is always the best solution, but the optimal dimension of the extension layer varies, depending on the target domain dataset.
- The highest concept detection accuracy for each network is always reached when LR classifiers are trained on features extracted from the last and the second last fully-connected layer using the FT3-ex strategy for TRECVID SIN and PASCAL VOC-2012 dataset (when examining each DCNN layer separately, i.e., excluding the fusion of features reported in column (e) of Tables 3.1 and 3.2), respectively. That is, features extracted from the top layers are more accurate than layers positioned lower in the network, but the optimal layer varies, depending on the target domain dataset.
- DCNN-based features significantly outperform the direct output alternative in the majority of cases. However, in a few cases, the direct network output works comparably well. The choice between the two approaches should be based on the application that the DCNN will be used, e.g., real-time applications' time and memory limitations would probably render using DCNNs as feature extractors in conjunction with additional learning (LR or SVMs) prohibitive. Furthermore, we observe that the features extracted from the final classifier of GoogLeNet-based networks outperform the other two auxiliary classifiers, in most cases.
- Finally, it is better to combine features extracted from many layers; specifically, performing late fusion on the output of the LR classifiers trained with each one of the last three fully-connected layers almost always outperforms using a single such classifier irrespective of the employed network (Tables 3.1 and 3.2: col. (e)). The above conclusion was also reached for the auxiliary classifiers of GoogLeNet-

based networks, but for space-limitations, we only present the fused output for each of these auxiliary classifiers (Tables 3.1 and 3.2: col. (g), (i)).

The interested reader can refer to [329] for an extensive experimental comparison with more DCNN architectures, different subsets of concepts and different DCNN and fine-tuning learning parameters.

Table 3.3 presents the results with respect to the MTL method presented in Sect. 3.2.2.2. In this case, we used features from four different DCNNs that were trained on ImageNet data [345]: (a) The 8-layer CaffeNet [210], (b) the 16-layer deep ConvNet [363], (c) the 22-layer GoogLeNet [377], (iv) the GoogLeNet-5k that was used for the fine-tuning experiments above. We will refer to these networks as CaffeNet1K, ConvNet1K, GNET1k, GNET5k, respectively. We applied each of these networks on the TRECVID keyframes and we used as a feature the network's direct output, that corresponds to the final class label prediction for 1000 ImageNet categories for CaffeNet1k, ConvNet1k, and GNET1k, and 5055 categories for GNET5k. All the feature vectors were finally reduced to 400 dimensions using principal components analysis (PCA), as this was shown to improve the performance for all the methods in our experiments by around 2% (in terms of MXinfAP). To improve the results, we also experimented with fine-tuning (FT) the above methods on various subsets of the 346 TRECVID SIN concepts using the extension strategy presented in Sect. 3.2.2.1 and evaluated above. This resulted in 5 FT networks that differ in the number and dimension of the extension layers and in the number of output categories. Subsequently, we again applied these FT networks on the TRECVID keyframes. To train our base classifiers, for each concept, a training set was assembled that included all positive annotated training examples for the given concept, and negatives to a maximum of 15:1 ratio.

Table 3.3 presents the results of our experiments in terms of MXinfAP. ELLA_QP is an intermediate version of the ELLA_LC that solves the objective function of ELLA [121] with respect to $\mathbf{s}^{(t)}$ using quadratic programming (QP), instead of solving the Lasso problem [121], but does not use the label constraint of ELLA_LC. Starting from the upper part of Table 3.3, which refers to features extracted from ImageNet DCNN networks, we can see that the ELLA_QP and ELLA_LC perform better than the STL alternatives both when LR and when LSVM is used as the base learner. In addition, solving Eq. (3.2) with QP (ELLA_QP) outperforms the original ELLA [121]. Adding also the label constraint (ELLA_LC) further improves the ELLA_QP method for all of the feature types. The ELLA_LC with LSVM is the best-performing method, reaching a MXinfAP of 26.10%. Similar conclusions can be reached if we look in the lower part of Table 3.3, where features extracted from the FT networks are used. Furthermore, we observe that fine-tuning is a procedure that significantly improves the retrieval accuracy of all the compared methods, with ELLA_LC reaching once again the highest performance (MXinfAP equal to 32.10%). To investigate the statistical significance of the difference of each method from the best-performing method we used a paired t-test as suggested by [43]; in Table 3.3, the absence of * suggests statistical significance. We found that differences between the ELLA_LC and all the other methods are significant (at 5% sig-

Table 3.3 MXinfAP for 38 concepts using different features or combinations of them: (a) using networks that have been trained on ImageNet data, (b) using ImageNet networks that have been fine-tuned on the TRECVID SIN 2013 training set. After the "-" symbol we indicate the number of concepts for which the network has been fine-tuned. For 4×DCNN and 5×DCNN FT the direct output of the four ImageNet and five FT networks, respectively, was fused, in terms of arithmetic mean, and served as input to the learning algorithms. The * symbol indicates that the difference in MXinfAP between the denoted method and the best-performing method in the same row of the table is not statistically significant

R#	Features	Direct output	Single-task learning			Joint concept learning				Proposed multi-task learning			
			LR	LSVM	KSVM	LP [268]	AMTL [376]	CMTL [438]	ELLA [121]	ELLA_QP LR	ELLA_QP LSVM	ELLA_LC LR	ELLA_LC LSVM
	(a) Using the output of ImageNet-based networks as features												
1	CaffeNet1k	-	13.00	14.20	12.81	11.77	12.90	11.56	13.14	13.99	16.27*	14.28	**16.36**
2	ConvNet1k	-	17.58	19.29	15.62	1608	17.58	16.09	17.88	18.45	21.02*	18.94	**21.10**
3	GNET1k	-	16.10	17.73	14.17	15.00	16.34	14.43	15.79	17.07	19.86*	17.48	**19.98**
4	GNET5k	-	20.89	22.68	20.73	20.54	21.01	19.99	15.65	21.88	24.05*	22.16	**24.14**
5	**4×DCNN**	-	21.77	24.29	22.64	19.58	22.96	21.42	21.17	23.66	25.97*	24.18	**26.10**
	(b) Using the output of networks fine-tuned on different subsets of the TRECVID SIN 2013 training set as features												
6	CaffeNet1k-345	20.29	22.21	24.16	23.00	21.29	24.22	24.03	16.63	23.09	25.47*	23.51	**25.88**
7	GNET1k-60	19.77	24.51	24.30	23.07	25.06*	22.56	22.25	23.71	24.56	**26.05**	24.51	25.90*
8	GNET1k-60	19.90	24.71	24.78	22.90	25.20*	23.87	22.87	24.57	24.69	**26.24**	24.52	**26.24**
9	GNET1k-323	23.97	26.67	28.65	27.79	27.22	28.67	28.09	25.75	27.56	29.86	28.19	**30.23**
10	GNET5k-323	22.78	27.13	29.32	28.53	28.21	29.47	29.27	27.15	28.61	30.80*	28.90	**31.01**
11	**5×DCNN FT**	25.35	28.56	30.60	29.93	30.27	30.94	30.15	28.19	29.89	31.82*	30.32	**32.10**

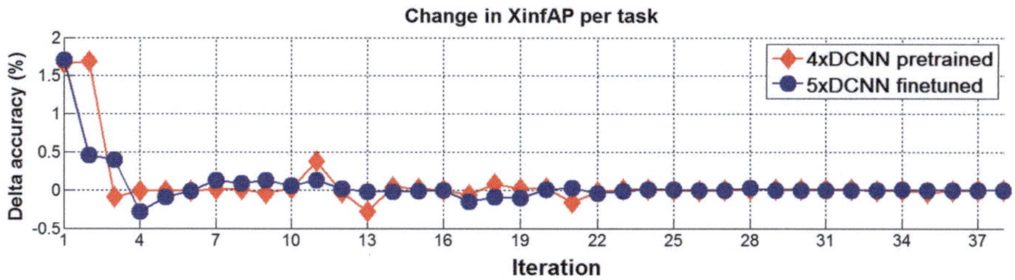

Fig. 3.4 Change in XinfAP for each task between the iteration that the task was first learned and the last iteration, (where all tasks had been learned), divided by the position of the task in the task sequence

nificance level) except for two runs based on LP (Table 3.3: R7-8) and all but one of the ELLA_QP LSVM runs (Table 3.3: R9). We note that although the differences between ELLA_QP and ELLA_LC are in most cases not significant, ELLA_LC exhibits better results consistently across the different runs (R1-11, except R7,8).

ELLA_LC updates the value of $\mathbf{s}^{(t)}$ only when it receives new training data for task t. This online characteristic of ELLA makes it faster than the batch MTL methods. At the same time, the update of $\mathbf{L}$ benefits the previously learned tasks by introducing new knowledge acquired from the last learned task. To assess whether the latter occurred, in Fig. 3.4, for each task we computed the change in XinfAP from when the task was first learned and the task's XinfAP in the last iteration (where all tasks had been learned. We normalize this quantity by the task's position in the task sequence. We can see that reverse transfer occurred, i.e., a positive change in accuracy for a task indicates this, mainly for the tasks that were learned early. As the pool of tasks increases, early tasks get new knowledge from many more tasks, which explains why the benefit is bigger for them.

3.3 Photo and Video Aesthetic Quality Assessment

Photo and video aesthetic quality assessment are two emerging and challenging fields of research. In the relevant literature, there are a few methods that examine the re-ranking, search, and retrieval of photos based on their aesthetic quality, including [193, 228, 307]. Aesthetic assessment methods are in great need for enhancing multimedia content management in various applications, such as personal photo collection management [362], food photo aesthetics assessment [231], and online fashion shopping photo assessment [409]. In the video domain, the automatic assessment of each video's aesthetic value could further improve the users' experience in multimedia content distribution channels, since videos could be retrieved or recommended by also taking their aesthetic quality into account.

In this chapter, we present our recent developments on a comprehensive and effective photo aesthetic assessment method based on the basic photographic rules [276], and an extension of this method to the video domain [395]. The latter, besides exploiting the information derived from both low- and high-level analysis of video layout, leading to a photo- and motion-based video representation scheme, also uses a kernel SVM extension, the KSVM-iGSU [397]. This classifier takes the inherent uncertainty of the input representation into consideration, in order to classify the videos and retrieve those of high-aesthetic value.

3.3.1 Related Work

The aesthetic quality assessment of photographs is a challenging field of research where a variety of methods have been proposed over the past few years. Many of the proposed methods detect the high aesthetic value photos by exploiting the information derived from low-level visual features, such as brightness, texture, and color distribution [110, 259, 382]. These methods are mainly based on the low-level feature extraction. High-level features refer to photo layout analysis. In [115], the photo aesthetic value is predicted based on the composition attributes, such as salient objects and the rule of thirds; content attributes, which express the concepts and objects depicted in the photo; and sky illumination attributes, which distinguish between photos taken in clear, cloudy, or sunset sky. The spatial distribution of edges, the color, and hue distribution, as well as the blurriness, brightness, and contrast are used in [200] in order to identify high-quality professional photos. In addition, in [246] the authors focus on the design of color and spatial features which are not computationally expensive. In [264], it is shown that generic image descriptors can sometimes outperform the aesthetic assessment methods that are based on the features specifically designed for this task. Web-based applications exploiting some of the above techniques have also appeared in [111, 247, 424]. Finally, in the relevant literature, there are also several works, which assess the aesthetic quality of a photo based on the features extracted from specific regions of the photo or for specific content. For example, in [379] the authors present a set of regional features that measure the clarity and the complexity of the subject areas and a set of global features that capture the color and spatial composition of photos using the hue wheel and the Hough transform.

Each of the above techniques uses low-level visual features and often some high-level features that allow the method to take into account up to three of the basic rules of photography. In this chapter, we present our recent developments [276] on the use of five representative feature vectors that correspond to five basic rules of photography, along with the pattern feature, which can effectively capture patterns and symmetry in natural photos. We assess the photo aesthetic quality using these five comprehensive feature vectors which can be used individually to capture the simplicity, the colorfulness, the sharpness, the existence of a pattern, and the layout composition of the photo. We also concatenate them into one vector, serving as the overall aesthetic quality assessment feature in our method, and we use it in combination with an SVM classifier to estimate whether a given photo exhibits high aesthetic quality or not.

Concerning the extension of the problem to the video domain, only a few methods for video aesthetic quality assessment have been proposed so far. The first methods in this domain tried to estimate the video aesthetic value by extracting mostly low-level features from video frames. For instance, in [302], a set of low-level features, such as sharpness, colorfulness, luminance,s and "blockiness" quality, and certain motion features, are extracted. Then, an SVM using the radial basis function (RBF) kernel is trained for assessing the aesthetic quality of videos. In [259], the authors treat the video as a sequence of still photos to which they apply a set of visual-based features together with two additional motion-based features, i.e., the length of subject region motion and motion stability, so as to distinguish professional videos from amateurish ones. They also applied a set of learning approaches, such as kernel SVM, Bayesian classification, and Gentle AdaBoost.

A more elaborate method that introduces a set of features ranging from low- and mid-level attributes to high-level style descriptors, combined with a kernel SVM learning stage, is presented in [411]. In [423], an RBF SVM is applied to a set of "semantically independent" features, such as camera motion and stabilization, and frame composition, along with a set of "semantically dependent" features, such as motion direction entropy, color saturation, and lightness. The semantic dependency of a feature refers to whether this feature relates or not to the semantic content of each frame. Moreover, in [42], low- and high-level visual and motion features are extracted at cell-, frame-, and shot-level and a low rank late fusion (LRLF) scheme is used for fusing the scores produced by a set of SVMs, each of which was trained with one specific aesthetic feature. More motion features are introduced in [426], where the authors evaluate the effectiveness of motion space, motion direction entropy and handshaking (i.e., camera stabilization) on VAQ assessment tasks. They also use naive Bayesian, SVM, and AdaBoost classification techniques. Finally, in [311], a variety of aesthetic-related features for video are designed, such as visual continuity and shot length, and their performance in retrieving professional videos in conjunction with a kernel SVM classifier is examined.

The video aesthetic assessment techniques in the literature are typically evaluated on different datasets, including the NHK "Where is beauty?" dataset [154], the Telefonica dataset [426], the dataset of [311], etc. The NHK dataset consists of 1000 professionally produced video segments that last about 1 min each. The Telefonica dataset consists of 160 short consumer videos (each being 11 to 60 s long), for which the mean opinion scores (MOS) in terms of aesthetic quality are provided. The dataset of [311] includes 1000 professionally generated videos, and 1000 amateur videos. Most of these datasets are not publicly available. In this chapter, we experiment with a new dataset for the problem of video aesthetic quality assessment, which was first presented in [395] and is publicly available.[1]

[1] http://mklab.iti.gr/project/certh-iti-vaq700-dataset.

3.3.2 Method

3.3.2.1 Photo Aesthetic Quality Assessment

In photography there is a number of generally accepted rules or guidelines, which, although cannot guarantee a perfect photo, if applied during the capturing process, can usually enhance the aesthetic appeal of the photo. In our approach [276] we try to describe each photo according to such a set of photographic rules. Therefore, we select five representative photographic rules under which we extract the appropriate image features in order to classify the photos as aesthetically pleasing or not. Below, we briefly present the rules in accordance with which we design our features.

1. Simplicity: In photography, the notion of simplicity ideally means the capturing of a single subject on a neutral background, avoiding distractions. By adopting this technique, the photographer highlights the subject, leading the eye directly on the desired point. The simplicity of photo composition plays a crucial role in aesthetic assessment and it depends on two basic rules, the color difference between the main subject and the background, and the spatial arrangement of the main subject. We start by making the assumption that the main subject is the least-uniform portion of the photo, and based on this, we identify our main subject by edge detection (using the photo gradient magnitude and orientation), followed by the application of simple morphological operations on a binarized edge mask, so as to result in a limited number of connected regions. Subsequently, in order to capture color differences, we (a) compute the HSV histogram of the main subject and background separately, and we estimate the mean value, the standard deviation, the kurtosis, the skewness and the Kullback–Leibler divergence of both distributions for each color component, and (b) considering two color regions of the photo, the main subject and the background, we estimate a 5-bin histogram of the color-difference formula, CIE 1976, which is presented in [289]. In parallel, in order to capture the spatial arrangement of the main subject, we compute for it the percentage of its pixels that appear in each of the nine patches of the rule of thirds grid.
2. Colorfulness: Capturing photographs with vibrant colors and intense contrast are among the most powerful ways to arouse viewers' attention. There are several photographic techniques involving the usage of color such as the complementary colors rule, the neighboring colors rule or the photo-shooting of a colorful object on an otherwise monochromatic background, as described in [39, 293]. To evaluate the colorfulness of photos we design a comprehensive color feature vector. At first, we perform k-means clustering in order to detect three basic color regions on photo. Subsequently, we exploit the RGB and HSV color spaces, as well as an emotion-based color space consisting of activity, weight and heat dimensions, which is presented in [371]. For each component of the three aforementioned color spaces we estimate a 5-bin histogram; these histograms are then concatenated into one color vector, capturing the color distribution on the three corresponding regions. Then, we aim to find which color characterizes each of

these three regions, and for this, we use the aforementioned color vector which is mapped onto a color description matrix of ten dominant colors. In order to define the importance of each area we also store the percentage of pixels that each color region occupies. For each of the nine patches of the rule of thirds grid we additionally estimate a 5-bin histogram for each color component of the HSV color space and the Correlated Color Temperature (CCT), which is proposed in [282]. Finally, we also extract a feature to measure contrast and darkness.

3. Sharpness: This is arguably one of the most important factors that affect the quality of photos. A clear, sharp subject automatically attracts the attention of the eye to the right point, while a blurred subject usually has an adverse aesthetic effect on photos. To this end, we perform the no-reference photo blur detection scheme described in [275] so as to extract features that can describe the blurriness of the photo, resulting in a 500-element sharpness feature vector. In addition, in order to detect more complicated forms of blur, such as motion blur, which is difficult to be captured on the power spectrum of Fourier transform, we use the Haar wavelet transform.
4. Pattern: The world is full of patterns, symmetry and textures. Photographers seem to appreciate this kind of beauty that surrounds us, as patterns and symmetry exude a sense of harmony and rhythm which makes the photographs appealing. In order to extract the appropriate information to describe the aforementioned characteristic of photos, we divide the photo in multiple half-photo parts. For every pair of half-photo patches we detect SURF interest points and subsequently, we perform keypoint matching, capturing the similarities of these patches. In addition, our aim is to examine the presence of intense edges and if these edges are distributed in the same manner in both half-photo patches, for each of the four pairs. In order to achieve this, we estimate the mean value, the standard deviation and the Kullbak–Leibler divergence after applying the Haar wavelet transform on both half-photo patches of each pair.
5. Composition is also an important aesthetic factor, since the appropriate arrangement of the objects on the photographic canvas can add balance and harmony, while a poor composition can distract the viewer's eye out of the intended point of interest. In the presented approach we examine three composition rules: the "fill the frame" (Fig. 3.5a), the rule of thirds (Fig. 3.5b) and the "landscape" composition (Fig. 3.5c), as presented in [171, 220]. To achieve this, we use the objectness measure, presented in [9], in order to detect eight objects on each photo. Then, our aim is to estimate the relative position of each object with respect to the center of each of the shaded photo patches, that is marked with a cross in Fig. 3.5. For assessing the "fill the frame" composition, we compute the euclidean distance and the angle of the object's center with respect to the center of the shaded patch depicted in Fig. 3.5a, as well as the spatial overlap between the shaded patch and the detected object's area (as an example, the latter area is marked with a dashed line in Fig. 3.5a). For the rule of thirds and the "landscape" composition we similarly estimate the euclidean distance, the angle and the spatial overlap of the object with respect to the shaded patches presented in Fig. 3.5b, c. For the

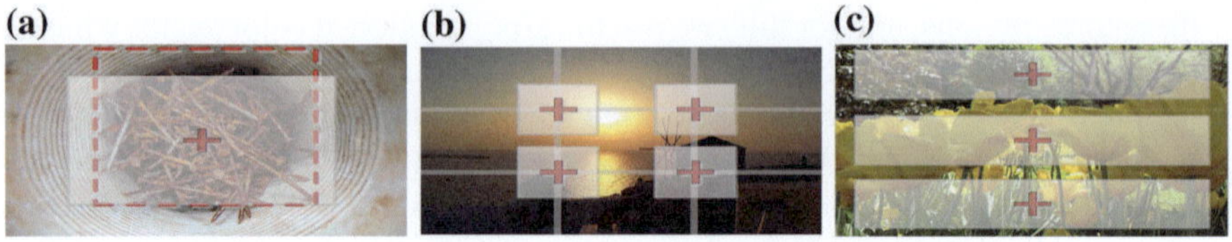

Fig. 3.5 Composition rules: **a** "fill the frame", **b** rule of thirds, **c** "landscape"

"landscape" composition, we additionally estimate the color distribution on the three patches of the "landscape" grid (Fig. 3.5c), based on the HSV color format.

Having computed the aforementioned feature vectors, we concatenate them in one final, comprehensive, 1323-dimensional vector. The overall procedure of the presented aesthetic quality assessment method is presented in Fig. 3.6. The code for our method is publicly available.[2]

3.3.2.2 Video Aesthetic Quality Assessment

For the problem of video aesthetic quality assessment, since video is typically treated as a sequence of still photos that gives the impression of motion, both the visual and motion modalities need to be exploited in order to effectively evaluate its aesthetic quality. That is, each video is described according to a set of rules borrowed from photography (as in the case of photo aesthetic quality assessment discussed above) and cinematography. Initially, each video is divided into its shots using the shot detection method of [16]. Then, for each video, we estimate the mean duration of its shots, and, considering that the shot transitions can be either abrupt or gradual, we estimate for each of these transition types their duration as a percentage of the whole video's duration. This procedure results in a 3-element video-level vector.

Subsequently, one keyframe per second is extracted from the original raw video sequence (irrespective of shot boundaries), and photo- and motion-based features are extracted for each one of them. Photo-based features include the simplicity, colorfulness, sharpness, pattern, and overall aesthetic quality values, which are extracted based on the still-photo aesthetic quality assessment method proposed in [276] and is discussed in detail above. Motion-based features, adopted from [426], include: (a) a measure of similarity between successive frames (cross-correlation between these frames), (b) a measure of the diversity of motion directions (motion direction entropy), (c) a measure of the stability of the camera during the capturing process (handshaking), and (d) a measure which can distinguish the difference between three categories of shots: focused shots, panorama shots, and static shots (shooting type). The above result in a 44-element keyframe-level feature vector. Concatenating with it the video-level feature vector, we end up with a 47-element vector as the final representation for each keyframe.

---

[2]The CERTH photo aesthetic method, http://mklab.iti.gr/project/IAQ.

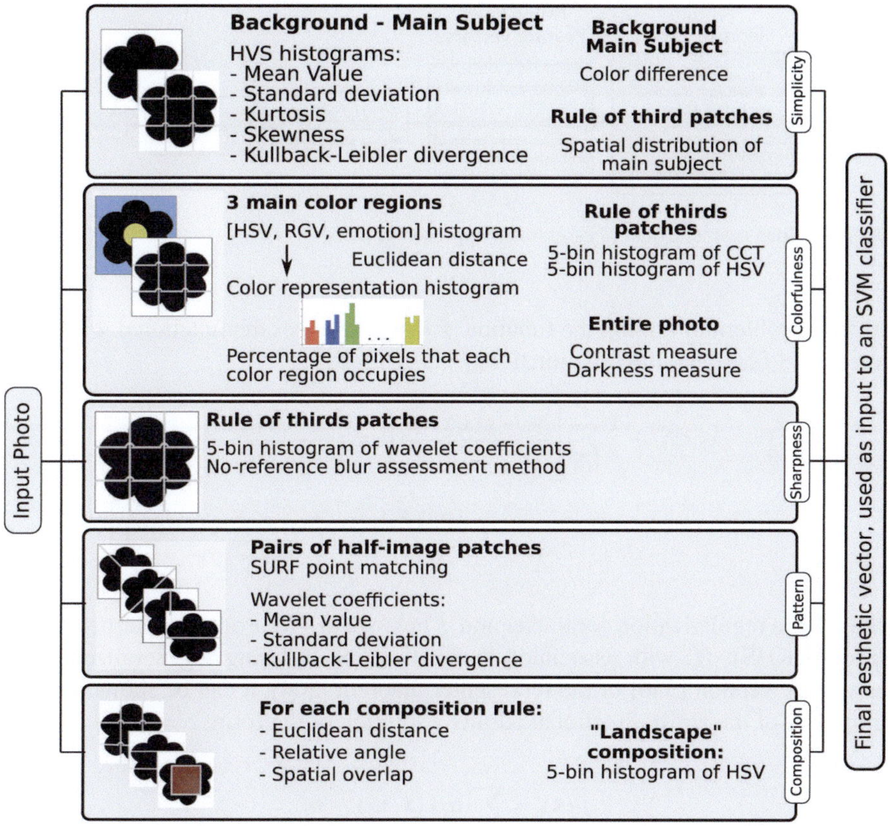

Fig. 3.6 Overview of the presented method

A challenge in the video aesthetic quality assessment problem, similarly to many video classification tasks, is that video representation techniques usually introduce uncertainty in the input that is subsequently fed to the classifiers. Thus, uncertainty needs to be taken into consideration during classifier training. The kernel SVM with Isotropic Gaussian Sample Uncertainty (KSVM-iGSU), proposed in [397], is an extension of the standard kernel SVM that exploits the uncertainty of input data in order to achieve better classification results. The overall method of the presented video aesthetic quality assessment method, originally proposed in [395], is shown in Fig. 3.7.

The uncertainty of the ith input example is modeled as an isotropic Gaussian distribution with given mean vector $\mathbf{x}_i \in \mathbb{R}^n$ and an isotropic covariance matrix, i.e., a scalar multiple of the identity matrix, $\sigma_i^2 I_n \in \mathbb{S}_{++}^n$, where n denotes the dimensionality of the input feature space, $\mathbb{S}_{++}^n$ denotes the convex cone of all symmetric positive definite $n \times n$ matrices with entries in $\mathbb{R}$, and I_n denotes the identity matrix of order n. The optimization problem of KSVM-iGSU can be cast as a variational

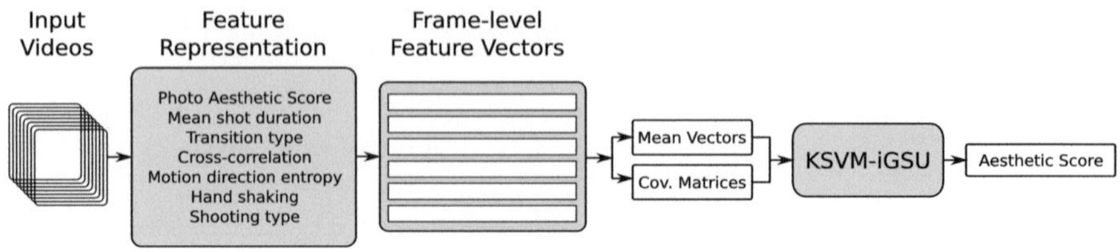

Fig. 3.7 Video aesthetic quality assessment approach of [395]

calculus problem of finding the function f that minimizes the functional $\Phi[f]$, i.e., $\min_{f\in H}\Phi[f]$, where the functional $\Phi[f]$ is given by

$$\Phi[f]=\frac{1}{2}\lambda\|f\|_H^2+\frac{1}{\ell}\sum_{i=1}^{\ell}\left[\frac{y_i-f(\mathbf{x}_i)-b}{2}\left(\operatorname{erf}\left(\frac{y_i-f(\mathbf{x}_i)-b}{\sqrt{2\sigma_i^2\|f\|_H^2}}\right)+y_i\right)\right.$$
$$\left.+\frac{\sqrt{\sigma_i^2\|f\|_H^2}}{\sqrt{2\pi}}\exp\left(\frac{(y_i-f(\mathbf{x}_i)-b)^2}{2\sigma_i^2\|f\|_H^2}\right)\right], \tag{3.7}$$

where λ is a regularization parameter and f belongs to a Reproducing Kernel Hilbert Space (RKHS), H, with associated kernel function k. Using a generalized semi-parametric version [356] of the representer theorem [204], it can be shown that the minimizer of the above functional admits a solution of the form

$$f(\mathbf{x})=\sum_{i=1}^{\ell}\alpha_i k(\mathbf{x},\mathbf{x}_i)-b, \tag{3.8}$$

where $b\in\mathbb{R}$, $\alpha_i\in\mathbb{R}$, $i=1,\ldots,\ell$.

We define the kernel matrix $\mathbf{K}$ as the symmetric positive definite $\ell\times\ell$ matrix given as $\mathbf{K}=\left(k(\mathbf{x}_i,\mathbf{x}_j)\right)_{i,j=1}^{\ell}$. If we set $\boldsymbol{\alpha}=(\alpha_1,\ldots,\alpha_\ell)^\top$ and let $\mathbf{k}_i$ denote the ith column of the kernel matrix $\mathbf{K}$, the objective function of KSVM-iGSU, $J_H\colon\mathbb{R}^\ell\times\mathbb{R}\to\mathbb{R}$, can be rewritten as follows

$$J_H(\boldsymbol{\alpha},b)=\frac{1}{2}\lambda\boldsymbol{\alpha}^\top\mathbf{K}\boldsymbol{\alpha}+\frac{1}{\ell}\sum_{i=1}^{\ell}\left[\frac{y_i-\mathbf{k}_i^\top\boldsymbol{\alpha}-b}{2}\left(\operatorname{erf}\left(\frac{y_i-\mathbf{k}_i^\top\boldsymbol{\alpha}-b}{\sqrt{2\sigma_i^2\boldsymbol{\alpha}^\top\mathbf{K}\boldsymbol{\alpha}}}\right)+y_i\right)\right.$$
$$\left.+\frac{\sqrt{\sigma_i^2\boldsymbol{\alpha}^\top\mathbf{K}\boldsymbol{\alpha}}}{\sqrt{2\pi}}\exp\left(-\frac{(y_i-\mathbf{k}_i^\top\boldsymbol{\alpha}-b)^2}{2\sigma_i^2\boldsymbol{\alpha}^\top\mathbf{K}\boldsymbol{\alpha}}\right)\right], \tag{3.9}$$

where the sum above expresses the total loss. We (jointly) minimize the above convex objective function with respect to $\boldsymbol{\alpha}$, b using the Limited-memory BFGS (L-BFGS) algorithm [243]. L-BFGS is a quasi-Newton optimization algorithm that approximates the Broyden–Fletcher–Goldfarb–Shanno (BFGS) [56] algorithm using a limited amount of computer memory. Since J_H is a convex function on $\mathbb{R}^\ell\times\mathbb{R}$

(see [396, 397]), L-BFGS leads to a global optimal solution; that is, at a pair $(\boldsymbol{\alpha}, b)$ such that the decision function given in the form of (3.8) minimizes the functional (3.7).

3.3.3 Experimental Results

3.3.3.1 Photo Aesthetic Quality Assessment Experimental Results

Most of the photo aesthetic assessment techniques evaluate the performance of their features on publicly available datasets which consist of photos acquired from online photography communities. There are hundreds of amateur and professional photos uploaded and rated by the community members. These photos are appropriate for aesthetic assessment tasks due to their content and the diversity of the ratings submitted by both amateurs and professionals. The former tent to judge the photos based on the emotion while the latter pay more attention to technical details.

To evaluate the presented approach we use three different datasets, CUHKPQ [379], CUHK [379] and AVA [306]. The CUHKPQ dataset is divided into seven thematic categories, and each photo has been classified by members of the photography community as a high-aesthetic or low-aesthetic quality photo. Similarly to the methodology of [246], we randomly partitioned ten times the photos of each category, assigning half of them as training, and the rest as testing set. Afterwards, we train a single SVM classifier for each individual category and the average results are reported. In addition, the contributors of [379] collected 12,000 photos from all categories (this subset is denoted as the CUHK dataset), on which we also perform experiments following the same experimental design. On the other side, the AVA dataset contains photos derived from a photo contest community[3] which are associated with their mean aesthetic scores. This dataset has already been divided in training and testing set by the authors of [306], so for both of these sets, following the experimental design of [200], we choose the 10% and 20% top ranked photos as high-aesthetic ones and the 10% and 20% bottom ranked as low-aesthetic photos, respectively. In this way, the photos with score in the middle of the score range are excluded as in [200], since they could introduce noise in the classification process. In all datasets, the performance of our aesthetic assessment approach is evaluated calculating the classification accuracy and the Area Under the ROC Curve (AUC) measures [158].

At first, we test the performance of the presented method on each of the seven categories of the CUHKPQ dataset [379] and we compare our features with previously presented methods. Moreover, in order to demonstrate that our results do not depend a lot on the photo subject, we further evaluate our method over all categories. For comparison we use the aesthetic assessment method proposed by Lo et al. in [246], for which the corresponding code has been released, the region-based

[3]www.dpchallenge.com.

and global aesthetic features proposed by Tang et al. in [379], the subject-oriented method proposed by Luo et al. in [259] and the high-level attributes proposed by Ke et al. in [200]. The corresponding results of the last three methods are taken from [379]. The performance evaluation using the AUC measure is shown in Table 3.4. As can be seen, our method achieves the best results, both for each of the different subject categories and overall, followed by the algorithm of Tang et al. and in some categories by the method of Lo et al. Furthermore, our individual features present promising performance in comparison to similar features of the other methods.

We continue with experiments on the CUHK dataset [379], consisting of 6000 high-aesthetic and 6000 low-aesthetic photos. In this case, we compare with the related methods [110, 200, 246, 264, 315], whose corresponding results were presented in [264]. The feature dimensionality and the accuracy of these methods are presented in Table 3.5, where we can see that our method outperforms most of the others. The generic photo features with Fisher Vector encoding and spatial pyramidal decomposition of [264] provide the highest accuracy, but these features exhibit extremely high dimensionality and, consequently, also excessive computational complexity, when it comes to using them for training an SVM classifier. Also, all results of [264] are obtained using a more elaborate SVM with a hinge loss using the primal formulation and a stochastic gradient descent algorithm [50], instead of the simpler linear SVM that is used in all other methods and our own method. At this point, we also implemented the most efficient generic descriptor of [264], the FV-Color-SP, and tested it with a linear SVM, to demonstrate that the combination of our photographic-rule-based features with generic descriptors can boost the overall performance. For the FV-Color-SP feature vector, we employ dimensionality reduction to 4000 elements, for computational efficiency purposes. It is clear from the experimental results shown in Table 3.5 that our features can indeed improve the results obtained using generic low-level features, when combined with the latter.

Finally, the performance of our method in comparison with the algorithm provided by Lo et al. on the "overall" category of the AVA [306] dataset is presented in Table 3.6. The corresponding results demonstrate that our method achieves good performance on another challenging dataset and that its results are consistently better than the results of [246]. In addition, in this dataset, which includes mostly professional photos, we can see that the pattern feature is one of the most effective individual features.

3.3.3.2 Video Aesthetic Quality Assessment Experimental Results

For the problem of video aesthetic quality assessment, we experiment with the publicly available[4] dataset presented in [395], i.e., the CERTH-ITI-VAQ700 dataset. This dataset includes 350 videos that are rated as being of high-aesthetic quality and another 350 as being of low aesthetic quality. Indicative frames of such videos are

[4]http://mklab.iti.gr/project/certh-iti-vaq700-dataset.

Table 3.4 Experimental results (AUC %) on the CUHKPQ dataset

	Features	Animal	Architecture	Human	Landscape	Night	Plant	Static	Overall
Lo et al. [246]	**Concatenated**	91.60	84.14	92.09	90.65	86.33	93.30	89.72	89.74
Tang et al. [379]	Dark channel	83.93	88.69	79.87	85.75	70.62	78.58	83.35	81.89
	Complexity combined	82.12	72.19	78.15	75.16	72.84	89.72	74.91	78.17
	Hue composition	78.61	83.76	79.09	89.36	72.14	83.16	83.67	81.65
	Scene composition	70.03	67.81	79.23	69.79	74.77	59.66	70.57	70.56
	Concatenated	87.12	90.04	96.31	92.73	83.09	91.47	88.90	90.44
Luo et al. [259]	Clarity contrast	80.74	53.48	66.67	53.79	62.97	74.39	73.09	67.38
	Lighting	75.51	64.60	76.12	62.26	53.11	77.52	74.30	70.32
	Geometry composition	74.25	58.06	68.28	43.93	60.75	73.08	59.20	63.93
	Simplicity	64.78	55.82	77.52	74.54	69.18	74.50	78.49	68.65
	Color combination	80.52	71.94	65.13	72.80	58.73	78.46	75.13	72.44
	Concatenated	87.12	90.04	96.31	92.73	83.09	91.47	88.90	77.92
Ke et al. [200]	Blur	75.66	79.81	73.81	77.85	66.65	79.63	76.62	75.92
	Brightness	69.93	81.38	78.01	78.48	72.44	73.37	69.76	74.64
	Hue count	62.60	70.82	70.27	59.64	55.37	69.20	55.11	63.53
	Concatenated	77.51	85.26	79.08	81.70	73.21	80.93	78.29	79.44
Proposed method	Simplicity	85.47	81.55	89.24	87.87	78.39	89.61	83.23	82.06
	Colorfulness	82.15	86.61	91.12	91.82	79.47	90.84	86.05	84.07
	Sharpness	94.51	87.21	96.15	86.74	90.42	92.48	90.66	90.85
	Pattern	89.66	83.12	86.14	85.62	89.54	89.50	81.84	84.34
	Composition	88.31	88.59	88.45	92.10	89.32	90.63	87.78	86.10
	Concatenated	**95.42**	**92.08**	**97.31**	**94.10**	**94.26**	**96.03**	**94.07**	**94.60**

Table 3.5 Classification accuracy (%) on the CUHK dataset

	Feature dimensionality	Accuracy
Datta et al. [110]	56	75.85
Ke et al. [200]	7	76.53
Lo et al. [246]	24	77.25
GIST [315]	512	67.96
BOV-SIFT-SP [264]	8192	81.36
BOV-Color-SP [264]	8192	82.13
FV-Color-SP [264]	2,62,144	**89.90**
Our features	1323	82.41
FV-Color-SP	4000	78.16
FV-Color-SP+Our	5323	85.02

Table 3.6 Overall classification accuracy on the AVA dataset

	Features	Accuracy (%) at 10%	Accuracy (%) at 20%
Lo et al. [246]	**Concatenated**	66.60	62.14
Proposed method	Simplicity	63.61	60.05
	Colorfulness	65.03	63.48
	Sharpness	75.94	72.42
	Pattern	76.92	71.80
	Composition	72.64	69.83
	Concatenated	**77.08**	**74.35**

shown in Fig. 3.8. We first randomly split the dataset into a training subset (50%) and an evaluation subset (50%), each maintaining a positive–negative ratio of 1:1. That is, each of the training and evaluation subsets includes 175 positive (high aesthetic) and 175 negative (low aesthetic) video examples. As discussed above, for video representation, 1 keyframe per second was extracted at regular time intervals from each video, and each keyframe was represented using our photo- and motion-based features.

The aforementioned keyframe-level video representations can be seen as observations of the input Gaussian distributions that describe the training videos. That is, let $\mathscr{X}$ be a set of ℓ annotated random vectors representing the video-level feature vectors. We assume that each random vector is distributed normally; i.e., for the random vector representing the ith video, $\mathbf{X}_i$, we have $\mathbf{X}_i \sim \mathscr{N}(\mathbf{x}_i, \Sigma_i)$. Also, for each random vector $\mathbf{X}_i$, a number, N_i, of observations, $\{\mathbf{x}_i^{(t)} \in \mathbb{R}^n : t = 1, \ldots, N_i\}$ are available; these are the keyframe-level feature vectors that have been computed. Then, the mean vector and the covariance matrix of $\mathbf{X}_i$ are computed respectively as follows

$$\mathbf{x}_i = \frac{\sum_{t=1}^{N_i} \mathbf{x}_i^{(t)}}{N_i}, \quad \mathbf{\Sigma}_i = \frac{\sum_{t=1}^{N_i} (\mathbf{x}_i^{(t)} - \mathbf{x}_i)(\mathbf{x}_i^{(t)} - \mathbf{x}_i)^\top}{N_i - 1} \tag{3.10}$$

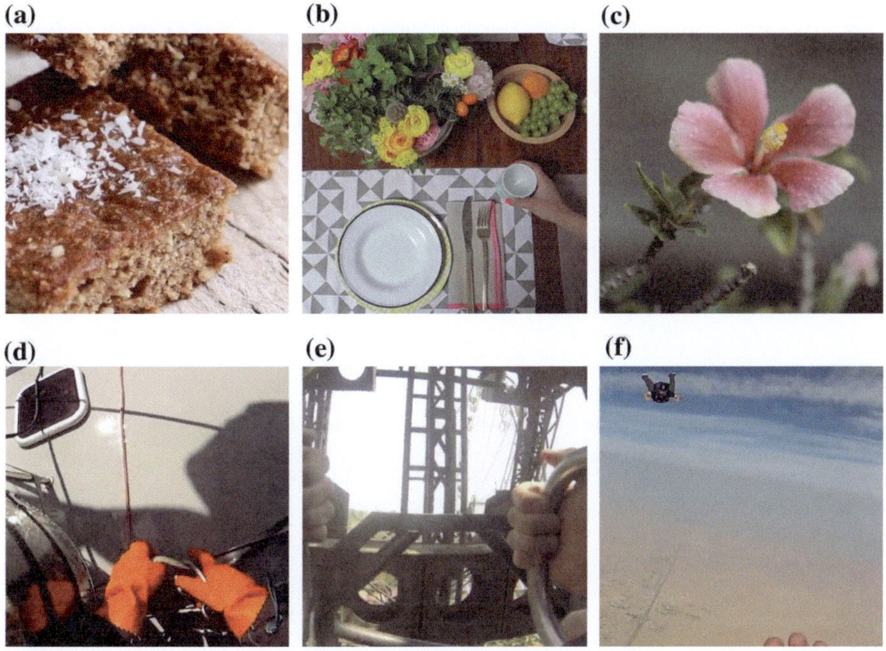

Fig. 3.8 Indicative examples of videos of high (**a**, **b**, **c**) and low (**d**, **e**, **f**) aesthetic value, available in the CERTH-ITI-VAQ700 dataset

Now, due to the assumption for isotropic covariance matrices, we approximate the above covariance matrices as multiples of the identity matrix, i.e., $\widehat{\mathbf{\Sigma}_i} = \sigma_i^2 I_n$. As discussed in [395], it suffices to set σ_i^2 equal to the mean value of the elements of the main diagonal of $\mathbf{\Sigma}_i$.

Since the problem of video aesthetic quality assessment can be naturally seen as a retrieval application, where a user queries for videos of high-aesthetic quality within a dataset, for assessing the performance of our method we use retrieval-oriented evaluation measures: the average precision (AP) [340], as well as the precision at depth n (where $n \in \{5, 10, 15, 20\}$) and the accuracy, which are measures that are typically used in the VAQ assessment literature [259, 276, 311, 423, 426].

The presented KSVM-iGSU-based method [395] is tested and compared to the standard kernel SVM (KSVM). KSVM is the state-of-the-art classifier for the problem of VAQ assessment [276, 302, 311, 423, 426]. For both KSVM-iGSU and KSVM, the radial basis function (RBF) kernel was used. Training parameters C, γ were obtained via a 3-fold cross-validation procedure (grid search) with C being searched in the range $\{2^{-4}, 2^{-3}, \ldots, 2^6, 2^7\}$ and γ in the range $\{2^{-7}, 2^{-6}, \ldots, 2^3, 2^4\}$. Each of the above experiments was repeated 10 times using different random training/evaluation subsets, similarly to [276].

Table 3.7 shows the average performance of KSVM-iGSU compared to the standard KSVM in terms of precision for the top-n retrieved videos, where $n =$

Table 3.7 Performance of our method (using KSVM-iGSU) compared to the standard KSVM in terms of precision at top-n retrieved videos ($n = 5, 10, 15, 20$), accuracy (AC), and average precision (AP) using CERTH-ITI-VAQ700 dataset

	KSVM (as in [311, 423, 426])	KSVM-iGSU (Proposed)
P@5	64.00	**82.00**
P@10	63.00	**82.00**
P@15	61.33	**83.33**
P@20	61.50	**81.50**
AC	67.87	**68.14**
AP	61.67	**69.97**

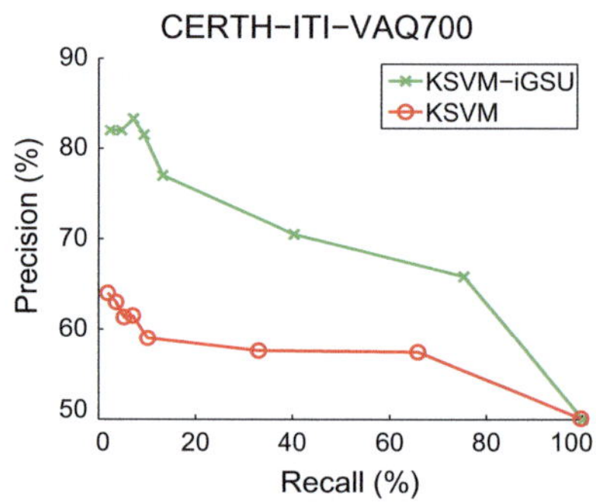

Fig. 3.9 Precision-recall curves for our VAQ assessment method (KSVM-iGSU) compared to the state-of-the-art KSVM approach using CERTH-ITI-VAQ700 dataset

5, 10, 15, 20. We see that our VAQ assessment method leads to considerably better results in terms of retrieval precision. Furthermore, the mean values of accuracy (AC) and average precision (AP) are also reported for 10 repetitions of the experiment. We see that, in terms of accuracy, our method slightly outperforms the state-of-the-art KSVM (68.14 over 67.87, respectively), but in terms of average precision, which is a more meaningful measure for retrieval tasks, our method reaches 69.97 as compared to KSVM's 61.67, leading to a 13.45% relative boost. Finally, Fig. 3.9 shows the recall-precision curves of our method (KSVM-iGSU) and standard KSVM.

3.4 Near-Duplicate Detection

Near-duplicates are defined as sets of media items which show the same event or object of interest (e.g., a monument) under slightly different conditions (e.g., illumination, camera parameters) or viewpoints (e.g., view angle, partial obstruction of object of interest). Two media items can also be defined as near-duplicates if one of them was created by postprocessing the other. A wide range of postprocessing operations were studied in the relevant literature (indicatively see [420]), such as storage of photos using a different compression format or with different encoding parameters, application of photometric variations (color and lighting changes) or other editing operations (e.g., caption, logo, and border insertion, or spatial cropping so as to remove such distinguishing marks). For a representative set of near-duplicate item examples, see Fig. 3.10.

In the literature, methods that deal with the identification of near-duplicates in media collections are categorized to near-duplicate retrieval and near-duplicate detection [244]. Near-duplicate retrieval refers to the situation, where a collection is established, the user inputs a query and the system matches the query with items in the collection, returning a ranked list, with descending order by similarity. Near-duplicate detection aims at identifying any near-duplicates within a given collection (not driven by a query).

Near-duplicate retrieval and detection present certain challenges; (a) Different capture conditions can result in photos of substantially different visual content despite depicting the exact same object of interest. Human vision is able to quickly identify a pair of near-duplicate photos, but it is not a trivial task for a single computer vision method to compensate for all possible variations and distortions that may appear in near-duplicate photos. (b) It is difficult to make reliable assumptions about which semantically similar photos should be considered as near-duplicates [406, 432]. (c) Most real-world applications demand detection in huge volumes of data; for a solution to be useful, it must be both fast and accurate.

3.4.1 Related Work

Most commonly, a photo near-duplicate retrieval or detection framework represents photos by extracting feature vectors and creates an index on these vectors to allow faster access. The near-duplicates of a photo are then retrieved by assessing the visual similarity between the query photo and the stored data with a help of a nearest neighbor search applied on the indexed descriptor vectors. The visual features that are usually extracted can be categorized in three groups: (a) global handcrafted features, (b) local handcrafted features and (c) features extracted with the use of DCNNs. Most near-duplicate detection approaches (such as [230]) employ sets of local descriptors (e.g., SIFT, SURF) or binary local descriptors (e.g., ORB and BRISK) which can produce a fine-grained but also a quite complex representation of the visual content. In order to create a coarser representation (ideally one that uses a single vector with relatively few elements) of the photo, an encoding method, such as Bag-of-Words [101], Fischer Vectors [323] or the most recent VLAD [180], must be applied to the aforementioned local descriptors. These techniques quantize the space of descriptor vectors and assign them to one or several words of a visual vocabulary that typically contains thousands of elements. Such methods are computationally demanding (feature extraction, encoding, matching of high-dimensional feature vectors), and the resulting representation vectors for each photo are quite large. This size is prohibitive for large-scale search applications due to memory and search efficiency constraints [372]. To address these issues, hashing techniques (e.g., Locality-Sensitive Hash-

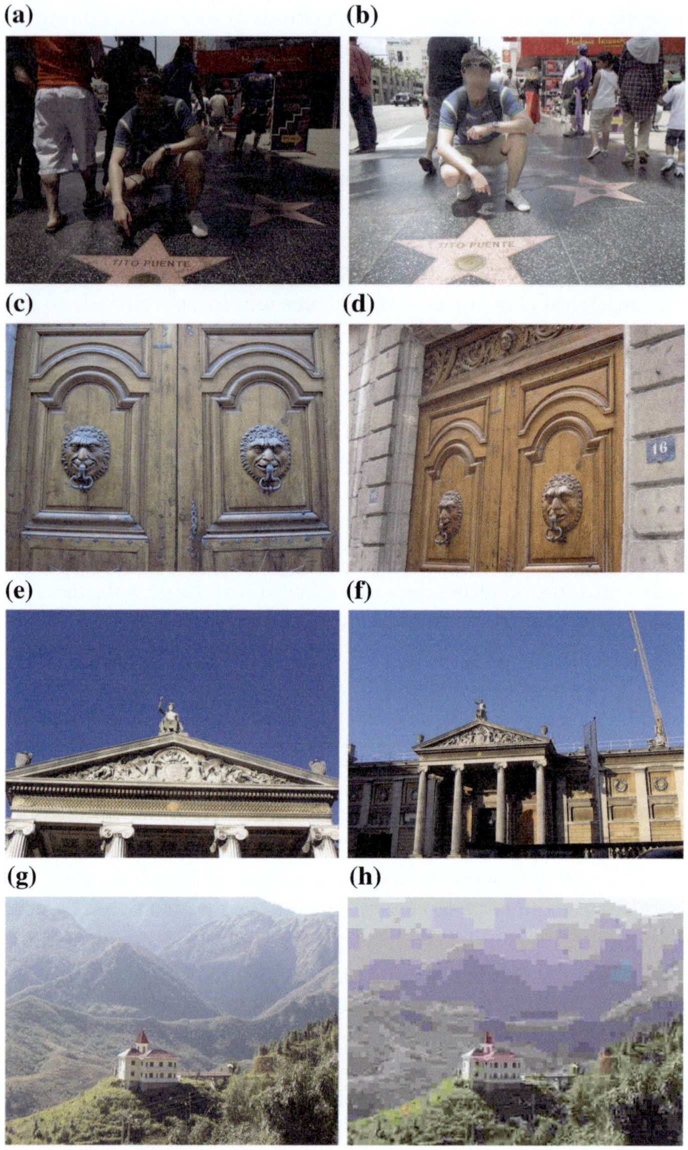

Fig. 3.10 Indicative examples of near-duplicates: **a**, **b** a pair of near-duplicate photos with photometric variation due to camera flash use (from the California-ND dataset), **c**, **d**: a pair of near-duplicate photos depicting the same object from a different viewpoint (from the Holidays dataset), **e**, **f** a partial near-duplicate pair of photos (from the Oxford Buildings dataset), and **g**, **h** a pair of near-duplicate photos resulting from the use of extreme JPEG compression settings (from the Copydays dataset)

ing [15], Spectral Hashing [414]) which improve the speed of search, are usually employed [120, 422]. Dimensionality reduction methods may also be utilized for shortening the length of the descriptor vectors in a near-duplicate retrieval or detection framework (such as the methods described in [178, 401]). Yet, these methods add an extra stage in the whole process and favor either speed or memory efficiency, but rarely both.

Especially in scenarios where time and space efficiency is a key factor, relying on high-dimensional feature vectors renders the use of such methods prohibitive. There are approaches found in the literature which are based on the global descriptors (e.g., color and texture), which directly extract a single fixed-size vector to represent the visual content of the whole photo under consideration. Such methods are computationally less expensive compared to the local descriptor-based ones, due to the faster feature extraction and the omission of constructing a visual vocabulary, but offer a coarser description of photos and therefore are not robust to certain photo-transformations (e.g., affine transformations, as discussed in [134]). Differently to the approaches discussed above, and driven by the success of DCNNs in large-scale image classification and concept detection tasks (as discussed in Sect. 3.2.2.1), DCNN-based visual representations are also used in image retrieval tasks, exhibiting state-of-the-art performance [309] on the standard benchmark datasets.

In the following, three different approaches to near-duplicate detection are presented; the first one using a fast global descriptor to assess the visual similarity of photos, which is destined for fast near-duplicate retrieval and detection in large collections of media items but only considering a specific set of photo alterations; a second one using local descriptors, which is robust to a wider variety of photo alterations and suitable for partial near-duplicate detection; and finally, a third one that uses DCNNs as feature generators (as discussed in Sect. 3.2), aiming to come up with a higher level description of the photos' content. Most related to the global descriptor-based algorithm, in terms of feature complexity, are the approaches described in [174, 226], which represent visual content with the help of global descriptors (e.g., color histograms, color moments, GIST). The local descriptor-based approach is similar to [372], while the presented DCNN-based approach is based on the method of [309]. All of the three presented approaches function in a offline/online fashion. That is, the main part of the methods (the offline processing of the media collection, which is agnostic of the queries that may be submitted) aims at indexing the collections' items and detecting the prior existence of any near-duplicates among them. The processing in offline mode is carried out only once and always precedes that of the online mode. During the online mode, any query to the preindexed collection can be answered swiftly utilizing the index constructed during the offline processing. Thus, the discussed approaches can serve both in near-duplicate retrieval and near-duplicate detection scenarios, i.e., the offline mode suffices for near-duplicate detection, while the online mode can answer near-duplicate retrieval queries.

Looking beyond still photos, a common framework of methods for near-duplicate retrieval of videos can be summarized in four stages [244]: (a) extracting features from videos, (b) constructing a compact and robust signature from the features for each video, (c) constructing an index on the signatures for fast similarity search and,

(d) comparing the signatures to retrieve near-duplicate videos. In [436], the features extracted are categorized in global features (color histograms, ordinal signatures), and local features (keypoint-based approaches). More recently, the authors of [244] used a finer categorization of features, namely video-level global signatures, frame-level global signatures, frame-level local signatures, spatiotemporal signature, and visual-temporal network signatures. Generally, global signatures are fast to compute and compact but they lack robustness to geometric and photometric transformations (similar to the case of photos). On the other hand, local signatures are computationally costly, especially frame-level local signatures, where descriptor keypoints are matched and their geometric information is also used to verify the scene similarity. Such signatures are usually extracted only on representative frames of shots, or the computations take place last in a coarse-to-fine framework.

3.4.2 Method

Aiming to cover several diverse cases where near-duplicate detection methods are applied, and as discussed in the previous section, we describe in this section three approaches: (a) a global descriptor-based approach, which is very light computationally wise. This approach is suitable for very large collections of photos, but can only detect a specific set of photo alterations; (b) a local descriptor-based approach, that can detect more complex near-duplicates (e.g., partial duplicates) at the expense of being more computationally and memory expensive; (c) a DCNN-based approach, that assesses the content in a high-level manner, being able to discover semantically similar photos that may have similar but also somewhat different visual content.

3.4.2.1 Global Descriptor-Based Approach

For the global descriptor-based near-duplicate photo retrieval and detection (denoted DCT-NDD in the sequel) we consider a set of photo alterations that include: (a) changes in illumination, (b) noise addition, (c) differences in JPEG compression, (d) scaling operations, (e) overlay of text labels, and (f) moderate cropping. Our aim is the development of a method that ensures robustness to the aforementioned photo alterations while being efficient in terms of processing space and time, thus enabling the swift analysis of large content collections. This method utilizes the well-known Discrete Cosine Transform (DCT), which has been used and exhibited good performance in a variety of different computer vision tasks, such as fingerprint matching [364] and digital watermarking [203].

The processing of the media collection during the offline mode starts with extracting the feature representation of the photos. The following process is performed on each photo of the collection. The algorithm initially resizes it to $m \times m$ pixels and represents it as a sum of cosine functions oscillating at different frequencies via a two-dimensional DCT. The outcome of this process is an $m \times m$ matrix where the top-left element corresponds to the DC (zero-frequency) coefficient and every other element moving from left to right and from top to bottom corresponds to an increase in the horizontal and vertical frequency by a half cycle, respectively. Then, we keep only the top-left $r \times r$ area ($r < m$) of the computed matrix, discarding high-frequency coefficients and thus removing information that contributes to the details of the photo. Consequently, the extracted $r \times r$ submatrix is reshaped and the DC-coefficient is removed in order to form a vector with length $r^2 - 1$. Finally, the dimensionality of the resulting vector is reduced from $r^2 - 1$ to d using Principal Component Analysis, so at the end of this process each photo of the collection is represented by a d-element feature vector.

For initially detecting the existence of near-duplicates among the items of the collection (i.e., during the offline mode and still prior to the receipt and processing of any query photo), the computed feature vectors are stored in a matrix with dimensions $n \times d$, denoted $\mathbf{X}$ in the sequel (where the jth row of this matrix contains the feature vector of the jth item). For the rest of this subsection we apply the following rule for math notations: a superscript to a matrix symbol denotes the specific row of this matrix (e.g., $\mathbf{X^j}$ denotes the jth row of matrix $\mathbf{X}$), while a subscript to a matrix symbol denotes the specific column of this matrix (e.g., $\mathbf{X_i}$ denotes the ith column of matrix $\mathbf{X}$). Consequently, X_i^j denotes the item of the $\mathbf{X}$ matrix in the jth row and the ith column. Matrices and vectors symbols are in bold font. The similarity of each pair of media items of the collection is stored in a matrix with dimensions $n \times n$, denoted $\mathbf{S}$. The element S_l^j of this matrix captures the similarity between the jth and lth media items and is computed as follows:

$$S_l^j = \frac{{\mathbf{X}^j}^\top \mathbf{X}^l}{\|\mathbf{X}^j\| \|\mathbf{X}^l\|} \tag{3.11}$$

By introducing an L_2-normalization of all feature vectors prior to the above calculations (so that $\|\mathbf{X}^j\| = 1, \forall j \in 1 \ldots n$), Eq. (3.11) becomes:

$$S_l^j = {\mathbf{X}^j}^\top \mathbf{X}^l = \sum_{i=1}^{d} X_i^j \cdot X_i^l \tag{3.12}$$

In this way, the cosine similarity is transformed to the dot product of the given vectors. Despite this computation being very fast, an exhaustive nearest neighbor search on the available data (i.e., computing $s_l^j \ \forall j, l \in 1 \ldots n$) would be highly time-demanding, therefore, we perform an accelerated search via pruning the number of pairwise similarities that need to be assessed. In particular, during the media collection's indexing process:

- We compute and store in a row-vector $\mathbf{R} \in \mathbb{R}^n$ the maximum value among all elements of each photo feature vector (i.e., $R_j = i_{max}(X_i^j)$).
- We compute and store in a row-vector $\mathbf{R}' \in \{1 \ldots n\}^n$ the order indicators for the elements of $\mathbf{R}$ if the corresponding R_j values were sorted in descending order

(i.e., $R'_j = 1$ shows that R_j is the largest value in $\mathbf{R}$, $R'_l = 2$ shows that R_l is the second-largest value in $\mathbf{R}$, etc.).

- We compute and store in a row-vector $\mathbf{N} \in \{1 \ldots d\}^n$ the number of positive elements contained in each feature vector.
- We compute and store in a row-vector $\mathbf{C} \in \mathbb{R}^d$ the maximum value of each DCT-coefficient for all feature vectors, and in a row-vector $\mathbf{C}' \in \{1 \ldots d\}^d$ the order indicators for the elements of $\mathbf{C}$ if the corresponding values were sorted in descending order.

The pruning of similarity calculations is performed based on the following rules:

- By utilizing the dot product upper-bound equation from [11],

$$S_l^j = \mathbf{X}^{j\top}\mathbf{X}^l \leq min(N_j, N_l) \cdot R_j \cdot R_l \tag{3.13}$$

we calculate the dot product of two feature vectors, only if the following Eq. (3.14) is satisfied, with t being a predefined threshold value:

$$min(N_j, N_l) \cdot R_j \cdot R_l > t \tag{3.14}$$

- For a given value of j, the order in which Eq. (3.14) is evaluated for the different X^l feature vectors is the one specified by $\mathbf{R}'$ (i.e., starting from the photos with the highest R_l values). Once we find a value of l for which Eq. (3.14) is not satisfied, we stop the procedure and omit the similarity estimation for the rest of the media items.
- During the calculation of the dot product between the DCT coefficients of $\mathbf{X}^j$ and $\mathbf{X}^l$ feature vectors, the order in which DCT coefficients are selected to be multiplied and accumulated is specified by $\mathbf{C}'$. Consequently, we check if the accumulated product of the first q DCT coefficients (with $q < d$) is above a predefined threshold t', as:

$$\sum_{i=1}^{q} X_i^j \cdot X_i^l > t' \tag{3.15}$$

If Eq. (3.15) is not satisfied, we do not apply any further similarity calculations for feature vectors $\mathbf{X}^j$ and $\mathbf{X}^l$ and we set $S_l^j = 0$.

Finally, we determine the items that satisfy the condition $\mathbf{X}^j \cdot \mathbf{X}^l > t$ and keep only the top-k of them for constructing a sparse similarity matrix.

The formed sparse similarity matrix $\mathbf{S}$ is treated as the weight matrix of a graph representing the similarities between all media items in the collection, and is used for detecting the strongly connected components (SCCs) of this graph using the established Tarjan method [380]. Each SCC is a subgraph in which every node is connected to every other node in the subgraph, i.e., a group of near-duplicates. The final output of this offline processing of the media collection is a graph such as the example one shown on the left side of Fig. 3.11.

Having completed the offline processing of the given collection, we can now efficiently respond to any request for detecting if this collection contains near-duplicates

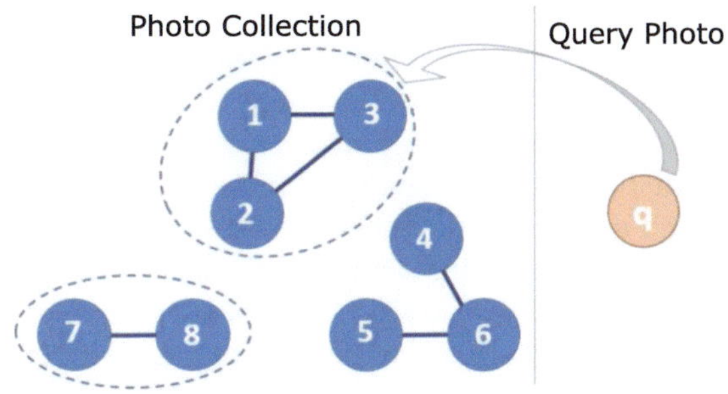

Fig. 3.11 Time-efficient near-duplicate detection based on the strongly connected components (SCCs) of the similarity graph. SCCs are denoted here with dashed ellipses

of any new (previously unseen) query photo during the online mode. Given the query photo, the described feature extraction process is performed. The most similar item in the collection for the given photo is detected by computing the cosine similarity of the latter to all the items in the collection; the set of rules for pruning the number of required similarity calculations that was introduced above is again used for speeding up the process. Finally, all items of the collection that belong to the same SCC as the detected nearest neighbor (based on the previously applied SCC detection), if any, are also retrieved as near-duplicates of the query photo. The latter is illustrated in Fig. 3.11, where the query photo is matched with media item #3, but media items #1 and #2 are also known to be near-duplicates of the query photo since they are included in the same SCC of the constructed graph. Thus, media items #1, #2 and #3 are all returned as detected near-duplicates of the query photo in this example. This approach restricts the number of pairwise similarities that need to be assessed in both the offline and online modes, and reduces the space complexity of the offline procedure.

3.4.2.2 Local Descriptor-Based Approach

In this section, we present the local descriptor-based approach for near-duplicate retrieval and detection (denoted SIFT-NDD in the sequel). Due to the heavy computational complexity of local descriptors and/or keypoint matching for each possible pair of photos in a collection, we follow a coarse to fine scheme, where candidate near-duplicate photos are first selected and then further refined in two stages: (a) the descriptor matching refinement stage and (b) the keypoints matching refinement stage.

The pipeline of the SIFT-NDD approach is as follows: SIFT keypoints [255] are detected in each photo of the collection. The detected keypoints are sorted based on their response metric and the respective SIFT descriptors are computed just on the top-n selected keypoints. All descriptors of the collection are clustered to k clusters, using the k-means method. The k centers of the clusters form a visual vocabulary, which in turn enables the descriptor-based representation of each photo using VLAD encoding [180]. A component-wise mass normalization and square-rooting is performed on the VLAD vectors to address the problem of "burstiness" (as discussed in [19]). A randomized KD forest index is constructed on VLAD vectors so as to compute the k-nearest neighbors of each photo VLAD vector, which are considered as potential near-duplicates of each photos.

In the first refinement stage, for each potential near-duplicate pair we proceed to match the SIFT descriptors by checking for each descriptor if the ratio of distance from the closest neighbor to the distance of the second closest is greater than 0.7 (as suggested by Lowe in [255]). We discard the near-duplicate pairs for which the ratio of matched descriptors to the total extracted descriptors is lower than an empirically set threshold. During the second refinement stage, the remaining near-duplicate candidates of the first stage are further trimmed by checking the geometric consistency of SIFT keypoints using the Geometric Coding method of [439]. Optionally, we can further check (a) the total photo area to matched area ratio, to exclude partial duplicates, (b) the query matched area to neighbor matched area ratio, to exclude scaled duplicates. Finally, we proceed to construct the graph of similarities between all media items in the collection, as discussed in Sect. 3.4.2.2, to conclude the offline mode processing and be able to respond to queries during the online mode.

3.4.2.3 DCNN-Based Descriptor Approach

Deep convolutional neural networks (DCNNs) exhibit hierarchical learning, a natural progression from low-level to high-level structure [223]: the most-bottom layers detect the presence of characteristics such as edges at particular location and orientation, the middle layers detect motifs formed by particular arrangements of edges, and the most-top layers detect high-order combinations that have a certain semantic meaning (e.g., complex motifs of edges that constitute a face).

To identify similar photos in a collection using a DCNN-based approach (denoted DCNN-NDD in the sequel), we adopt the method of [309]. Specifically, we selected the GoogLeNet pretrained ImageNet network [377] that was also used as a source DCNN in Sect. 3.2 for concept-based annotation. The structure of the network is illustrated in Fig. 3.2 (excluding the extension layers), i.e., GoogLeNet is a 22-layer network consisting of nine inception layers that are connected sequentially. GoogLeNet takes as input a 224 $\times$ 224 photo which is then forward propagated through the network. In order to perform near-duplicate detection we select a specific GoogLeNet convolutional layer and use its responses (which are L_2-normalized) to describe the different input image regions. This results in a collection for all regions of all photos, and all filters of the chosen layer. Then, we perform k-means clustering in this collection in order to obtain a vocabulary of k words. Then, each filter response vector is assigned to its nearest visual word, enabling the subsequent encoding of all the filter responses from all regions into one feature vector using VLAD encoding [180]. Finally, the VLAD descriptors are normalized by intra-normalization [19]. Taking into consideration the evaluation carried out in [309], we choose to extract the features from the "inception3a/output" layer as this layer scored the best results in various datasets. Furthermore, differently from [309] we choose to construct a visual vocabulary with $k = 256$ words, and reduce the dimensionality of the convolutional responses features from 256 to 192 using PCA prior to VLAD encoding, to reduce the size of the resulting VLAD vectors. Finally, we proceed to construct the graph of similarities between all media items in the collection, as discussed in Sect. 3.4.2.2, similarly to what was done in the previous two approaches (DCT-NDD, SIFT-NDD).

3.4.2.4 Near-Duplicate Detection for Video Collections

In this section, we present a near-duplicate technique for collections of videos. The video near-duplicate retrieval (denoted VNDR in the sequel) method can detect near-duplicate videos under various transformations/distortions, and videos which are fractions of others in a large corpus. The VNDR method has three main stages: (a) feature extraction, (b) coarse similarity assessment and (c) fine similarity assessment and temporal alignment. In the first stage, we select 2 frames per second and we follow the same procedure described in Sect. 3.4.2.3 to extract a DCNN-based feature vector from the "loss3/classifier" layer for each selected frame. The row vectors of each analyzed frame are horizontally concatenated to create the signature matrix of each video. The height of the signature matrix is equal to the length of the feature vector, while the width is variable and proportional to the videos length. In the second stage, for each video we compute the mean value of each prediction class of GoogLeNet by averaging the rows of the signature matrix, producing a signature vector for the video. This signature vector can roughly indicate the presence of certain concepts throughout the video. Constructing an index on the signature vectors using Randomized KD forests, and performing a kNN search we can quickly discover potential near-duplicate videos and exclude non-near-duplicates videos from the more computationally expensive third stage. In the third stage, we employ a 2-dimensional normalized cross-correlation method on signature matrices of a pair of near-duplicate candidate videos to compute a similarity time-series. If the maximum value of this time-series is above an empirically set threshold, the videos are considered as near-duplicates and the position of this maximum value in the time-series denotes the temporal position in which the pair of videos contain a near-duplicate segment.

3.4.3 Experimental Results

We conducted a series of experiments, to test the accuracy and efficiency of the developed global, local and DCNN-based descriptor approaches for photo near-duplicate detection, as well as the near-duplicate detection approach for video collections. All these techniques tackle the problem of near-duplicate detection, yet, as discussed in their respective sections, each of them deals with certain cases of near-duplicate detection and has special merits, and thus, to fairly evaluate each method, we used the most appropriate datasets, i.e., for the global descriptor-based method we use datasets that consider the specific set of alterations discussed in Sect. 3.4.2.1, adding a large number of distractor photos, while for the local descriptor-based and DCNN-based methods we use datasets that contain partial duplicates and more complex cases of near-duplicates.

The DCT-NDD algorithm's performance was compared against state-of-the-art methods of the literature, using the mean average precision (MAP) metric. The employed datasets are listed below:

- The Copydays dataset [118] contains 157 photos and considers three different alterations (cropping, JPEG compression and "strong" attacks such as printing, hand-painting and scanning).
- The Copydays1 dataset is a variation of the Copydays dataset, described in [226].
- The Feature Detector Evaluation Sequences dataset [296] contains the photo sequences Leuven, UBC, Bikes, Graffiti, Wall, Bark, Boat, where in each sequence different alterations were applied (i.e., illumination, JPEG compression, blur, viewpoint changes, rotation).
- The Copydays Overlay dataset was created by the authors after resizing the 157 photos of the Copydays dataset to 1000 pixels height, and overlaying a text banner at the top-left, top-right, center, bottom-left, and bottom-right areas of these photos, using a 72pt font size.
- The Flickr100k dataset [327] consists of 1,00,071 photos collected from Flickr by searching popular Flickr tags. This dataset was used for adding distractors to the aforementioned datasets.

Table 3.8 reports the MAP scores of the evaluated approaches on the considered datasets. Column 1 lists the alterations found in each dataset or subset thereof, column 2 specifies the corresponding datasets, column 3 lists the applied methods, and columns 4 and 5 report the MAP score without or with using additional distractor photos, respectively. According to these results, the DCT-NDD approach performs the best in the cases of noise addition, scaling and JPEG compression. This performance is slightly reduced, although still remaining high, when distractor photos are included in the dataset. Concerning the case where the original photos were postprocessed by applying illumination changes, the DCT-NDD technique is the best among three considered literature approaches on the Leuven dataset (also achieving MAP score equal to 1.00 when no distractor photos were used), while it performs slightly worse than the method of [226] on the Copydays1 dataset. Similar findings about the algorithm's performance are observed for the blur alteration, where the MAP score of the DCT-NDD method is the highest among all compared techniques on the Bikes dataset, and close to the best one on the Copydays1 dataset. Finally, our algorithm's performance, when photo cropping is applied, varies for the Copydays (Crop) and Copydays1 datasets. This variation is explained by the fact that the first dataset is created by gradually cropping the original photos, removing from 10 up to 80% of their surface (which is extreme variation). Under such conditions, methods based on the local features and geometric constraints (such as [440]) are more capable of identifying small cropped parts of the original photos. In contrast, the Copydays1 dataset is constructed by cropping the original photos' surface by up to 25% (i.e., it

Table 3.8 Performance of the evaluated methods for the considered photo alterations

Photo alterations	Dataset	Method	MAP (%)	MAP (%) (+100k distractors)
Photometric - illumination change	Leuven	[138] (SIFT)	35	
		[138] (CNN)	62	
		[138] (U.CNN)	58	
		DCT-NDD	**100**	91
	Copydays1	[226]	**96**	
		DCT-NDD	86	74
Noise addition	Copydays1	[226]	94	
		DCT-NDD	**100**	91
JPEG compression	Copydays (JPEG)	[440]		91
		DCT-NDD	**100**	91
	UBC	[138] (SIFT)	55	
		[138] (CNN)	65	
		[138] (U.CNN)	70	
		DCT-NDD	**100**	91
	Copydays1	[226]	99	
		DCT-NDD	**100**	91
Scale	Copydays1	[226]	96	
		DCT-NDD	**100**	91
Blur	Copydays1	[226]	**93**	
		DCT-NDD	85	79
	Bikes	[138] (SIFT)	30	
		[138] (CNN)	55	
		[138] (U.CNN)	61	
		DCT-NDD	**83**	75
Crop	Copydays (Crop)	[440]		**93**
		DCT-NDD	43	32
	Copydays1	[226]	**89**	
		DCT-NDD	86	72
Overlay	Copydays Overlay	DCT-NDD	**94**	91

does not apply extreme cropping), in which case the DCT-NDD approach performs competitively to the examined literature approaches. Last but not least, the developed DCT-NDD algorithm exhibits robustness to the insertion of overlaying text labels in the original photos (Copydays Overlay dataset).

In the next set of experiments, aiming to assess the SIFT-NDD and DCNN-NDD methods, the following datasets were used.

- The California-ND dataset [184] contains 701 photos taken directly from a real user's personal photo collections. As a result, it includes many challenging non-identical near-duplicate cases without resorting to the use of artificial photo transformations. In order to deal with the subjectivity and ambiguity that near-duplicate cases exhibit, the dataset is annotated by 10 different subjects, including the photographer. These annotations can be combined into a nonbinary ground-truth, representing the probability that a pair of photos is considered a near-duplicate.
- The Holidays dataset [179] is a set of photos contains personal holidays photos. The photos were taken to test the robustness to various attacks: rotations, viewpoint and illumination changes, blurring, etc. The dataset includes a very large variety of scene types (natural, man-made, water and fire effects, etc.), and contains 500 photo groups, each of which represents a distinct scene or object. The first photo of each group is the query photo and the near-duplicates of it are the other photos of the group.
- The University of Kentucky benchmark dataset (UKBench, [265]) contains 10200 photos of (2550 groups with four photos each), at size 640×480. The photos are rotated and blurred.
- The Oxford Buildings dataset [327] consists of 5062 photos collected from Flickr by searching for particular Oxford landmarks. The collection has been manually annotated to generate a comprehensive ground-truth for 11 different landmarks, each represented by 5 possible queries. This gives a set of 55 queries over which an object retrieval system can be evaluated. The queries are a cropped portion of a photo in the collection, therefore, this dataset is oriented toward partial near-duplicate photo retrieval.

Table 3.9 reports the MAP scores of the evaluated approaches on the selected photo datasets. Column 1 specifies the tested method, column 2, 3, 4, and 5 list the achieved mean average precision score (MAP) of each tested method on California-ND, Holidays, UKBench, and Oxford Building datasets respectively. According to these results, the SIFT-NDD method performs better than the DCNN-NDD method on UKBench and Oxford Buildings datasets which are oriented toward partial near-duplicate photo retrieval. This due to the use of local descriptors that incorporate spatial information into the feature vector that describes the photo. Inversely, the DCNN-NDD method performs better than the SIFT-NDD method on the California-ND and Holidays datasets.

Table 3.10 reports the mean extraction time per photo for all the near-duplicate retrieval and detection methods discussed here. We tested the SIFT-NDD standard approach (SIFT-NDD/serial) and an approach running the feature extraction in parallel (SIFT-NDD/parallel) using the Intel OpenMP library. For the DCNN-NDD

Table 3.9 Evaluation of SIFT-NDD and DCNN-NDD approaches against near-duplicate detection methods from the literature

Dataset	California-ND MAP (%)	Holidays MAP (%)	UKBench MAP (%)	Oxford buildings MAP (%)
SIFT-NDD	76.3	81.6	84.3	79.3
DCNN-NDD	**93.2**	**91.2**	73.2	63.9
[434]	85.2	–	–	–
[421]	–	89.9	–	–
[23]	–	–	**95.0**	–
[410]	–	–	–	**82.80**

Table 3.10 Feature extraction times for each of the proposed near-duplicate detection approaches. For the local descriptor-based approach (SIFT-NDD/serial) the feature extraction time for a parallel implementation is also presented (SIFT-NDD/parallel), while for the DCNN-based approach (DCNN-NDD/CPU), we also present the feature extraction times when using a GPU (DCNN-NDD/GPU) and when using a GPU and the NVIDIA CUDA Deep Neural Network library (DCNN-NDD/GPU+cudNN)

Approach	Mean feature extraction time per photo (ms)
DCT-NDD	**0.08**
SIFT-NDD/serial	405
SIFT-NDD/parallel	58
DCNN-NDD/CPU	124
DCNN-NDD/GPU	28
DCNN-NDD/GPU+cudNN	14

method, we test the performance using the Caffe deep learning framework running on CPU, GPU, and finally utilizing the NVIDIA cuDNN library, which provides highly tuned implementations for standard routines and can offer an up to 2.2x speed-up on most NVIDIA GPU cards. The DCNN-NDD on GPU (DCNN-NDD/GPU) and DCNN-NDD on GPU using cuDNN (DCNN-NDD/GPU+CUDNN) mean feature extraction times are calculated using a batch size equal to 24. All experiments discussed in this section are executed on a Windows 7 64-bit PC with Intel Core (TM) i7-4790K CPU @ 3.50GHz, 16GB RAM, and an NVIDIA Geforce GTX 1060 GPU. According to these results, the DCT-NDD which is suited for application where specific photo alterations are considered (as discussed in Sect. 3.4.2.3) is the faster one by a large margin. As expected, we can also see how the use of a GPU can drastically reduce the feature extraction time for DCNN-based methods.

To evaluate the video near-duplicate retrieval method (VNDR) we used the CC_WEB_VIDEO dataset [420], which consists of 13,129 videos related to 24 distinct text queries. Each text query was issued to YouTube, Google Video, and Yahoo! Video. The videos gathered include exact- and near-duplicate videos under various photometric variations (color/lighting change), editing changes (logo

Table 3.11 Evaluation of video near-duplicate retrieval methods

Method	MAP (%)
VNDR	91.3
SIG_CH of [420]	89.2
HIRACH of [420]	**95.2**

insertion, borders addition around frames, superposition of text), and content modifications (unrelated frames' addition with different content). We conducted experiments comparing the proposed method against the method of [420], using the mean average precision (MAP). Table 3.11 reports the results. We observe that the proposed method performs better than the SIG_CH approach of [420]. The HIRACH approach of [420] performs the best, however, this technique is based on the local handcrafted features, therefore, it presents higher computational complexity compared to using global handcrafted features (as discussed in Sect. 3.4.1) or DCNN-based features, which are used in VNDR.

3.5 Event-Based Photo Clustering and Summarization

Clustering algorithms partition a collection of items into groups called clusters, such that similar items are assigned into the same group. Using clustering algorithms large collections can be handled in such a way that items can be organized, and subsequently summarized by selecting a representative item from each different cluster to construct a summary. Regarding photo collections, a clustering algorithm may segment the photos of the collection to visually similar clusters or semantically similar clusters. In this section, we deal with clustering algorithms that group together photos with close capture times.

3.5.1 Related Work

There is a variety of works in the literature that deal with the management of photo collections (such as [437]), but very few deal with the explicit problem of event-based photo clustering. In an early work, the authors of [145] propose the use of capture date/time (timestamps) found in photos' metadata, in order to cluster a photo collection to events. They perform an analysis on consumer media capture behavior to show that the temporal distribution of photos is not well described by a Poisson model and propose a fractal process, to perform the temporal clustering. However, this method only makes use of the timestamps, not taking into consideration the visual content of the photos. In [254], various algorithms for the management of photo collections, and among them, an automated event clustering method, are proposed. The clustering technique is based on the timestamps as well as color information. In [94] several variants of an automatic unsupervised algorithm to partition a collection of digital photographs are presented, based either on temporal similarity alone, or temporal and content-based similarity. The authors quantify inter-photo similarity at multiple temporal scales to identify likely event clusters, and the final clusters are determined according to three clustering goodness criteria. The use of multiple temporal scales and multiple clustering criteria helps to convey meaningful results, yet, the computational complexity is $O(N^2)$. In [291], a probabilistic approach is presented that fuses multimodal data for event-based home photo clustering, which include time, visual content as well as camera settings. The clusters are discovered through the Expectation–Maximization algorithm.

3.5.2 Method

The event-based clustering method presented here concerns photo collections about a specific event. The event depicted in such a collection typically consists of several subevents, namely groups of photos that constitute a distinct action within a bounded time and space, and the discovery of these subevents' bounds is the objective of the method proposed here. Furthermore, selecting a representative photo from each detected subevent, we can construct a storyline of photos that summarizes the whole collection. To give an example, suppose that a person attends a public event such as some competitions of the Olympic games of London 2012 and takes a number of photos. The individual sports competitions (e.g., first day of men's tennis, women's weightlifting final, etc.) can be considered as sub-events of the entire London 2012 summer Olympic event. Our event-based photo collection clustering method would detect all photos of each sport competition (subevents). Selecting the most appropriate photo of each subevent, it would construct a summary of this Olympics event.

The main stages of the photo collection event-based clustering and summarization method are: (a) feature extraction from photos, (b) employing an event-based clustering algorithm to cluster the photos using the extracted features, (c) selection of representative photos for summarizing the whole photo collection. The type of features used to describe the visual content of photos in the first stage can vary: a fast global descriptor (such HSV color histograms, or the features used in Sect. 3.4.2.1) or a more robust aggregation of local descriptors (extracted similarly to the approach described in Sect. 3.4.2.2) could be used. We choose to extract DCNN-based features using again the Caffe deep learning framework [210] and the 22-layer GoogLeNet DCNN pre-trained model [377]. The GoogLeNet model, besides the main classifier, uses two auxiliary classifiers, with softmax loss as the classifier, predicting the same 1000 classes as the main classifier (see Fig. 3.2). For the specific problem of event-based photo collection clustering and summarization, we choose to extract the "loss1/classifier" and "loss3/classifier" layers due to the semantic nature of these layers output, resulting in two 1000-dimensional vectors. The 2000-dimensional concatenated feature vector is used to represent each photo. We then perform PCA to reduce its dimensionality to 300.

During the second stage, the employed event-based clustering algorithm used can be one of the following:

- Cascaded Event-based Clustering approach (CEC): consists of three stages: (a) time-based splitting, (b) geolocation-based splitting, and (c) merging. In the first stage, we sort the photos based on their capture time and the temporal distance of each photo to the next one is computed. The timeline of the temporally sorted photos is split where consecutive photos have temporal distance above the mean of all temporal distances. During the second stage, geolocation information is used to further split clusters of photos, considering the case of concurrent subevents at different locations. We compute all photos pairwise capture location distances using the haversine distance [341]. Using k-means, we cluster the pairwise capture location distances into two clusters. The cluster with the lowest mean of distances (m_1) presumably signifies photos captured in the same subevent while the cluster with the highest mean of distances presumably corresponds to photos captured in different subevents. We check the pairwise capture location distances for the photos within each cluster of the first stage, and photos with distance more than m_1, are moved to a new cluster. In the third stage, clusters are merged using time and geolocation information. If the temporal distance of two clusters (i.e., the temporal distance between the last photo of one cluster and the first photo of the next cluster) is smaller than the mean of the intracluster temporal distances then these two clusters are merged. We also merge temporally neighboring clusters whose geolocation difference is less than m_1. For the clusters that do not have geolocation information, the merging is continued by considering the concept scores similarity, essentially checking if pairwise distances of photos of two clusters are below an empirically set threshold. If none of the photos in the collection has geolocation information, then the second stage of geolocation-based splitting is omitted.
- Event-based clustering utilizing the Potential-based Hierarchical Agglomerative algorithm (PHA): We normalize the capture times information of photos in the collection in the $[0 \ldots 1]$ range. We concatenate the features extracted during the first stage with the normalized capture time of photos, if this information is available, or with a zero-values attribute for the photos with no capture time information available. We then construct a similarity matrix of the augmented feature vectors. We weight the similarity matrix with the inverse of the photos physical locations distance, so that similarity is increased for photos with close capture locations. We finally apply the clustering method of [256] on the weighted similarity matrix.
- Baseline method: In the conducted experiments for event-based clustering (see Sect. 3.5.3), we included an additional method, denoted as "baseline", in which we consider only temporal metadata for the clustering to subevents (similarly to [145]). This is included for showcasing the merits of the aforementioned CEC and PHA methods.

Table 3.12 Evaluation of event-based clustering methods for photo collections

	Vancouver		London	
	FI (%)	JI (%)	FI (%)	JI (%)
Baseline	19.2	24.3	28.1	42.6
CEC	**24.6**	**31.1**	**34.3**	**51.6**
PHA	24.3	30.7	31.2	45.5

Finally, to summarize the photo collection we select a photo from each cluster. The photo to be selected can be the one that is the most similar to rest of the photos in the same cluster; this computation is fast, considering that we already have a similarity matrix of all photos in the collection constructed in the second stage of the method. Alternatively, the summarization algorithm may rely on aesthetics assessment: the aesthetic quality of all photos in each cluster can be evaluated, as discussed in Sect. 3.3, and the highest scoring one can be selected as the representative of a specific cluster. Additionally, a summarization algorithm may rely on near-duplicate detection (Sect. 3.4): the presence of numerous near-duplicates about an object/scene of interest in a cluster may signify the importance of this specific object/scene to the user, and thus, one of these near-duplicates can be selected to represent the cluster. Note here, that such a summarization method solely concerns event-centered photo collections; for a discussion on the automatic selection of important photos from personal collections, based on the insights emerging from a user study, see Chap. 8.

3.5.3 Experimental Results

The aforementioned approaches of photo collection event-based clustering are evaluated on the datasets of the MediaEval 2014 SEM [82] task:

- The Vancouver dataset, which consists of 1351 photos and captures various subevents of the Vancouver 2010 Winter Olympic Games
- The London dataset, which consists of 2124 photos and captures various subevents of the London 2012 Olympic Games.

For the evaluation of the methods against the ground-truth event-based clustering, we used two measures: (a) the F-measure (F1), and (b) the Jaccard Index (JI), which is defined as the number of unique elements common to both sets divided by the total number of unique elements in both sets.

Table 3.12 reports the F-measure and Jaccard Index scores of the presented methods on the Vancouver and London datasets. According to these results, the CEC method performed marginally better than PHA on the Vancouver dataset, while on the London one the CEC method performed the best by a large margin. The baseline method performed poorly in both datasets, since it exploits only the temporal metadata of the photos. An indicative example is shown in Fig. 3.12, where a subset of the

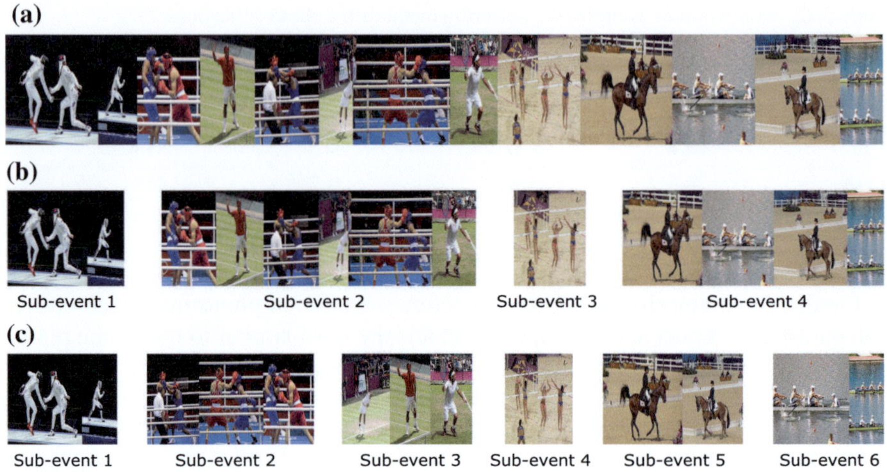

Fig. 3.12 **a** A subset of the photo collection of the London 2012 Olympic games (London dataset), captured by multiple users and depicting concurrent subevents. **b** The result of applying the baseline event-based clustering method. **c** The result of applying the PHA or CEC method (their results were identical for this specific subset of the London dataset)

London dataset is used. In the top row, the photos of this subset are displayed, sorted according to their capture time. Note that the photos of this dataset are captured by multiple users and therefore they depict concurrent subevents. In the middle row, the result of applying the baseline event-based clustering method is depicted, while the bottom row shows the result of applying either the PHA or the CEC methods (the results were identical for this specific subset of the London dataset). We notice that the baseline method included both boxing and men's tennis in the same subevent (subevent-2 of the middle row), since these were concurrent subevents (same applies for the case of fencing and rowing being included in the same subevent-4 of the middle row). Both of the proposed event-based clustering techniques managed to assign the photos of these sport events to different subevents (subevent-2 and subevent-3 of the bottom row for boxing and men's tennis, respectively, and subevent-5 and subevent-6 of the bottom row for fencing and rowing, respectively). As a final note, and taking into consideration that the CEC method relies heavily on the capture time of photos, while the PHA method uses this just as auxiliary information, we conclude that the PHA method is ideal for the scenarios where temporal information is partially or fully unavailable.

3.6 Conclusions

In this chapter, we surveyed the literature and presented our developed methods that can be used for photo/video annotation, photo/video quality assessment, near-duplicate detection, and event-based photo clustering and summarization. These methods are valuable tools in implementing a digital preservation and forgetting strategy.

For the problem of photo/video annotation, we presented a deep learning two-step process that can be used both for photo and video shot annotation and we focused on important directions for improving concept detection accuracy. Experiments performed on two datasets show that the method of increasing the depth of a pretrained network with one fully-connected layer and fine-tuning the rest of the layers on the target dataset can improve the network's concept detection accuracy, compared to other fine-tuning approaches. Using layers' responses as feature vectors for a learning model can lead to additional gains, compared to using the direct network's output. Using more elaborate methods (such as the presented ELLA_LC model instead of simple models) can further improve concept detection accuracy, reaching a 32.10% of MXinfAP when evaluated on the TRECVID SIN 2013 dataset. This number is among the state-of-the-art results for this specific dataset and, although seemingly low (since it is much lower than 100%), a qualitative analysis shows how good results it represents. For example, considering the concept chair that reaches an infAP of 32.84%, we observe in the resulting ranked list of concept-based retrieval results that among the top-20 retrieved keyframes all of them are positive; among the top-50 retrieved keyframes 46 are positive; and among the top-100 ones 86 of them are positive samples.

We also discussed the literature about the problems of photo/video aesthetic quality assessment and presented our developed methods. We presented a comprehensive photo aesthetic assessment method, which exploits five basic photographic rules ("simplicity," "colorfulness," "sharpness," "pattern," and "composition") to extract rule-specific low- and high-level visual features. The experimental results of this approach, and of the combination of these features with previously proposed generic ones, demonstrated the importance of taking basic photographic rules into account when designing an aesthetic quality assessment method. Regarding the problem of video aesthetic quality assessment, we presented a method that combines a comprehensive set of video features with a new learning approach, which takes the video representation's uncertainty into consideration. Experimental results of our approach on a dataset constructed by us, demonstrated considerable performance improvement in comparison to the state-of-the-art learning methods used for video aesthetic quality assessment. Applying these techniques, we can assess the aesthetic quality in an automatic way, with no user interaction, and help the detection of items of poor quality which are more likely to be archived or "forgotten" (i.e., deleted) in a PoF framework.

Furthermore, we reviewed the most commonly used approaches in the literature for near-duplicate detection and retrieval. We presented three approaches based on the different types of features. The experimental results demonstrated the merits of each tested approach. More specifically, a global descriptor-based approach is the fastest but is more suited when a specific set of photo alterations is considered. A local descriptor-based approach performed the best when employed for partial near-duplicate detection. A DCNN-based approach presented very good overall performance. We also described and evaluated a video near-duplicate retrieval method, which is able to detect segments of a near-duplicate video in another.

Finally, we presented and compared two event-based clustering methods that partition the photo collection to different subevents under the assumption that a photo collection concerns a single event. Taking into consideration the subevent clusters created and various other results, such as the aesthetic quality of the photos/videos or the presence of near-duplicates in each cluster, we are able to construct a summary for the whole collection. Near-duplicate detection and summarization algorithms can assist the condensation of large photo/video collections.

The methods presented in this chapter are used in subsequent chapters in this book. For instance, in Chap. 4 they are used for automatically predicting the long-term importance of a photo; in Chap. 5 they are exploited in a pre-processing step for the contextualization of photo collections; in Chap. 7 they are integrated in the Semantic Desktop infrastructure; and, in Chap. 8 they are used in a method for preservation-centered automatic photo selection.

Part II
Multimedia Preservation Theory

Chapter 4
Preservation Value and Managed Forgetting

Claudia Niederée, Nattiya Kanhabua, Tuan Tran and Kaweh Djafari Naini

Abstract In the cognitive processes of humans, forgetting is a very effective way for focusing on the important things, while unstressing things, which are (currently) less important. The translation of *forgetting* into the digital world is, thus, a promising approach for better dealing with the increasing problem of information overload. Information overload is not only caused by the mere volume of information, it is also triggered by the fact that all information is seemingly on the same level of importance. In the ideal case, a perfect dynamic assessment of importance could restrict the information space strictly to the information currently needed, thus dramatically reducing information overload. The role of a digital memory including digital forgetting is to support, not to replace or to hinder human memory. Therefore, a useful approach for "managed forgetting"—a controlled form of digital forgetting—in a digital memory has to be carefully designed, such that it complements human memory. A core ingredient of managed forgetting is the assessment of the importance of information items. Furthermore, forgetting actions are required that go beyond the binary decision between keep and delete. For the short-term perspective, managed forgetting replaces the binary decision on importance by a gradually changing value: Information sinks away from the user with a decreasing value, which we call "Memory Buoyancy". The transition from short-term value to long-term importance brings a variety of new challenges. When we look into the "Preservation Value" of an information item, we have to estimate the future importance of a resource. This challenging task is further complicated by the facts that (a) preservation looks into very long time frames (e.g., decades rather than months) and (b) the importance of information items may change over time. The Preservation Value provides the basis

C. Niederée (✉) · T. Tran · K. D. Naini
L3S Research Center, Hannover, Germany
e-mail: niederee@L3S.de

T. Tran
e-mail: ttran@L3S.de

K. D. Naini
e-mail: naini@L3S.de

N. Kanhabua
NTENT Inc., Barcelona, Spain
e-mail: nkanhabua@ntent.com

V. Mezaris et al. (eds.), *Personal Multimedia Preservation*, Springer Series on Cultural Computing, https://doi.org/10.1007/978-3-319-73465-1_4

for making preservation decisions, e.g., how much to invest for ensuring that a media item such as a photo will survive the next years or decades. We, furthermore, investigate into methods for information value assessment in support of managed forgetting. For this purpose, we analyze existing methods for information value assessment and discuss their usefulness in the context of computing the Preservation Value. We also outline methods for Preservation Value computation for different exemplary settings. This will also point to the more in-depth discussion of computing Preservation Value in the semantic desktop and photo preservation as it is discussed in later chapters of the book. Finally, we discuss managed forgetting beyond assessing the importance of information items. We study a portfolio of forgetting methods, i.e., methods that can be used to implement managed forgetting on top of the values for information importance. This includes methods such as information hiding, forgetful search, summarization and aggregation as well as deletion.

4.1 Effective Information Management with Managed Forgetting

The idea of "managed forgetting" is to systematically deal with information that progressively decreases in importance, in order to enable the user to focus on the things that are important. At first glance, digital forms of forgetting seem to contradict the idea of preservation, which is about keeping things, not about throwing them away. However, if no special actions are taken for long-term preservation, we already face a rather random digital forgetting process in the digital world today in the private as well as in the professional information management context as has already been discussed in Chap. 1 of this book. Furthermore, from a more global perspective, there is a growing understanding that a systematic support for digital *forgetting* [278] has to be considered as an alternative to the dominating "keep-it-all" paradigm and the often random survival of information, e.g., in the public space of the web.

We suggest to replace such random forgetting processes with managed forgetting. Here, users are supported in their explicit decisions about what information to keep, and how such information should be organized and preserved. In particular, we envision an idea of "gradual forgetting", where complete digital forgetting is just the extreme and a wide range of forgetting actions including different levels of condensation is foreseen. This concept is expected to help in preservation decisions. It is also expected to create immediate benefits for active information use by helping to keep the active information spaces more focused. The aim is to strike a balance between preservation and managed forgetting, also taking into account constraints for digital forgetting (e.g., legal regulations).

To support managed forgetting, it is essential to evaluate the information resources with respect to their importance. This embraces current importance as well as "preservation-worthiness" in the long term. Such assessment methods need to be flexible enough to cope with the inherent heterogeneity and temporal dynamics of resources over time. For coping with short-term and long-term importance, we define two complementing parameters to assess information values of resources for managed forgetting.

The first parameter, "Memory Buoyancy" (MB), is inspired by the metaphor of information objects sinking down in the digital memory with decreasing importance, usage, etc., increasing their distance from the user. This type of information value is highly associated to **short-term** interests [416]. MB is influenced by a variety of factors such as usage of a resource or importance of the resource's topic in the current context.

The second information assessment value is "Preservation Value" (PV). It is used for making preservation decisions, i.e., deciding on whether the resource under consideration should be preserved or how much should be invested in preserving it. The PV will use an overlapping but different set of parameters for its computation, compared to MB. PV is more related to long-term interests and to more objective types of assessment, e.g., diversity and coverage.

Beyond information value assessment, managed forgetting also requires methods that act upon those values. We call this actions "forgetting actions". A wide variety of actions is possible here. For MB, i.e., short-term importance, the target of such actions is mainly to support the user in keeping focused, to make dealing with information spaces more delightful, and to reduce information overload. This implies methods such as information hiding (based on MB threshold) and forgetful search which punishes search results with low MB value. For PV, i.e., long-term value, actions related to long-term management and preservation are important. This includes preservation decisions such as what to preserve and how much to invest into preservation. In addition, this includes actions such as summarization, aggregation, and elimination of near duplicates as more refined forgetting actions.

Finally, deletion or suggestion for deletion is also a possible forgetting action both for short-term as well as for long-term importance.

4.2 Short-Term Value and Memory Buoyancy

MB indicates the short-term importance of a digital object reflecting some type of "closeness" to current human memory processes and current activities. MB is inspired by the metaphor of information objects sinking down in the digital memory with decreasing importance, usage, etc., increasing their distance from the user.

Our discussions of the topic in this book are based on the following definition of MB:

Definition 4.1 Memory Buoyancy (MB) is a value attached to a resource reflecting the expected benefit from bringing this resource digitally close to the user in the current context. Here, bringing the resource digitally close to the user means reducing the cognitive effort of the user for finding and accessing the resource.

This idea embraces the concept of resource importance as well as the idea of complementing human memory. Following the idea of complementing human memory, MB is related in a nontrivial way to the interaction with resources and to the degree to which memories and an image of a digital object fade in human brain over time, either as a result of interference in human memory, or because of other factors intervening in the remembering or recall process. On the one hand, it is important to identify the objects that are currently important or will be important in the near future, i.e., which have a high probability to be (re-)accessed. On the other hand, for complementing human memory, it is also important to consider both (a) how easy is it to find the identified important resources (access effort) and (b) how probable is it that the actor needs to rehearse the information from the resource (vs. he still remembers the content and, thus, will not re-access). Only when considering both aspects, benefits can be created for the user by bringing the resource closer to him or her. For identifying important resources as well as for assessing re-access effort, it is important to not just consider a resource and the action on this resource in isolation, but to understand the interaction with related resources.

Based on the systematic review of existing practices in human-assisted digital mementos, as well as on cognitive aspects of complementing human memory discussed thus far, we propose a general framework as a basis for incorporating MB and short-term managed forgetting into digital memories with a special focus on personal information management (PIM) [106]. In PIM, an ever-growing information space tends to clutter with information which is irrelevant in given situations and thus is in danger to become unmanageable and useless both for technical reasons (e.g., resource limits on smart phones) and for cognitive reasons (information overload). Therefore, managed forgetting can play an important role in accessing and managing personal information space.

Following the above considerations, we developed an initial conceptual framework for managed forgetting and contextualized remembering in digital systems. While we are aware of the importance of contextualization in the framework, we focus on the aspects of contexts that are relevant and useful for managed forgetting. Our proposed conceptual framework is inspired by an integrated and contextual perspective on Information Retrieval (IR) presented in [175]. As illustrated in Fig. 4.1, the conceptual framework consists of three main parts:

- A virtual "information space" which is composed of human and digital memory;
- A "context" which defines a social, societal, and organizational environment into which the information space is embedded;
- A "human actor" accessing and interacting with the information space.

We decided to conceptually split the human actor from his/her memory and to rather consider the human and the digital memory as an integral system. There are two reasons for this: (a) we are especially interested in what we can learn from human memory for creating effectively accessible digital memories (time-aware information access) and (b) the boundaries between human and digital memory are in flux due to an increased delegation to digital memory.

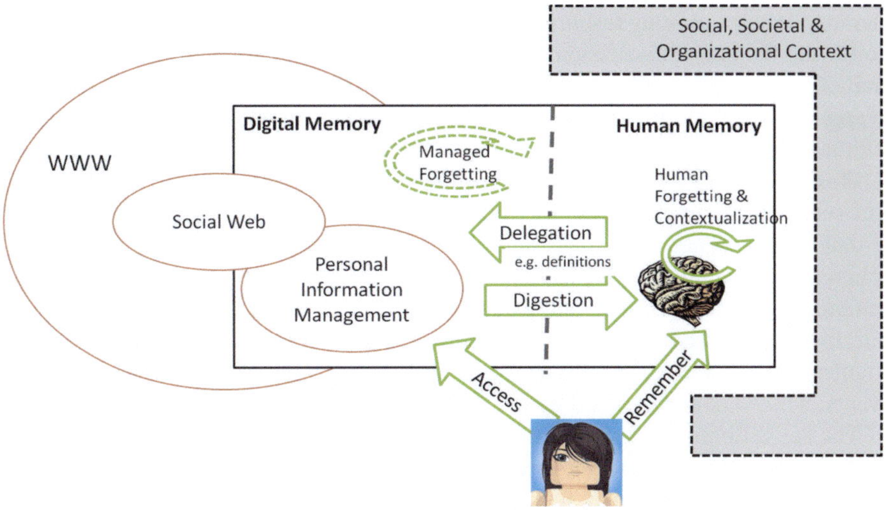

Fig. 4.1 Conceptual framework for managed forgetting and contextualized remembering in digital systems with special focus on personal information management

In this framework, we introduce three main concepts for describing central processes in this framework: “resources”, “interactions”, and “human actors”.

Resource is the abstraction of information artifacts in the information space. A resource can refer to data objects stored in the digital systems, but it can also refer to the image of such objects as encoded and stored in the human brain, or as shared by human actors in three overlapping spheres of digital memory—personal information management (organizing resources on local devices such as mobiles or personal computers), the social web (online storage and sharing still of personal information), and the web in more general (see Fig. 4.1).

Interaction refers to actions within the information space that resemble or are relevant to human memory processes (i.e., information encoding, storing and recalling [13]). We consider three main types of interaction: (a) delegation and digestion, (b) forgetting and contextualization, and (c) access and remembering. By “delegation”, information is moved into outer spheres (e.g., from human memory to things that can be looked up, or from personal information management to the social web). This happens increasingly, triggered by improved access strategies and increased availability of information via the web (e.g., via smart phones). An example is looking up definitions instead of learning them. “Digestion” is the counterpart to delegation at the boundary between human and digital memory. Closely related to this, the human actor conceptually has two choices, when he needs information: he can try to find it in his memory (“Remember”), where forgetting and contextualization are important processes; or he tries to find them in the digital space (“Access”). Of course, using digital resources again implies cognitive processes, before they can be used. Managed forgetting now comes in as an additional process in the digital memory. It helps to bring resources, which are important to the user closer to the user. Following the above discussion about complementing human memory, the ultimate goal of managed forgetting is to bring resources closer to the user, that are expected to create a benefit to him in the current situation. This would not enclose resources with information, which is useful or important but already memorized by the user.

Human actor can "access" his/her information space through access interfaces and such "direct interactions" can be, for instance, search, lookup or exploration of data objects. There also exist "indirect interactions" between actors and external contexts, for example, relevance of resources as background information, topic and general importance of topic, and external constraints, which also play an important role in the proposed framework. "Remembering" can be (roughly) considered as counterpart of "access" for human memory. It is typically triggered by external events, which are experienced by the human actor.

The key difference between our proposed model and the previous work [175] is to explicitly introduce "managed forgetting" into the framework. Managed forgetting creates immediate benefit by focusing on relevant content in a time-aware fashion, "forgetting" (unfocusing) things that are no longer important.

Managed forgetting for the short-term perspective is based on assessing the value of a resource in the current context. This type of information value is highly associated to short-term interests [416], which is influenced by a variety of factors that can be roughly grouped in the following categories: usage parameters (such as frequency and recency of use, user ratings, recurrent pattern), type and provenance parameters (information object type, source/creator), context parameters (such as relevance of resources as background information, general importance of topic, external constraints), and temporal parameters (age, lifetime specifications). In order to support managed forgetting, various factors influencing MB need to be investigated as well as approaches for learning most effective factor combinations.

Furthermore, approaches for enabling the user to explicitly and implicitly influence the values for MB (and for PV) have to be considered, e.g., explicit expiry dates and lifetime specifications or tagging objects as non-forgettable.

4.3 Preservation Value and Its Drivers

In contrast to MB, which has been discussed in the previous section, PV is related to long-term information management considering time frames of decades. PV is crucial to preservation decisions, since it aims to estimate the expected long-term benefit of a resource.

In this section, we discuss PV in more detail, present a working definition for PV, and discuss a set of dimensions for drivers of PV as a foundation for a systematic way of determining PV. Furthermore, we relate PV assessment and managed forgetting to the field of content appraisal known from research and practical work in the area of preservation.

4.3.1 Preservation Value

In particular, PV is used to determine the amount of investment to be made for ensuring the long-term survival and understandability of the resource under consideration. This can refer to preservation decisions such as how many copies to keep or to investment in semantic preservation, which also takes into account context evolution aspects. In the extreme case, PV can also be used to make keep or delete decisions.

Our discussions of the topic in this book are based on the following definition of PV:

Definition 4.2 Preservation Value (PV) is a value attached to a resource reflecting the benefit expected from the long-term survival of it.

The computation of PV, obviously, is a challenging task. The definition already highlights one of the major challenges in assessing PV: it is linked to the expected future value of a resource. This encompasses predicting the future value of a resource. Since neither future value nor future uses of a resource can be fully known at a given point in time, it is clear that PV can only be an estimate of the expected future value. Overall, automatic computation of PV is a very novel field. Such assessments are typically done by humans.

4.3.2 Preservation Value Dimensions

In addition, PV is influenced by a variety of partially setting-specific factors. Therefore, it is not expected that there will be one single method, which can compute PV of resources for all possible settings and types of content, even if we just restrict to personal and organizational preservation. For example, the decision, if I want to keep a photo or an email on the long run, is influenced by other factors. It has to be noted here again that preservation refers to very long time frames.

However, we have identified eight high-level dimensions that can be used to categorize the evidences used for computing PV. They provide a basis for developing a more systematic approach to PV assessment. The list of dimensions has been compiled based on content selection work from literature [408, 418], own studies in content selection for preservation [69, 70], and a study of work on appraisal in the archival domain [93, 355]. In the following, we describe those dimensions together with examples for illustrating the concept of each dimension:

Content Type This dimension refers to the type of the content to be assessed. Types might be considered on several levels ranging from image versus text formats to more semantic types, e.g., distinguishing a holiday photo from a food picture.

Investment In a wide sense, this dimension refers to the investment, which has been made into the resource and its improvement/change. For a photo collection, such investment might be the annotation of photos, the improvement of photos in photo software, or the creation of multiple photos of the same scene.

Gravity This dimension refers to the relationship or closeness of a resource to important events, processes, and structures in the domain under consideration. For personal photos this might be the closeness to an important event such as a wedding or an important life situations such as the first years of one's child.

Time Although the age of the content and time-related properties in more general are less important for long-term information management than for the decision about short-term interests, temporal aspects still play an important role for assessing Preservation Value. For social web content, for example, there is a trend to be more selective, when the content gets older.

Social Graph This dimension describes the relationship of the resource to the relevant social graph, i.e., the persons related to the resource, their roles, and relationships. This might refer to the creators and editors of a resource as well as to persons related to the content of the resource.

Popularity This dimension refers to the usage and perception of the resource. For the case of social web content, this might refer to shared and liked content.

Coverage and Diversity This dimension refers to factors, which consider the resource in relationship to other resources in the same collection. This includes, for instance, diversity or coverage of sub-events, which are also used in making preservation decisions and, thus, influence PV. It can, for example, be taken into account by trying to cover all the sub-events of a holiday, when selecting the most important photos to preserve from a holiday photo collection.

Quality This dimension refers to the quality of the resource. Obvious examples for content quality is photo quality assessing, e.g., if the photo is blurred or exhibits good contrast. More advanced quality aspects are, for example, photo composition and aesthetics.

From the consideration of the dimensions, a better understanding of the PV itself as well as of the importance of those dimensions for the computation of PV is expected. They also help in abstracting from the individual case.

4.3.3 Preservation Value and Appraisal

In this book, we are mainly focusing on preservation in the personal setting. However, so far little work exists in the field of personal preservation (see also Sect. 2.4.5). We, therefore, in this section, also look into preservation practices from the organizational setting, because we can learn from organizational practices for personal preservation. We are especially interested in the idea of "appraisal", which is linked to our concept of "managed forgetting". There is a general understanding in the preservation community that (digital) preservation is also a selection process [93, 160, 222], since it is neither useful nor possible to preserve everything [222]. This introduces the task of *appraisal* into the preservation process [93, 355]. Formally, appraisal is the process of determining the value of records, which are estimated based on their legal or financial meaning, or other factors. These values will assist archivists in deciding which record is worth to be preserved and how long they should be retained.

In assessing the value of a resource, two types of value are considered: primary value and secondary value [355]. Roughly speaking, primary value refers to the value that a resource has for the organization that created it. It is typically related to ongoing business value. The secondary value can target a wider audience beyond the creating organization. It refers to a broader historical and societal value of a resource. This, for example, embraces the ability of a resource to reflect historical developments and situations.

Functional appraisal and macro-appraisal [93], as alternative appraisal methods suggest not to start the appraisal process by looking into individual resources. They suggest to look into an organization's purpose and processes (functions), and then identify which records reflect those functions best. For breaking this down, first some broad functions can be identified for an organization and each function can be further divided into a set of sub-functions.

In the following, we will link the Preservation Value dimensions proposed above to appraisal methods and criteria used in archives. An obvious link can be made from the approach of functional appraisal and macro-appraisal [93] to the dimensions of **gravity** and the **social graph**. As in the case of **gravity**, macro-appraisal looks into the importance of information items for the institution, looking into the structure and processes of the institution. Functional appraisal looks at "the functions carried out by the record creator"[1] and uses this information in appraisal instead of content criteria, which is related to the dimension of the **social graph**, which has a broader scope enabling its application in personal and organizational settings. Another aspect, which is linked to the dimension of **gravity** is the aspect of long-term historical importance, which is often used as a criteria for assessing secondary value in appraisal.

For the dimension of **investment**, our approach refers to the preparation of resource and the corresponding improvement. However, archivists would also take the legal risks or administration efforts into account. The dimension of **popularity** is linked to the idea of "Social Significance" as named as appraisal criteria in [160]. Popularity can be seen as the measurable part of social significance, but does not fully cover this aspect. The dimension **coverage and diversity** is not directly related to an appraisal criterion. However, it is implicitly linked to the idea of the macro-appraisal approach, which by its strategy aims to cover the big picture of the content to be preserved.

The dimension **time** is important in both appraisal and in our approach. For example, the need of a reappraisal process [92] is emphasized and there is a general understanding that in the digital age preservation decisions have to be taken in a timely fashion [160].

---

[1] http://www.paradigm.ac.uk/workbook/appraisal/appraisal-approaches.html.

For the dimension **content type**, we focus on the semantic type of a content object rather than on its format as a decision criterion for preservation. This is again linked to a functional approach to appraisal.

4.4 Methods for Information Value Assessment

4.4.1 Existing Methods for Information Value Assessment

An important field embracing the distinction between important and less important information is Information Retrieval (IR). In this field, importance or more precisely relevance of an information resource for the information need of a user is underlying the selection and ranking process of IR components. In addition to the pure content of the documents, which are core in classical IR approaches [262], further factors are used in modern IR approaches for information value assessment. This especially includes the link structure of the information space, which is exploited in the popular PageRank algorithm [318]. Additional factors are also used for information value assessment in IR such as diversity [4] of the top results aiming for coverage and complementarity of the search results.

A more socially oriented form of information value assessment is used in recommender systems or collaborative filtering [151]. In this proactive form of information filtering, the assessment of the value of a new item for a user is learned from the behavior of "similar" users for this item. This can for example be perceived interest (e.g., user bought this item) or ratings given for this item.

Other more efficiency-driven methods of information value assessment are memory caching and index pruning. In index pruning [61, 76], the value of information in the index is assessed based on its potential to contribute to relevant results. Here, the assessment is used to decide about cutting off parts of the index, which are not very productive aiming for smaller and more efficient indices. In memory caching, information value assessment is used to dynamically decide, which information items remain in a limited fast memory structure, the cache, and which are replaced by more promising items. Caching memory plays an important role for efficient web search by caching frequent results [30, 133]. Index pruning and web caching can also be combined [366].

Memory caching is just one of an entire class of methods, which uses usage patterns for analyzing the importance/value of information. In [416], for example, usage and activity patterns are used to predict users short-term interest or intent while in [22], usage patterns are used to predict navigation behavior.

Another method used in information value assessment is spreading activation, a concept adopted from cognitive science. Similar to the aforementioned PageRank algorithm, resources are not considered in isolation, but rather as parts of (semantic) networks. Along the paths created by such networks, activation can be propagated (spread), also raising the importance of resources related to an activated (e.g., used or accessed) resource. Spreading activation is, for example, used in the context of search [99, 342] and in the context of Personal Information Management [196] for improving results.

4.4.2 *Exemplary Methods in Support of Managed Forgetting*

Managed forgetting is a very novel field, where no established methods exist yet. In addition, the computation of information value, which is in the core of managed forgetting, depends upon the respective setting and upon the type of content considered. In the following sections, we present four case studies and the related methods for computing information value in support of managed forgetting. We start from the computation of MB in the context of desktop data, followed by PV computation also for semantically enriched desktop data, which is discussed in more detail in Chap. 7. In addition, we look into PV computation for personal photo collections as an important type of personal content, which is discussed in more detail in Chap. 8 of this book. Finally, we investigate the retention preferences in social media, which addresses a mid-term information value. We thus illustrate information value assessment for a variety of content types and for different time frames (from short-term importance to long-term value).

4.4.3 *Computing Memory Buoyancy with Semantic Information*

Taking up the idea of complementing human memory discussed above, the presented method is inspired by a re-access model of human effort in (re-)finding a resource for accessing it. The effort of re-accessing a resource depends on a variety of factors and is related to MB. For example, if a human actor accesses a photo every day, it will take him or her nearly no time to recall the location of the photo in his computer. In line with existing approaches, such models must take into account the usage activities of information resources in the past, and devise a salient way to predict the accessibility probability of the item in the future [77, 300].

Actually, the task of computing a MB value for resources is framed as a ranking problem. The ranking process consists of two steps. In the first step, we mine the activity history and devise a MB scoring function based on the recency and frequency of access, so that more recently and frequently accessed documents get higher MB scores. This step embraces a time-decay component for taking into consideration that the effect of having accessed a document fades over time. This is actually true for human brain re-access models as well as for models, which predict access based on previous document interactions. Different time-decay models have been considered for this purpose including polynomial decay and the Weinbul distribution.

In the second step, a propagation method is used to propagate the activation of documents along selected connections based on a semantic network defined for the considered information space. From experiments, we have seen that a simple propagation model does not perform very well, since it fails to distinguish the different contributions of individual types of resource relationships to MB propagation. Therefore, the revised approach introduces a machine learning framework that can learn the contributions of individual relationship types and can combine them automatically.

4.4.3.1 Activity-Based Memory Buoyancy

In order to compute the scores for MB, we use the access times of the document from the access history. We estimate the score of a document through the distances of previous access time points and the time of interest. For this purpose, we start from an activity-based MB scoring function. This is a function that takes as input the time t and document d, and based on the access sequence $T_{d,t}$ computes an MB Score as an output. If no other evidence (i.e., access of document) is present, the function is purely driven by the decay effect. An access at time t_i resets the score to its original value. In Table 4.1, we present different activity-based scoring functions studied in this work, each corresponding to one decay function. Each of these functions only considers the most recent access at time t_d, and can be used as a basic **recency-based** method.

Frequency In [12], Anderson et al. suggest that the frequency of interactions also plays an important role in the human recall of a resource, as by the relearning effect. Hence, for each of the functions in Table 4.1, we introduce a "frequency"-based variant, which aggregates the effect of decays in different time points:

$$v_f(d, t) = \sum_{t_i \in W} v_r(d, t_i) \tag{4.1}$$

where $v_r(d, t_i)$ can be any of the recency-based functions in Table 4.1. The sequence $W \subseteq T_{d,t}$ represents the time window in which all time points are taken into con-

Table 4.1 List of activity-based ranking functions

Method name	Function	Parameters
Most recently used	$MRU(\text{d, t}) = \frac{1}{t-t_d+1}$	None
Polynomial decay	$\text{PD(d, t)} = \frac{1}{(t-t_d)^{\alpha}+1}$	α: Decay rate
Ebbinghaus curve	$\text{Ebb(d, t)} = e^{\frac{(t_d-t)}{S}}$	S: Relative memory strength
Weibull distribution	$\text{Wei(d, t)} = e^{-\frac{\alpha(t-t_d)^s}{s}}$	s: Forgetting steepness, α: volume of what can be remembered

sideration for the ranking. For instance, if $W = T_{d,t}$ and $v_r = MRU$, we have the well-established *most frequently used* method in cache replacement policies. If $W = T_{d,t}$ and $v_r = PD$, we have the decay ranking model in [320]. The *Frequency* algorithm used in Mozilla Firefox [84], on the other hand, constructs W from only the last ten items of $T_{d,t}$, in order to avoid the convolution of too old accesses into the current rank. In this work, we follow this idea, and only aggregate from the last ten time points of accesses for each document.

4.4.3.2 Memory Buoyancy Propagation

Before we can discuss our propagation learning framework, we introduce some formal notations. A semantic information space is a collection of documents or resources and is denoted as D. A document or a resource d can be of different types (photos, office documents, folders, web pages, etc.) and has different attributes (e.g., titles, authors, and creation time). Given any two documents d_1 and d_2, there can exist multiple relations with different semantics. For instance, d_1 and d_2 are both created by the same author, d_1 is the containing folder of the file d_2. Relations can be associated with some scores indicating the strength of their relation, for instance, the cosine score for content similarity. Let R denote a set of all semantic relations. For each pair (d_i, d_j), we have an $|R|$-dimensional vector $X_{ij} = (x_{ij1}, x_{ij2}, \ldots, x_{ij|R|})^T$, where $x_{ijk} \geq 0$ represents the score of the k-th relation between d_i and d_j, $x_{ijk} = 0$ if d_i and d_j are not connected by the relation. Usually, the number of relations is small compared to the number of all documents in the information space. The collection of relation scores $X = \{X_{ij}\}$ forms the weights of edges in a multi-graph, where nodes are all documents in D, and each edge corresponds to a semantic relation. With these notations, the problem can be formalized as follows. Given a collection of documents D, a set of relation scores X, time of interest t, and an activity history L_t corresponding to a user u, or to a group of users U, identify documents with highest importance with respect to u's or U's task and interest at time t.

Propagation Process In this new version of propagation model, we treat the process that the user finds the important documents as a Markov process, when she recalls and searches for important documents via the related resources. For each pair of connected documents (d_i, d_j), we define the transition probability from document d_i to d_j as

$$p_{ij}(w) = \begin{cases} \frac{\sum_k w_k x_{ijk}}{\sum_l \sum_k w_k x_{ilk}} & \text{if } X_{ij} \neq \emptyset \text{ and } L_{d_j,t} \neq \emptyset \\ 0 & \text{otherwise,} \end{cases} \tag{4.2}$$

where w is the weighting vector for the semantic relations in R. The condition $L_{d_j,t} \neq \emptyset$ ensures that the propagation has no effect on the documents that have not been created before the time t, i.e., no propagation to the future. Similarly, the indices l's run only over the documents d_l with $L_{d_l,t} \neq \emptyset$. Consequently, we have $\sum_j p_{ij} = 1$ for all documents d_i. In practice, to avoid rank sink when performing the propagation, if a document has no relation, we assume a dummy edge from it to all other documents with zero probability.

Next, we describe our propagation framework. Let P be the transition matrix of documents in D. We follow the PageRank model to define the propagation as an iterative process

$$\mathbf{s}^{(n+1)} = \lambda P^T \mathbf{s}^{(n)} + (1 - \lambda)\mathbf{v}, \quad (4.3)$$

where $\mathbf{s}^{(n)} = (s(d_1, t), s(d_2, t), \ldots, s(d_m, t))$ is the vector of documents' MB values at iteration n, (m is the number of documents appearing in L_t), $\mathbf{v}$ is the vector of values obtained by an activity-based scoring method, and λ is the damping factor.

Learning Framework: The learning aim is to identify the weights $w_1, \ldots, w_{|R|}$ of the semantic relations which results in the best prediction of document rankings. In this work, we propose to exploit the activity history to learn the optimal w. In particular, we simulate the navigation of the user at each time point t' in the past, and compare the computed ranks of the documents with the ranks based on the frequency of access in the time point $t' + 1$. The idea is to learn w in a way, which minimizes the number of mis-ranked pairs (d_1, d_2), i.e., it minimizes the situations where $s(d_1, t') > s(d_2, t')$, although document d_1 has been accessed less than d_2 until time point $t' + 1$.

Formally, we define the label $y_{ij} = s(d_i, t') - s(d_j, t')$ and the ground-truth $\hat{y}$, $\hat{y}_{ij} = -1$ if d_i has less access than d_j at $t' + 1$ and $\hat{y}_{ij} = 1$ otherwise. We learn w by solving the following optimization problem:

$$\min_w F(w) = \|w\|^2 + \theta \sum_{(d_i,d_j)\in A} h(y_{ij}), \quad (4.4)$$

where A is the training data, θ is the regularization parameter that controls the complexity of the model (i.e., $\|w\|^2$), while minimizing the mis-ranked pairs in A via the loss function h. In this work, we apply the simple hinge loss function: $h(y) = \max(0, 1 - \hat{y}.y)$. Equation 4.4 then can be solved using the well-known supervised PageRank framework [24] employing the gradient-descent-based learning paradigm for efficiency. More details can be found in our paper at [390].

4.4.3.3 Evaluation Results

The methods for computing MB described above have been evaluated in experiments, in order to assess their effectiveness. The following baselines have been used in the evaluation:

Recency–Frequency: These baselines use values of the activity-based scoring functions to provide the final ranking without propagation. This includes the two recency-based methods MRU and Ebb, and their frequency-based variants, denoted as FMRU and FEbb (details in [390]).

PageRank: This baseline ranks the documents by their authority scores, estimated in a graph of documents relations. The scores of documents are initialized equally. It can be thought of as the propagation method without the activity-based rankings and without a differentiation based on relationship types. In our case, we adapt the PageRank algorithm by aggregating all relations between two documents into one single relation, with the weighting score obtained by averaging out all the individual relation weights.

SUPRA: Papadakis et al. [320] proposed combining the activity-based ranking results with a one-step propagation in a layered framework. The relations are constructed simply by identifying documents accessed in the same sessions. In our scenarios, we define the "sessions" to be one unit time step, which is one hour.

The results of the evaluations are reported in detail in [390] and relevant findings are summarized in what follows.

The first experiment aims to evaluate how well the system performs in the revisit prediction task, i.e., predicting the likelihood that a document will be accessed by the user in the subsequent time point. This is the well-established task in research on web recommendation [84], personal file retrieval [139], etc. We evaluate the correlation between the predicted rank of a document at a time point t and the real document accesses at the time point $t + 1$.

Inspired by [197], we have employed the following evaluation metrics:

- Success at 1 (**S@1**): It quantifies the fraction of time points t (from all time points of study) at which the first-ranked documents according to a ranking method are truly accessed at $t+1$. This resembles the Precision at 1 (P@1) metric in traditional IR tasks.
- Success at 10 (**S@10**): It quantifies the fraction of documents truly accessed in the next time point, from all documents ranked at top 10, averaging over all time points of study in the micro-average manner (i.e., per-document average).
- Average Ranking Position (**ARP**): This metric starts from the subsequent document access backwards. It computes the average ranking position of accessed documents as produced by a ranking method. The lower the value, the better the performance of the corresponding ranking system.

From the results of the experiments with the revisit prediction task, some interesting insights can be gained. Among the ranking methods, PageRank has the worst predictive performance. This is because it ignores the recency and frequency signals of the documents. Another interesting observation is that for activity-based ranking methods, adding frequency into the ranking function did not really help in revisit prediction: FMRU performs worse than MRU and FEbb performs worse than Ebb in all metrics, although the differences are not significant. At the first glance, this contradicts somewhat to previous findings on the influence of frequency in document ranking [322]. However, after a deeper analysis, we believe that the cause stems from the fact that a revisiting action typically involves very recent documents, as also argued in [197]. Aggregating recency scores over a time span (10-day window as in our case) can introduce some documents belonging to different tasks and thus bring more noise to the ranking results. One direction for future work is thus to design a more flexible time window size which adapts to the user's task.

Compared to the sole activity-based ranking methods, adding propagation shows clear improvements in prediction, starting from the baseline SUPRA. Bringing semantic relations into the propagation improves even further, producing significantly higher performance for all cases of temporal priors. Our best performing method, propagation with polynomial decay prior, improves the results by 60% as compared to SUPRA. In addition, in contrast to the observed trend in the activity-based ranking, here the combination of frequency and recency with the propagation actually produces better results than the combination between only recency and the propagation.

We also evaluate the effectiveness of our proposed system with respect to the user perception and appreciation. We do this by simulating the way users re-access and reassess the documents in their collections. For this purpose, we performed an experiment with a desktop data set of selected users. Actually, the Semantic Desktop, as discussed in more detail in Chap. 7 was used for this purpose.

In the dataset Person, each assessor chose 4 weeks to evaluate. For the dataset Collaboration, two assessors are asked to choose 3 weeks per each, all are related to joint events they participated in. The activity history is constructed according to the activities of to this pair of users. The ranking methods are configured to provide the ranks of document with respect to the same time step of the user's evaluations. The same trend as in the prediction task can be observed here: The activity-based ranking methods perform better than PageRank but worse than SUPRA and our propagation variants. Similarly, the frequency-based functions perform worse than the recency ones as isolated methods, but improve the results when combined with the propagation. All propagation methods except the MRU prior-based give higher results than SUPRA. In addition, the performance of all methods in the user-perceived study is slightly higher than in the prediction task. This suggests that many of the suggested documents, although not accessed subsequently, are still deemed "important" by the user.

4.4.4 Computing Preservation Value for Desktop Data

For computing PV for desktop data, the Semantic Desktop [273] has been used—a desktop system, which relies on semantic annotation of content and an ontology representing the conceptual information model of the user. The Semantic Desktop is a powerful approach to support organizational as well as personal knowledge management. In computing PV, evidences are used along the PV dimensions of content, type, investment, gravity, social graph, popularity, coverage, and quality. For example, number of annotations and text related to a resource are used to measure investment, the closeness of resources and the importance of some resources (also dependent on their type) are used to consider gravity as well as content type, and image quality is used for the quality dimension. This method for preservation computation is discussed in more detail in Chap. 7.

4.4.5 Computing Preservation Value for Photo Selection

When considering preservation, photos are an important type of content to be preserved for the long run. For photo selection, a user study on this topic has been performed for understanding user expectations with respect to photo collection preservation. An important finding from the user study is that the objective quality of photos is rated as the second least important selection criterion, after the sharing intent. This shows that quality and aesthetics, although being important and used for "general purpose" photo selection, is not considered very important in the case of selecting images for preservation. In contrast, criteria more related to reminiscence, such as event coverage, typical image, and "the picture evokes (positive) memories" are all rated high, with highest ratings for memory evocation.

Exploiting modern multimedia analysis methods as they are described in Chap. 3 of this book and using the results of the user study, an automatic method for predicting long-term importance of photos within a collection has been developed and evaluated. It relies on a number of the aforementioned PV dimensions including the dimensions coverage (in the form of event coverage and the consideration of near duplicates), investment (e.g., when multiple photos are taken of the same situation), and quality (looking into photo quality). The user study and its results as well as the developed photo selection method are discussed in more detail in Chap. 8 of this book.

4.4.6 Investigating Retention in Social Media

In this case study, we looked into the idea of PV or the wish for retention in a social media context. Preservation of human generated content in social media is another important scenario for preservation of personal content. In our study, we took into account the different dimensions of PV by using not only the content itself but also different types of features, e.g., for the popularity of content and the social graph and the relationship of the persons relevant to the content. In this study, we analyzed relevant features for content retention. In addition, we also investigated a method for the automatic recognition of memorable posts based on an adequate training set and a machine learning approach.

4.4.6.1 User Study on Social Media Content Retention

In order to better understand human expectations and build a ground-truth of memorable social network posts, we set up a user study on top of the Facebook platform.

The main goal of this evaluation was to collect participants' opinions regarding retention preferences for their own Facebook posts, shares, and updates of Facebook posts from different time periods. For facilitating the participation, we prepared an intuitive evaluation in a form of Facebook apps. We took extra care regarding the participants' privacy and to comply with Facebook's Platform Policies.[2] A summary of the user study can be found in [117].

In the study, each participant had to judge their own posts on a 5-point Likert scale answering the following question: *Which posts do you think are relevant and worth keeping for the future needs?* Once a post is rated using a 5 points scale starting from 0 (irrelevant) to 4 (extremely relevant), it fades out providing more space for posts to scroll up.

We asked participants to judge about 100–200 of their posts. It is important to note that we are not judging participant's memory skills, but instead we are collecting their personal opinions. Due to that, we presented participants' posts in a chronological order starting from the latest. In this case, for more active users, 100 posts may date back to just a few days, reaching up to months for less active ones.

In order to not only get ratings for the most recent posts shown to users (as it can be biased in displaying posts), we picked starting time points differently among participants in our user study. We defined three distinct groups of participants with respect to the recency of the posts they evaluated. Each participant was randomly assigned to one of the groups at the beginning of evaluation (according to his/her Facebook id). Participants in Group 1 (*recent*) were assigned to evaluate posts starting from the most recent ones (February 2014) in their timelines. Participants in Group 2 (*mid-term*) were assigned to evaluate posts starting from January 2011 and back to this date. Finally, Group 3 (*long-term*) received posts from January 2009 and before (if available). This results in rated posts spanning from 2007 to 2014.

The study was performed between the second week of November 2013 and the third week of February 2014. We had 41 participants, 24 males, and 17 females, with age ranging from 23 to 39 years. In total, there are 8494 evaluated posts. Additionally, once the users provided us authorization to access their data, we were able to collect general numbers that help us to depict the general use of Facebook social network. From 2008 to 2014, on the average, there are about 30 to 100 posts annotated per year and user. For 2007, only three participants evaluated posts, thus we discarded posts from this year for most of the analysis.

Facebook defines seven types of posts, namely, link, checkin, offer, photo, question, swf, and video. This basically describes the type of content that is attached to a post. In the dataset, we found the following distribution among these categories: 42.5% of evaluated posts consists of status updates, followed by shared links (33%), photos (19%), and videos (4%). We disregarded *swf*, *offer*, and *checkin* types, which do not have sufficient occurrences to be significant. We also investigated the distribution of different content types over years. Our observation is that there is a clear increase in the use of videos and photos over time. Several factors help us to explain this change in behavior. First, the catch up of broadband connection allowed users

---

[2] https://developers.facebook.com/policy/.

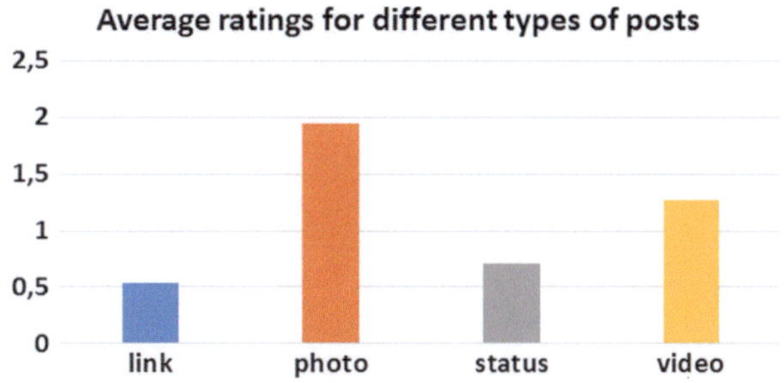

Fig. 4.2 Average ratings of social media content by content type

to quickly upload large amounts of data (photos and videos). Second, the dissemination of smart phones with embedded cameras played an important role. Nowadays, anyone can quickly take a snapshot and upload it on the web. Statistics from photo sharing website Flickr[3] show that the most used cameras are, by far, embedded smart phone cameras.[4] The rate of links and status information changes over years, however, there is no clear trend seen.

In addition, the second characterizing field (so-called *status_type*) defines predefined actions taken by the user. For example, the type 'photo' can have *status_* type 'added_photos', 'tagged_in_photo', or 'shared_story'. Due to space limitation, we left out the analysis of these types, nevertheless, we use these features in our experiments. The distribution of ratings in the full dataset shows a clear dominance (57%) of irrelevant posts (with rating 0). This is followed by 16% of posts with rating 1; 13% with rating 2; 8% with rating 3 and 6% of top-rated posts (with rating 4). This results in an average rating of 0.92 with standard deviation 1.58 and variance 1.26.

When looking into the individual content types (see Fig. 4.2), we found out that *photos* have the highest average rating of 1.94 followed by *videos* with an average rating of 1.27. The average ratings of *status* updates (0.71) and *links* (0.54) are much lower suggesting a dominating role of photos and videos for memorable posts.

Besides other features relevant for identifying memorable posts, we are interested in the role of time in deciding about content retention, i.e., whether older content on the average is rated lower than more recent content. For this purpose, we analyzed the dependency between content ratings and the age of content.

In Fig. 4.3, the dash line shows the average rating for the different years of content creation.

The image shows a clear trend where participants in the evaluation assigned higher ratings to more recent posts. This is in line with the idea of a decay function underlying the content retention model. The decrease in the average rating with growing age of content is especially steep in the first year (2013/2014). However, we also see an increase in the rating values in 2008, where we leave this for further investigation. In Fig. 4.3 (solid lines), we see the development of the average ratings for individual content types (videos have only been included starting in 2010, because

[3]http://www.flickr.com.

[4]http://www.flickr.com/cameras.

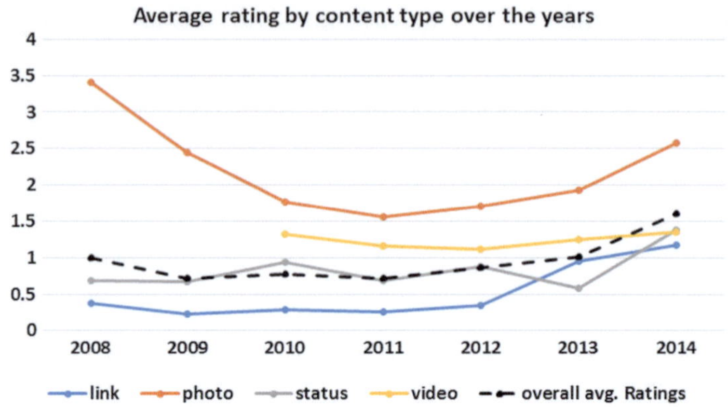

Fig. 4.3 Observed average ratings for increasing content age (the dash line), and the average ratings for individual content types over increasing content age (solid lines)

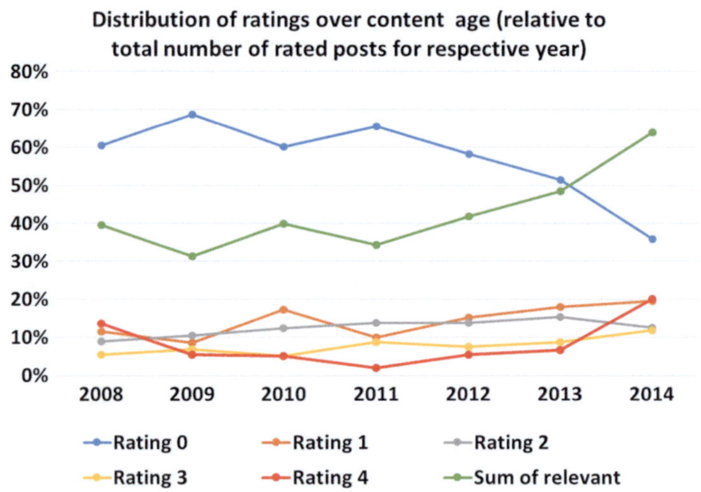

Fig. 4.4 Distribution of the ratings per content types over years

the number of videos in the dataset before 2010 is very small). Once more, we observe an increase of ratings for the most recent content. However, we also see very high average ratings for older photos (older than 5 years). Thus, we assume that seeing these older (already forgotten) photos again caused some positive surprise, which resulted in higher ratings. This perception would support the idea of creating Facebook summaries for reminiscence. However, this still would require further investigation, since unfortunately only a rather small number of photos was available for rating in 2008 and thus the observation is only based on a rather small data set.

For analyzing the temporal behavior in more detail, Fig. 4.4 shows the distribution (ratio) of ratings 0–4 among the content categories over years (content age).

Besides the dominance of content rated as irrelevant (blue line, rating 0), we can see a clear decrease of content rated as irrelevant for the more recent content. Accordingly, there is an increase of content rated *relevant*, which is shown in the green line as an aggregation of content rated from 1 to 4. An increase of positively rated posts can especially be seen for content rated as very relevant (red line, rating 4), which increases its rating by a factor of 4 from 2010 to 2014. Figure 4.4 also supports the idea of a decay function (forgetting) when assessing the memorability of older posts.

On Facebook, users are able to *comment* or *like* a particular post. *Comments* are a very common feature on the web. Any user (with a adequate permission) is able to express her opinion on a subject. *Like* is a particular feature of Facebook where users vote to show their appreciation on a given post. Both actions have a limited audience that is imposed by the author of the original post. In the most common case (default setup), a user's post is visible for her network of friends, and those are the ones that are able to comment and like the post. Our first analysis of results already suggests that the average number of comments and average number of likes for the evaluated posts have an impact on the rating of the post: the higher the number of likes and number of comments, the higher the rating.

From these statistics, one can deduce first ideas for determining features that have a high impact in the identification of memorable posts. Roughly speaking, recent photos with high number of likes and high number of comments seem to be the best evidence.

User Feedback: To further complement our user studies, we asked the participants to fill a short survey in order to give us qualitative feedback to understand people's Facebook habits. All participants stated that the main use of Facebook is for communication, 83% claimed using Facebook in private life matters and 50% for business. Additionally, 58% of the participants claimed to use Facebook as a personal archive.

Regarding this preservation aspect, half of the participants claimed to have deleted (at least once) older posts. Almost 74% of the participants also stated that they have removed their tag (once or more) associated to a particular picture. Interestingly, when asked if they "care" about their profiles and timelines, only 50% answered yes, contradicting with the fact that they sometimes "clean" their profiles.

To summarize this section, we performed a user study in order to collect a ground-truth for memorable posts. The primary data analyzes show that most of the posts (around 60%) are considered expendable and, temporal aspects have significant impact on memorability perception. In this light, in the following sections, we present a series of experiments in order to empirically uncover the best features that identify memorable items.

4.4.6.2 Features for Retention

The annotated dataset provides the basis for building models for ranking memorable items. Feature selection experiments allow to identify a compact core feature set for the task at hand.

For capturing factors that might influence retention decisions of users, we compiled a broad set of 139 features. They can be categorized in five groups: temporal, social interactions, content-based, privacy, and network. The inclusion of temporal features is inspired by the idea that retention preferences are influenced by a decay function as it was also confirmed by the data analysis in the previous section.

For temporal features, we consider the temporal aspect of the post in terms of creation date, age, and lifetime. While "age" is the time between the evaluation and creation date, "lifetime" is measuring the active time of a post starting at the time it was created to the last update. We also use variants of the age feature, which use the time of the last update and the time of the last commenting, respectively, instead of the creation time.

The social features capture core signals of social interaction in a social web application, covering the features that are typically used in Facebook analysis: number of likes (No.Likes), number of comments (No.Comments), and number of shares (No.Shares).

The next group of features are content-based features. We use the type of the post and some specific meta data about the post. This is based on the content-based features offered by Facebook and includes, for example, features such as status type, type, hasLink, hasIcon, app type, etc. We map each categorical feature (like status type) to multiple binary features. To respect user privacy and the privacy policies, the only text-based feature in our set is the length of text included in posts and comments. In other words, we do not utilize the textual content of posts.

The privacy features are based on the privacy options offered by Facebook, which are used to restrict the access to a post to a particular set of user.

Furthermore, for each post, we compute standard network measures, such as, cluster coefficient, density, diameter, path length, and modularity. The network features are extracted from the network of all users involved in a post, and also on the networks of likes and comments.

We also use a personalized normalization (Pers.) for the social and network features based on the average values of the collections of individual users. This better adapts the features to the individual characteristics and behavior of individual users. Including the normalized version of the features, we use 5 temporal, 6 social features, 47 content-based, 13 privacy, and 68 network features. The number of network features is relatively high since we analyze the typical network features for the different types of social graphs that are implied by Facebook interactions separately (e.g., likes, messages, and comments), and also include a normalized version of each of these features.

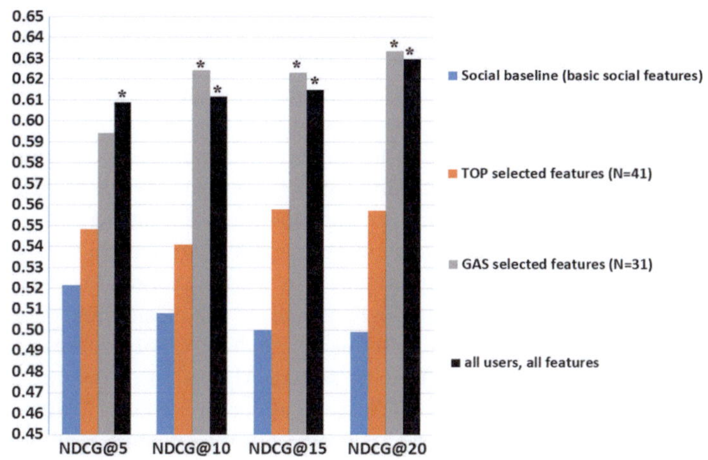

Fig. 4.5 Effectiveness of ranking

4.4.6.3 Learning Models for Ranking with Feature Selection

Based on the candidate features, our goal here is ranking a user's posts to identify the most memorable ones as it is a crucial stage for various interesting applications, such as constructing targeted summaries. To this end, we adopt strategies from the web search domain, where machine-learned rankers are heavily investigated and, as far as we know, incorporated into commercial search engines [245]. If we make an analogy, a user in our case corresponds to a query in the search setup, and user's posts correspond to the documents retrieved for the query. During the training stage, for a given user u, we construct an m-dimensional feature vector F for each post of this user, and augment the vector with the label r assigned to this post (obviously, labels are the ratings collected in the user study, after a mapping to a range 0–4 as the posts rated as 1 are not at all considered memorable). For the testing, we feed vectors in the form of $< u, F >$ to the learnt model for each user in the test set; and the model outputs a ranked list of posts for each user. We evaluate the success of the ranking using a typical metric from the literature, namely, Normalized Discounted Cumulative Gain (NDCG), which is a rank sensitive metric that takes into account graded labels. We report NDCG scores at the cutoff values of $\{5, 10, 15, 20\}$.

In the experiments, we employ a well-known algorithm, namely RankSVM, from learning-to-rank literature [185]. Instead of single data instances, RankSVM considers pairs of instances (posts of a user, in our case) while building a model. We apply leave-one-out cross validation.

Figure 4.5 reveals the performance of RankSVM for ranking posts using all the proposed features. As a baseline, we also train a model using three basic social features, namely, the number of likes, comments, and shares. We choose the latter features for the baseline ranker as they are the most intuitive popularity signals in social web and very likely to be involved in practical applications, such as the

Facebook's post ranking applications. The results show that our proposed features are actually very useful, and using these features for training a ranker yields relative effectiveness improvement of up to 26% over the baseline ranker trained with the basic social features (i.e., comparing the first and last bars for each metric in Fig. 4.5).

The next question we address is: Can we identify a subset of the proposed features that has the highest impact in ranking memorable posts? While feature selection methods are widely applied for various classification tasks, only a few works have investigated their performance in a learning-to-rank framework [108, 116, 146]. Here, we adopt two filtering-type approaches: In the first approach, so-called TOP, we use each feature on its own to rank the posts of the users, and then choose top-N features with highest effectiveness in terms of the NDCG@10 scores [108]. Second, we adopt the so-called GAS (Greedy search Algorithm of Feature Selection) introduced by Geng et al. [146]. In GAS, we again compute each feature's isolated effectiveness, but additionally, we also compute pairwise feature similarity, i.e., to what extent the top-10 rankings generated by two different features correlate. To compute the similarity of two ranked lists, we use Kendall's Tau metric. Then, the feature selection proceeds in a greedy manner as follows: In each iteration, first the feature with the highest effectiveness score is selected. Next, all other features' effectiveness scores are discounted with their similarity to the already selected feature. The algorithm stops when it reaches the required number of features, N. We experiment for all possible values of N, from 1 to 138 (as $N = 139$ is the case with all features), and evaluate the performance. Figure 4.5 also demonstrates that feature selection with TOP strategy (for the best performing value of N, which is found to be 41) cannot outperform models trained with all available features. However, using GAS strategy and with only 30 features we can achieve the same effectiveness as using all 139 features (i.e., compare the third and last bars for each metric in Fig. 4.5).

For this latter case, we analyze the features selected by GAS in each fold to identify the most promising features for the task of ranking posts. As the absolute value of the weights assigned to features by the RankSVM model (built using a linear kernel) can reflect the importance of features [72], we average these absolute values for the features appearing in the learnt model in each fold. Table 4.2 shows the features with the highest average scores in the models built after feature selection with GAS.

We see that the most discriminative features cover all four feature categories except the privacy. Regarding top-10 features in the list, content-based and social categories, with 4 and 3 features respectively, are the most influential ones. We also observe that features that are adapted to the behavior pattern of individual users such as pers.no.likes play an important role for ranking memorable posts. Interestingly, the feature content type is outperformed by the feature status type. Our explanation is that status type can be considered as a refined form of content type, which captures what has been done with the content (e.g., "added photo"). This more fine grained information has proven to be more important for the ranking task than the information on the content type alone. Network features computed from the graphs in the social network have less impact for the characterization of memorable posts. And finally, the temporal feature age is also among the top-10 features, a finding in line with our earlier claims on the relationship of the time and human retention preferences.

Table 4.2 Best features selected by GAS—core social features (baseline) denoted by*

Category	Feature	Weight
Content-base	Pers.Length Description	1.676
Social	No.Shares*	1.190
Social	Pers.No.Shares	0.471
Social	No.Likes*	0.453
Network	Overlap.No.Friends (all)	0.392
Content-base	Status_Type	0.329
Temporal	age (created time)	0.327
Content-base	Pers.Length.Story	0.326
Network	Cluster Coefficient	0.320
Content-base	Length Message	0.269
Social	Pers.No.Likes	0.260
Content-base	APP_Type	0.259
Content-base	hasMessage	0.200
Content-base	Length Story	0.199
Content-base	hasDescription	0.167
Content-base	hasStory	0.151
Content-base	Type	0.140
Content-base	Length Comments	0.140
Content-base	Pers.Length Message	0.115
Temporal	CreatedTime	0.112
Network	Density (all)	0.091
Social	Pers.No.Comments	0.065
Content-base	Length Description	0.063
Network	Overlap.No.Friends (likes)	0.059
Network	Path length (like)	0.023
Network	Overlap.No.Friends (tagged)	0.009
Social	No.Comments*	0.006

The results summarized in Fig. 4.5 are encouraging, because, even in a relatively small setup with 41 users in total, our approach considerably improves the NDCG@5 and NDCG@15 scores in comparison to using a single ranking model (i.e., compare the first and last bars in the figure for each metric). Finally, we also experimented with feature selection in this setup, where we applied Top-N and GAS strategies. In Fig. 4.5, we only report the results for the better performing GAS strategy. It turns out that feature selection using GAS strategy is outperforming the basic social features significantly, denoted with ⋆ in Fig. 4.5, as well as the set of all features for NDCG@10, NDCG@15, and NDCG@20.

4.5 Forgetting Actions—Leveraging Information Value

The raw information value, as it has been discussed in the previous sections is only part of the managed forgetting approach, although a very central one. It describes the short or long-term value of an information object. In this section, we investigate how information value—PV as well as MB—can be used as part of the managed forgetting approach. There are different ways of leveraging those types of information values.

First of all those values can be made accessible to users for supporting users' decisions (see Sect. 4.5.1). This is especially helpful if it is combined with an adequate form of visualization or categorization. Second, such values can be used by other information management and information access methods such as search for reflecting the forgetful approach, such as implementing a forgetful version of search (see Sect. 4.5.2). Finally, those information values can be used for supporting and/or partially automating decision making. This is especially relevant in the context of preservation decisions (see Sect. 4.5.3).

4.5.1 *Informing the User*

The value coming from information value assessment can be directly used to inform the user about the current value or importance of an object. Such numeric values are, however, difficult to interpret. Therefore, a translation into categories using adequate thresholds might be helpful and ease decision-making based on the information values MB and PV.

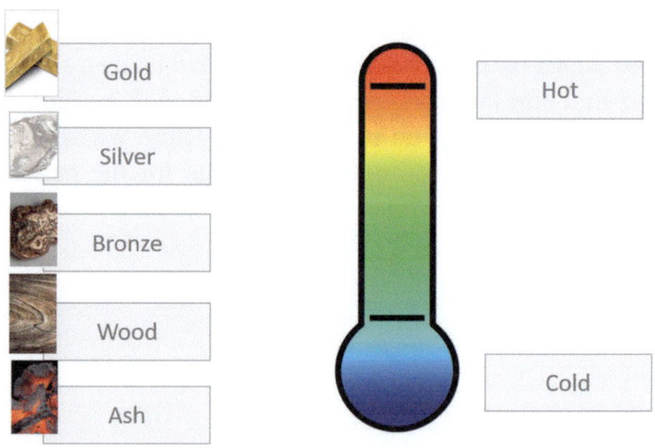

Fig. 4.6 Visualization options/logical categories for Preservation Value (left) and Memory Buoyancy (right)

This is especially important for decisions with respect to preservation. Information objects can for example be grouped into the categories such as *gold*, *silver*, *bronze*, *wood*, and *ash* based on their PV as shown in Fig. 4.6. Similar category sets can be imagined for MB values, where "temperature" might serve as an adequate metaphor for short-term importance. A possible category set for short-term importance, thus, could be *hot*, *warm*, *lukewarm*, and *cold*. Such human-readable labels make it easier for the user to interpret the respective information value.

Those categories can also be used in visualization of the respective information objects. This may include visual highlighting of important items, e.g., framing in strong colors, marking, etc. At the opposite site of the range, less important items can be visually unstressed up to hiding information objects, which are currently not important. This leads directly to the use of information value in information access methods as it is discussed in the next subsection.

4.5.2 Forgetful Methods

Information value can also be incorporated into other methods used for information access and information management. The aforementioned visualizations, which support highlighting and/or hiding selected information objects, are already a first example incorporating information values, e.g., in a file management system.

More demanding ways of incorporating information value are possible, when combining forgetting and search into what we call forgetful search. Here, the relevance assessment of an information objects based on its content and the query can be combined with the current importance of the object according to the information value assessment.

The easiest way of combination is by use of a threshold. Only information objects with a information value above a specific information value (the threshold) are incorporated into the search result, i.e., information objects below the threshold although relevant to the queries are hidden in the search or excluded from the search result. More advanced forms of forgetful search can be achieved by flexibly combining the impact of relevance and information value in a mixed formula.

Other forms of forgetful methods refer to different forms of reduction and aggregation. Less important information items might be summarized or condensed in other ways (e.g., for images). Furthermore, redundancies in the form of duplicates or near duplicates can be reduced by just keeping one or a smaller number of the (near) duplicates. This aspect has already been raised in the context of the PV dimensions and is further elaborated for the photo section method presented in Chap. 8.

4.5.3 Supporting Preservation Decisions

The most obvious way of using the PV is to make decisions about preservation. A threshold can be set and only resources with a PV above this threshold will be considered for preservation (i.e., sent to the preservation system). Such a process can be automated or the resources above the threshold can be presented to the user for final decision.

One possible time point for preservation decisions, is when the respective resource goes out of active use (decreased MB for a specified time period). Before this point in time, it might be expensive to keep track of the changes of the resource in the active system and to synchronize them with the resource copy in the preservation store. Waiting until long after the active life of the resource will put resources with high PV at risk. Other scheduling options would be a regular (e.g., monthly) computation of PV with preservation decisions or a manually triggered PV computation (e.g., for a collection of photos or the resources of a project, which has been completed).

The Preservation Value cannot only be used for binary preservation decisions: preserve or not preserve. It has to be noted again that "not preserve" does not mean "delete". It just means the resource is not sent to the preservation system. It might still reside in the active system or any type of backup system. The PV or a category inferred from this value can also be provided to the preservation system as an indication of the effort to be invested for the respective resource. As mentioned above, human-readable categories such as "gold", "silver", "bronze", etc., can help the user in getting an intuitive understanding of PV. The PV (or PV categories) can be used by the preservation system to select the adequate preservation levels (e.g., how much redundancy, how much effort to put into conversions to new formats etc.). In addition, the PV can also be used for deciding about other preservation options such as just preserving a summary of a collection of images with low PV or storing more context information for a resource with high PV (see discussion on redundancy above). Such actions on top of the PV can be build into a preservation system for achieving more intelligent, value-aware preservation systems.

4.6 Conclusions

In this chapter, we have introduced the concept of managed forgetting as an alternative to the currently dominating keep-it-all-(and-live-with-random-survival) strategy. We have presented its opportunities and challenges as well as first steps towards its implementation.

Information value assessment, which is in the core of managed forgetting, has been considered from a short-term and a long-term perspective resulting Memory Buoyancy (MB) as an information value linked to current importance of a resource and Preservation Value (PV) related to expected long-term benefit, respectively. Assessing information value especially with a long-term perspective is a challenging and setting-dependent task, since it implies anticipating future uses of a resource. In the chapter, we also presented first methods for computing MB and PV for different settings such as social media content and personal desktop data with further methods being discussed in Chaps. 7 and 8. The discussion of information value assessment has been complemented by the presentation of various forgetting actions, i.e., methods for leveraging the computed information value for achieving a full implementation of managed forgetting in support of more effective information management and preservation solutions.

It is, however, clear that further research is still required for a full realization of the novel approach of managed forgetting. This includes for example methods for information value assessment for further settings, the implementation and evaluation of further forgetting actions, and an improved understanding of the interaction and possible synergies between human forgetting and digital forgetting.

Chapter 5
Keeping Information in Context

Mark A. Greenwood, Nam Khanh Tran, Konstantinos Apostolidis and Vasileios Mezaris

Abstract Without context, words have no meaning, and the same is true for documents, in that often a wider context is required to fully interpret the information they contain. For example, a family photo is practically useless if you do not know who the people portrayed in it are, and likewise, a document that refers to the president of the US is of little use without knowing who held the job at the time the document was written. This becomes even more important when considering the long-term preservation of documents, as not only is human memory fallible, but over long periods the people accessing the documents will change (e.g. photos passed down through generations), as will their understanding and knowledge of the world. While preserving the context associated with a document is an important first step in ensuring information remains useful over long periods of time, we also need to consider how information evolves. Over any significant time period, the meaning of information changes. This evolution can range from changes in the meaning of individual words to more general terms or concepts, such as who holds a specific position in an organization. In this chapter, we look in detail at all of these challenges and describe the development of a conceptual framework in which context information can be collected, preserved, evolved and used to access and interpret documents. A number of techniques are presented showing real examples of context in action that fit within the framework, and applying to both text documents and image collections.

M. A. Greenwood (✉)
The University of Sheffield, Western Bank, Sheffield S10 2TN, UK
e-mail: m.a.greenwood@sheffield.ac.uk

N. K. Tran
L3S Research Center, Leibniz Universität Hannover, Appelstrasse 9a,
30167 Hannover, Germany
e-mail: ntran@l3s.de

K. Apostolidis · V. Mezaris
Information Technologies Institute (ITI), Centre for Research
and Technology Hellas (CERTH), 57001 Thermi, Greece
e-mail: kapost@iti.gr

V. Mezaris
e-mail: bmezaris@iti.gr

V. Mezaris et al. (eds.), *Personal Multimedia Preservation*, Springer Series
on Cultural Computing, https://doi.org/10.1007/978-3-319-73465-1_5

5.1 What Is Context?

You shall know a word by the company it keeps. J. R. Firth, 1957

In its simplest form, context is external information which is either required or aids in understanding an 'item'. This extra information may just be a few words to help disambiguate a single word [137] (is a bulb a light bulb or the root of a plant; without context you cannot be sure) or it might be large quantities of extra information (understanding a document on geopolitics, for example, may require a lot of extra background information). Time also plays an important factor in what context is needed. Terms that are unambiguous in today's world can easily fall out of use or their use change over time. A good example of this is the word computer which used to refer to a person employed to do computations, a meaning which many people today are unaware of. This means that while many concepts might not need to be explained now, their meaning would need to be captured as context information and preserved so that they could be unambiguously interpreted in the future.

Broadly speaking, there are two main types of knowledge, world and personal, that can provide context for a document. World knowledge is usually the same for everyone and describes the world in which we live. This kind of knowledge is already collected and encoded in a number of successful projects, such as DBpedia and Wikidata. Barring a large-scale digital dark age [212], this general knowledge will continue to be accessible even in the distant future. Personal knowledge, however, is often never written down, and once lost cannot be recreated, so it is exceedingly important that this information be captured and archived if personal documents are to be preserved and kept useful over long periods of time. Personal knowledge does not, of course, have to refer simply to an individual. Organizations also have a world view and internal domain knowledge that is unique to them. When preserving company documents, capturing this organizational memory is just as important as capturing world knowledge and the personal knowledge of the person who authored the document.

The rest of this section gives an overview of different types of context and shows how it might be gathered and used through an illustrative example, before the more technical aspects are discussed later in the chapter.

5.1.1 An Illustrated Example

Rather than focusing on the technical details, we shall start by looking at an example illustrating the main concepts, which paved the way for the development of many of the components documented in the rest of this chapter. This revolves around a diary entry and a photo covering a single event that occurred during a meeting held in Luleå, Sweden.

If we assume that this diary entry is the first document (text or image) that we are preserving, then we will have no existing personal store of world knowledge

Jörgen had offered to take Elaine, Maria, and Robert out to Gammelstad this morning before the meeting started as they are looking at running a memory study there over the summer. When Jörgen arrived to pick them up I decided to be cheeky and ask if there was room in the car for one more. There was so I got to do the touristy thing of looking around while everyone else did some actual work. A large snow pile made an excellent back drop for Robert to take a group photo which hopefully I'll get a copy of at some point. It was certainly an interesting place to look around and you can understand why it is a UNESCO world heritage site.

Diary Entry 5.1 File metadata list the author as 'Mark A. Greenwood' and the creation data as the 12th of February 2014

to call upon. The first stage of contextualization will therefore be to link the document to a source of world knowledge, which for this example we will assume is Wikipedia (implementations of this idea are more likely to use DBpedia, but for a *handworked* example, Wikipedia makes more sense). In this instance, that would involve generating links to the pages for Gammelstad[1] and UNESCO,[2] as they are the two *famous* entities within the text. This leaves five entity mentions (Jörgen, Elaine, Maria, Robert and I) which, if not well known, must fall within the user's personal knowledge.

With no pre-existing store of personal knowledge available to act as context, the only information we have is the file metadata, which allows us to map the first person pronoun *I* to the document's author *Mark A. Greenwood*. This leaves us with four unknown people for which the system would need to prompt the user for additional data. At a minimum, this additional data should probably consist of a person's full name and their relationship to the user (i.e. Robert Logie is a collaborator on the ForgetIT project and works at The University of Edinburgh). Alternatively, such information could be available from the user's own information sources, such as (electronic) address book, email account or calendar.

Having gathered this information, the next step would be to store the current personal knowledge in an archive. The diary entry could then be contextualized by storing not only the entry itself but also links to both the world and personal knowledge.

In addition to allowing us to store extra context information alongside the diary entry, this has also started the process of building up a repository of personal knowledge which can in turn be used to contextualize new documents more accurately and with less user intervention. It would be beneficial if this linking process were part of an interactive feedback loop [150] so that users could see the benefit of existing data being used to enhance their output (e.g. links to Gammelstad and UNESCO appearing *magically*) as this would encourage them to provide personal data when prompted.

Having now fully contextualized the diary entry, let us turn our attention to the task of contextualizing and preserving Photo 5.1. The first thing to note is that the photo and the diary entry clearly act as context for one another. If both were archived

[1] http://en.wikipedia.org/wiki/Gammelstad_Church_Town.

[2] http://en.wikipedia.org/wiki/UNESCO.

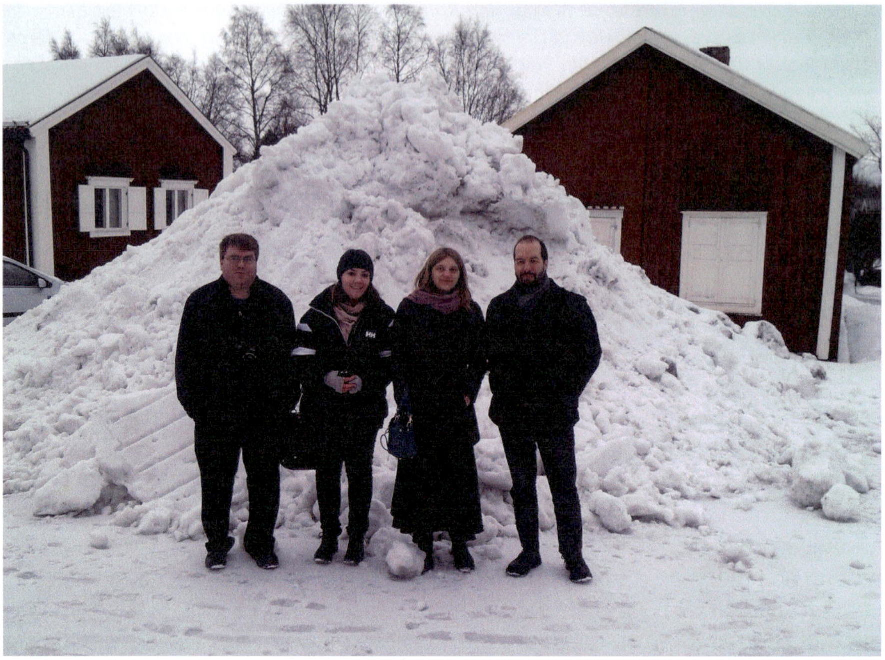

Photo. 5.1 Metadata associated with this photo show that it was taken at 7:48:33 UTC on the 12th of February 2014 at N65°38′42.75′′ E22°1′38.573′′ at a magnetic bearing of 171.5°. Copyright © Robert Logie

at the same time, this context would be obvious, but as we are assuming that the photo is being preserved at a later date than the diary entry, then this link needs to be made clear. This highlights the fact that one important source of contextual information is the documents which have already been archived. Previously archived documents can act as context in two ways:

- An item being preserved can refer to previously preserved items. In this case, a link between Photo 5.1 and Diary Entry 5.1 could be explicitly recorded to provide contextual information that explains both the occasion of the photo and its content (i.e. the people and location).
- The processing of each new item adds to what we know about the individual user's personal knowledge. In this example, contextualizing the diary entry will have led to four previously unknown people being added to the user's personal knowledge.

It is likely that the explicit linking of the diary and photo would be a manual action taken by the user. It may, however, be possible to suggest the relationship to the user based on the associated metadata and context information generated when the diary entry was preserved. First, the photo and the diary were both created, according to the metadata, on the same day (the 12th of February 2014), which at least suggests a common context. Furthermore, the GPS information can be used to search for

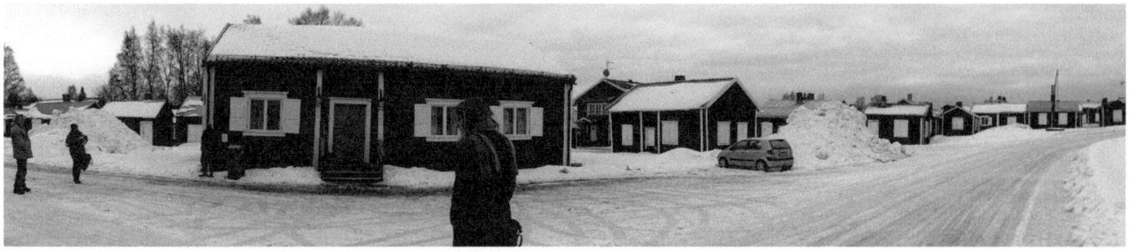

Photo. 5.2 A *wider* context? Copyright © Mark A. Greenwood

Wikipedia pages describing nearby places which would link the photo to the same page describing Gammelstad[3] as used to provide world knowledge for the diary entry. Combining the GPS data with magnetic bearing (if available) and the focal length of the shot, a list of places that may be visible can also be extracted and proposed to the user. An example of place information for Photo 5.1 (based on the GPS info listed in the caption) is given below:

Visible	Name	Type(s)	Distance
No	Luleå V	Sublocality level 1 Sublocality Political	13626 m
No	Äldreboende Ingridshem	Establishment	290 m
No	Snickare Anders Viklund i Luleå AB	Establishment	225 m
No	Öhemsvgen	Bus station Transit station Establishment	225 m

The GPS metadata associated with the photo could also be used to select other photos which could act as context. In this example, Photo 5.2 has almost identical GPS metadata, but clearly shows a wider view than the original photo and would help to provide a larger visual context.

In a similar way to textual documents, images can be contextualized based on their content as well as their associated metadata. In this example, face detection would highlight the four people in the photo and could be used to prompt the user to identify the people. If the link to the diary entry had already been formed, then the names of the people associated with it could even be suggested. Also, face clustering can detect similar (already named) faces in existing archived images and suggest them to the user. As all the personal knowledge needed for contextualizing the photo was already gathered and stored for the diary entry, the previously preserved personal knowledge can be referenced to avoid duplication of information within the preservation system.

[3]https://en.wikipedia.org/w/api.php?action=query&list=geosearch&gscoord=65.6452|22.0274.

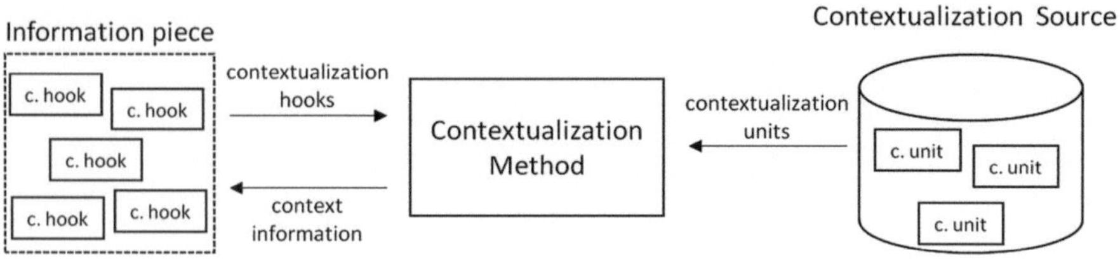

Fig. 5.1 A general overview of contextualization

5.1.2 A Generalised Approach to Contextualization

While the aforementioned example shows how context information can be gathered and used in order to aid in preserving documents in an unambiguous form, a slightly more abstract description of how we view the process of contextualization will help set the scene for the more technical details which make up the rest of this chapter.

Our view of the process of contextualizing a document can be summarized as in Fig. 5.1. We have an 'information piece' (a document or image) which needs contextualizing. This item contains a number of 'context hooks' which refer to information possibly recorded elsewhere, or about which more information should be captured as part of the process of contextualization. As we will see later in this chapter, these hooks could be named entities or phrases in a text document, or concepts visible in an image. As well as the document being processed, there is a store of information that can be used as a 'contextualization source' which contains information, referred to as 'context units', which can provide information about one or more 'context hooks'. The job of any 'contextualization method' is therefore to link a 'context hook' to one or more 'context units' and to preserve this association along with the 'information piece'.

5.2 Techniques for Contextualization

As with any complex task, there are many ways to approach solving the contextualization problem. Approaches will clearly differ depending on the type of document being processed: text versus images, long documents versus short documents, etc. It is also possible, of course, to have multiple competing and/or complementary approaches that can be tested on the same set of documents. Put simply, there is no single solution to contextualization. The rest of this section is devoted to a number of different approaches to contextualization that aim to cover a broad range of document types. The first section focuses on text documents, followed by approaches for contextualizing image collections.

5.2.1 Contextualizing Text

As with many techniques that process textual information, the genres, writing styles and lengths of the documents play an important part in the effectiveness of a given contextualization technique. Specifically, we found that document length plays a highly significant role, which is understandable given that a longer document contains more information and therefore is likely to be more self-contained. We have therefore developed separate techniques for processing long versus short documents [71, 384, 385, 387].

5.2.1.1 Temporal Contextualization of Short Texts

With the continued growth and adoption of Twitter and other microblogging platforms for the dissemination of news, there has been a parallel increase in Natural Language Processing (NLP) research aimed specifically at this style of short texts. This work ranges from those approaches which aim for a deep understanding of the information within a tweet (or similar sized posts on any other microblogging platform), often using semantic annotation to link entities within a tweet to a knowledge base [152, 157, 292], to work on adopting underlying techniques, such as Part-of-Speech tagging and tokenization, to the style of language usually seen in these short posts [45, 317, 339].

Much of this work focuses on processing each tweet in isolation, but tweets usually form part of a larger conversation, either through replies or the use of hashtags. The occurrence of the same hashtag in a large body of tweets from a single time period (usually referred to as a trending hashtag) clearly suggests a connection that can be used, at least in part, as clues to context, but to date, this data has largely been left unexplored.

In this section, we study the problem of annotating trending hashtags on Twitter using entities derived from Wikipedia. Instead of establishing a static semantic connection between hashtags and entities, we are interested in dynamically linking the hashtags to entities that are closest to the underlying events during the time period the hashtag is trending; hence, we allow the context to evolve over time. For instance, while '#sochi' refers to a city in Russia, during February 2014, the hashtag was used to report the *2014 Winter Olympics* (cf. Fig. 5.2); therefore, it should be linked more to Wikipedia pages related to the event than to the location.

Compared with traditional domains of text (e.g. news articles), associating hashtags with known entities poses additional challenges. Hashtags' surface forms (i.e. the sequence of characters) are very ad hoc, as they are chosen not in favour of the text quality but to be short and memorable. In addition, the rapid evolution of the semantics of hashtags (e.g. in the case of '#sochi') makes them more ambiguous. Furthermore, a hashtag can encode multiple topics at one time period. For example, in March 2014, '#oscar' refers to the *86th Academy Awards*, but at the same time also to the *Trial of Oscar Pistorius*. Sometimes, it is difficult even for humans to understand a trending hashtag without knowledge about what is happening with the entities in the real world (such as the trial of Oscar Pistorius). Automatic processing of hashtags can also be complicated by the use of multi-word expressions, which can be difficult to interpret [280]. A famous example, #nowthatcherisdead, saw many people on Twitter misinterpreting the death of Margaret Thatcher as the death of the pop star Cher.

In this work, we describe a novel solution to these challenges by exploiting temporal knowledge about entity dynamics derived from Wikipedia. We hypothesize that a trending hashtag indicates an increase in public attention to certain entities which can also be observed on Wikipedia. For example, in Fig. 5.2, we can identify *2014 Winter Olympics* as a prominent entity for '#sochi' during February 2014, by observing the change of user attention to the entity, for instance, via the page view statistics of Wikipedia articles. We exploit both Wikipedia edits and page views for annotation. We also propose a novel learning method, inspired by the information spreading nature of social media, to suggest the optimal annotations without the need for human labelling.

For this work, we have chosen to study hashtags at the daily level, i.e. we only consider the creation day of the tweet (from its timestamp). A hashtag is classified as 'trending' at a point in time if the number of tweets it occurs in is significantly higher than on other days [221, 225]. Each trending hashtag can be associated with one or more 'burst time periods' surrounding the trending time points, where the user's interest in the underlying topic remains stronger than during other periods. The problem is formally defined as follows: *Given a trending hashtag h and the burst time period $T(h)$ of h, identify the top-k most prominent entities e for h.*

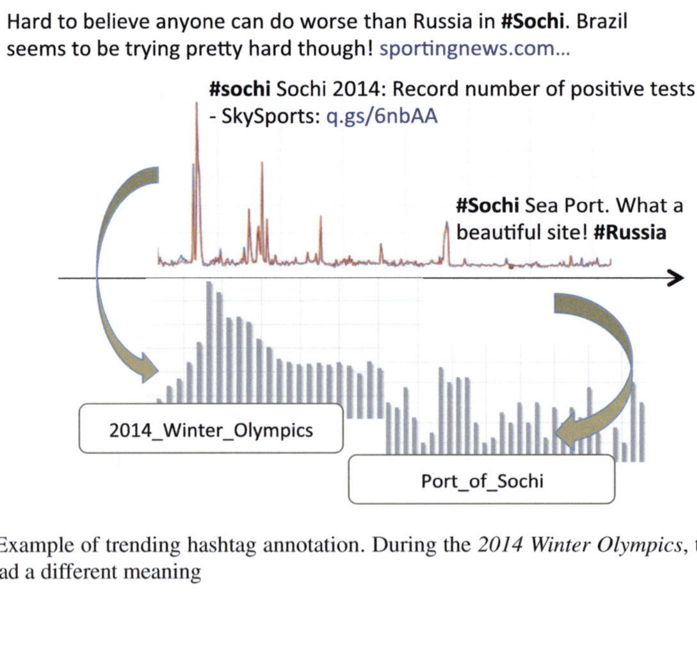

Fig. 5.2 Example of trending hashtag annotation. During the *2014 Winter Olympics*, the hashtag '#sochi' had a different meaning

It is worth noting that not all trending hashtags are mappable to Wikipedia entities, as the coverage of topics in Wikipedia is much lower than on Twitter, a limitation common to all systems which rely on Wikipedia, and we therefore focus on precision over recall. Our approach breaks down into three main components. The first step is to identify all entity candidates using the text of the tweets associated with a hashtag. In the second step, we compute a number of similarity scores between each candidate and the hashtag, based on different types of contexts. Finally, we learn an unsupervised, unified ranking function for each hashtag-entity pair and choose the top-k entities with the highest scores.

The most obvious resource to identify candidate entities for a hashtag is via its tweets. We follow common approaches that use a lexicon to match each textual phrase in a tweet to a potential entity set [135, 361]. Our lexicon is constructed from Wikipedia page titles, hyperlink anchors, redirects and disambiguation pages. We generate textual phrases by generating all n-grams ($n \leq 5$) from the input tweets within $T(h)$. We apply the longest match heuristic [292]: we start with the longest n-grams and stop as soon as an entity set is found; otherwise, we continue with the constituent, smaller n-grams.

While lexicon-based linking works well for single tweets, applying it on the hashtag level has subtle implications. Processing a huge amount of text, especially during a hashtag trending time period, incurs expensive computational costs. Therefore, to guarantee a good recall in this step while still maintaining a feasible computation, we apply entity linking only on a random sample of the complete tweet set, $T(h)$. For each candidate entity e, we also include all entities whose Wikipedia article is linked with the article of e by an outgoing or incoming link.

To rank the entity by prominence, we measure the similarity between each candidate entity and the hashtag. We evaluate three types of similarities. The first type, *mention similarity*, relies on the explicit mentions of entities in tweets and assumes that entities directly linked from more prominent anchors are more relevant to the hashtag. It is estimated using both statistics from Wikipedia and tweet phrases and turns out to be surprisingly effective in practice.

For entities that are not directly linked to mentions (the mention similarity is zero), we exploit external resources instead, such as web pages linked from tweets, or entities' home pages. By exploiting the content of entities from these external sources, we can complement the explicit similarity metrics based on mentions. We refer to this as *context similarity*.

The first two metrics rely on the textual representation and are degraded by the linguistic difference between the two platforms. To overcome this drawback, we incorporate the temporal dynamics of hashtags and entities, which serve as a proxy to the change of user interests towards the underlying topics [79]. We employ the correlation between the time series of hashtag adoption and the entity view as the third similarity measure (*temporal similarity*).

While each similarity measure captures one aspect of the prominence of an entity, we unify the scores to obtain a global ranking function. In this work, we combine the individual similarities using the following linear function:

$$f(e,h) = \alpha f_m(e,h) + \beta f_c(e,h) + \gamma f_t(e,h) \tag{5.1}$$

where α, β, $and \gamma$ are model weights and f_m, f_c, and f_t are the similarity measures derived from mentions, context and temporal information between the entity e and the hashtag h. We further constrain $\alpha + \beta + \gamma = 1$ so that the ranking scores of entities are normalized between 0 and 1. The *Influence Prominence Learning* (IPL) algorithm we have developed, which automatically learns the parameters without the need of human-labelled data, is explained in detail in [387].

Experimental Setup

Unfortunately, there is no standard benchmark dataset available for this problem. Available datasets on microblog annotation (such as the Micro-posts challenge [36]) often skip global information, and hence, we cannot infer the social statistics of hashtags. Therefore, we created our own dataset using the Twitter API to collect a sample of 500,551,041 tweets from January to April 2014. We removed hashtags that were adopted by fewer than 500 users, had no letters or had characters repeated more than four times (e.g. '#oooommgg'). We identified trending hashtags by computing the daily time series of hashtag tweet counts, and removing those for which the time-series variance score was less than 900. To identify the hashtag burst time period $T(h)$, we computed the outlier fraction [225] for each hashtag h and day t: $p_t(h) = \frac{|n_t - n_b|}{\max(n_b, n_{\min})}$, where n_t is the number of tweets containing h, n_b is the median value of n_t over all points in a 2-month time window centred on t and $n_{\min} = 10$ is the threshold to filter low activity hashtags. The hashtag was skipped if its highest outlier fraction score was less than 15. Finally, we define the burst time period of a trending hashtag as the time window of size w, centred at day t_0 with the highest $p_{t_0}(h)$.

For the Wikipedia datasets, we processed a snapshot from 3rd May 2014, which covers all events in the Twitter dataset, using Hedera [386], a scalable tool for processing the Wikipedia revision history dataset based on the Map-Reduce paradigm. In addition, we make use of the Wikipedia page view dataset, which details how many times a Wikipedia article was requested on an hourly level. We processed the dataset for the 4 months of our study and used Hedera to accumulate all view counts of redirects to the relevant articles. A statistical break down of this dataset is given in Table 5.1.

Table 5.1 Statistics of the evaluation dataset

Total tweets	500,551,041
Trending hashtags	2,444
Test hashtags	30
Test tweets	352,394
Distinct mentions	145,941
Test (entity, hashtag) pairs	6,965
Candidates per hashtag (avg.)	50
Extended candidates (avg.)	182

From the trending hashtags, we sample 30 distinct hashtags for evaluation. Since our study focuses on trending hashtags that are mappable to entities in Wikipedia, the sampling must cover a sufficient number of ‘popular’ topics that are reflected in Wikipedia, and at the same time rare topics in the long tail. To do this, we apply several heuristics in the sampling. First, we only consider hashtags where the lexicon-based linking results in at least 20 different entities. Second, we randomly choose hashtags to cover different types of topics (long-running events, breaking events, memes, etc.). Instead of inspecting all hashtags in our corpus, we follow [225] and calculate the fraction of tweets published before, during and after the peak. The hashtags are then clustered in this 3-dimensional vector space. Each cluster suggests a group of hashtags with a distinct semantics [225]. We then pick hashtags randomly from each cluster, resulting in a total of 200 hashtags. From this rough sample, three inspectors carefully checked the tweets and chose 30 hashtags where the meanings were clear.

The parameters for the linear function to combine the similarity scores are set as follows: we initialize the similarity weights to $\frac{1}{3}$, the damping factor to $\tau = 0.85$, and the weight for the language model to $\lambda = 0.9$. The learning rate μ is empirically fixed to $\mu = 0.003$.

As results of a system in isolation are fairly meaningless, we present our approach in comparison with a number of other entity annotation methods. Our first group of baselines includes Wikiminer [298], an entity linking system for general text, and TagMe [136] which is for short text. For each method, we use the default parameter settings, apply them for the individual tweets and take the average of the annotation confidence scores as the prominence ranking function. The second group of baselines includes systems specifically designed for microblogs. For the content-based methods, we compare against Meij’s system [292], which uses a supervised method to rank entities with respect to tweets. We train the model using the same training data as in the original paper. For the graph-based method, we compare against KAURI [361], a method that uses user interest propagation to optimize the entity linking scores. To tune the parameters, we picked four hashtags from different clusters, randomly sampled 50 tweets for each, and manually annotated the tweets. We also compare three variants of our method, using only local functions for entity ranking (referred to as M, C and T for ‘mention’, ‘context’ and ‘time’, respectively).

In total, there are 6,965 entity-hashtag pairs returned by all systems. We employed five volunteers to evaluate the pairs in the range from 0 to 2, where 0 means the entity is noisy or obviously unrelated, 2 means the entity is strongly tied to the topic of the hashtag and 1 means that although the entity and hashtag might share some common contexts, they are not involved in a direct relationship (for instance, the entity is too general a concept, such as *ice hockey*). The annotators were advised to use search engines, the Twitter search box, or Wikipedia archives whenever applicable to get more background on the stories. Inter-annotator agreement under Fleiss score is 0.625.

Table 5.2 Experimental results on the sampled trending hashtags

	TagMe	Wikiminer	Meij	Kauri	M	C	T	IPL
P@5	0.284	0.253	0.500	0.305	0.453	0.263	0.474	**0.642**
P@15	0.253	0.147	**0.670**	0.319	0.312	0.245	0.378	0.495
MAP	0.148	0.096	0.375	0.162	0.211	0.140	0.291	**0.439**

Results and Discussion

Table 5.2 shows the performance comparison of all these approaches using the standard metrics for a ranking system (precision at 5 and 15 and MAP at 15). In general, all baselines perform worse than reported in the literature, confirming the higher complexity of the hashtag annotation task as compared with traditional tasks. Interestingly, using our local similarities already produces better results than TagMe and Wikiminer. The model f_m derived from mentions significantly outperforms both the baselines in all metrics. Combining the similarities improves the performance even more significantly; all significance tests are done against both TagMe and Wikiminer, with a p-value < 0.01. Compared to the baselines, IPL improves the performance by 17–28%. The time similarity achieves the highest result compared with other content-based mention and context similarities. This supports our assumption that lexical matching is not always the best strategy to link entities in tweets. The time-series-based metric incurs lower cost than others, yet it produces a considerably good performance. Context similarity based on Wikipedia edits does not yield much improvement. This can be explained in two ways. First, information in Wikipedia is largely biased to popular entities, so that it fails to capture many entities in the long tail. Second, language models are dependent on direct word representations, which are different between Twitter and Wikipedia. This is another advantage of non-content measures such as f_t.

For the second group of baselines (Kauri and Meij), we also observe the reduction in precision, especially for Kauri. This is because the method relies on the coherence of user interests within a group of tweets to be able to perform well, which does not hold in the context of hashtags. One surprising result is that Meij performs better than IPL in terms of P@15. However, it performs worse in terms of MAP and P@5, suggesting that most of the correctly identified entities are ranked lower in the list. This is reasonable, as Meij attempts to optimize (with human supervision effort) the semantic agreement between entities and information found in the tweets, instead of ranking their prominence as in our work. To investigate this case further, we re-examined the hashtags and divided them by their semantics, according to whether the hashtags are spurious trends of memes inside social media (endogenous, e.g. '#stopasian2014'), or whether they reflect external events (exogenous, e.g. '#mh370').

The performance of the methods in terms of MAP scores is shown in Fig. 5.3. It can be clearly seen that entity linking methods perform well in the endogenous group, but then deteriorate in the exogenous group. The explanation is that for endogenous hashtags, the topical consonance between tweets is very low; thus, we can barely annotate further than identifying just individual concepts. In this case, topical annotation is trumped by conceptual annotation. However, whenever the hashtag evolves into a meaningful topic, a deeper annotation method will produce a significant improvement, as seen in Fig. 5.3.

Finally, we study the impact of the burst time period on the annotation quality. For this, we expand the window size *w* and examine how different methods perform. The result is depicted in Fig. 5.4. It is obvious that within the window of 2 months (where the hashtag time series is constructed and a trending time is identified), our method is stable and always outperforms the baselines by a large margin. Even when the trending hashtag has been saturated, hence introducing more noise, our method is still able to identify the prominent entities with high quality.

In summary, we have shown that our approach performs well at the task of linking hashtags to entities described in Wikipedia. This linkage allows us to provide extra context to a tweet containing a hashtag by providing one or more links to Wikipedia. This is especially useful with short texts such as tweets, where often all useful context is excluded due to the space constraints. Added to this, our approach also takes into account the evolution of concepts, ensuring that the right meaning is used, thereby further reducing ambiguity and providing a more useful context.

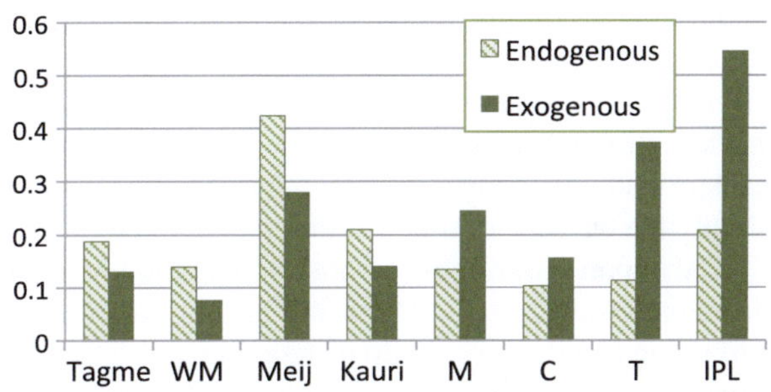

Fig. 5.3 Performance of the methods for different types of trending hashtags

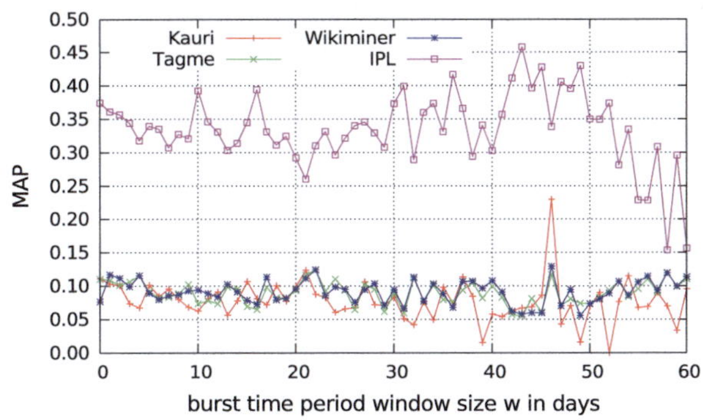

Fig. 5.4 IPL compared to other baselines on different sizes of the burst time window *T*

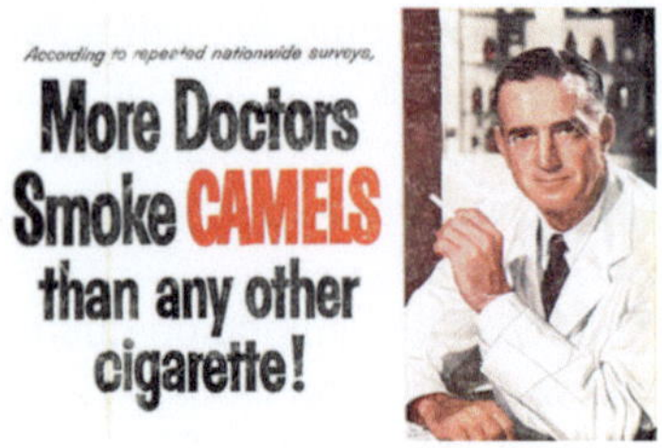
According to repeated nationwide surveys,
More Doctors Smoke CAMELS than any other cigarette!

Contextualization
Prior to 1964, many of the cigarette companies advertised their brand by falsely claiming that their product did not have serious health risks. A couple of examples would be "Play safe with Philip Morris" and "More doctors smoke Camels". Such claims were made both to increase the sales of their product and to combat the increasing public knowledge of smoking's negative health effects.

Fig. 5.5 Camel advertisement (left) and contextualization information taken from Wikipedia (right)

5.2.1.2 Time-Aware Re-contextualization

In the previous section, we described an approach to contextualizing very short documents. In this section, we turn our attention to longer documents, specifically focusing on news articles as these contain many entities that can be linked to an external source of world knowledge.

Reading a current news article about your own country is typically straightforward as your own world knowledge allows you to unambiguously understand the text. Things are different if you read an article from say the 60s or the 70s as can be found in news archives such as the New York Times Archive.[4] In this section, we are especially interested in time-aware *re-contextualization*, where explicit context information is required to bridge the gap between our current understanding of the world and the situation at the time of content creation. This includes changes in background knowledge, the societal and political situation, language, technology or simply the passage of time leading readers to forget.

The importance of time-aware re-contextualization is well illustrated by the advertisement poster from the 1950s in Fig. 5.5. From today's perspective, it is more than surprising that doctors would be recommending smoking. It can, however, be understood from the context information at the right side of Fig. 5.5, which has been extracted from the Wikipedia article on tobacco advertising.

Dealing with content from former times is not restricted to expert users such as journalists, historians or researchers. With the growing age of the web, general web users are increasingly confronted with content which requires time relevant context to be properly interpreted.

Basic forms of contextualization have already been suggested in earlier works such as [168, 295, 298]. The Wikify! system [295], for example, enables an automated linkage of concept mentions with Wikipedia pages. Pure linkage to the Wikipedia article is, however, not sufficient for the re-contextualization task we are targeting. First, Wikipedia pages on popular concepts, events and entities tend to contain large amounts of content, while the concrete aspect of the text to be contextualized might be covered only marginally or not at all, and relevant information might be distributed

[4]http://catalog.ldc.upenn.edu/LDC2008T19.

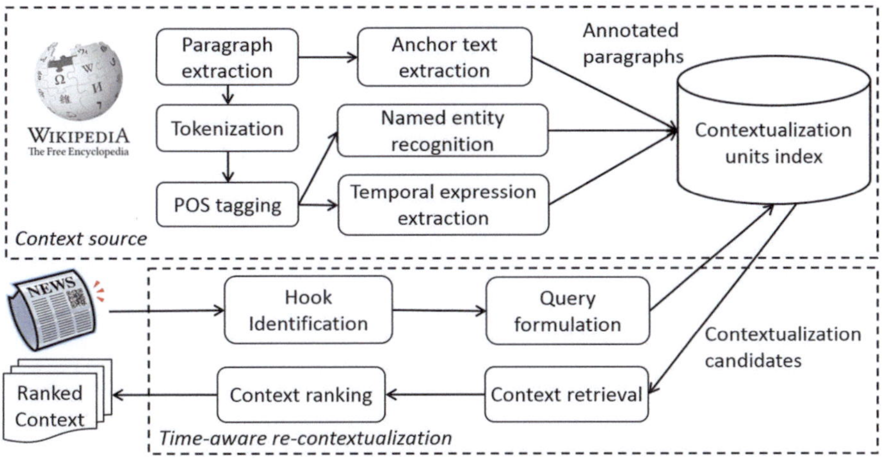

Fig. 5.6 Overview of our approach to time-aware re-contextualization

over various articles. Furthermore, the crucial temporal aspect is also missing in pure linking approaches.

Time-aware re-contextualization, that is, the association of an information piece i (such as a phrase in a text) with additional context units c_i for easing its understanding is a challenging task. Several sub-goals of the information search process have to be combined with each other: (1) c_i has to be relevant for i, (2) c_i has to complement the information already available in i and the surrounding document, (3) c_i has to consider the time of creation (or reference) of i and (4) the set of collected context information for i should be concise to avoid overloading the user.

The work presented in this section automates the process of time-aware re-contextualization and provides advanced approaches for retrieval and ranking of contextualization candidates by taking into consideration complementarity. In more detail, we follow a two-step process. In the first step, we identify contextualization candidates based on contextualization hooks, i.e. the parts of document that require contextualization, such as entity or concept mentions. For this purpose, we explore and analyse different methods for formulating (generating) queries, which are used for retrieving adequate contextualization candidates from an underlying knowledge source. In the second step, we rank the candidates. Similarly to diversification approaches (e.g. [435]), this requires balancing two goals: high content-based and temporal relevance for the text to be contextualized, on the one hand, and complementarity for providing information that cannot already be found in the text, on the other hand. For our contextualization approach, we use Wikipedia as the knowledge source (because of its worldwide topical and temporal coverage).

In the general contextualization model underlying our approach, we distinguish the information piece d to be contextualized and the contextualization source, where the information for the contextualization comes from. Within d a context hook h is an aspect or part of d that requires further information for its time-aware interpretation.

The contextualization source is organized into contextualization units cu. In our approach, we have pre-processed a Wikipedia dump as the contextualization source resulting in annotated and indexed Wikipedia paragraphs as contextualization units (see Fig. 5.6). For information items d to be contextualized, we use articles from the New York Times Archive[5] with manually annotated contextualization hooks, i.e. we assume that a reader has marked the places he/she finds difficult to understand.

Starting from the context hooks, the next process is to retrieve a ranked list of contextualization units from the contextualization source. In time-aware re-contextualization, the time gap between the creation and reading time of d imposes additional challenges. In our approach, the contextualization process consists of two main steps: (1) formulating queries that are able to retrieve contextualization units, which are good candidates for contextualization; (2) retrieving and ranking the candidates from the contextualization source using the queries from step (1). For step (1), we explore document-based and hook-based query formulation methods and present a procedure that selects good queries based on recall-oriented query performance prediction. For step (2), we employ a retrieval method based on language modelling and re-rank the retrieved contextualization candidates based on a variety of features and a learning to rank approach for ensuring complementarity. These steps are described in detail below.

The goal of the query formulation phase consists of generating a set of queries Q_d for a given document d to retrieve contextualization candidates as input for the re-ranking phase. We explore two families of query formulation methods: one using the document to be contextualized itself as a 'generator' of queries and the other using contextualization hooks as generators. Since some of these methods can generate more than one query from an input document, we also discuss two procedures to merge the ranked result lists.

The first family of query formulation methods exploits the document content and structure. Similarly to [388], we use three methods to formulate queries from documents: *title*, *lead* and *title* + *lead*. *Title* formulates a query consisting of the document title, which is indicative of the main topic of the article. *Lead* uses the lead paragraph of a document, typically representing a concise summary of the article and including its main actors. *Title* + *lead* is a combination of the previous two methods which formulates a query consisting of both the title and the lead paragraph of the document. All the queries are pre-processed by tokenization, stop-word removal and stemming. We did not investigate further information extraction approaches for query formulation, since it has already been shown that these methods perform better than more complex information extraction techniques, e.g. key phrase extraction [388].

Documents in our model are assumed to contain a set of hooks explicitly representing the information needs of the reader or, more precisely, what requires contextualization to be understood and interpreted. The analysis done in [71] showed that context hooks are not only entity or concept mentions but can also be general terms and short phrases. We consider two basic hook-based query formulation methods: *all_hooks* and *each_hook*. *All_hooks* includes all the hooks for a document in a single

[5]http://catalog.ldc.upenn.edu/LDC2008T19.

query, representing a tailored perspective of the user's combined information needs for the document. *Each_hook* queries each hook separately, focusing on specific information about single actors, aspects, or sub-topics of the document. The queries generated by these methods are augmented with the title of the document, under the assumption that it is a good representative of the document's topic. We also experimented with more advanced methods based on identifying hook relationships, for instance, considering their co-occurrence in a document collection. However, since these approaches did not perform better than the *all_hooks* method described before, we will not discuss them further.

Different methods based on ranking and selection of query terms from an initial query might be employed [37, 224, 277], considering the entire set of hooks for a document as the initial query. We explore an adaptive method which formulates queries based on the characteristics of the input document and hooks. Our approach consists of predicting the performances of candidate queries representing subsets of hooks for a given document, ranking them according to the predicted performance, and selecting the top-m to be performed for the document. The value of m is identified through experiments. In contrast to previous works in query performance prediction, the prediction model is trained on recall performances instead of precision. Furthermore, we define novel features for query performance prediction that explicitly take the temporal dimension into account. Finally, our method assesses performances of subsets of query terms (hooks) and can generate more than one query (subsets of hooks).

Given a document d and the set of its hooks H_d, we compute its power set $\mathscr{P}(H_d)$ and create a candidate query for each set of hooks $p \in \mathscr{P}(H_d)$. Again, candidate queries are augmented with the title of the document. We measure the performance of each candidate query in terms of its recall because, as already explained, at retrieval phase we are interested in retrieving as many contextualization candidates as possible. In this work, we predict query performance with a regression model learned via Support Vector Regression (SVR) [119]. In this model, each learning sample $s = (\mathbf{f}_q, r_q)$ consists in a feature vector $\mathbf{f}_q$ describing query q (as well as the document it refers to) and its recall r_q, i.e. the label to be predicted. Note that different numbers of top l results can be used to compute the recall. The feature set that we use to represent queries and the document it belongs to are described in the rest of this section. It is composed of novel temporal features for query performance prediction, along with more standard features [62, 162, 304].

We compute a family of *linguistic features* [304] for a query by considering its text and the document it refers to. This results in a set of features both at query and document level: the length of the query, in words; the number of duplicate terms in the query; the number of entities (people, locations, organization and artefacts) in the query; the number of nouns in the query; the number of verbs in the query; the number of hooks in the query; the length of the document's title; the length of the document's lead paragraph; the number of entities in the document (title and lead paragraph); the number of nouns in the documents; the number of verbs in the document; the number of hooks for the document; and the number of duplicates in the document.

The *document frequency* of a hook h represents the percentage of contextualization units in the corpus containing h, and it is computed as

$$df(h) = \log \frac{N_h}{N} \tag{5.2}$$

where N_h is the number of contextualization units in the corpus containing h and N is the size of the corpus. At document level, we compute the document frequency for every hook of the document the query belongs to, i.e. $df\ (h)\ \forall h \in H_d$, and then we derive aggregate statistics like average, standard deviation, maximum value and minimum value. Similarly, at query level, we compute $df\ (h)$ for every hook in the query, and we derive the same aggregate statistics as before. In the following, we will refer to average, standard deviation, maximum value and minimum value simply as *aggregate statistics*.

In order to restrict the popularity of a term to a particular time period $T = [t_0 - w; t_0 + w]$, we compute Eq. 5.2 only for those contextualization units having at least one temporal reference contained in T. This can be done efficiently since contextualization units in our corpus have been annotated with the temporal references mentioned in them. The time period we are interested in is centred around the publication date of the document, i.e. $t_0 = p_d$, and the parameter w determines the width of the interval. After experimenting different values of w, we set $w = 2$ years for our dataset.

The *scope* of a query has been defined in [162] as the percentage of documents (contextualization units in our case) in the corpus that contain at least one query term. Besides the scope of the query itself, we also compute the scope of the document title and the scope of the document hooks H_d when queried together.

We define the *temporal scope* of a query as the percentage of contextualization units in the corpus that contains at least one query term and at least one temporal expression within a given time period. The time period that we consider is the same as the one considered for the computation of temporal document frequency, i.e. a period centred around the publication date of the document and with temporal window equal to $2w$. Again, we experimented different values of w and we set $w = 2$ years.

For a given query q, we retrieve the top-k contextualization units and we compute aggregated statistics of their relevance scores given by the underlying retrieval model. The value of k has been empirically set to 100 after experimenting different candidate values. We also computed relevance features at document level, using both document's title and document's hooks as queries.

For a given query q generated from a document d and every retrieved contextualization unit c in its top-k result set (again, $k = 100$), we compute the *temporal similarity* between q and c, and we derive aggregated statistics over the elements in the result set. Temporal similarity between time points t_1 and t_2 is computed through the time-decay function [192]:

$$TSU(t_1, t_2) = \alpha^{\lambda \frac{|t_1 - t_2|}{\mu}} \tag{5.3}$$

where α and λ are constants, $0 < \alpha < 1$ and $\lambda > 0$, and μ is a unit of time distance. The temporal similarity between a query q and a result c is computed as $\max_{t \in T_c}\{TSU(t, p_d)\}$, where T_c is the set of temporal references mentioned in c, and p_d is the publication date of the document q refers to. This can be done efficiently since temporal references mentioned in contextualization units have been extracted and stored at indexing time.

We also computed temporal similarity features at document level, using both document's title and document's hooks as queries. The computation of the features is the same as the one described above.

We observed that changing the function parameters did not affect the correlation capabilities of the feature, and we set $\lambda = 0.25$, $\alpha = 0.5$, and $\mu = 2$ years in our experiments.

We now describe the methods used in addressing the second part of the re-contextualization process: retrieving and re-ranking context. For the retrieval step, given the queries generated from the different methods for each document described above, we use a retrieval model based on language modelling to create a ranked list of contextualization candidates. Later, learning to select relevant context items is applied to this ranked list.

For the retrieval step, we use query-likelihood language modelling [330] to determine the similarity of a query with the context. In particular, given a query q generated by using one of the query formulation methods for the document d, we compute the likelihood of generating the query q from a language model estimated from a context c with the assumption that query terms are independent.

$$P(c|q) \propto P(c) \prod_{w \in q} P(w|c)^{n(w,q)} \tag{5.4}$$

where w is a query term in q, $n(w, q)$ the term frequency of w in q, and $P(w|c)$ is the probability of w estimated using Dirichlet smoothing:

$$P(w|c) = \frac{n(w, c) + \mu P(w)}{\mu + \sum_{w'} n(w', c)} \tag{5.5}$$

where μ is the smoothing parameter, $P(w)$ is the probability of w in the collection.

To combine the rankings produced by each query of a document, we exploited two combining methods, namely, round-robin, which chooses one result from each ranked list, skipping any result if it has occurred before, and CombSUM, which sums up a result's scores from all ranked lists where it was retrieved. In the experiment, we observed that round-robin method achieves better performance than CombSUM especially in terms of recall, which is also reported in [388]. Therefore, we decided to use round-robin method for combining different ranked lists.

Once we have obtained a ranked list of contextualization candidates for each document, we turn to context selection (re-ranking) where we need to decide which of the context items are most viable. Our ranking algorithm needs to balance two goals, high topical and temporal relevance for the document and complementarity for providing additional information. In this work, we use supervised machine learning that takes as input a set of labelled examples (context to document mappings) and various complementarity features of these examples similar to diversity features [435].

The first class that we employ is *topic diversity*, which aims to compare the dissimilarity between document d and context c on a higher level by representing them using topics. We use Latent Dirichlet Allocation (LDA) [44] to model a set of implicit topics distribution of the document and context. We define this feature as follows:

$$R_1(c, d) = \sqrt{\sum_{k=1}^{m}(p(z_k|d) - p(z_k|c))^2}$$

where m is the number of topics, and z_k is the topic index.

We also considered *text difference* as a feature: in this case, we represent the document and context as a set of words. The novelty of context c is measured by the number of new words in the smoothed set representation of c. If a word w occurred frequently in context c but less frequently in document d, it is likely that new information not covered by d is covered by c. For computation, document and context are represented by a set of informative words (removing stop words, stemming) denoted by $Set(d)$ and $Set(c)$, respectively. We compute this feature as follows:

$$R_2(c, d) = \|Set(c) \cap \overline{Set(d)}\|$$

The way of computing *entity difference* is similar to the one for text difference, with the difference that document and context are represented by a set of entities. The feature is denoted as $R_3(c, d)$.

Anchor texts can be regarded as a short summary (i.e. a few words) of the target document and capture what the document is about. This feature can be computed similarly as text and entity features and is denoted as $R_4(c, d)$. We extract anchor texts using WikiMiner [298] with a confidence threshold γ.

The next feature we use is *distribution similarity*, which is denoted as $R_5(c, d)$.

$$R_5(c, d) = -KL(\theta_c, \theta_d) = -\sum_{w_i} P(w_i|\theta_c) \log \frac{P(w_i|\theta_d)}{P(w_i|\theta_c)}$$

where θ_d and θ_c are the language models for document d and context c, respectively, and are multinomial distributions. We compute θ_d (and similarly for θ_c) using maximum likelihood estimation (MLE) given as

$$P(w_i|d) = \frac{tf(w_i, d)}{\sum_{w_j} tf(w_j, d)}$$

The problem with using MLE is that if a word never occurs in document d, its probability will be zero ($P(w_i|d) = 0$). Thus, a word in context c but not in document d will make $KL(\theta_c|\theta_d) = \infty$. In order to solve this problem, we make use of Dirichlet smoothing method.

$$P_\lambda(w_i|d) = \frac{tf(w_i, d) + \lambda p(w_i)}{\sum_{w_j}(tf(w_j, d) + \lambda p(w_j))}$$

There are several ways to compute geometric distance measure, such as Manhattan distance and Cosine distance. We leverage Cosine distance because of its robustness to document length.

$$R_6(c, d) = \cos(c, d) = \frac{\sum_{k=1}^{n} w_k(c) w_k(d)}{\|d\| \; \|c\|}$$

In our experiment, we used each unique word as one dimension and the *tf.idf* score as the weight of each dimension.

In order to retrieve high topical and temporal relevant contextualization candidates for the document, we also consider the relevance and temporal features. For the former, we exploit the retrieval scores of context returned by our retrieval model. For the later, we apply temporal similarity measurement, i.e. TSU which has been described previously.

Experimental Setup

In our experiments, we used the New York Times Annotated Corpus, which contains 1.8 million documents from January 1987 to June 2007, as the document collection to be contextualized and Wikipedia as the contextualization source. We obtained a copy of Wikipedia as of 4 February 2013 and considered *paragraphs* as contextualization units. In this particular snapshot, we have 4,414,920 proper articles that contain 25,708,539 paragraphs. For each paragraph, we used Stanford CoreNLP [263] for tokenization, entity annotation and temporal expression extraction. In addition, *anchor* texts found in the paragraph hyperlinks are also extracted. We used Apache Solr[6] to index the annotated paragraphs.

In order to obtain a ground-truth dataset (both for training and evaluation), we ultimately picked a set of 51 articles that spanned a wide range of topics (business, technology, education, science, politics and sports) focusing on older articles (29 articles published in 1987, 2 articles in 1988, 6 articles in 1990, 7 articles in 1991 and 7 articles in 1992) and recruited six human annotators to manually annotate those articles.

The annotators were presented with an annotation interface in which they can evaluate article/context pairs (relevant or non-relevant). The annotation guidelines specified that the annotators should assign relevance to the context that provides *additional information* which complements the information in the article and which helps to understand the article. For each article, we retrieved up to 20 candidate contexts with each query formulation method and then removed duplicates.

[6]https://lucene.apache.org/solr/.

In total, our annotated dataset consists of 9,464 article/context pairs, where the annotators evaluated 26.9 relevant contexts per article on average. To foster further research on this challenging task, our ground-truth dataset is publicly available.[7] We averaged the pairwise kappa values of all possible combinations of annotators that had overlapping candidates they had annotated and we obtained a reasonable agreement of $\kappa_c = 0.37$ given the high complexity of this contextualization task.

The parameters are set as follows. For query performance prediction, the regression model was built using the Support Vector Regression implementation of LibSVM.[8] In particular, we trained an n-SVR model with Gaussian Kernel through tenfold cross validation. The open parameters were tuned via grid search to $C = 3$, $\gamma = 0.5$ and $\nu = 0.75$. Linguistic features were extracted using Stanford CoreNLP [263].

For re-ranking context, we performed fivefold cross validation at document level. We conducted experiments using several machine learning algorithms to confirm the robustness of our approach, i.e. it does not depend on any specific algorithm. Specifically, we employed Random Forests (RF), RankBoost (RB) and AdaRank that are implemented in RankLib.[9] In order to compute topic-based features, we employed the topic modelling tool, Mallet[10] by specifying the number of topics to 100, for this task. In addition, we set the confidence threshold to $\gamma = 0.3$ for extracting anchor texts using WikiMiner. For smoothing, we set $\mu = 2000$ and $\lambda p(w_i) = 0.5$.

For the evaluation metrics, we consider precision at rank 1, 3, 10 (P@1, P@3, P@10, respectively), recall, and Mean Average Precision (MAP). These measures provide a short summary of the quality of the retrieved context. In our experiment, a context is considered relevant if it is marked as relevant by an annotator; otherwise, we consider it as non-relevant. We used the top-20 returned context suggestions for evaluation because we do not expect that readers would consider more than 20 contextualization units. Statistical significance was performed using a two-tailed paired t-test and is marked as $^\blacktriangle$ and $^\vartriangle$ for a significant improvement (with $p < 0.01$ and $p < 0.05$, respectively), and significant decrease with $^\blacktriangledown$ and $^\triangledown$ (for $p < 0.01$ and $p < 0.05$, respectively).

As a comparison to our proposed approach, we also investigated three competitive baselines. Proposed by Milne and Witten [298] our *M&W* baseline represents the state of the art in automatic linking approaches. We use the algorithm and best performing settings as described in [298]. In order to apply this method to our task, we consider all paragraphs of all linked pages as a candidate set. A standard query-likelihood language model, *LM*, is used for the initial retrieval which provides the top retrieved documents as a candidate set for the contextualization task. Since our aim is to contextualize old articles, the temporal dimension is important and so for our final baseline. For our final baseline, *Time-aware Language Model (LM-T)*, we selected a state-of-the-art time-aware ranking method, which has previously been shown to be very effective at answering temporal queries. It assumes the textual and

[7] http://www.l3s.de/~ntran/contextualization/.

[8] http://www.csie.ntu.edu.tw/~cjlin/libsvm/.

[9] http://sourceforge.net/p/lemur/wiki/RankLib/.

[10] http://mallet.cs.umass.edu/topics.php.

temporal part of the document d are generated independently from the corresponding parts of the context c, yielding

$$P(d|c) = P(d_{text}|c_{text}) \times P(d_{time}|c_{time}) \tag{5.6}$$

where d_{time} is the document's publication date, c_{time} is the set of temporal expressions in the context c.

The first factor $P(d_{text}|c_{text})$ can be computed by Eqs. 5.4 and 5.5. The second factor in Eq. 5.6 is estimated, based on a simplified variant of [38], as

$$P(d_{time}|c_{time}) = \frac{1}{|\ c_{time}\ |} \sum_{t \in c_{time}} P(d_{time}|t) \tag{5.7}$$

If the document has zero probability of being generated from the context, Jelinek-Mercer smoothing is employed, and we estimate probability of generating the document's publication date from context c as

$$P(d_{time}|c_{time}) = (1-\lambda)\frac{1}{|\ C_{time}\ |} \sum_{t \in C_{time}} P(d_{time}|t) + \lambda \frac{1}{|\ c_{time}\ |} \sum_{t \in c_{time}} P(d_{time}|t) \tag{5.8}$$

where $\lambda \in [0, 1]$ is a tunable mixing parameter which is set to $\lambda = 0.5$ in our experiment (changing this parameter does not affect our results), and C_{time} refers to the temporal part of the context collection treated as a single context and $P(d_{time}|t)$ is estimated by using time-decay function, i.e. TSU computed as in Eq. 5.3.

We evaluate and compare the performances of the different query formulation methods focusing on recall metric. The results reported in the rest of this section are averaged over the 51 documents in our dataset.

In order to fairly evaluate and compare the recall capabilities of the different methods, which can generate different numbers of queries, and we allow each method to retrieve the same number of results k. The round-robin method is used to create a single result set of k elements from different ranked lists.

The query formulation methods are based on predicting the performance (recall in our case) of candidate queries, ranking them according to the prediction, and then using the top-m queries to retrieve results. Thus, the quality of the query performance prediction itself has to be evaluated before assessing and comparing the performance of the whole query formulation method.

A regression model has been trained via 10-fold cross validation, and the results reported hereafter have been averaged over the 10 folds. The correlation coefficient is equal to 0.973, the root mean squared error equal to 0.056 and the mean absolute error equal to 0.037. The low error values and high correlation value, if compared

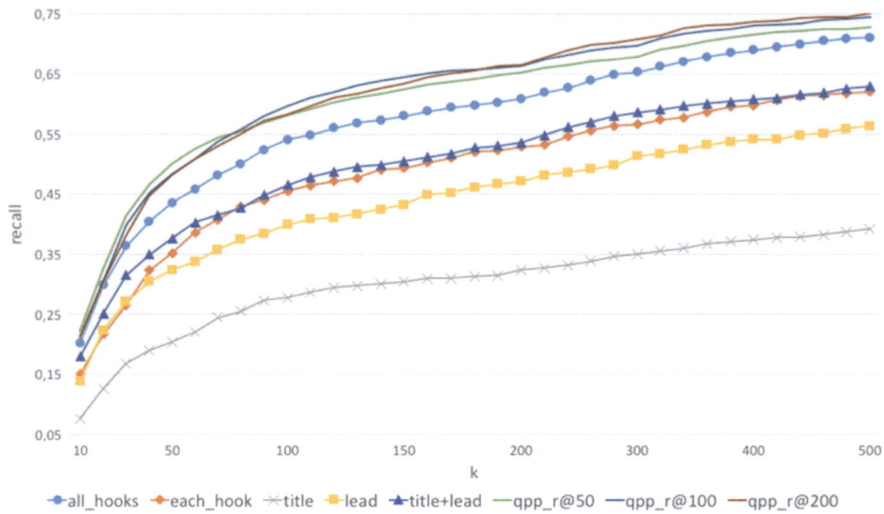

Fig. 5.7 Recall curves of document-based and hook-based methods

with the performance in predicting query precision reported in previous works (e.g. [63, 334]), show that the recall of queries in our task can be predicted quite accurately using the proposed features.

In order to analyse which are the most important features in our model, we identified the top-10 features according to their absolute correlation coefficient. These features include the following: *max query relevance*, *number of hooks in document*, *min document's hooks df*, *max document's hooks temporal df*, *document's hooks scope*, *avg query temporal similarity*, *document's title temporal scope*, *std query relevance*, *avg document's title temporal similarity* and *std query temporal similarity*. The presence of temporal document frequency, temporal similarity and temporal scope shows that the temporal features that we identified play an important role in the model. We can also note that both query-level and document-level features are important, since the set is made of four features from the former and six features from the latter. Finally, there is only one linguistic feature in the set, namely, the number of hooks in the document, confirming that this class of features alone does not correlate well with query performance [62].

We now compare recall values for the document-based methods (*title*, *lead* and *title* + *lead*), the basic hook-based methods (*each_hook*, *all_hooks*), as well as the method based on query performance prediction, hereafter called *qpp*. For the latter method, we report the performances achieved when using prediction models trained with different labels: we experimented with different l values, namely, $l = 50, 100, 200$, for the computation of the recall at l to be used as label.

These three methods will be called *qpp_r@50*, *qpp_r@100* and *qpp_r@200*, respectively, in the rest of the experiments. Note that each *qpp* method considered here uses the top-2 queries, according to their predicted performances, to retrieve the results. The choice of selecting $m = 2$ queries will be explained and motivated later in this section.

The recall curves of the different methods, for different values of top-k results, are shown in Fig. 5.7. The curves of $title$ and $lead$ are the lowest ones, while their combination ($title + lead$) becomes comparable with *each_hook*. Querying using all the hooks of a document together, i.e. *all_hooks*, exposes higher recall values than all the aforementioned methods, showing that performing hook-based queries does lead to better performances in terms of recall with respect to document-based methods. The difference in performances between *each_hook* and *all_hooks* is due to the fact that querying all the hooks together prefers contextualization candidates that contain many hooks. These are potentially more relevant, as they refer to different aspects (hooks) of the same document.

Regarding the qpp methods, for $k > 20 - 30$, the recall values achieved are between 3 and 7% higher than the ones obtained by *all_hooks*. For larger values of k, e.g. $k > 400$, the difference between the qpp methods and *all_hooks* reduces because the prediction models used by the qpp methods have been optimized for lower values of k (recall that $l = 50, 100, 200$).

This means that, if the number of k results to be retrieved for the re-ranking phase is known and fixed in advance, this information can be exploited early in the training of the query performance prediction model by setting $l = k$, leading to higher recall values for that particular k.

Another comparative analysis between qpp methods and *all_hooks* can be done by categorizing the documents according to their *difficulty*, which we define in terms of the amount of relevant context that can be retrieved for a given document. This means that difficult documents are those for which little relevant context can be retrieved, before the re-ranking phase. We categorize documents as 'easy' or 'hard' with respect to the *all_hooks* method, since it represents a baseline in this comparative analysis with qpp methods.

The splitting of the documents into easy and hard was performed by considering the recall at $k = 200$ achieved by *all_hooks* for the different documents. Since the recall values associated to the different documents exhibited a uniform distribution, we split the document set into two equal parts, one representing easy documents and the other representing hard documents.

Table 5.3 shows the performances of *qpp_r*@50, *qpp_r*@100 and *qpp_r*@200 compared to the ones of *all_hooks* for the different categories of difficulty. The comparison between each qpp method and *all_hooks* is done considering the recall at the k value used to train the prediction model (i.e. $k = l, l = 50, 100, 200$). Besides *qpp_r*@50, *qpp_r*@100 and *qpp_r*@200 are on average better than *all_hooks* both for easy and hard documents, their improvements are greater for hard documents. In case of *qpp_r*@100, for instance, the relative improvement with respect to the recall value achieved by *all_hooks* is 5.6% for easy documents and 18.3% for hard documents. We believe that the capability of getting higher recall improvements for documents whose relevant context units are difficult to retrieve is a considerable characteristic for the qpp methods.

Table 5.3 Recall of *all_hooks* and *qpp* methods over different classes of documents (based on their retrieval difficulty)

	R@50		R@100		R@200	
	qpp	*all_hooks*	*qpp*	*all_hooks*	*qpp*	*all_hooks*
Easy	**0.6208**	0.5666	**0.7361**	0.6969	**0.7951**	0.7686
Hard	**0.3837**	0.3094	**0.4606**	0.3892	**0.5391**	0.4550

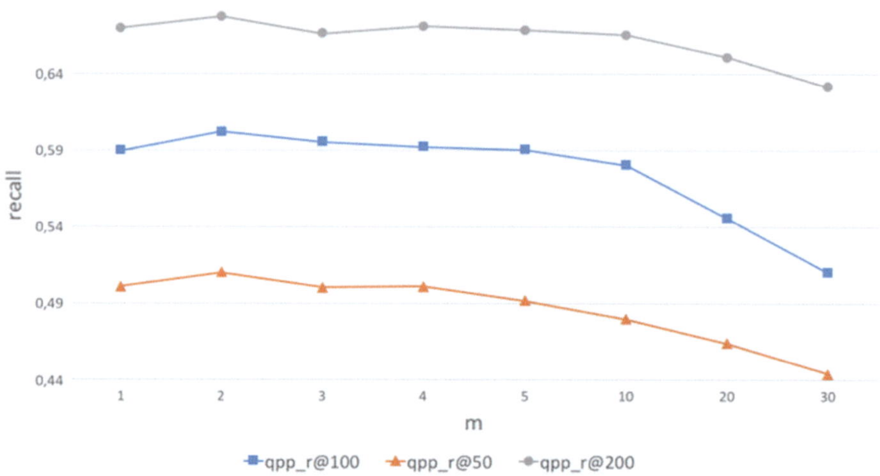

Fig. 5.8 Recall values of *qpp_r*@50, *qpp_r*@100 and *qpp_r*@200 by varying the number of top-*m* queries

As a conclusion, in this section, we showed that exploiting hooks in query formulation is more effective, in terms of recall, than document-based query formulation methods. Moreover, we showed that learning to select candidate hook-based queries can be better, again in terms of recall, than the basic hook-based query formulation methods.

The number of top-ranked queries that *qpp* methods perform is an open parameter, which we tuned via an empirical analysis observing the recall performances when selecting different numbers of top-*m* ranked queries. Recall that, for sake of fair comparison, we allow each method to pick the same number of results k from the result lists retrieved by the queries that it generated for a given document. This means that increasing the number of queries to be selected and performed does not necessarily lead to higher recall.

Figure 5.8 shows the recall values achieved by *qpp_r*@50 (computed at top-50 results), *qpp_r*@100 (computed at top-100 results) and *qpp_r*@200 (computed at top-200 results) for different numbers of top-*m* queries selected. A common trend over the different curves can be observed: they stay quite stable for small values of m, exhibiting a little peak for $m = 2$, and then they decrease for increasing values

Table 5.4 Retrieval performance of document-based and hook-based query models. The significance test is compared with Row 1 (within the first group) and Row 3 (for the second and third groups)

	P@1	P@3	P@10	MAP	Recall
Document-based query models					
title	0.2156	0.1895	0.1745	0.2446	0.1211
lead	0.4902▲	0.4641▲	0.3333▲	0.4908▲	0.2603▲
title + lead	0.5294▲	0.4705▲	0.3901▲	0.5161▲	0.2723▲
Basic hook-based query models					
each_hook	0.3333	0.3464	0.2745	0.4003	0.1969
all_hooks	0.5490	0.5098	0.4137	0.5640	0.2979
Query performance prediction model					
qpp_r@100	**0.5882**	**0.5490**▲	**0.4529**▲	**0.5802**▲	**0.3097**▲

Table 5.5 Retrieval performance of *all_hooks* and *qpp_@100* on a set of difficult documents

	P@1	P@3	P@10	MAP	Recall
all_hooks	**0.5000**	0.3462	0.2885	0.4487	0.2217
qpp_r@100	**0.5000**	**0.4743**△	**0.3730**△	**0.5048**△	**0.2357**

of m. After observing this behaviour, we decided to fix the number of performed queries to $m = 2$.

Results and Discussion

We report the retrieval performance of different query formulation methods and analyse the effectiveness of our context ranking methods trained using different machine learning algorithms. First, we investigated the performance of the standard, well-known Wikification technique, i.e. the M&W method, in retrieving contextualization candidates. Our experiment considered all paragraphs of all linked pages as candidates. The results obtained using the M&W method achieve the low recall value of 0.2290, thus indicating that current semantic linking approaches are not appropriate for the contextualization task.

Table 5.4 shows the results of the different query formulation methods. The first group (top) reports results for candidate retrieval based on document-based query models in which the best performing model is *title + lead* that uses content from the article's title and lead paragraph. Table 5.4 shows that the *qpp_r@100* model is the best performing among the hook-based query models and significantly improves over *title + lead* on all metrics.

Similar to the previous experiment, Table 5.5 reports the results of *all_hooks* and *qpp_@100* retrieval baselines on a subset of difficult documents (here recall is computed on top-20 candidates). On this subset, *qpp_r@100* also shows significant improvement over *all_hooks* in terms of precision. In short, the results on different query formulation methods indicate that using hook-based approaches outperform

Table 5.6 Retrieval performance of different machine-learned ranking methods compared to the best performing retrieval baselines

	P@1	P@3	P@10	MAP	Recall
title + lead					
LM	0.5294	0.4705	0.3901	0.5161	0.2723
RF	**0.7672**▲	0.5757△	**0.4909**▲	**0.6170**▲	**0.3522**▲
RB	0.6036	**0.5945**△	0.4694▲	0.5945	0.3417▲
Adabank	0.6254	0.5406	0.4143	0.5457	0.3249
all_hooks					
LM	0.5490	0.5098	0.4137	0.5640	0.2979
RF	**0.8272**▲	**0.6630**▲	**0.5014** ▲	**0.6427**△	0.3611▲
RB	0.7855▲	0.6593▲	0.5009▲	0.6475△	**0.3637**▲
AdaRank	0.6472	0.5836	0.4687	0.6034	0.3372△
qpp_r@100					
LM	0.5882	0.5490	0.4529	0.5802	0.3097
RF	**0.8054**▲	**0.6993**▲	0.5140▲	0.6498▲	**0.3951**▲
RB	0.7218	0.6915▲	**0.5300**▲	**0.6632**▲	0.3792▲
AdaRank	0.6072	0.6139	0.4895	0.6109	0.3479▲

the document-based approach that based on merely article internal structure. Using the query performance prediction method obtains the highest performance on all metrics, followed by *all_hooks*.

We now present the results of our re-ranking approach when using a set of innovative complementarity features to further improve performances of the context ranking step, especially in terms of precision. We select *title + lead* for the document-based approach and *all_hooks, qpp_r@100* for the hook-based approach.

The first (top) group in Table 5.6 shows the results when applying machine learning to the *title + lead* retrieval baseline. All three algorithms are able to improve precision at rank k, MAP and recall. RF and RB obtain significant improvement where RF achieves the highest score on most metrics, except precision at rank 3 where RB is the best. The second (middle) group reports the results of *all_hooks* retrieval baseline, augmented by the re-ranking step. In this case, RF and RB are again able to significantly improve over *all_hooks* on all metrics while AdaRank is also performing significantly better than *all_hooks* in terms of recall. Among three algorithms, RF achieves the highest results, except for recall. Similarly, all three machine learning algorithms perform significantly better than the *qpp_@100* retrieval baseline. Again, in this case, RF obtain the highest performances, closely followed by RB.

In order to compare our approach to time-aware language model which takes into account temporal information, we use the queries derived from query performance prediction method, i.e. *qpp_@100* that obtain the highest results among our query formulation methods. Table 5.7 shows that using time-aware language models is not efficient in our case. This is possibly because lots of relevant context (paragraphs in

Table 5.7 Retrieval performance of our proposed ranking method and the state-of-the-art time-aware language modelling approach. The significance test is compared against LM-T

qpp_@100	P@1	P@3	P@10	MAP	Recall
LM-T	0.5882	0.4967	0.4176	0.5446	0.2796
LM	0.5882	0.5490	0.4529	0.5802	0.3097$^{\triangle}$
RF	**0.8054**$^{\triangle}$	**0.6993**$^{\blacktriangle}$	**0.5140**$^{\blacktriangle}$	**0.6498**$^{\blacktriangle}$	**0.3951**$^{\blacktriangle}$

News article - *Maj. Gen. Richard V. Secord, a main organizer of the Iran arms sales and the contra supply operation, testified today that he had been told that President Reagan had been informed that proceeds from the sales to Iran had been diverted to the Nicaraguan rebels.*

Context - *Speaking of the Iran-Contra affair, a Reagan administration scandal that involved the diverting of funds being shipped to Iran to the contras in Nicaragua, Reagan says, "None of the arms we'd shipped to Iran had gone to the terrorists who had kidnapped our citizens." Of the scandal, Reagan writes, " and, I presume, knew how deeply I felt about the need for the contras' survival as a democratic resistance force in Nicaragua. Perhaps that knowledge... led them to support the contras secretly and saw no reason to report this to me." He also says of himself, "As president, I was at the helm, so I am the one who is ultimately responsible." Also, Reagan discusses his political rivalry and personal friendship with former Speaker of the House Tip O'Neill.*

Fig. 5.9 Example of contextualization candidate for a given document with no explicit temporal information

our case) do not have any temporal information as shown in Fig. 5.9. Consequently, these candidates are ranked low (e.g. higher than 20) in the ranked list returned by LM-T. This result indicates that purely using the time dimension in context retrieval is not sufficient in the contextualization task. It also confirms the importance of complementarity that is used in our re-ranking step.

These results link nicely back to the general model of contextualization we presented towards the beginning of this chapter (see page xxx), in so far as they rely on extracting 'context hooks' from a document (referred to as an 'information piece' in our model) and linking them to 'context units' to provide a state-of-the-art time-aware contextualization approach.

5.2.2 Contextualizing Photo Collections

In this section, we discuss the application of contextualization on photo collections. A previously processed set of personal photo collections or photos from the web can be considered as the pool of 'context units', while photos of this pool that are semantically similar to photos of a new collection can be considered as 'context hooks' (see Sect. 5.1.2). The additional information provided, about the situation in which the photos of the user collection were captured, results in a more complete view of the event, and ultimately helps the formation of well-preserved semantic memories of an event (as discussed in Chap. 2). In the following, we discuss in more detail two characteristic methods for photo collection contextualization: (a) a personal photo collection contextualization method, and (b) a photo collection contextualization method that acquires 'world knowledge', taking advantage of information found on the web.

An approach for a personal photo collection contextualization is to enrich an event-centred user collection by retrieving additional content (i.e. photos covering different aspects of the same event) from other resources. This can be applied in cases where an individual attends either public events (e.g. sports competitions, concerts) or personal events (e.g. a professional meeting, a birthday party and a family trip) and captures photos, and also has access to photo collections of different users that attended the same event. To give a more specific example, suppose that a person attends a public event such as the London 2012 Olympic Games and takes photos. At the end of the event, what remains to the user are the memories and photos. A large number of people attended the same event capturing the sports, and more specifically the moments which they considered interesting. The information collected by individuals is diverse, covering the overall event. By combining this information and sharing it, we can provide a more holistic description of the event.

The event depicted in a photo collection to be contextualized will typically consist of several sub-events, i.e. groups of photos that constitute a distinct action within a bounded time and space. For the Olympic Games, the individual sports competitions (e.g. first day of men's tennis, women's weightlifting final) can be considered as sub-events of the entire London 2012 summer Olympic event (see Fig. 3.12 in Chap. 3 for an example). We argue that such sub-events related to the overall photo collection can play a major role in the contextualization process.

In light of the above considerations, it is no surprise that photo collection contextualization relies on techniques for event-based clustering, multi-user galleries temporal synchronization, and sub-event matching. A variety of such collection analysis methods has been proposed in the literature for tackling the problems of organizing and visualizing personal photo collections (e.g. [75, 254]), selecting representative photos out of a photo collection [321], event-based clustering (e.g. [17], also discussed in Sect. 3.5) and temporal synchronization of multi-user collections (e.g. [347]). However, very few works deal explicitly with photo collection contextualization. One example is the method of [383], which compares events at collection level instead of taking into account individual photo features. Given an event described by a set of photos, this method can retrieve photos from the same event captured by different users, utilizing visual, temporal and geolocation information (although the authors do not test the latter in their experiments).

An alternative approach for photo collection contextualization is to use the web as a pool of 'context units', discarding this way the restrictive need for photo collections coming from different known users that attended the specific event. Both of the aforementioned methods are discussed in the following sections.

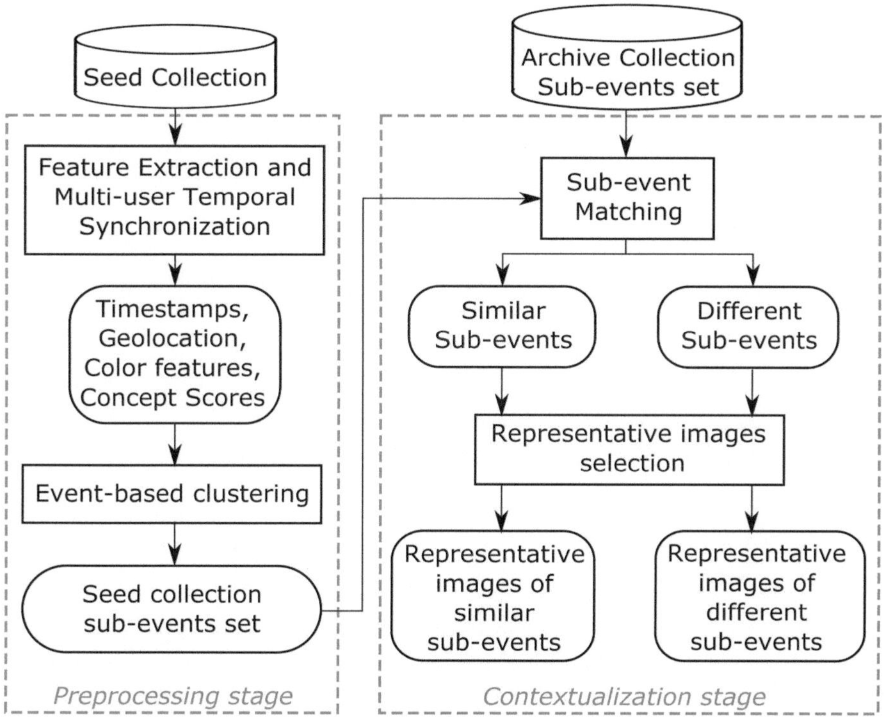

Fig. 5.10 Overview of the personal photo collection contextualization method

5.2.2.1 Personal Photo Collection Contextualization

We present a personal photo collection contextualization method (originally proposed in [18]) that enriches the content of a user collection with additional photos extracted from collections of different users who attended the same event. This method adopts the notions of a single 'seed' collection (the user collection to be contextualized) and 'archive' collections (the collections of other users from which contextual information will be drawn). 'Seed' and 'archive' collections are assumed to belong to the same event; thus, this particular method does not deal with recognizing the event or deciding whether two collections depict the same event.

Figure 5.10 shows the framework of this method, which consists of two stages: the pre-processing stage of the user collection and the actual contextualization stage. During the first stage, the photos of the 'seed' collection are analysed and the collection is split into sub-events using a clustering method (such as the method in [17]). During the actual contextualization stage, similar and different sub-events of the event are detected within the 'archive' collection and matched to 'seed' collection sub-events, while a selected representative subset of their photos is used for enriching and contextualizing the 'seed' collection. The 'archive' collections are considered to

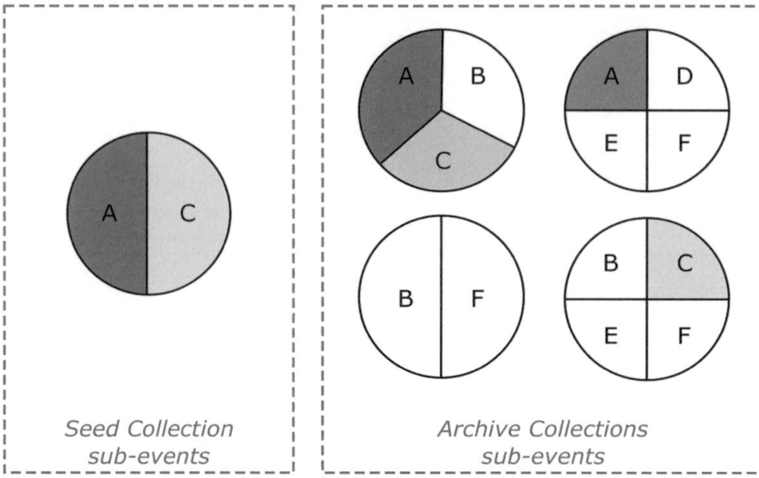

Fig. 5.11 An example of 'seed' and 'archive' collections sub-events. The symbols A to F denote different sub-events of the overall event

be already analysed and organized in sub-events since this stage is performed iteratively as each new collection of photos is added to the 'archive' collection. Thus, as depicted in Fig. 5.10, the event-based clustering is executed only when a new 'seed' collection is submitted.

An example of the event-based clustering and matching stages of the contextualization procedure is depicted in Fig. 5.11, during which all collections (circles) are split into sub-events (circle sectors). During the sub-event matching stage, the sub-events of the 'archive' collections are matched to those of the 'seed' collection (A and C sub-events are common between 'seed' and 'archive' collections, while B, D, E and F sub-events are unique in the 'archive' collection). Depending on the user needs, the photos that are used for contextualizing the 'seed' collection can be selected from both similar sub-events (A and C sub-events) and different sub-events (B, D, E and F sub-events of the 'archive' collections) with the percentage of photos taken from similar and different sub-events being user-defined.

Photo Analysis and Event-Based Clustering

We stress the importance of using multiple features for representing a photo, to support the later stages of the event-based clustering and sub-event matching, particularly in the case of events with sub-events in multiple locations and/or temporally overlapping. To this end, the following photo visual content features and metadata are employed:

1. time information, i.e. the capture date and time of the photo;
2. geolocation, i.e. the GPS coordinates of the location at which the photo was captured;
3. colour information, extracted using HSV colourspace histograms; and

4. concept detection scores, extracted by applying a concept detection algorithm [269] resulting in a 346-dimensional vector, where each value is a score indicating the probability of a particular concept being depicted in the photo.

Although time information can often be easily extracted from the EXIF metadata of the photos, there are cases where it is not available (e.g. photos are captured using an old camera, and no metadata are saved) or not directly exploitable (e.g. when photo capture devices of different users are not synchronized or are set to different time zones). In the latter case, and in order to render time information usable, a multi-user time synchronization method must be used (such as [347]) to estimate the temporal offset of each of the 'archive' collections to the 'seed' collection. Additionally, geolocation information might be missing from some photos, since not all photo capture devices are able to include this type of information in a photo's EXIF metadata. Therefore, we cannot rely on such geolocation information, but only use it as auxiliary information when available.

Sub-event Matching

Let S be the 'seed' collection that is clustered in N_S sub-events $S^i, i = 1, \dots, N_S$. Each sub-cluster S^i contains N_{S^i} photos $s^{i,j}, j = 1, \dots, N_{S^i}$. For each photo $s^{i,j}$, we can use the capture time $s_T^{i,j}$ information, the GPS location $s_{GPS}^{i,j}$, the HSV histogram $s_{HSV}^{i,j}$ and the concept detection scores $s_{SC}^{i,j}$. Similarly, $A_k^j, j = 1, \dots, N_{A_k}$ is the jth sub-event of the 'archive' collection of user k denoting the corresponding photo information as $a_{k,\{HSV/GPS/SC/T\}}^{i,j}$. To match a 'seed' collection sub-event to sub-events of the 'archive' collections, four sub-event distance measures are introduced.

1. Temporal distance (*time*): this baseline approach utilizes the time information of the photos. The distance between a 'seed' sub-event and an 'archive' one is the minimum pairwise temporal distance of their photos, and is given by

$$D_T(S^i, A_k^j) = \begin{cases} \min\limits_{m,n}\{|(s_T^{i,m} - a_{k,T}^{j,n}|)\}, & \text{if sub-events are not temporally overlapping} \\ 0, & \text{otherwise} \end{cases}$$

where $1 \leq m \leq N_{S^i}$ and $1 \leq n \leq N_{A_k^j}$.

2. Colour information distance (*HSV*): in this approach, sub-event distance is defined as the minimum pairwise distance between the HSV colour histograms of the sub-events photos:

$$D_H(S^i, A_k^j) = \min_{m,n}\{d_{\cos}(s_{HSV}^{i,m}, a_{k,HSV}^{j,n})\}$$

where $d_{\cos}$ is the cosine distance.

3. Semantic distance (*scores*): in this case, we use the minimum pairwise distance between vectors of concept detection scores:

$$D_{SC}(S^i, A_k^j) = \min_{m,n}\{d_{cd}(s_{SC}^{i,m}, a_{k,SC}^{j,n})\}$$

where d_{cd} is a distance used for concept detection scores, given by Eq. 6 in [294].

4. Signature distance (*signature*): while the aforementioned approaches employ pairwise photo-based distances, an approach that calculates the distances among entire sub-events without calculating pairwise photo distances can be adopted, in which each sub-event is described by a single vector, namely, its signature. To construct the signature vector of a sub-event, we calculate the mean and variance of vectors of concept detection scores. We then keep the u concept indices with the highest mean, and finally, we sort them in ascending order of their variances. The signature vector is representative of the entire sub-event, since it contains concepts that attained a high score (top u), while at the same time their position in the vector shows the significance of the specific concept (low variance).
The indices of the concept c of sub-events S^i and A_k^j are denoted as $S^i_{SIG_c}$ and A^j_{k,SIG_c}, respectively. If the concept c does not belong to the top u concept indices, then its value is set to 0. The distance of two sub-event signatures equals the sum of the distances D_C of the signatures for all concepts.

$$D_{SIG}(S^i, A_k^j) = \sum_{c=1}^{N_C} D_C(S^i_{SIG_c}, A^j_{k,SIG_c}) \tag{5.9}$$

If a concept c belongs in both signatures, then distance D_C equals the $\mathrm{W}(p) \cdot p$ where $p = |(S^i_{SIG_c} - A^i_{k,SIG_c})|$. As a result, concept indices with low variance have more impact on the distance calculation. The intuition of this distance measure is that two sub-events are close if they contain more common concepts having high score and same positions. If a concept index exists only in one signature, then D_C is set to $W(i)(u+1)$, where i is the index of concept c in this signature. Finally, if a concept index does not exist in any of the signatures, then D_C is set to $\mathrm{W}(p+1) \cdot (u+1)$. Therefore, the distance measure based on the signatures of sub-events is defined as

$$D_C(S^i, A_k^j) = \begin{cases} \mathrm{W}(p)\cdot p, & \text{if } S^i_{SIG_c} > 0 \text{ and } A^j_{k,SIG_c} > 0 \\ \mathrm{W}(p)\cdot(u+1), & \text{if } S^i_{SIG_c} > 0 \text{ xor } A^j_{k,SIG_c} > 0 \\ \mathrm{W}(p+1)\cdot(u+1), & \text{otherwise} \end{cases}$$

The *time* measure can be combined with other sub-event distance measures. The weighted sum of *time* and *HSV*, *scores* or *signatures* ($D_{T,x} = w \cdot D_T + (1-w) \cdot D_{\{x\}}$) where $x \in \{HSV, SC, SIG\}$) is tested in later experiments. Furthermore, geolocation information is employed only to further refine the matched sub-events. A t_{GEO} distance threshold is calculated that denotes if two sub-events are considered spatially close or not. For the estimation of t_{GEO} we cluster all pairwise 'archive' photo spatial distances using the k-means clustering algorithm, setting the number of clusters $k = 2$. Threshold t_{GEO} is set equal to the value of the lowest cluster centre. Pairs of photos with capture location distance larger than t_{GEO} are excluded from the matching procedure. Finally, we select a subset of 'archive' sub-events whose distance to a 'seed' sub-event is below the corresponding thresholds $(t_T, t_{T,x}, t_x)$, where $x \in \{HSV, SC, SIG\}$.

Seed Collection Enrichment

Having matched each 'seed' user sub-event to an 'archive' sub-event, we select the photos of the matched 'archive' sub-events that are either similar or dissimilar to the 'seed' user collection photos, depending on the user needs. To achieve this, two user-controlled parameters, a and b, are established. Parameter a $(a > 0)$ controls the total number of photos that will be used for contextualizing the 'seed' collection. Parameter b $(0 \leq b \leq 1)$ specifies what percentage of these photos should belong to sub-events that are also contained in the 'seed' collection. We select the $a \cdot b \cdot N$ 'archive' sub-event photos (where $N = \sum_{i=1}^{N_S} N_{S^i}$ is the total number of 'seed' collection photos) that are most similar to the 'seed' collection sub-events, and from each 'archive' sub-event, we pick one photo which is the most dissimilar to the photos already contained in this sub-event of the 'seed' collection. The set of the $a \cdot b \cdot N$ photos is the set of photos that contextualizes the sub-events of the event that were originally contained in the 'seed' collection. The remaining $a \cdot (1 - b) \cdot N$ photos that enrich the 'seed' collection are collected from the most dissimilar sub-events. In the case of $b \approx 0$, the user requests the contextualization of their collection to be performed by considering only different sub-events, and the selection is based on a measure of photo significance. In [109], a method that detects significant events in personal photo collections is presented. More specifically, the number of photos captured by a user within a temporal window is modelled as a time series, which is subsequently analysed to detect potential significant events. We follow a simpler approach in which the significance of each photo is calculated according to the temporal distance from the rest of the sub-event's photos. The significance SG of a photo $a_k^{j,l}$ which belongs in sub-event A_k^j is given by

$$SG(a_k^{j,l}) = \sum_{p=1}^{N_{A_k^j}} \exp\left(-g|a_{k,T}^{j,l} - a_{k,T}^{j,p}|\right)$$

By tuning parameter g, the exponential can become significant only for photos that are temporally close, while for the rest, the exponential is negligible. As a result, the above sum depends also on the number of temporally close photos to $a_k^{j,l}$. Given a sub-event, the significance of all photos is initially calculated, and then, the one having the highest significance is selected. If the 'archive' sub-event is dissimilar to the 'seed' collection sub-events, then this photo is used as the representative one for the 'seed' collection enrichment. If the 'archive' sub-event is similar to one of the 'seed' collection sub-events and the selected photo is temporally far from the 'seed' collection photos, the photo is selected as the representative one for the 'seed' collection. Otherwise, the photo with the second highest significance is examined. This procedure is continued until a temporally distant photo is detected.

Evaluation of Personal Photo Collection Contextualization Method

We used the two datasets[11] of the MediaEval 2014 SEM task [83] for evaluating the personal photo collection contextualization method proposed here. The goals of this task are as follows: the temporal alignment of a series of photo galleries that relate to the same event but have been collected by different users; the alignment of the photos on a common timeline; and the detection of the sub-events attended by the users. The *Vancouver* dataset consists of 1351 photos capturing various sub-events of the Vancouver 2010 Winter Olympic Games, split into 35 user collections. The *London* dataset consists of 2124 photos capturing various sub-events of the London 2012 Olympic Games, split into 37 user collections. We used the *Vancouver* dataset to estimate the threshold values (t_T, $t_{T,x}$, t_x, where $x \in \{HSV, SC, SIG\}$) for each sub-event distance calculation approach and used their estimated values on the *London* dataset, which are $t_T = 0.10$, $t_{T,HSV} = 0.27$, $t_{T,SC} = 1.05$, $t_{T,SIG} = 0.69$, $t_{HSV} = 0.05$, $t_{SC} = 0.8$ and $t_{SIG} = 0.27$.

In the experiments conducted on the *London* dataset, we consider the collection of the first user ($user1$) as the 'seed' collection, while the remaining 36 user collections form the 'archive' collections which are pre-processed. For the pre-processing method of clustering to sub-events, we used the ground truth of MediaEval 2014 SEM task [83] in order to test the actual contextualization part of our method. We also performed a set of experiments considering a subset of user collections (specifically those which contain at least two sub-events) as 'seed' collections and averaged the results. Finally, it is worth noting that geolocation information is available for a small portion of photos in this dataset.

We evaluate the results of our approaches on sub-event matching using the established precision (P), recall (R) and F-measure (F1) measures. Table 5.8 shows the results for each matching approach, using the first user of the London dataset as 'seed' and the rest of the users as the 'archive' collections, since the first user has the most extended collection of sub-events.

We observe in Table 5.8 that the baseline method does not perform well, due to the London dataset containing temporally overlapping events. Combining time information with the other features, a significant boost is achieved (compare *time+HSV*, *time+scores* and *time+signatures* to *HSV*, *scores* and *signatures* approaches, respectively). Specifically, *time+HSV* approach achieved the highest F1 measure. Furthermore, in the case where the time information is not available, the *scores*-based approach can distinguish sub-events better than the other proposed approaches. These observations using the first user as the 'seed' collection are confirmed for the case where we use the union of several user collections as the 'seed' collection, in Table 5.9. The selection of user collection to be used as the 'seed' was based on the number of sub-events included to be at least 5.

We numerically evaluate the impact of using these photos for contextualization by examining the sub-events that they contain. Specifically, we establish and use three evaluation measures:

[11] The datasets are publicly available at http://mmlab.disi.unitn.it/MediaEvalSEM2014/.

Table 5.8 Different sub-event matching methods evaluation using $user1$ collection as the 'seed'

Method	P	R	F1
Time	0.466	0.872	0.607
Time + HSV	**0.894**	0.764	**0.824**
Time + scores	0.765	0.750	0.757
Time + signatures	0.677	**0.880**	0.765
HSV	0.840	0.568	0.677
Scores	0.659	0.763	0.707
Signatures	0.773	0.425	0.548

Table 5.9 Different sub-event matching methods evaluation using multiple users' collections as the 'seed' and averaging the results

Method	P	R	F1
Time	0.399	**0.872**	0.536
Time + HSV	**0.702**	0.724	**0.702**
Time + scores	0.685	0.681	0.666
Time + signatures	0.587	0.675	0.611
HSV	0.567	0.447	0.462
Scores	0.624	0.549	0.525
Signatures	0.544	0.323	0.392

- Percentage of Similar (PoS): out of the photos of the 'archive' collections that were selected on the basis of representing similar sub-events; we measure the percentage that truly belongs to such sub-events. This measure ranges from 0 to 1, where 1 is the optimal.
- Percentage of Dissimilar (PoD): out of the photos of the 'archive' collections that were selected on the basis of representing dissimilar sub-events; we measure the percentage that truly belong to such sub-events. This measure ranges from 0 to 1, where 1 is the optimal.
- Cluster Recall (CR): here we measure the coverage increase after contextualization. The initial coverage of the 'seed' collection is calculated based on the number of different sub-events of the total number of sub-events contained in the overall event. By contextualizing the collection, we attempt to include more sub-events into the 'seed' collection and increase the coverage.

Figure 5.12 illustrates the values of these measures when varying the values of parameters a and b, while indicative results for selected values of a and b are shown in Table 5.10. As far as the CR measure is concerned, the $user1$ 'seed' collection consists of 46 sub-events out of the 238 total sub-events before contextualization, which is equal to 0.1932. As parameter a increases, meaning that the user selected to increase the number of photos that are used for contextualizing the 'seed' collection, the CR measure also increases and reaches almost 0.3. This indicates that the

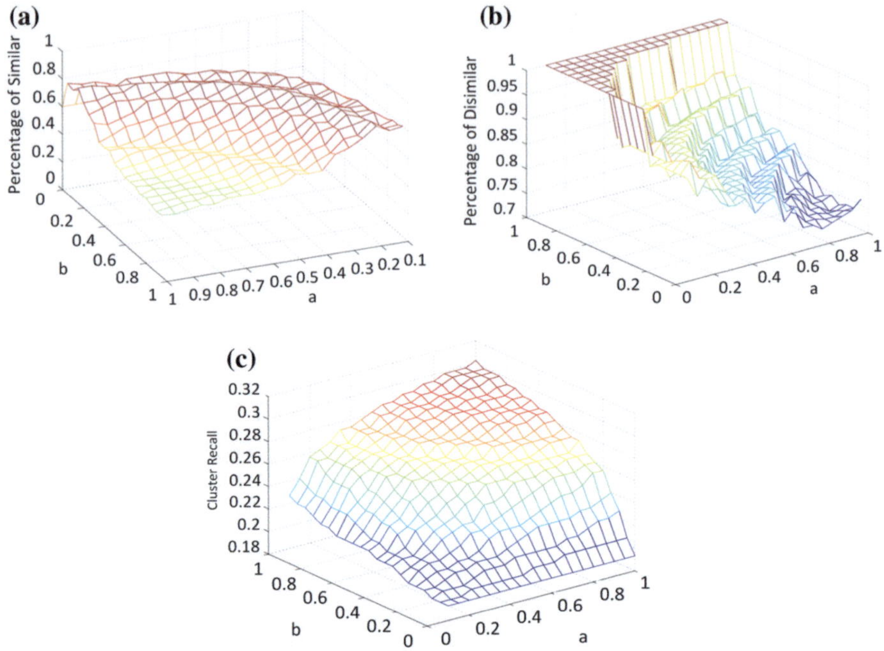

Fig. 5.12 Evaluation results using the three defined evaluation measures, for different a and b parameters **a** percentage of similar, **b** percentage of dissimilar and **c** cluster recall

contextualized 'seed' collection offers a broader coverage of the event, in comparison to the information contained in the 'seed' collection prior to contextualization.

An example of the contextualization results, for both similar and dissimilar sub-events, is shown in Fig. 5.13. These sub-events were selected by applying the personal photo collection contextualization method on the *London* dataset. This example shows how the 'seed' collection is contextualized with different photos. In Fig. 5.13a, the 'seed' collection photos are illustrated, grouped in sub-events using ground truth. It seems that this collection contains photos from a part of the opening and award ceremonies, and the rowing (coxless pair, eight, single scull, quad scull), weightlifting, soccer, marathon, long jump, track, wrestling, tennis, beach volley and judo competitions. Figure 5.13b shows the photos of similar sub-events that were chosen from the 'archive' collections for contextualization. Finally, Fig. 5.13c shows the photos that were selected from the sub-events not present in the 'seed' collection. These include photos from the taekwondo, cycling, fencing, basketball and horse riding competitions, as well as different parts of the opening and award ceremonies.

Table 5.10 Percentage of Similar (PoS), Percentage of Dissimilar (PoD) and Cluster Recall (CR) clustering evaluation measures for different *a* and *b* parameters

Method	a = 0.5			a = 1		
	b = 0.2	b = 0.5	b = 0.8	b = 0.2	b = 0.5	b = 0.8
PoS	**0.8**	0.76	0.57	0.83	0.58	0.46
PoD	0.82	0.84	**0.90**	0.72	0.81	0.88
CR	0.22	0.26	0.27	0.25	0.28	**0.29**

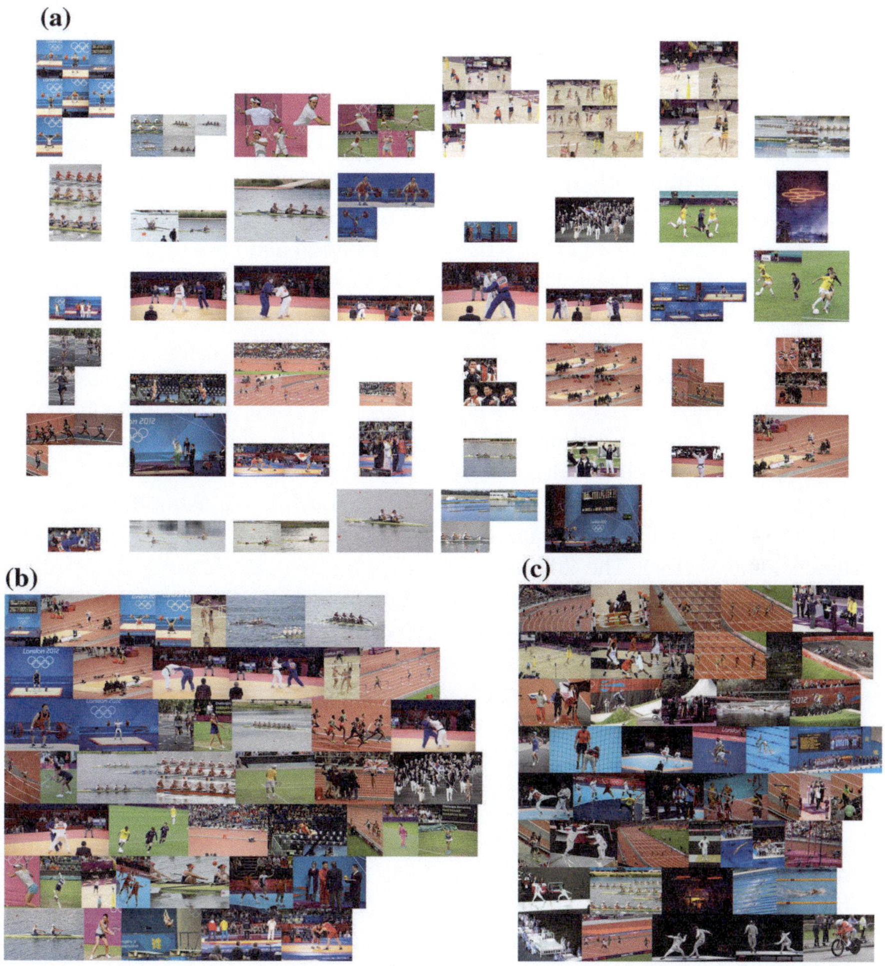

Fig. 5.13 **a** 'seed' collection sub-events. **b** Photos added through contextualization that belong to sub-events already contained in the 'seed' collection. **c** Photos added through contextualization that belong to different sub-events of the same event

5.2.2.2 Photo Collection Contextualization Using Web Data

The personal photo contextualization method discussed in Sect. 5.2.2.1 has two limitations: (a) The collection to be contextualized must be about a single event that several other users have also attended and created their own photo collections for, and (b) the other users that attended the event must have their collections (the 'archive' collections) submitted and pre-processed by the method, i.e. they must have been temporally aligned using a time synchronization algorithm (e.g. [347]) and split into sub-events using an event-based clustering algorithm (see Sect. 3.5) prior to the actual contextualization. The photo contextualization method presented in this section draws information using the web as a 'world knowledge' pool, thus overcoming the aforementioned limitations. The need for other photo collections from different users attending the same event is substituted with the input of a short textual description of the event.

An overview of this method is illustrated in Fig. 5.14. This method takes as input a photo collection that has been captured by a user attending an event and a textual description of the event that contains the name, location and time of the event. Web photos that are related to the event are retrieved and downloaded, their visual content is analysed and a selection of them is provided to the user as additional contextual content.

First, the user's photo collection is fed into an image analysis component. Using the Caffe framework [181] and the 22-layer GoogLeNet Deep Convolutional Neural Network (DCNN) pre-trained model [377], the loss1/classifier and loss3/classifier layers' output is extracted (resulting in two 1000-dimensional vectors). The L*a*b* colourspace colour histogram of each photo is also calculated, using 8 bins for the L* plane, 32 bins for the a* plane and 32 bins for the b* plane (resulting in a 72-dimensional vector). The 2072-dimensional concatenated feature vector of the DCNN layers output and the L*a*b* histogram are used to represent each photo in the user collection. The textual description that must be provided by the user consists of the name of the event (e.g. Olympic Games), the location (e.g. London) where the event took place and the date that the event took place (e.g. 2012). This information is then used to create a set of queries which are sent to web search engines, and a pool of data is collected, from which the contextual information will be selected. The following three web queries are performed:

1. A query to the Google text search engine; the P first web pages and the Y first YouTube links of the search results are kept. Moreover, the photos contained in the returned web pages are also collected. The query to the Google text search engine is formed by combining the textual description provided by the user, using AND (&) (i.e. event & location & time).
2. A query is sent to the Bing search engine; the B top-ranked photos are collected. The query is generated similarly to the previous one.
3. A query is sent to the Flickr search engine; the F top-ranked photos are collected. In the case of Flickr, the Flickr API allows us to add constraints to the queries. Thus, apart from the initial query (i.e. event & location & time), we also send

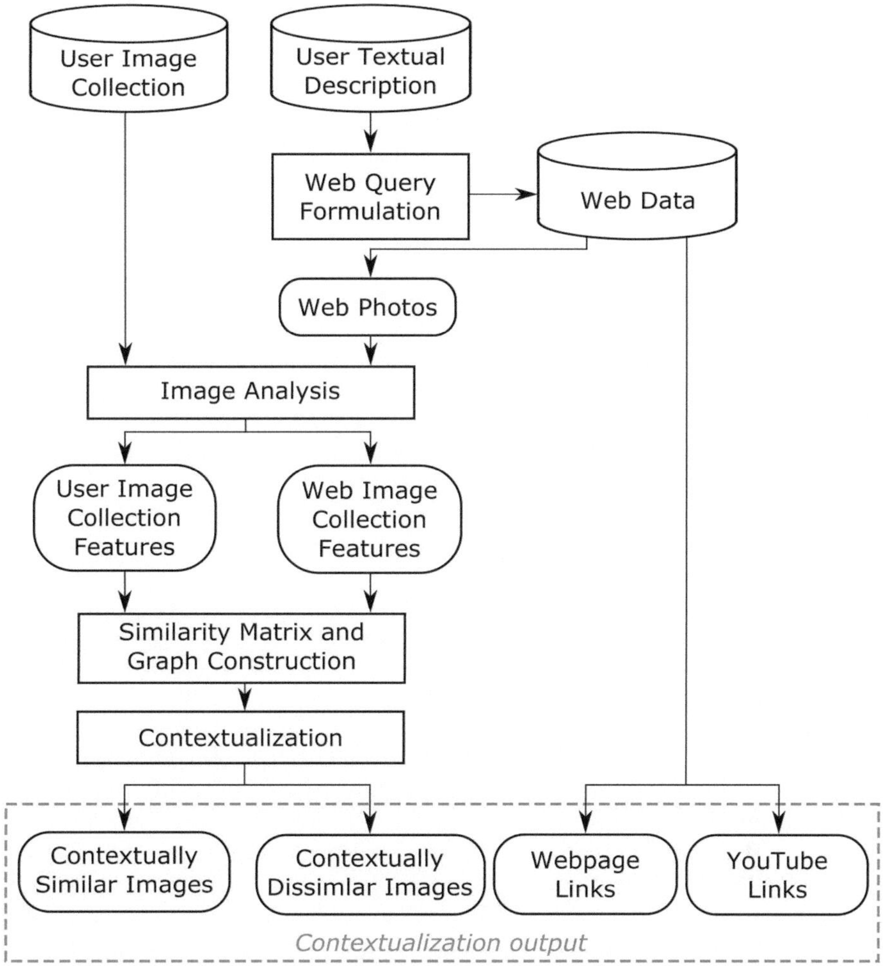

Fig. 5.14 Overview of the photo collection contextualization method that uses web data

two additional queries; one limiting the location of the place where the photos are taken (assuming that they contain location coordinates) and the other limiting the time that the photos have been taken (assuming that this information is available at the photo's metadata). In case of limiting the location, the query is formulated using the event and location terms (i.e. event & location), while for limiting the time, only event and time terms are used (event & time).

The number of returned items for each query (P, Y, B, F thresholds) is selected empirically. The links of web pages and YouTube videos are directly returned to the user as contextual information. The set of photos collected in the above steps is used as the pool of data from which the contextualization information is retrieved. This pool, denoted as web photos from now on, serves a similar purpose to the archived collection set of the method discussed in Sect. 5.2.2.1. Specifically, these web photos are fed into the image analysis component, and the same features as in the case of the user-supplied photo collection are extracted.

To perform the actual contextualization step, we construct a similarity matrix $\mathbf{W}$ between the N_w web photos and N_u user photos, so that $W_{i,j}$ denotes the similarity between the ith photo of the web photos to the jth photo of the user data ($i \in [1 \dots N_w]$, $j \in [1 \dots N_u]$). Four thresholds t_1, t_2, t_3 and t_4 are established, with $t_1, t_2, t_3, t_4 \in [0 \dots 1]$ and $t_4 < t_3 < t_2 < t_1$. All pairs of web photos and user photos are examined:

- An (i,j) pair with $t_2 < W_{i,j} < t_1$ is considered contextually similar. These photos are similar to those of the user photo collection but not identical and are used to describe in more detail a sub-event that the user has also captured.
- An (i,j) pair with $t_4 < W_{i,j} < t_3$ is considered contextually dissimilar. These photos are from the same event, but quite different from those of the user photo collection, and are used to describe the event from a different aspect to the user.
- An (i,j) pair with $W_{i,j} > t_1$ is considered as a pair of duplicates, and these photos are discarded.
- An (i,j) pair with $W_{i,j} < t_4$ is considered irrelevant, and these photos are discarded.
- An (i,j) pair in the interval $t_2 < W_{i,j} < t_3$ is omitted to get more accurate results, since it is not clear if these photos should be considered contextually similar or dissimilar to the user photo collection.

In order to make sure that no identical or near-duplicate photos are selected from web photos, a similarity matrix of all photos in the web photos collection is constructed, using the Euclidean distances of their features. This similarity matrix is considered as the weight matrix of a graph, and subsequently, the strongly connected components of the graph are found. Each strongly connected component is a sub-graph in which every node is connected to every other node in the sub-graph. Therefore, a strongly connected component is a group of very similar photos in the web photos collection. Each time a photo from the web photos is selected for contextualization, the strong component of the web photos graph in which this photo belongs is marked as used, and no other photos are selected from it.

The values of internal parameters t_1, t_2, t_3 and t_4 are set empirically to, respectively, 0.95, 0.89, 0.76 and 0.70. The implemented method requires only two user-controlled input parameters $a (a > 0)$ and $b (0 < b < 1)$. Similar to the personal photo collection contextualization method presented in Sect. 5.2.2.1, a controls the number of web photos that will be used for contextualizing the user collection, while b specifies the percentage of the latter photos that should belong to the contextually similar set; the rest of the web photos that will be used for contextualizing the user collection are drawn from the contextually dissimilar set.

Evaluation of Photo Collection Contextualization Using Web Data Method

The method is tested again using the *London* dataset of the MediaEval SEM task [83]. We randomly selected 129 photos covering all sub-events of the dataset and

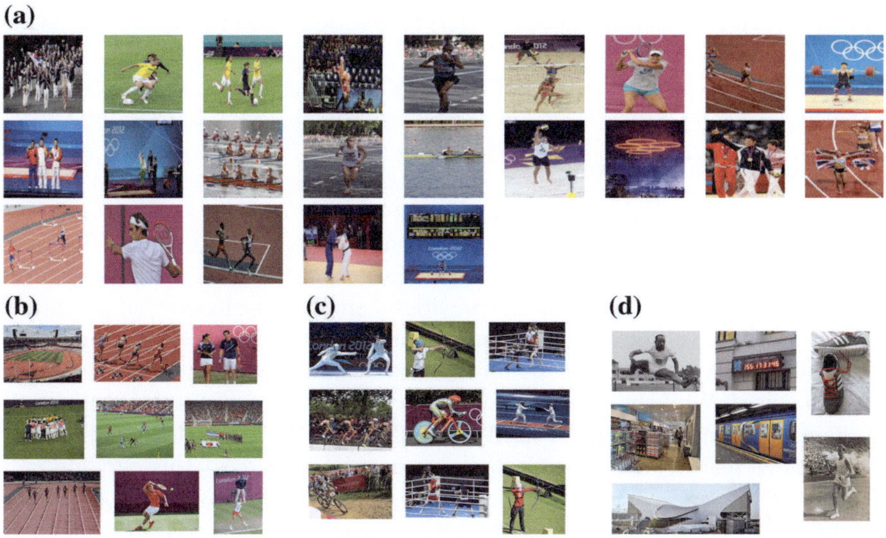

Fig. 5.15 **a** User collection. **b** Contextually similar web photos. **c** Contextually dissimilar web photos. **d** Irrelevant web photos

created the event name of the textual description as Olympic Games, the location as London and the year as 2012. 588 photos were downloaded from the web and served as the web photos collection.

Due to lack of ground-truth data for the photo collection gathered from the web, we evaluate the results of this contextualization method visually. A subset of the user collection is shown in Fig. 5.15a, and the retrieved web photos collection is shown in Figs. 5.15b–d. Figure 5.15b contains the contextually similar photos and we observe that these depict sub-events that are contained in the user collection, but from different aspects. On the other side, Fig. 5.15c contains the contextually dissimilar photos, depicting sub-events that are not contained in the user collection. Finally, the rest of the photos retrieved from the web, in Fig. 5.15(d), are the photos that were not used for contextualization.

Additionally, the following web page links are returned by the web queries and provided as contextual information:

- http://www.olympic.org/london-2012-summer-olympics
- https://en.wikipedia.org/wiki/2012_Summer_Olympics
- https://en.wikipedia.org/wiki/London_Olympics
- http://www.miniclip.com/games/london-2012-olympic-games/en/

In conclusion, we can see how the resulting contextualized collection includes complementary information for the events that were attended by the user that submitted the original collection which should help to aid the better understanding of those events. It also includes additional information about events the user did not attend, in order to give a more complete view of the whole Olympics. Both of these aspects fit perfectly with the general model of contextualization detailed at the beginning of this chapter.

5.3 Context Evolution

The idea behind context evolution is to give some sense of how the world (your own personal sphere as well as the world in general) changes over time. Such changes clearly affect our ability to understand previously archived documents, as our current world view may well be very different to that when the document was originally produced. For the purpose of modelling context evolution, context can be structured or unstructured. While both forms evolve over time, we believe that this happens in different ways, and we therefore need differing approaches to modelling this.

Structured data, by their very nature, are curated resources. This curation may be an active process where an ontology or data source is knowingly updated and maintained, or an unintended side effect, such as adding a new contact to an email client, which provides structured data that could be used for contextualization. In both cases, changes in the data are handled by an existing process. This applies equally to large sources of world knowledge (such as the fairly frequent updated releases of DBpedia) and to personal data. In structured resources, the evolution of context information is often already handled as new data supplements, rather than replaces existing information.

In contrast, unstructured context is entirely lacking in information relating to how it might have evolved over time. For example, this context may take the form of topics relevant to preserved documents, which give a sense of what a document might be talking about, but as they may not be linked to any other information, it is not clear exactly what they refer to and how that meaning might change from one document to another. Thus, extra information that can be extracted about the terms and how they evolve would be beneficial. This may involve explicitly determining the evolution of a term/topic or it might revolve more around the way the information is presented, allowing users to easily infer the evolution aspects.

Imagine that the data contain a simple statement: ‘the situation in Iran is obviously worrying and the Foreign Office is keeping a close watch on events’. It is likely that both ‘Iran’ and ‘Foreign Office’ would be linked to a structured source of context information (world and organizational in turn) and while useful, neither gives a sense of what the ‘situation in Iran’ might refer to. The date of the document will, however, give some sense of what this might be; for the late 1970s to early 1980s, it would most likely be referring to the revolution, while since the late 1990s, it is likely to refer to their nuclear research programme, and it may well refer to human rights issues regardless of the time period. We therefore need to know how the world has evolved to set the document in the correct context.

In the rest of this section, we detail a number of approaches to context evolution that are able to process either structured or unstructured context.

5.3.1 Structured Context

In most cases, structured knowledge which could be viewed or used as context is produced and maintained by some form of manual process. This process may be specifically aimed at producing structured knowledge, such as the construction and maintenance of an ontology, or just a side effect of using an application. For example, adding the contact details for a new employee to the address book in an email client has the side effect of producing structured knowledge that could be used for contextualization. Regardless of the approach, the result is the same; the issues are how the data evolve over time, how we can capture this information and how the changes can be reported or explained to the user.

Our approach to modelling the evolution of context revolves around being able to track how structured information changes over time. We take a similar approach to [124] and adopt the idea of *Valid Time*: a set of points or intervals of time in which a single fact is known to be true. Ideally, this would involve having accurate timestamps associated with every piece of information, but this is not always feasible. For example, an ontology does not allow properties on relations, making it impossible to timestamp the addition of a relation between two existing entities. In the worst-case scenario, there may only be periodic updates of the data with only a single timestamp on the entire knowledge repository. In such an extreme case, the changes would need to be determined via finding all differences, and each change could not be individually assigned an accurate *Valid Time*. For the purpose of further discussion, we will assume that some intermediate situation holds in which the evolving data, but not necessarily all data, have a *Valid Time* associated with it.

We have previously assumed that information useful for contextualization will be stored as an ontology, and so the first step in handling the evolution of this information is to specify how information on *Valid Time* should be encoded within it. Since relations within an ontology cannot have properties, in a standard ontology it is only possible to associate timestamps with instances. Fortunately, this only really affects datatype properties (i.e. those that lead to a value such as a string or number rather than an object property that leads to another instance in the ontology), and it is always possibly to rewrite a datatype property as an object property if required.

With the focus now on recording *Valid Time* for object properties, it is a simple case of adding new datatype properties to each instance that records the period for which they are valid. This could use the standard `xsd:datetime` format to allow timestamps to be accurate to the minute (i.e. 2014-05-23T10:20:13+05:30), or could be a simpler integer representation of a date if accuracy only to the day is required (i.e. 20140523).

Let us assume that we are working with an organizational ontology that includes people and the jobs they hold. Stored as triples, this may give us information such as the following (using an oo prefix to stand for organizational ontology):

```
<oo:Employee1> <rdfs:label> "Joe Bloggs"
<oo:Employee1> <oo:jobTitle> "Cleaner"
```

While simple, this approach does not allow for changes in job title over time to be recorded. Switching from a datatype property to an object property allows us to extend the data with *Valid Time* information, stored as an integer in the form yyyyMMdd, as follows:

```
<oo:Employee1> <rdfs:label> "Joe Bloggs"

<oo:Employee1> <oo:jobTitle> <oo:Job1>
<oo:Job1> <rdfs:label> "Cleaner"
<oo:Job1> <oo:fromdate> 20080305
<oo:Job1> <oo:todate> 99991231
```

This extended ontology now shows that the employee was hired as a cleaner on the 3rd of May 2008, while the far future date, in the `todate` property, shows that they are still working in that role at the time of the ontology creation. Now let us assume that after just over 2 years, Joe is promoted to a supervisory role, and that his change in job title is added to the ontology.

```
<oo:Employee1> <rdfs:label> "Joe Bloggs"

<oo:Employee1> <oo:jobTitle> <oo:Job1>
<oo:Job1> <rdfs:label> "Cleaner"
<oo:Job1> <oo:fromdate> 20080305
<oo:Job1> <oo:todate> 20100607

<oo:Employee1> <oo:jobTitle> <oo:Job2>
<oo:Job2> <rdfs:label> "Cleaning Supervisor"
<oo:Job2> <oo:fromdate> 20100607
<oo:Job2> <oo:todate> 99991231
```

This approach also allows multiple overlapping pieces of information. For example, let us assume that cleaning was not a full-time job, and so after working for the company for a year, up until the time he was promoted to supervisor, Joe was also employed as a porter.

```
<oo:Employee1> <rdfs:label> "Joe Bloggs"

<oo:Employee1> <oo:jobTitle> <oo:Job1>
<oo:Job1> <rdfs:label> "Cleaner"
<oo:Job1> <oo:fromdate> 20080305
<oo:Job1> <oo:todate> 20100606

<oo:Employee1> <oo:jobTitle> <oo:Job2>
<oo:Job2> <rdfs:label> "Cleaning Supervisor"
<oo:Job2> <oo:fromdate> 20100607
<oo:Job2> <oo:todate> 99991231

<oo:Employee1> <oo:jobTitle> <oo:Job3>
<oo:Job3> <rdfs:label> "Porter"
<oo:Job3> <oo:fromdate> 20090305
<oo:Job3> <oo:todate> 20100606
```

Notice how each change to the ontology is now non-destructive. The only changes made are additions or setting the `todate` data property to a valid date stamp rather than the far future filler value. This means that no information is ever lost, and so a single current snapshot of the ontology contains all the information related to documents written at any time during the organization's history (or at least since they adopted this approach to data storage).

One potential problem with using such an ontology for contextualization is that it now includes information which was true but is no longer so. For example, in the last ontology snippet given above, we can see that information on Joe Bloggs being both a cleaner and porter is present, although at the current time he is only employed as a cleaning supervisor. That means that we need to be careful to restrict the parts of the ontology used for contextualizing a document to only those which are valid at the time the document was created. Fortunately, it is easy to add a filter to any SPARQL query to extract specific elements of an ontology. The following query extracts a list of employees and their job titles on the 1st April 2009.

```
select ?e ?j where {
?e <oo:jobTitle> ?j .
?j <oo:fromdate> ?f .
?j <oo:todate> ?t
FILTER (?f <= 20090401 && ?t >= 20090401)
}
```

Using our example ontology, this query would return Joe Bloggs employed as a cleaner. If we are only interested in the current status, then we can utilize the far future date to select just those items that are currently valid (avoiding the filter, in this case, should increase the performance):

```
select ?e ?j where {
?e <oo:jobTitle> ?j .
?j <oo:fromdate> ?f .
?j <oo:todate> "99991231"^^<http://www.w3.org
    /2001/XMLSchema#int>
}
```

With this ability to determine the state of the ontology at any point in time, it is possible to track changes over time. A timeline showing the jobs held by a given person over a given time period is now easy to produce. The problem is that, even in short documents, a lot of context information may be present, and if a long time has elapsed since the document was originally written, then its context could have evolved significantly. While it may be possible to display all the changes to the user in some fashion, it is likely to simply lead to information overload. The solution, although not ideal, is to manually weight domain-specific properties in order to focus on showing the evolution of the most important concepts and relationships within the ontology.

While this approach to handling context evolution within a structured knowledge source is quite easy to adopt and use, it should be noted that having information and it being useful are two separate concepts. As with many of the techniques detailed in this chapter, a good user interface would be required to surface this information in a usable fashion. User applications are, however, outside the scope of this chapter.

5.3.2 Unstructured Context

As explained earlier, unstructured context is entirely lacking in information relating to how it might have evolved over time. In this section, we focus on the evolution of topics, illustrated via the following problem: *Given a topic or entity of interest q, such as Iran or Germany, determine the context evolution of that entity over a given period of time*. The problem contains two subtasks: (i) identify the context that the entity is involved in at a specific time, and (ii) determine the evolution of the context over time.

To tackle this problem, we propose an approach which consists of three main steps: *Document Gathering* that collects relevant documents for each topic (where a topic is a 'context hook' as defined on page 136) used as a query q, *Context Extraction* extracts associated topics from those documents and *Context Evolution* determines which topics are relevant at a particular point in time.

The first step is to gather relevant documents from a time-stamped collection for a given query. The time-stamped corpus contains a set of articles with specific publication dates; e.g. New York Time articles published from 1987 to 2007, and UK Parliament debates spanning from 1935 to present. In order to obtain relevant documents, we use a query-likelihood language model that determines the similarity of the query q with documents from the corpus (as described in Sect. 5.2.1.2). The likelihood of the query q from a language model estimated from a document d with the assumption that query terms are independent is calculated as follows:

$$P(d|q) \propto P(d) \prod_{w \in q} P(w|d)^{n(w,q)}$$

where w is a query term in q, $n(w, q)$ is the term frequency of w and q, and $P(w|d)$ is the probability of w estimated using Dirichlet smoothing:

$$P(w|d) = \frac{n(w, c) + \mu P(w)}{\mu + \sum_{w'} n(w', c)}$$

where μ is the smoothing parameter, and $P(w)$ is the probability of each term w in the collection.

In order to extract context in which a given entity is involved, we consider topics mentioned in documents as context and make use of Latent Dirichlet Allocation (LDA) to accomplish this task. LDA is a generative model of documents. Assuming that we have a corpus D containing a set of documents, and each document d is represented by a bag of words. LDA assumes that every word in a document is generated by first picking a latent topic and then sampling from the distribution of words conditioned on the selected topic. Probability distributions obtained after training an LDA model include $P(w|z)$, the probability word w given topic z, and $P(z|d)$, the probability of topic z given document d.

When attempting to determine context evolution, the first task is to determine the significant years for a given entity. This can be estimated in a straightforward way, by counting how many times each year has been mentioned in the documents in the time-stamped corpus. In addition, we want to see the reason why a particular year has been mentioned frequently and how the context that the entity involved in changes during the time. For this purpose, we estimate the topic distribution of each significant year. Let $P(z|d)$ be the topic distribution of each document returned by LDA, and let D_y be the set of documents mentioning y as their publication dates. We can estimate the topic distribution of each year, i.e. $P(z|y)$ using the following equation:

$$P(z|y) = \frac{1}{|D_y|} \sum_{d \in D_y} P(z|d)$$

Using the probability $P(z|y)$, we can determine a set of topics that the query entity is heavily associated with for a given year y. This information can be represented as context evolution timelines.

In order to determine the evolution of a specific topic over time, we can compute the probability $P(y|z)$ as follows:

$$P(y|z) = \frac{P(z|y) \times P(y)}{P(z)} P(y|z) \propto P(z|y) \times P(y)$$

where $P(z|y)$ is computed as described above, and $P(y)$ is estimated as

$$P(y) = \frac{\sum_{d \in D; y_d == y} 1}{|D|}$$

where $|D|$ is a total number of documents in the collection.

To illustrate the effectiveness of the proposed approach, we qualitatively analyse the results using several entity queries on the UK Parliament Debate corpus.[12] Let us consider *'Iran'* as the entity of interest. Our method first identifies a list of most important years, based on how frequently the entity was discussed in each year. In this example, 1991, 2010 and 2014 are determined significant years for the entity *'Iran'* in the corpus. For each significant year, a set of related contexts is then extracted, where each context is represented by a list of correlated words, as shown in Table 5.11.

The proposed method can also analyse the evolution of extracted contexts over time. For example, the *'iraq war saddam'* topic was mostly discussed in 1991 but was frequently mentioned again in 1999. It reflects the conflict between Iran and Iraq during such years. Similarly, the topic of Russia's relation with Iran occurred in the debate corpus in 1980, but received high attention again in 2014.

These results clearly show that the set of topics related to a given 'context hook' changes over time, and that visualizing those changing topics can give an insight into how the meaning of the context hook has changed over that time period.

---

[12] http://parser.theyworkforyou.com/hansard.html.

Table 5.11 Example of significant years and related topics for the entity Iran

Year	Topics
1991	Iraq war saddam hussein
	House debate government statement
	Israel middle east peace
2010	Afghanistan pakistan security force
	Iran russia sanction foreign
	European europe union minister
2014	Syria minister government libya
	Iran russia sanction foreign
	Afghanistan pakistan security force

5.4 Practical Uses for Context Information

While the main aim of contextualization is to provide a context in which previously archived documents can be interpreted, this does not prohibit the information from being utilized to provide an immediate benefit to those adopting contextualization within their applications and frameworks. One place where context can play an important role is within a search system, by allowing related information to be used to answer search queries. Adoption of the approaches we have outlined can thus have an immediate as well as long-term benefit. In fact, such an approach often allows relevant documents that would never be found by a conventional text search engine to be retrieved and highly ranked. In the rest of this section, we describe one such search system, GATE Mímir, which can make use of context information to provide a rich search experience.

GATE Mímir[13] [104] is an open source, multi-paradigm information management index and repository which can be used to index and search over text, annotations and context information. It allows queries that arbitrarily mix full-text, structural, linguistic and context queries, and that can scale to gigabytes of text. To support such queries, a GATE Mímir index allows combinations of text (to enable full-text search); annotations (linguistic metadata associated with the text, e.g. 'Person', and including wildcards, standard binary operators, etc.); and context data (world and personal knowledge stored in an ontology, which allows the system to perform generalisations based on knowledge that a city is located in a particular country).

It is worth noting that in our example, the related data (organizational or personal depending on the application) are actually used both during the annotation of the documents and at search time, although the two uses differ substantially. The data are used to both contextualize the documents (i.e. to annotate them with instance data) and then again at search time where related information can be utilized to fulfil the search query. The main advantage of this approach over existing text search engines is that there are interesting questions which can only be answered using

[13]http://gate.ac.uk/family/mimir.html.

the additional data. The combination of text, annotations and context data allow, for example, us to find documents using queries such as:

```
{Person sparql = "SELECT ?inst WHERE
{?inst :birthPlace <http://dbpedia.org/resource/
   Sheffield>}"
} [0..4] root:say}}
```

This query basically says: *find all the places at which a Person annotation, who is mentioned in DBpedia as being born in Sheffield, occurs within at most five words of the verb 'to say'*. It is important to note that few, if any, of the documents which would match this query mention place of birth; that information would be present in the ontology used for contextualization.

While we have shown just a single complex query that includes context, this has demonstrated how powerful combining information in this way can be. This approach allows us to provide an immediate benefit to users adopting our approaches to contextualization as part of a preservation strategy, rather than the focus being purely on how the data can be used in some distant future to look back at old data, a situation that might, initially at least, seem less interesting to potential adopters. For many more examples of how useful this approach, see [281].

5.5 Summary and Discussion

We started this discussion of contextualization with the quote *You shall know a word by the company it keeps* [137], and throughout the chapter have introduced a number of concepts, ideas and approaches which embody this notion, while extending it beyond a single word to encompass textual documents and images.

The techniques we have described are based on our general approach to contextualization (detailed on page 136) in which a 'contextualization method' attempts to associate extra information, referred to as 'context units', with specific elements of a document, which we call 'context hooks'. While we have not detailed approaches for all document types, we have presented algorithms for contextualizing short social media posts, longer text documents (such as newspaper articles) and two approaches for contextualizing image collections, which together cover a large proportion of the documents encountered on a daily basis. Context information, as with any other type of information, is only useful if it is kept up to date, and for this, we have introduced two approaches to context evolution: one that handles structured context information, and one which attempts to determine the evolution of unstructured information.

Taken together, these approaches generate a potentially vast trove of context information that can be preserved alongside documents to enable them to be unambiguously interpreted at a later date. The information can, however, have an immediate use in providing data for search and other document navigation tasks. While such tools are primarily UI related, and so outside the scope of this chapter, we have presented one possible search use case to illustrate this point more clearly.

To conclude, information is defined by the context, both world and personal, in which it was first created. That context needs to be captured, stored and presented back to users if we stand any chance of ensuring the information stays fully understandable over long periods of time. The techniques described in this chapter are important steps in this direction and should allow others to take us further down this road.

Chapter 6
Bridging Information Management and Preservation: A Reference Model

Francesco Gallo, Claudia Niederée and Walter Allasia

Abstract The idea of the Preserve-or-Forget (PoF) approach introduced in this book is to follow a forgetful, focused approach to digital preservation, which is inspired by human forgetting and remembering. Its goal is to ease the adoption of preservation technology especially in the personal and organizational context and to ensure that important content is kept safe, useful, and understandable in the long run. For this purpose, it stresses the smooth interaction between information management and preservation management. Leveraging the PoF approach, in this chapter we introduce a reference model, which will be referred to in the following as PoF Reference Model. The model pays special attention to the functionality which bridges between Information Management System (Active System) and Digital Preservation System (DPS), such as the selection of content for preservation and the transfer of content between the systems. The model aims to encapsulate the core ideas of the PoF approach, which considers Active System and DPS as a joint ecosystem into a re-usable model, and is inspired by the core principles of this approach: synergetic preservation, managed forgetting, and contextualized remembering. The design of the PoF Reference Model was driven by the identification of five required characteristics for such a reference model: it has to be integrative, value-driven, brain-inspired, forgetful, and evolution-aware. The PoF Reference Model consists of a functional part (Functional Model) and of an associated Information Model. The Functional Model is made up of three layers: Core Layer, Remember and Forget Layer, and Evolution Layer. For each layer, we discuss the main functional entities and the representative workflows, also relating them to existing standards and practices in digital preservation. The functionality required to mediate between the Active System and the DPS has been encapsulated into the PoF Middleware, which has been designed

F. Gallo (✉) · W. Allasia
EURIX Srl, Torino, Italy
e-mail: gallo@eurixgroup.com

W. Allasia
e-mail: allasia@eurixgroup.com

C. Niederée
L3S Research Center, Hannover, Germany
e-mail: niederee@L3S.de

V. Mezaris et al. (eds.), *Personal Multimedia Preservation*, Springer Series on Cultural Computing, https://doi.org/10.1007/978-3-319-73465-1_6

and implemented as part of the ForgetIT project. The Information Model describes the preservation entities and their relationships, also discussing the interoperability with existing digital preservation standards.

6.1 Introduction

In this chapter, we present a model and an implementation for the novel approach to intelligent preservation management propagated in this book, which is inspired by the three principles: synergetic preservation, managed forgetting, and contextualized remembering— the PoF approach, for short. The model discussed here will be referred to in the following as PoF Reference Model. We follow a forgetful, focused approach to digital preservation, which is inspired by human forgetting and remembering. Its goal is to ease the adoption of preservation technology especially in the personal and organizational context and to ensure that important content is kept safe, useful, and understandable in the long run.

The PoF Reference Model leverages the ideas of the approach to a conceptual level: required conceptual functionalities, core processes, and relevant concepts are collected in a systematic way and are related to each other. The model aims to encapsulate the core ideas of this approach into a re-usable model. Similar to the OAIS Reference Model [67], the model described here defines the terminology and concepts for the approach, which can be used as a basis for the implementation of the approach as well as for the further discussion and development of a forgetful approach to preservation.

The PoF Reference Model targets personal as well as organizational preservation settings, which are not covered by legal regulations such as deposit laws. The focus is not on supporting memory institutions, although parts of the approach (e.g., contextualization) might be applicable in this area as well. The selected settings can especially benefit from the PoF approach, since (a) there is a big gap to preservation adoption in those fields, (b) there are explicit preservation choices to be made, and (c) there is a need for automation of the processes, in order to reduce the amount of investment required for preservation.

Since our approach stresses the smooth interaction between the so far mainly separated worlds of information management and preservation management, the PoF Reference Model pays special attention to the functionality which bridges between the Information Management System (which we call Active System) and the Digital Preservation System (DPS). This includes the selection of content for preservation, the transfer of content between the systems, contextualization for easing long-term interpretation, processing during preservation time in reaction to changes, as well as access to the joint information space populated both by preserved content and content in active use.

In order to support a smooth transition between the Active System and the DPS, in the PoF Reference Model we are considering active information use and preservation as part of a *joint ecosystem*, stressing the smooth transitions and the synergetic interactions rather than the system borders. This is also a core distinction from the OAIS model, which is restricted to the DPS.

It is worth noting that the PoF Reference Model does not intend to replace the OAIS model and other preservation standards. As mentioned above, it has a different focus than OAIS and can interact with OAIS compatible approaches.

In the following, we discuss a functional and an information part of the PoF Reference Model, which are referred to in the following as Functional Model and Information Model, respectively.

In this chapter, we also present a possible mapping of this joint ecosystem onto three separate systems, i.e., the Active System (in the form of adapters and/or system extensions), the DPS (typically OAIS based), and a middleware component, named PoF Middleware, which couples both systems in a flexible way. The PoF Middleware is the core part of the exemplary implementation of the PoF approach.

6.2 Foundations of the PoF Reference Model

The goal of the PoF Reference Model is to ease the use of preservation systems.

In a nutshell, it should be easy to get things preserved, the right things should be preserved and the things should stay useful in the long term. Thus, we have to consider the full cycle of getting things into the DPS, managing them there for a considerable time and bringing them back into use.

This raises three questions: (1) how do we get content easily from the Active System into the DPS? (2) which content should be put into the DPS? (3) how can we keep the content useful in the long run and bring it back in a reasonable form, when needed? Here, it has to be considered that we speak of time frames of several decades in the context of preservation.

For answering question (1) it is important that the gap, which actually exists between an Active System and a DPS, has to be bridged. Thus, the PoF Reference Model should support an *integrative* approach. For question (2) on which content to select, it makes sense to follow the idea of appraisal typically followed in an archive, i.e., having a decision process for which content to keep. Since we want to ease the use of DPS, it is desirable that this process is automated, performing information value assessment for identifying important content to be preserved: this opts for a *value-driven* approach. Finally, question (3) implies that evolution, which takes place while the content is in the archival system, has to be carefully considered, in order to keep it accessible and useful in the long term. Thus, the approach taken by the model should be *evolution-aware*. In addition to these three characteristics, as already discussed in the previous chapters, our approach takes inspiration from the effectiveness of humans in remembering important things and forgetting irrelevant things. Therefore, our model is also supposed to be *brain-inspired* and *forgetful* in its preservation decisions.

Thus, five main characteristics have been identified for the proposed PoF Reference Model, supporting the PoF approach for a sustainable and smooth transition between information and preservation management. Those characteristics and their implications will be discussed in more detail in the following sections.

6.2.1 Integrative: Bridging the Gap Between Information and Preservation Management

It is the aim of the PoF approach to preservation to create a smooth transition between active information use and preservation of information, which so far are some quite separate worlds. For this purpose, the PoF Reference Model should be *integrative*, bringing the Active System and the DPS closer together.

However, due to the inherent long-term perspective of preservation-related solutions it is not the aim to build a strongly integrated, monolithic system. In the long run, it has to be foreseen that the used Active System and the employed DPS will both change [3]. The idea is rather a flexible integration, which enables smooth bidirectional transition of information between the Active System and the DPS and, at the same time, is also prepared for major changes in the overall environment [319].

A core part of integration is to enable the smooth transition of content to be preserved into the DPS and the meaningful reactivation of content back into the Active System after a (possibly very long) period in the DPS. An integrative solution should also embrace the idea of a *joint information space*, where the information in the DPS stays conceptually accessible, e.g., visible in search results, even if the content is only available in the DPS.

One part of achieving a smooth transition is to introduce a middleware system (the so-called PoF Middleware) to act as a pre-ingest system (or pre-access) and prepare information packages for delivery in either way. With highly automated procedures for preparation of these packages according to agreements or requirements, preservation technology becomes easier to use and the quality of the information packages becomes more consistent, which alleviate the burden of information package handling on both sides (see e.g. [164]). In addition, an integrative system should also support the decisions on what to preserve for easing the integration of preservation into the information management workflows, finally aiming for an integrated information and preservation management workflow.

6.2.2 Value-Driven: Acting upon Short-Term and Long-Term Information Value

As already discussed in Chap. 4 of this book in more detail, one of the core ideas of the PoF approach is to deviate from the general *keep it all* model, which makes the implicit assumption that all information has the same value with respect to being kept or for being important, in more general. The value of information is multifaceted and can be considered from different perspectives. We distinguish *short-term value*, i.e., value for current activities, from the *long-term value* of a resource, e.g., for an organization. For the combined information and preservation management system, both short-term value and long-term value of information have to be considered.

The short-term value refers to the value of content for the current focus of activity. Identifying the short-term value of a document is of high interest for creating immediate benefit in information management, e.g., by de-cluttering the desktop in Personal Information Management (see Chap. 7). For a more in depth discussion on short-term value and the related concept of Memory Buoyancy (MB) see Chap. 4.

The long-term value of a resource is obviously relevant in the context of preservation. It refers to the value a resource has in the long term. Such long-term value can be used to decide about the investment to be made into preservation for the respective resource [14]. For a more in-depth discussion on long-term value and the related concept of Preservation Value (PV) see Chap. 4.

6.2.3 Brain-Inspired: What Can We Learn from Human Forgetting and Remembering?

The model discussed in this chapter is inspired by a joint perspective on Human and Digital Memory as described in [310]. On the Human Memory side, three main types of memory are distinguished in such joint perspective, depicted in Fig. 6.1: *Working Memory*, *Episodic Memory* and *Semantic Memory*. For a discussion of the memory types see also Sects. 2.1.3 and 2.1.4. Together with the currently activated Episodic and Semantic Memory, the Verbal Short-Term Memory (things just heard) and the Visual Short-Term Memory (things just seen) form the Working Memory, which frames the current situation. Knowledge is activated on demand from the Semantic and Episodic Memory according to current needs via the so-called Executive Functions. Perception (depicted on top of Fig. 6.1) is one driver for such activation. It is worth noting that perceived signals do not directly become part of the Verbal or Visual Short-Term Memory, which are constantly updated, but they are rather filtered and interpreted by things already in the memory for making sense of the perceived signals.

Similarly, as shown in Fig. 6.1, we also foresee a Working Memory within the Digital Memory in our model. This is composed of the digital resources currently relevant, e.g., used or important for current tasks or activities. In an automated Digital Working Memory signals from resource usage, pattern of usage, and change as well as relationships between resources will be used to update the Digital Working Memory. For this purpose, in our model, we introduce Managed Forgetting functions which control the transitions between the different parts of the Digital Memory (see also Chap. 4).

Together, the Working Memory and the Digital Working Memory form the Virtual Working Memory. Clearly, there is an influence between both of them. In the ideal

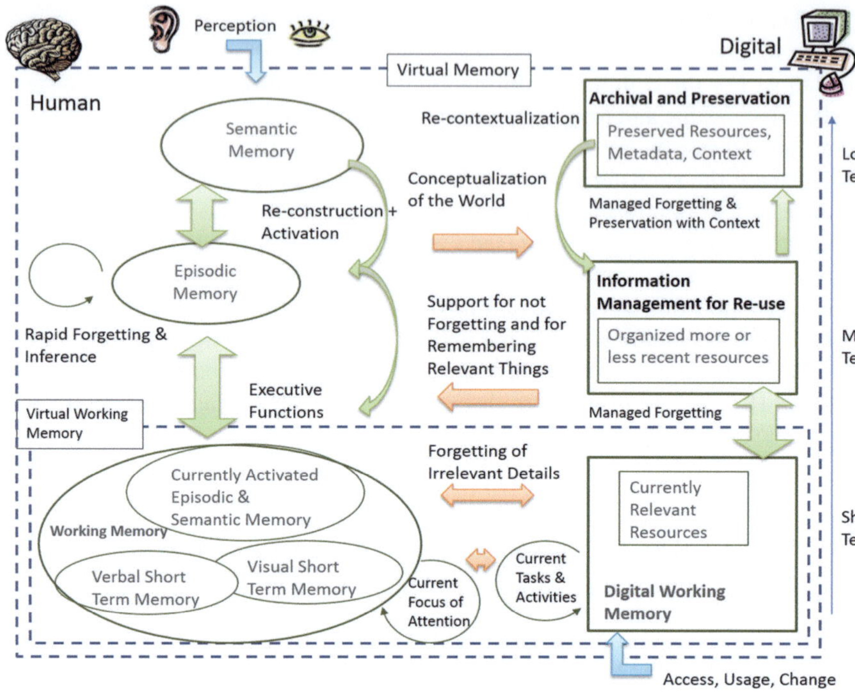

Fig. 6.1 Joint perspective on forgetful, interacting Human and Digital Memory (see also [310])

case, the Digital Working Memory would show to the user just all the information that the user needs in the current situation, but does not have in the Working Memory. Note that it is also possible that there is an influence of the way the Digital Memory works on the Human (Working) Memory (joint system perspective). For example, with the easy storage of phone numbers in mobile phones, humans no longer have to remember those numbers.

Managed Forgetting functions are also used to identify content that is of long-term value (see Sect. 6.2.2) and should, therefore, be preserved. In Fig. 6.1, we distinguish (a) Information Management for Re-use, as it is, e.g., done on a desktop computer or a server and (b) the system for Archival and Preservation (on top of Fig. 6.1). When content is transferred to Archival and Preservation, it makes sense to add context information to it (*contextualization*, see also Chap. 5). This prepares the content for re-contextualization which is required when preserved content is brought back at a (much) later time. The idea of re-contextualization as an active situation-dependent process of bringing back things "stored" in the memory is again inspired from Human Memory: when we as humans remember things this is also a re-construction process, which depends upon the current situation.

Episodic Memory is a detailed storage of events and is typically subject to fast forgetting as well as blurring between the memory of similar events due to interference. Here, Digital Memory complementing Human Memory, e.g., via photos, can serve as a reminder of things that are forgotten, but that one might want to remember or refresh at a later point in time. For this purpose, it is crucial to select the adequate content to preserve.

Semantic Memory is a more conceptual part of memory, which stresses on patterns, abstractions, and lessons learned and is directly connected to Perception (see top of Fig. 6.1). Here, the strongest interaction between Human Memory and Digital Memory is that the organization of digital resources does or should reflect the conceptualization of the world of the user, which is linked to the Semantic Memory. In Chap. 7 of this book, the Semantic Desktop approach is described as an example of more explicit modeling of the *Conceptualization of the World* with a richer annotation of resources. This knowledge about resources is used in the Information Management for Re-use and in the Archival and Preservation of the joint perspective outlined in Fig. 6.1.

6.2.4 Forgetful: Focus on the Important Things

As an alternative to the dominant *keep it all* approach, the PoF approach opts for conscious decisions about what is important and thus should be kept (and preserved). Since preservation comes at a cost, it is important to make such conscious decisions about what to preserve or how much to invest in the preservation of which part of the information space (see for example [49, 201, 335]). For this need, a forgetful approach based on Managed Forgetting is a good fit, as discussed in detail in Chap. 4.

A forgetful approach is based on *Information Value* assessment, i.e., computing and predicting the value of information resources (see e.g. [390]). Effective information value assessment, especially for long-term information value, is a complex task involving a variety of parameters and heuristics. Based on such value, preservation decisions can be taken. On a high level, these decisions could include choice of preservation provider and/or service as well as decisions about redundancy and transformations.

6.2.5 Evolution-Aware: Embracing the Long-Term Perspective

Since we are targeting integrated information and preservation management systems, we are operating in a long-lived context, covering a time perspective of several decades. Even things that are considered relatively stable in the current setting of an information system—such as the type or class of content management system in use—will change over time [3]. For sustainable operation, it is important to be prepared for such changes. It is one of the core ideas of the PoF approach to keep the important information accessible and usable even in case of large changes in the setting and context of operation. For incorporating *evolution-awareness* into our model, several types of evolution with different impacts on the model itself have to be considered:

1. *Changes in conceptual model of the Active System*: This could be due to, for example, changes in the organizational ontology underlying the content structuring as well as processes described in the content. This creates a semantic gap between the archived content (relying on the old implicit or explicit ontology) and the active content (structured by new ontology). This gap has to be bridged, at latest when preserved content is brought back into the active environment, in order to enable correct interpretation of the re-activated content (see Chap. 5);
2. *Active System evolution and exchange (Migration)*: The used Active System might be subject to major changes or might even be completely replaced by another system, if we look at time frames of several decades. In spite of such changes the content should stay accessible and usable [3];
3. *DPS evolution or exchange*: In the same way, the chosen DPS might evolve or could be exchanged over time. This implies the migration of content into a new DPS [173]. In the ideal case, this should have as little impact on the Active System as possible [3];
4. *Change in best practices and technology*: Formats as well as employed technologies might become obsolete over time. This requires the identification of such changes as well as adequate actions to react to those changes, such as format transformations.

The last item in the list above is a classical issue of any DPS. It is, therefore, not covered in too much detail here, since we focus on the things that go beyond current best practices in digital preservation.

6.3 PoF Functional Model

In the following we describe the functional part of the PoF Reference Model, which we refer to as PoF Functional Model or Functional Model for short, while the information part of the model (named Information Model) is described in Sect. 6.4.

The Functional Model is concerned with the main workflows of the PoF approach and the functionalities required for realizing those workflows. Special focus is given to the novel concepts introduced, namely the aspect of using Managed Forgetting in support of preservation, the role of contextualization and the impact of evolution. The PoF Functional Model is complemented by the PoF Information model presented in Sect. 6.4.

As in the case of the OAIS model, the functional view of the PoF Reference Model considers the main functional entities of the proposed reference model. Furthermore, we also describe the main workflows in the model and how the functional entities contribute to those workflows. Again the stress is on the parts which connect the two types of systems, Active System and DPS, with each other.

6.3.1 Layers, Workflows, and Functional Entities

The proposed PoF Functional Model is made up of three layers, which also represent different levels of compliance with the PoF approach:

- The **Core Layer** considers the basic functionalities required for connecting the Active System and the DPS;
- Building upon this layer, the **Remember and Forget Layer** introduces the brain-inspired and forgetful aspects into the PoF Reference Model implementing more advanced functionalities related to preservation preparation and re-activation;
- Finally, the **Evolution Layer** is responsible for all types of functionalities dealing with long-term change and evolution.

The different workflows and functional entities in the PoF Functional Model are associated with the three model layers above and are summarized in Table 6.1, where for each layer we list the associated workflows and the related functional entities.

The description of the layers, workflows, and functional entities is provided in the following. Some workflows are stepwise refined in the more complex layers.

Table 6.1 PoF Functional Model: layers, workflows, and functional entities

Model layers	Workflows	Functional entities
Core layer	Preservation preparation (*basic*) Re-activation (*basic*)	ID management Exchange support
Remember and forget layer	Preservation preparation Re-activation	Content value assessment
		Managed forgetting and appraisal
		De-contextualization
		Contextualization
		Preservation contract management
		Re-contextualization
		Search and navigation
		Metadata management
Evolution layer	Situation change	Content value re-assessment
	Setting change	Evolution monitoring
	System change (active system change and preservation system change)	Context evolution management
		Context-aware preservation management

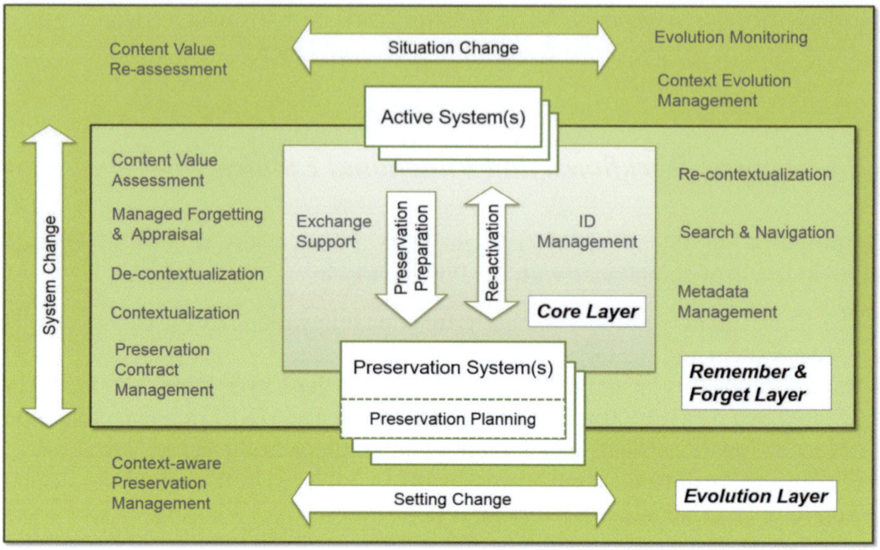

Fig. 6.2 High-level functional view of the PoF Reference Model

An overview of the PoF Functional Model components (layers, workflows, functional entities) is depicted in Fig. 6.2: within each layer box the relevant entities and workflows are shown. In the following sections, we provide a more detailed representation of each workflow with the steps associated to each process and the involved entities. It is worth noting that Fig. 6.2 already makes some assumptions about the functionalities implemented in the Active System and, especially, the DPS: those functionalities, which are part of one of the respective systems, are not explicitly listed in the PoF Reference Model.

For our purpose, we assume a OAIS compliant DPS implementing functionalities such as *Ingest*, *Data Management*, *Archival Storage* and *Access* of preserved content: in Fig. 6.2 we omitted all OAIS-compliant entities but the *Preservation Planning*, due to its relevance in the context of the Evolution Layer, as discussed in the following. Additional details about OAIS functional entities can be found in [67]. From OAIS model, we also take the concept of *Information Package* [67]: the Submission Information Package(SIP) and the Dissemination Information Package (DIP) in the PoF approach are enriched with context information to support synergetic preservation, while for what concerns the implementation of the Archival Information Package (AIP) the PoF approach leverages the specific solution adopted for the DPS.

The three layers are used in the following to describe the functional view of the PoF Reference Model in more detail.

6.3.2 *Core Layer*

The Core Layer embraces basic forms of two workflows connecting the Active System and the DPS, the **Preservation Preparation** workflow and the **Re-activation** workflow (see Fig. 6.2). In support of these two core workflows in their basic form, the Core Layer includes two types of functionality for managing resource identification and information exchange:

- **ID Management** is mainly responsible for mapping between the identifier (ID) of the resources in the Active System and the ID used in the DPS for identifying (and locating) the respective content resources. Since several versions of the same resource can be put in the DPS, the ID Management functionality also has to take care of resource versions and their mappings to archive IDs.
- **Exchange Support** is responsible for enabling the exchange of content and metadata between the Active System and the DPS. It adapts and maintains protocols for this purpose. The Exchange Support functionality handles both outgoing information and incoming packages that should be put back into active use. This includes basic functional activities for preparation of Information Packages, such as automatic identification and extraction of technical metadata providing input to the enrichment phase, and the creation of packages according to a given contract, the so-called preservation contract described in the following (see Table 6.3). The Exchange Support functionality can be considered as a client-side communication adapter and can, for example, be implemented in the form of a repository and related basic processes.

6.3.2.1 Basic Preservation Preparation

The Preservation Preparation workflow prepares content received from the Active System for preservation and transfers it to the DPS. For the pure transfer it relies on the functionality of the Exchange Support. On an abstract level, this workflow—in its basic form— consists of five steps (see Fig. 6.3): (1) *select* the content to be archived, (2) *provide* the content to the archival process, (3) *enrich* the content with

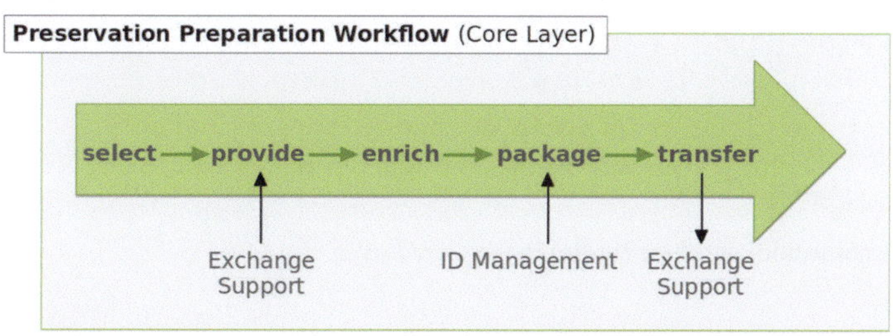

Fig. 6.3 Preservation Preparation Workflow (basic) in the Core Layer

context for preservation, (4) *package* the content according to the expectations of the DPS, and (5) *transfer* the content into the DPS. In terms of preservation terminology, the Preservation Preparation workflow can be considered as a pre-ingest workflow, which leads into the ingestion functionality of the DPS. This interaction is discussed in more detail in Sect. 6.5. Furthermore, it is worth noting that the enrich functionality is available on the Core Layer only in its basic form (e.g., to add technical information such as file format to the content to be archived). More advanced enrich functionality is discussed for the Remember and Forget Layer.

6.3.2.2 Basic Re-activation

The Re-activation workflow takes care of enabling the Active System to retrieve and re-activate content, which has been transferred to the DPS. Again on an abstract level, this workflow—in its basic form—consists of five steps (see Fig. 6.4): (1) *request* the content to be retrieved from the DPS (here via its identifier), (2) *search* requested content thus translating the request into archival ID(s) (in the basic workflow just involving the ID Management functionality), (3) *fetch* the respective content from the DPS, (4) *prepare* the content for delivery to the Active System, and (5) *deliver* content to the Active System.

In the Core Layer, the DPS is involved mainly in the fetch activity, which makes use of the Access functionality offered by the DPS to retrieve the content. As in the case of the Preservation Preparation workflow, some of the steps in the Re-activation workflow are only included in a very basic form on the Core Layer and are extended with more advanced functionalities on the Remember and Forget Layer.

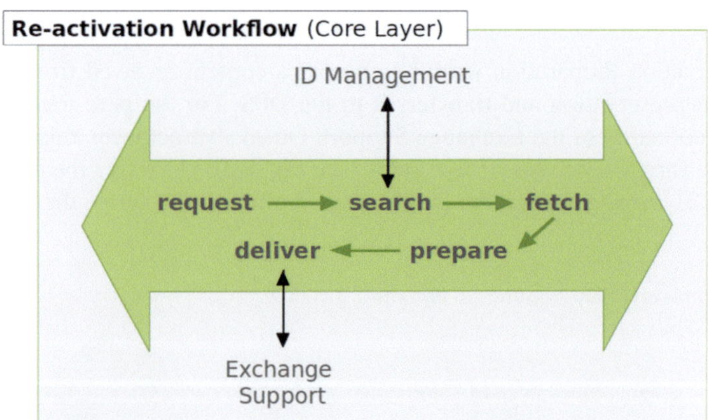

Fig. 6.4 Re-activation workflow (basic) in the Core Layer

6.3.3 *Remember and Forget Layer*

The Remember and Forget Layer introduces *brain-inspired* functionality into the PoF Reference Model, which targets the concepts of managed forgetting and contextualized remembering. For this purpose, the Remember and Forget Layer extends the two workflows **Preservation Preparation** and **Re-activation** from the Core Layer with further, more advanced functionalities related to contextualization and re-contextualization, to value assessment and to content access, which are described in the following. All of those listed functionalities create additional metadata, which have to be managed in a systematic way. Therefore, the Remember and Forget Layer also contains a functional entity for managing metadata. The workflows mentioned above define activities that contain rules, constraints, and settings, that should be agreed upon and that could be defined in a Preservation Contract. This contract is properly handled by a functional entity for contract management, which potentially relates to many, if not all, entities and is not drawn in the figures to avoid clutter.

6.3.3.1 Preservation Preparation

The Preservation Preparation workflow at the level of the Remember and Forget layer still consists of the same five steps defined for the Core Layer (*select*, *provide*, *enrich*, *package*, and *transfer*), as depicted in Fig. 6.5, but now uses two additional functionalities for the assessment of content value and for Managed Forgetting in the phase of selecting content for preservation, as described below:

- **Content Value Assessment** is based on the idea that understanding the value of content is in the core of content appraisal for preservation and managed forgetting. Content value assessment aims to determine the value of a resource. This value may change over time and there are different value dimensions, which reflect the value considering different purposes or perspectives and which may influence each other.

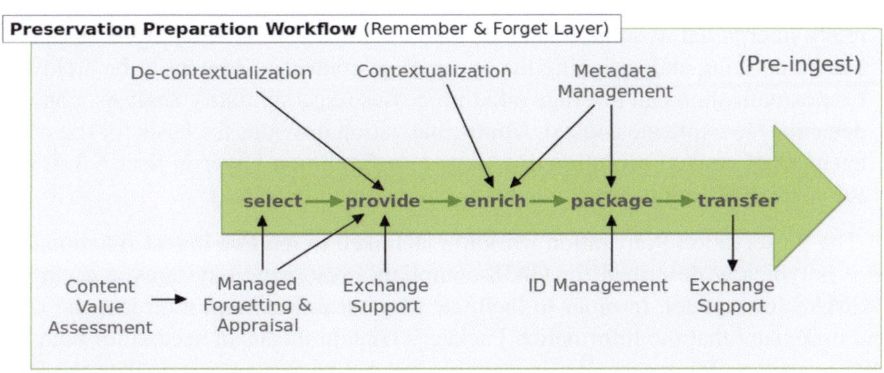

Fig. 6.5 Preservation Preparation workflow in the Remember and Forget Layer

There is, for example, a value dimension reflecting current importance, the MB, and a dimension reflecting the long-term importance or relevance of a resource, the PV. For assessing content value, the Content Value Assessment component takes evidence from the Active System, e.g., about information use, content creation, and further knowledge about the role of resources in the Active System. Content value can be used as a basis for making preservation decisions, e.g., whether a resource should be preserved or not, or how much should be invested in the preservation of a resource. Content value can also be used in the Active System, e.g., for especially highlighting resources with high content value.

- **Managed Forgetting and Appraisal** takes into account that with the dramatic growth of the amount of content, nowadays it becomes more and more important to make conscious decisions about preservation. Clear decisions on what to put into the DPS and explicit content appraisal have always been part of the processes of an archive [160], although not always as much in personal archiving [270]. The component for Managed Forgetting and Appraisal aims to help in automating such decisions, a need that has been identified earlier [161], for both personal archiving as well as organizational settings. This is encapsulated in the concept of Managed Forgetting, which uses the results of Content Value Assessment for deciding about preservation and forgetting actions. The effects of Managed Forgetting and Appraisal is not restricted to the preservation functionality only, it can also be used in the Active System for improved information access.

Furthermore, the steps of the Preservation Preparation are extended with two functionalities related to contextualization:

- **De-contextualization** refers to the extraction of an object from its Active System context in preparation of packaging it for archiving. Decoupling the object under preservation from its Active System context is nontrivial, since it has to be decided how much of its current context has to be taken for its future contextualization and where a cutting can and should be made. De-contextualization and Contextualization (see below) are conceptually closely related.
- **Contextualization** consists of providing sufficient additional information for the content to be preserved, in order to allow archived items to be fully and correctly interpreted at some undefined future date. This functionality is responsible for defining and assigning the appropriate context to content to be archived. Contextualization can leverage other processes (e.g., similarity analysis, concept detection) to explicate context. Contextualization provides the basis for the management of context evolution over time (see Evolution Layer in Sect. 6.3.4) and Re-contextualization (see Re-activation workflow in Fig. 6.6).

The Preservation Preparation workflow is linked to the **Pre-ingest** functionality as it is typically described for OAIS-compliant preservation systems, e.g., in the PAIMAS [66] model. In order to facilitate easy (seamless) ingestion into the DPS and make sure that the Information Packages contain metadata needed for both the DPS as well as for access, Pre-ingest aids the Active Systems as well as the DPS systems adhering to standard protocols and metadata, as defined in the Preservation

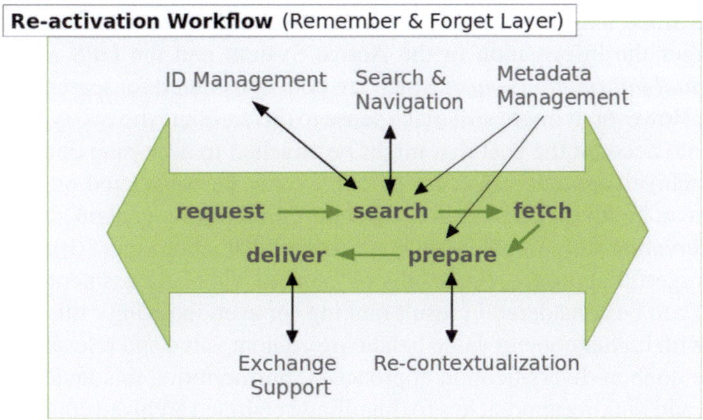

Fig. 6.6 Re-activation workflow in the Remember and Forget Layer

Contract. This also means that the Pre-ingest function puts up some requirements on the Active Systems to follow certain protocols (which can/should be domain specific). Our Preservation Preparation workflow, from the perspective of the DPS, serves as such a Pre-ingest function.

6.3.3.2 Re-activation

For the Re-activation workflow, two additional functionalities are used, with respect to the Core Layer, for the search and future access to the preserved content:

- **Re-contextualization** has the purpose of supporting the interpretation of a content object at the time of access (which might be a considerable time after archival). Re-contextualization occurs when a document is retrieved from the DPS at some future date. Once retrieved from the DPS and before it is put back into active use, the context information, which has been provided by the Contextualization functionality, stored together with the content object and possibly updated or extended over time, is retrieved. This context information is used for Re-contextualization, i.e., to relate the content object to the current usage context. Re-contextualization can also include the re-construction or extension of context information for content archived with no or insufficient original context.
- **Search and Navigation** is responsible to enable finding things that have been preserved. Various types of content search and navigation can be supported here. This includes search in the metadata, full-text search in the content (or more general content-based search also including non-textual content), search in the context information and in other types of annotation, exploratory search for understanding the archive content, etc. For our integrative and forgetful approach it is crucial (a) to manage the interaction between the search in the Active System and the search in the DPS and (b) to understand how the forgetful approach and search support

interact. Since we are following an integrative approach, it makes sense for (a) to consider the information in the Active System and the DPS as a type of a *joint virtual information space*, which are both considered for search in the Active System. However, it might still make sense to differentiate the two types of content taking into account the cost that might be attached to accessing content from the DPS. Archived content might, for example, only be considered on demand or if nothing can be found in the Active System. Furthermore, content stemming from the preservation store might be marked in result lists. For aspect (b), the influence of the forgetful approach, the results of Content Value Assessment (namely MB and PV) can be considered in result ranking (or even indexing): this would prefer results with higher content value balancing content value and relevance as it is for example done in diversification approaches. Furthermore, this includes adequate filtering and ranking approaches for handling versioned archived content. Situation search can also be used here. However, since it is especially relevant for Active System Change it is discussed in Sect. 6.3.4.

6.3.3.3 Metadata and Preservation Contract

In both workflows of the Remember and ForgetLayer, metadata are generated and used for different purposes. This metadata is taken care of by different functional entities also responsible for managing the Preservation Contract, the agreement concerning the preservation rules and strategy among all actors. The functional entities mentioned above are described in the following:

- **Metadata Management** is responsible for the different kinds of metadata that are created and exchanged by the aforementioned functional entities. This includes a variety of different types of metadata such as current and past values for MB and PV, information on the context of a resource, information extracted from resources for further processing as well as indexing information for Search and Navigation. Some of the metadata, which is collected here just remains in this middleware for supporting its operation. Other parts of the metadata such as the PV and the context information will be stored as part of the archived object in the DPS. The Metadata Management functional entity interacts with the respective components of the DPS by (a) providing input for enriching the metadata in the DPS for improved preservation management, (b) incorporating information coming from the DPS (e.g., for the joint indexing) and (c) by - as mentioned before - storing some of the metadata as part of the resources to be preserved.
- **Preservation Contract Management** is involved before transferring any digital items or collections from Active System to DPS, when a submission agreement has to be established between the participating actors, preferably following a standard approach, e.g., as described in PAIMAS [66]. In ForgetIT, we extended this to also include aspects of relevance to the re-activation of content and, therefore, labeled it *Preservation Contract* to signify that it does not only concern the submission phase. The Preservation Contract should contain accurate information about the type of

package content, structure, and metadata. It should also include requirements for security and privacy mechanisms at transfer and storage. Furthermore, it should be stated in the agreement if there is a need or requirement for migration at ingest. Other examples are a specification to what extent metadata should be obtained and generated during the Pre-ingest process, if there is a specific demand on storage, or rules regarding management of objects in the DPS including different preservation levels as forgetting options. There is also room for agreements about e.g. privacy requirements and exploitation rights.

6.3.4 Evolution Layer

A preservation framework per definition exists in a long-lived environment aimed to survive at least decades. Clearly, most of the involved parts widely ranging from formats, technology and systems to semantics, and relevant real-world situations (represented by the application) will not remain stable (i.e., unchanged) over such long period of times. This implies that adequately dealing with changes is a core property that is required from such a framework.

The purpose of the Evolution Layer is to adequately deal with the upcoming changes, such that the preserved content remains accessible and understandable. Clearly this means different things for different types of changes. Other types of actions are, for example, required in case a media format gets out of use as compared to the situation that an organization is re-organized.

The Evolution Layer, therefore, groups the changes considered in three classes, each handled by its own type of change workflow. Thus, the Evolution Layer contains three new workflows: the **Situation Change** workflow is responsible for monitoring semantic changes in the Active System and propagating them into the DPS, in order to keep the preserved content understandable; the **Setting Change** workflow deals with changes in practices, formats and technology in the environment of the preservation (setting); finally, the **System Change** workflow is responsible for situations, where one of the involved systems changes.

In support of the aforementioned workflows, the Evolution Layer includes additional functionalities which are described in the following.

6.3.4.1 Situation Change

Active Systems such as the Semantic Desktop (see Chap. 7) reflect real-world processes and situations and thus the content and structures in such systems are subject to change, which we capture under the notion of Situation Change. Since the preserved content coexists with such changes, this raises the question, if such changes have implications for the preserved content. Even if the content is not directly affected, changes such as re-structuring in an organization or change in life situation of an

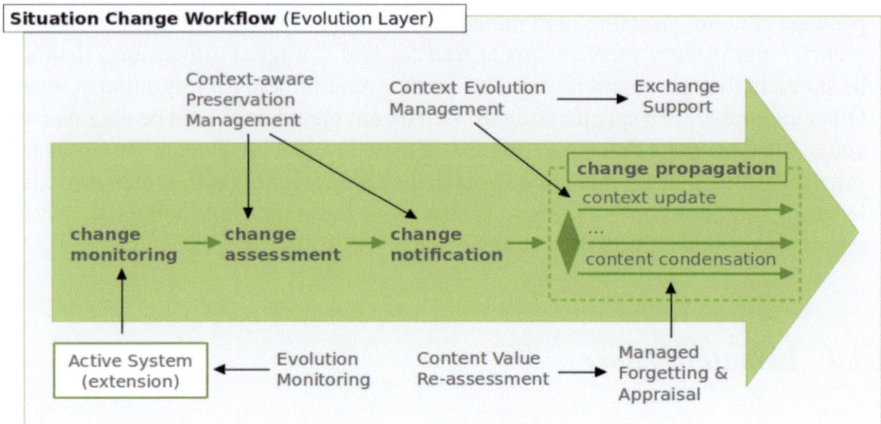

Fig. 6.7 Situation Change workflow in the Evolution Layer

individual might have implications for the interpretation and contextualization of preserved content.

For this purpose, a Situation Change workflow has been defined. This workflow consists of four steps (as depicted in Fig. 6.7): (1) *change monitoring*, (2) *change assessment* (assessment of detected changes), (3) *change notification* (notification of involved components such as the DPS on relevant changes), and (4) *change propagation*, which performs different types of actions depending on the observed change and the chosen change propagation strategy.

Change monitoring is responsible for detecting changes in the content and the content structuring of the Active System. This is typically best realized by an extension of the Active System. An important and more demanding step in the workflow is change assessment. The idea here is that changes are analysed with respect to their potential impact on the preserved content. It does not make sense to consider every small change that happens in the Active System. Rather Situation Change is only interested in the *larger* high-impact changes. One way of dealing with this idea is to distinguish more and less important concepts, instances, and relationships in the content structures of the Active System and to propagate this importance level to the changes affecting such entities. Alternatively or in addition, it is also possible to give different impact levels to different types of change operation, e.g., the deletion of a department will have higher impact than a smaller change of name. Change assessment is the basis for filtering out irrelevant changes and for performing change notification, i.e., informing relevant system components about the change. This will lead to change propagation, which can take different forms depending on the type of the change and the selected change strategy. A change might, for example, imply that the preserved context information is modified or extended, in order to capture the change and to be able to reflect it, when re-contextualization is performed. Another action that can be triggered by a change is the re-assessment of the content value: due to a change, e.g., a change in employment, an entity such as the former employer might cease in importance, which would lead to a decreased PV of content items related to such an entity.

For monitoring, assessing the changes and deciding about the consequences, in support to the Situation Change workflow, the following functionalities have been introduced in the Evolution Layer:

- **Evolution Monitoring** is required for the change monitoring step in the Situation Change workflow. This is mainly performed in an extension of the Active System, because this is the main place, where evolution in the conceptual model of the application becomes visible. Such changes might, for example, be changes in the ontology (implicitly) underlying the organization of the information triggered, e.g., by a major re-organization. Evolution Monitoring has to observe changes in the explicit representations of the conceptual model (such as taxonomies, information structures) in the Active System as well as more implicit signals of context evolution (e.g., newly upcoming topics, tags getting out of use, department sites no longer updated).
- **Context Evolution Management** is responsible for keeping up-to-date the context information which has been stored along with the archived content. This may include the storage of further context information, in case of larger changes in the Active System (e.g., major re-structuring of an organization). This also includes keeping track of such larger changes, which have happened in the Active System on a conceptual level. Such a change history can be used in Re-contextualization for making the content understandable in the changed new context.
- **Content Value Re-assessment** here serves a very similar purpose as the functionality Content Value Assessment described for the Remember and Forget layer. It revisits the value assessments originally provided by the Content Value Assessment based on observed evolution in context. It is considered separately in our model, since the resources that it works on are now already preserved, which has implications on the computation of the value (e.g., the role of usage data) as well as on where this functionality is performed. One option, which has been followed in the ForgetIT project, is to map it to in storage computation.

6.3.4.2 Setting Change

Although the DPS should have its own support for typical OAIS functionalities, such as Preservation Planning and Administration [67], the many-to-many relationship in the PoF Reference Model and the long-term perspective of those functions mean that at least parts of those functionalities need to be shared and communicated over several systems. The reference architecture of the model, described in Sect. 6.5, includes a middleware component, namely the PoF Middleware, which acts as a man-in-the-middle between Active Systems and DPS and therefore has a suitable position for capturing these bidirectional interactions. The OAIS Preservation Planning function could, for example, benefit from a component responsible for the technology watch and residing in the middleware, thereby gathering and aggregating information about,

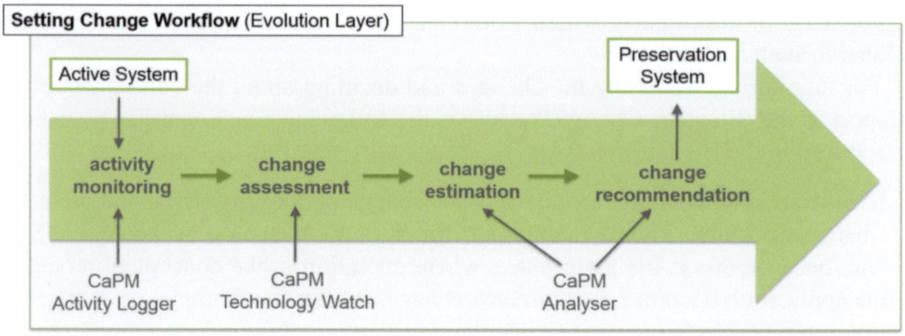

Fig. 6.8 Setting Change workflow in the Evolution Layer

e.g., usage of file formats in all systems connected to the same middleware. Another example would be when Preservation Planning in a DPS declare a file format as obsolete, this information could then be shared with the PoF Middleware which propagates this to Active System and DPS.

Based on such evidence, the PoF Middleware provides additional possibilities to summarize and analyze the usage and, e.g., storage quotas over several systems, thereby giving an overview of the holdings for a particular customer. Since a customer might use several Active Systems, as well as preserved content in several archives, such an overview is beneficial in locating objects that need preservation actions.

The Setting Change workflow consists of four different phases with two different starting points (as depicted in Fig. 6.8), involving the **Context-aware Preservation Management (CaPM)** entity, described below: (1) *activity monitoring*, which logs the bidirectional communication between the Active System and DPS including process activities, systems in action, and digital objects passing through; (2) *change assessment*, that detects and propagates change in usage; (3) *change estimation*, which suggests suitable change recommendations based on rules defined in Preservation Contract including, e.g., PV, and use statistics, and (4) *change recommendation*, which propagates recommended actions to DPS, which could be of different types, such as transformation of content or change of physical and logical content structure.

The Evolution Layer includes the CaPM functional entity, with three supporting functional entities, namely: Activity Logger, Technology Watch, and Analyser. Together they support the workflow described above:

- **Context-aware Preservation Management (CaPM)** functional entity externalizes and extends parts of OAIS Preservation Planning and OAIS Administration by keeping track of Active Systems as well as the (several) DPS that are involved. The main idea here is that it should be easy to seamlessly put back preserved information into active use in either the same system as it originates from, but even more importantly into other information systems (of the same type). Even the same system might have evolved to newer versions with different standards, and maybe even a different information structure or ontology. This must also be tracked by the CaPM functionality.

- **CaPM Activity Logger** provides support for monitoring of activities in PoF workflows. A typical example is to keep track of the execution of tasks executed by components in the workflows. This data will then serve as one input to the change assessment.
- **CaPM Technology Watch** gathers data on objects handled by the PoF workflows. This includes information on Active System and DPS, as well as technical metadata on the object, e.g., file format. This information combined with input from CaPM Activity Logger forms the basis for a change assessment, which, if needed, triggers a change estimation.
- **CaPM Analyser** supports the change estimation process, based on an initial assessment of the need for a setting change, by aggregating and processing data provided from earlier functions and should provide a graphical user interface for human interpretation and intervention. The CaPM Analyser may calculate a preferred setting change based on thresholds and rules, provided by, e.g., a Preservation Contract, but it can be interactively overridden by a human operator. The decision, be it automatic or manual, will then become a change recommendation that is handed over to the DPS to be implemented.

6.3.4.3 System Change

Within the Evolution Layer, System Change refers to the case, where one of the participating systems is replaced. This might be the Active System (e.g., because a new type of Active System is adopted for the same task) or the DPS (e.g., because a preservation provider goes out of business or the user wants to change the provider). Of course, it is also possible that the middleware is replaced with a middleware solution based on a different approach or technology. However, this case is out of the scope of this reference model.

The two cases, change of Active System and change of DPS have very different implications and are, therefore, considered separately.

Active System Change

The most interesting aspect for the change of Active System is how the content preserved with Active System A can still be accessed, if the system no longer exists or is no longer in use. This might mean to access the preserved content through a new Active System B or to access it via a lightweight access infrastructure such as a Web Interface. For covering those cases, we have identified a modified Re-activation workflow (see Fig. 6.9).

A prerequisite for accessing the content of Active System A is some type of an identifier (and credentials) for getting access to the content that has been connected to a user via Active System A. After *authentication* (1), the owner or another user on behalf of the owner can access the content. For not overwhelming the user with the

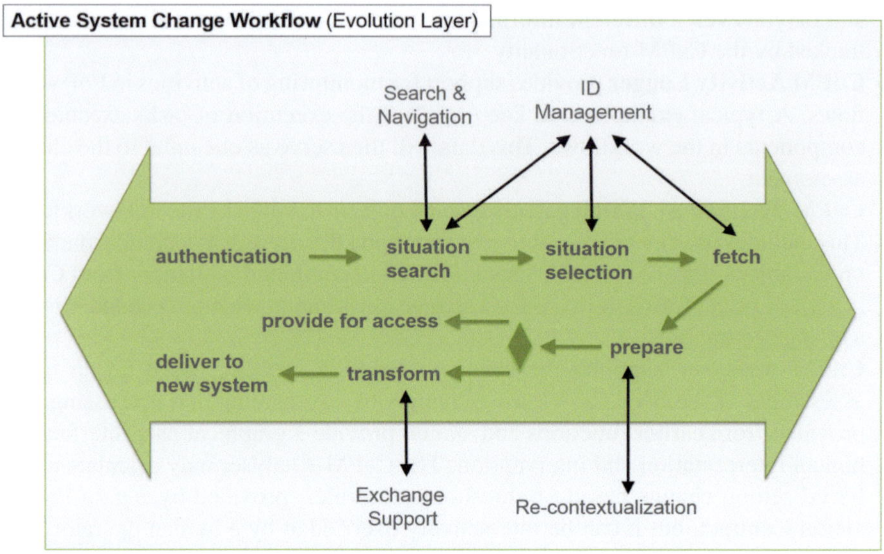

Fig. 6.9 Re-activation workflow for Active System Change

full content collection, which might have a considerable size, a high-level and user-friendly structuring principle is required. For this purpose, the concept of *Situations* has been introduced into the model (see Sect. 6.4.1 for details). Therefore, after authentication, the user can perform a *situation search* (2), which returns to the user a list of situations, for which there is content in the archive (or the list of situations fulfilling the user query). Search can be either offered as an integrated part of the new Active System B or separately (e.g., via a Web Interface). For each of the situations also a short description in the form of a profile is given (see Situation Profile in Sect. 6.4.1). The *situation selection* step (3) enables the user to select relevant situations, which subsequently during the *fetch* step (4) can be retrieved by the system via the mapping from situation to content objects provided by the ID Management functional entity. During the *prepare* step (5) as in the normal case of Re-activation, the content is prepared applying, e.g., Re-contextualization and made available via the Exchange Support. At this point, the *transform* step (6) might be necessary to transform the content and the context into a format that can be digested by the Active System B before the *deliver to new system* step (7) takes place. Alternatively, if no content transformation is required, the *provide for access* step (6) can be performed based on the content as it is provided by Exchange Support, e.g., for browsing the content.

Preservation System Change

A change of DPS can happen for various reasons including technology change, preservation provider change, etc. In each case, it will become necessary to get the preserved content out of the DPS to be discarded and to import it into a new

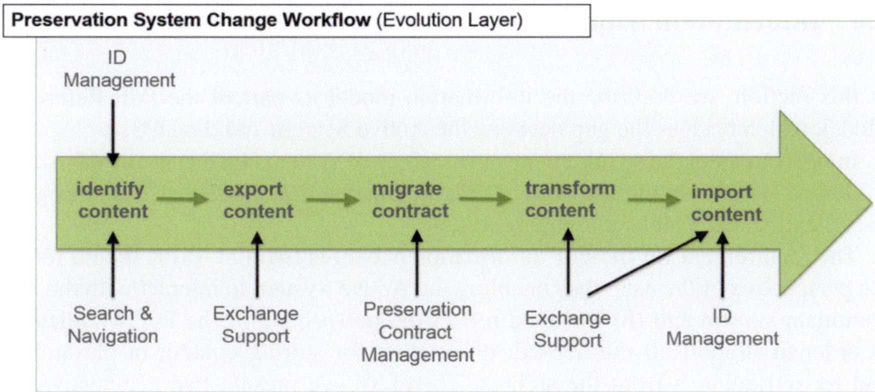

Fig. 6.10 Simple migration workflow for Preservation System Change

DPS. In addition to dealing with the content, it is also necessary to deal with the Preservation Contract associated with the content, as can be seen in the workflow shown in Fig. 6.10.

The workflow shows a high-level Preservation System Change process. During the (1) *identify content* step, all the content that belongs to the system instance or the user that wants to change the DPS is identified. In case of a technology change, this must be done for all the users or a bulk export function can be used; then the (2) *export content* step requires that all the content is fetched and exported together with the necessary metadata, e.g., linking content to situations or linking content to context. Also, since the middleware has information on what metadata and the format of metadata that is required from the new DPS it is possible to request the export to be in a suitable format; in addition, during the (3) *migrate contract* step, the Preservation Contract is migrated to meet the service offer, possibilities and practices of the new DPS; the migration might have implications that require re-negotiations with the user, therefore it is expected that contract migration is no fully automated process; it may be then necessary to (4) *transform content* (and metadata) in order to comply with the newly negotiated contract, depending on what was possible to achieve already during the export content phase. This would also lead to an update of the provenance metadata for the objects, since they have been handled by different actors during this process. Subsequently, content is imported, possibly after re-packaging according to the new Preservation Contract: this takes place during the (5) *import content* step, when the ID Management functionality is used to link the new archival IDs with the IDs known to the Active System and possibly internal IDs of the Middleware.

Under certain circumstances, a change of DPS might just concern a subset of the digital objects in the current DPS. In that case, it could be useful to utilize the CaPM Analyser and CaPM Technology Watch to support decision making on whether to make that change or not, based on, e.g., the number of objects concerned or the volume of those objects.

6.4 Information Model

In this section, we describe the information model as part of the PoF Reference Model, which bridges the gap between the Active System and the DPS.

In order to meet the requirements of a variety of systems on the site of the Active System as well as on the site of the DPS, the information model has been designed to be flexible, extensible, and inter-operable.

The requirement for the PoF Information Model is twofold: (a) it should reflect the perspective of the user, thus enabling the Active System to interact with the PoF compliant system and (b) it should reflect the perspective of the PoF Middleware in order to support all the needed information for storing content in the archive and for retrieving it from the archive. Therefore, we present two perspectives of the information model, the user perspective (see Fig. 6.11) and the PoF Middleware perspective (see Fig. 6.12).

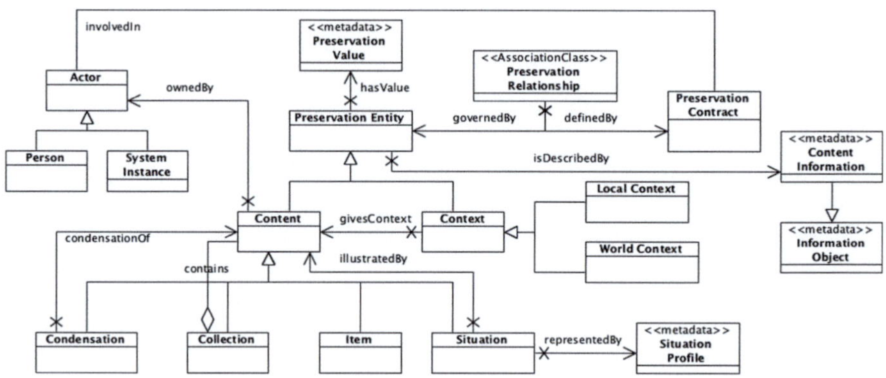

Fig. 6.11 Information Model from user perspective

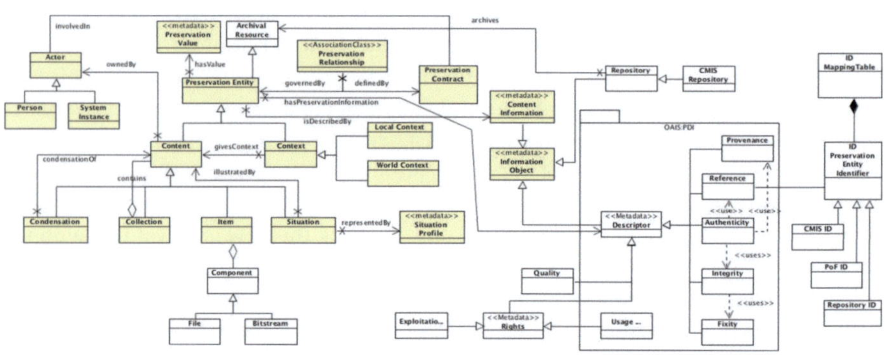

Fig. 6.12 Information Model from middleware perspective (user perspective in yellow)

Three core elements have been identified for the PoF Information Model:

- **Content**, obviously, representing the content to be preserved.
- **Context** provides additional information helping in the interpretation of the content, as required when considering the long-term perspective.
- **Situation** provides a novel, high- level structuring concept for archival content.

Due to its central role in the model, the concept of Situations and its meaning for preservation is discussed in more detail in the next section, before the information model as a whole is presented.

6.4.1 Situations as Units of Preservation

Users as well as organizations have to be able to incrementally store things and retrieve units of content from the archive even after long time periods. This should also be possible in the case, when the original Active System no longer exists. To this end, we have chosen a *situation-driven* approach: typically, content is created for (or in) a situation such as a holiday trip for personal context or is created in a project for organizational context and is also associated with this situation in memory, e.g., my photos of my trip to Paris. Therefore, we have decided to introduce Situations as an important high-level structuring concept into the Reference Model.

According to our definition, a **Situation** represents an event, a life situation, or an experience from the perspective of a user or an organization. For enabling a high flexibility, which fits many preservation settings a rather wide definition is chosen here. Examples for situations are: a holiday trip or a life event such a wedding in the personal context, a project or a project meeting in the organizational context.

In the archive, the content is associated with the situation (or rather a representation of it). This does not mean that all resources such as photos belonging to the same situation have to be archived at the same time or have to be stored at the same place in the archive. The purpose of introducing situations is to provide the user with a high-level notion for perceiving the structure of the potentially large and growing amount of content that is put into the archive over the time. Archive content will be associated with situations and can be accessed in terms of situations. In some way, situations are similar to the concept of collections as they are used in digital archives. However, we see an important difference. It is the purpose of the archive to enable the memorization of situations by storing content that enables remembering relevant aspects of the situation. The preserved content thus illustrates the preserved situations.

Similar to an event, a situation is associated with a time span, which describes the temporal dimension of the situation and with location information. Due to the wide definition of situation the considered time frame can vary widely. This is driven by the user's understanding of situation granularity. A Situation can be very short, but also can span several years. Nested Situations are also possible, allowing situations to be part of larger ones. Table 6.2 summarizes the core attributes of a *Situation Profile*,

Table 6.2 Core attributes of the Situation Profile

Attribute	Description
Id	Unique ID for the situation
Title	Name of the situation
Type	Type of situation
Time	Time range related to the situations
Locations	Location or locations related to the situation
Persons	Important persons related to the situation
Further entities	Important entities that are not persons, such as pets, buildings or organizations
Memory cues	Information that is expected to be useful in memorizing and retrieving the situation
Description	Optional short description of the situation
PV	Preservation value of the situation

which is the representation of a situation in the PoF Information Model. It provides a core set of metadata for describing a situation.

In order to enable interoperability among different Active Systems (if we need to migrate from one to another or in case of changes), an agreement upon or standardization of situation profiles would be desirable. This would ease the access to situations, which have been archive on behalf of one Active System and are supposed to be brought back in the context of another Active System.

An approach similar to the one used for Dublin Core (DC) [413] can be adopted, by identifying a core set of elements to be used as descriptive metadata associated to a given situation. Such attributes could be standardized, as done by the Dublin Core Metadata Initiative (DCMI), and further specified in order to cover a wide variety of situations. Subsequently, further attributes can be agreed upon for specific types of situations such as holidays, projects, etc., resulting in a more specific set of attributes comparable to the qualified DC elements.

Completing this section describing the Situations, we introduce some aspects related to the human memory behavior. The notion of the situations is related to concepts of cognitive science in two ways. First of all, the situation can be related to episodic memory. Following the current understanding of human memory behavior (see for example [25, 26]) and more precisely focusing the attention on the *Episodic Memory* (as discussed in [90]), our brain and *human archival system* have to store "*Situations*" with the associated and related *contents*. A *Situation* in some aspects can be compared to a *Episodic Memory Item* (EMI) (rather than being translated to a rigid OAIS-like *Information Package*). An EMI is:

- *complex*, because it is made up of several parts and concepts (or even sub-parts);
- *heterogeneous*, because its parts are of different kinds: we, for example, have associations, contexts, concepts, and images;
- *dynamic*, because an EMI can change over the time due to the changes of associated resources;

- *unstructured*, because even if some parts can be structured more or less rigidly (i.e., by concept hierarchies and semantics), many other parts can be completely unstructured such as images, contextual information (feelings, moods or environmental cues) and generally not classified information;
- *loosely coupled* with other EMIs.

Situations in our PoF Information Model can be considered in a similar way, in order to support and complement human memory with a digital memory. A second aspect of Situations that is inspired by cognitive processes is the inclusion of memory cues into the Situation Profiles.

6.4.2 Core Information Model: The User Perspective

From the point of view of the user or of the Active System, we can summarize the Information Model as shown in Fig. 6.11.

As stated above in the previous section, the three classes **Content**, **Context**, and **Situation** are the core elements of the Information Model. Both, **Context** and **Content** are **Preservation Entities**, i.e., they are elements, that the user can provide to the archival system for preservation. Content can be an individual content **Item** or a **Collection**, which will again contain content objects.

As another child of **Content**, the Information Model contains the concept **Condensation**, which is an object created from a content object such as a collection or an content item by condensation operations such as *text summarization*. *Information reduction* is an important concept in the *forgetting* environment and is one of the possible forgetting actions resulting in condensed objects that can replace or augment and improve the original projects.

Information on **Context**, the second core concept of the PoF Information Model, is kept in the archive for helping in the interpretation of content objects. Context can be provided in many different forms and for content on all levels of granularity, including individual items, collections as well as situations. In addition, we distinguish **Local Context** and **World Context** depending upon the scope of the respective information: this distinguishes information that is only known in the local scope and information considered as *world* knowledge.

The third core element, **Situation**, is also a child of **Content**. This provides a high flexibility allowing nesting of situations as well as for nested collections to be assigned to a *Situation*. A Situation is *represented by* a **Situation Profile**, an associated Profile storing the properties of the *Situation* (details of the Situation Profile are described in Table 6.2). As shown in Fig. 6.11, the Situations in Reference Model are linked by the association *representedBy* to the **Situation Profile**. As explained above, *Situation* and *Situation Profile* are *beyond* the OAIS approach.

A further important concept in the Information Model is ownership of the preserved content. This is modeled by introducing the concept of an **Actor**, which can be a **Person** or a **System Instance** of the **Active System**. For modeling ownership, the

Actor is linked to the **Content** element via the relationship *owned by*. This enables for flexible assignment of ownership.

Another important concept of the user's perspective of the information model, is the relationship to a preservation provider. This is modeled in the Information model by the associative class of a **Preservation Relationship**, which is attached (associated) to both the **Preservation Entity** and the **Preservation Contract**. Such a relationship is defined by a **Preservation Contract**, in which the preservation actions for the respective Preservation Entities are defined (see also [66]).

In addition, Preservation Entities are also associated with a **PV**, which reflects the expected benefit of preserving the respective entity and acts as a parameter for the preservation processes (mainly assessments and preservation planning activities).

All the information related to **Content** (such as title, type, etc.) is represented by **Content Information** which can be considered as a child of an **Information Object** according to OAIS.

The individual Model Entities are detailed in Table 6.3.

6.4.3 Extended Information Model: Middleware Perspective

In the previous section, we have described the PoF Middleware from the point of view of the *User*. Here, we describe the point of view of the Middleware. The Middleware has to manage the mapping between the Information Model as seen by the user (or organization) and the Information Model of the underlying DPS (or systems). Figure 6.12 shows the Extended information model, which reflects the perspective of the Middleware. For better comparison, the elements (classes) coming from the *User Perspective* have been highlighted (yellow background color) and can be considered as *core elements* of the model.

A core aspect of the Middleware perspective is shown at the right corner of the figure, the **ID Mapping Table**. Since the preservation entities as they are seen by the Active System are not mapped 1:1 to the DPS, it is necessary that the Middleware manages a mapping between the Preservation Entities and the Archival Resources in the respective repositories. For maximal flexibility an ID mapping is used for this purpose. The class **Preservation Entity Identifier**, which is a type of **Reference**, is the identifier of a preserved entity. This can be identifiers of different kinds. Therefore, there are at least three children, the **CMIS ID** is the identifier used for the resource in the Active System, **PoF ID** is an identifier used for internal purposes and **Repository ID** is the ID of the Resource in the Archive. All these IDs are related to each other by the **ID Mapping Table** that can be considered as their *aggregator* (represented by the black diamond in the diagram). This mapping table is also use to link archival resource to Situations.

A class specifically useful for the Middleware and not for the User, is the **Archival Resource**, a parent class of **Preservation Entity**. Actually the User has to deal only with **Preservation Entity**, while the Middleware has to store into archives the related resource as top level. Hence a further abstraction layer was needed in order

Table 6.3 Information Model entities for user and for middleware perspective (see Fig. 6.12)

Entity Name	Description
User Perspective	
Situation	A **Situation** is an event, a life situation, or an experience from the perspective of a user or an organization. It is introduced as a user-oriented structuring principle for the preserved content. A user can store, retrieve and access content in terms of situations. Situations are illustrated by content objects, typically collections of preserved content items. An example is the situation "My Holidays in Crete" illustrated by a selected set of photos from this trip with high PV
Situation profile	**Situation Profile** is a metadata record describing a situation. In its core, it consist of a set of attribute value pairs as described in Table 6.2. The information in the situation profile is kept simple and system independent, in order to ease finding and recognizing situations, even if the Active System no longer exists
Content	**Content** is an abstract concept for referring to different types of content that can be provided for preservation and can be part of content collections. This can be individual items (Item), collections of other content items (Collection) as well as condensed information objects (Condensation). Furthermore, also Situations are considered as Content
Context	**Context** is extra information, which is intended to help in the interpretation understanding the preserved content objects, especially, when re-accessed after a long time. Context can be collected in different ways, e.g., provided by the user, extracted or collected from external sources, and it can come in different forms, e.g., structured semantic information, extra images, text, links to external knowledge basis, etc
Local context	**Local Context** is context information associated with a content object based on local knowledge. In contrast to world knowledge, this is information, which is (mainly) only known in the environment of the content object (e.g., within the organization, or by a person and his/her family and friends
World context	**World Context** is context information associated with a content object based on "world knowledge". It is assumed that such world knowledge is generally known (not only in the local environment) and, thus, can be retrieved from external sources at the time of preservation, but also retrospectively at the time of later access. This property makes local context more important for preservation than world context
Collection	A **Collection** is a content object consisting of a set of content objects. Those contained content objects can either be individual content items such as an image or they can be again collections, thus allowing nested collections
Condensation	A **Condensation** is a content object, which has been obtained by a condensation operation from one or a set of other content objects. This can for example a text summary obtained by summarizing a text document or a set of text documents. Another example is a low-resolution image obtained by a transformation from a high-resolution image or a reduced image collection obtained by using a near-duplicate detection method. Condensation plays an important role in creating additional forgetting options beyond keep-or-delete

(continued)

Table 6.3 (continued)

Entity Name	Description
User Perspective	
Item	An **Item** is an individual content object, such as an image, a text file, or a video. An item may also consist of groups of sub-items and/or components that are bound to relevant Descriptors. The Item descriptor contains information about the Item. An Item that contains no sub-items can be considered a whole. An Item that does contain sub-items can be considered a compilation. Items may also contain annotations to their sub-parts [176]
Preservation entity	A **Preservation Entity** is an object to be preserved coming from the Active System. This concept provides an umbrella over the two core concepts Context and Context in the PoF Information Model capturing them both as preservable objects. Furthermore, it links such objects to be preserved with preservation-related information: It links such object to a preservation relationship, which defines the way the respective object is preserved, and to a PV, which act as a parameter to the preservation process
PV	**Preservation Value** is a value reflecting the expected benefit from keeping the related Preservation in the long run. Here numerical values as well as more user-friendly preservation categories such as gold, silver, bronze, etc., are possible. PV can be used both for deciding if something is preserved or not and for actually deciding about preservation options, e.g., the redundancy level
Preservation relationship	A **Preservation Relationship** is a relationship between an Actor and a preservation service provider, who takes care of the preservation actions. The Preservation actions and constraints are defined in a Preservation contract. The actions taken for a Preservation entity are governed by this Preservation Relationship and the associated Contract
Preservation contract	A **Preservation Contract** is an agreed upon contract between a preservation provider and a preservation client, which defines rules for digital preservation actions and communications to be undertaken within the middleware as well as within the DPS (see [66])
Actor	An **Actor** is an entity that takes an active role as a subject with respect to content to be preserved. This can for example be as the owner of a content object or as a preservation contract holder. An Actor is not restricted to be a person. It can also be a system instance acting on behalf of a person or an organization in the interaction with a preservation middleware. Indirectly, this will typically boil down to a person or a role in an organization, which, for example, has the ownership of the content
Person	A **Person** is a real person or a role within an organization that can be taken by several persons at the same time or over time. In the Information Model, persons come into play as owners of content objects and as actors involved in preservation contracts.
System instance	A **System Instance** is an instance of the Active System, which interacts with the Preservation Middleware on behalf of a user or a group of users. In this role, it might act as an intermediary between the user(s) and the DPS. However, since the Active System may go out of operation, it is important to define processes on how to deal with relationships such as content ownership in this case

(continued)

Table 6.3 (continued)

Entity Name	Description
User Perspective	
Information object	**Information Object** is defined according to OAIS specification and provides a set of attributes defining the semantics (meaning) of a content. In our model, it can be considered as the abstract element for **descriptors**
Content information	**Content Information** extends the Information Object and represents all the information related to a Preservation Entity, it may contain editorial information (such as title, author, editor, series, year, ID code, keywords, etc.), technical (such as format, length, size, etc.) and other descriptive attributes.
Middleware perspective	
Archival resource	An **Archival Resource** is a resource as it is archived in a DPS
Component	A **Component** is the binding of a digital resource to a set of Descriptors, i.e., the information concerning all or part of the specific resource instance. A Component itself is not an Item; Components are building blocks of Items [176]
File	A **File** is a Component materialized as a unit recognized by a computer system, subsystem, or application [176]
BitStream	A **BitStream** is a Component recorded as contiguous or non-contiguous data within a File. If metadata are specific to streams or tracks (e.g., audio and video tracks of a file), Bitstream shall be used and descriptors shall be added on Bitstream level [176]
Rights	**Rights** represent information concerning legal, regulatory or contractual provisions that affect ownership, control, access, or use of resources insofar as they impact the long-term preservation (e.g., intellectual property, copyrights, privacy, etc.). Actions or events in the preservation of resources need to respect such rights [176]
Exploitation rights	**Exploitation Rights** represent information specifically related to the ownership and commercial exploitation of the digital resource
ID mapping table	The **ID Mapping Table** provides a mapping among the different types of entities based on their IDs. The user only needs to know the ID generated in the user application and the DPS only makes use of a repository ID. The middleware bridges the gap between Active System and DPS by linking such identifiers, also using a PoF identifier for internal purposes. Note that the mappings can also be 1:N mappings. The mapping table can be implemented in different ways
Preservation entity identifier	A **Preservation Entity Identifier** represents the different identifiers associated to a given Preservation Entity in the different systems or for the different perspectives: the user perspectives requires a Active System identifier (**CMIS ID**), the middleware perspective makes use of a **PoF ID**, while a **Repository ID** represents the content identifier in the DPS. The way these identifiers are implemented and managed depends on the particular implementation. For the Active System identifier, we assume an ID based on the CMIS standard

(continued)

Table 6.3 (continued)

Entity Name	Description
User Perspective	
Repository	A **Repository** is a system used to store digital content and its associated metadata, providing methods to import, update, search and access content, exposing standard and application-independent interfaces. A digital repository can be part of a Content Management System used by a user application or be included in a Digital Preservation solution, where it is extended with long term preservation functionalities
CMIS repository	A **CMIS Repository** exposes interfaces based on the OASIS CMIS standard, to enable interoperability among different content management systems and to provide functionalities to import, update, search and access the content using CMIS standard
Usage rights	**Usage Rights** represent information related to the usage of the digital resource. They define if preservation actions can be undertaken by DPSs
Descriptor	A **Descriptor** associates information with the enclosing entity. This information may be a Component (e.g. image) or a textual statement [176]
Quality	**Quality** provides information related to the description of the technical condition of preserved items and resources. This information can at least partly be automatically extracted from content with specialized tools but often requires manual revision and validation. This manual work causes considerable costs, which is an additional reason for preserving it. Quality information includes digital defects (such as audio and visual) and characteristics, their collocation in time and space and their severity. Additionally, structural information and technical metadata of resources in relation to relevant standards are considered. It is worth to highlight that it is needed to preserve as wells the description of the hardware devices, tools, and agents used for extracting and reviewing that quality information [176]
Provenance	**Provenance** documents the chronology of events regarding the creation, modification, ownership, and custody of a resource, such as who produced it and who has had custody since its origination; it provides information on the history of the multimedia content (including processing history) [176]
Reference	**Reference** provides information that is used for identifying the digital resources. It provides one or more identifiers, or systems of identifiers, by which the resources may be uniquely and persistently identified. Reference information supports the linkage of identical or related resources that might be stored in separate repositories. These repositories may use different mechanisms for identifying resources (e.g., using different standards for representing local identifiers) [176].

(continued)

Table 6.3 (continued)

Entity Name	Description
User Perspective	
Authenticity	**Authenticity** provides information to enable any User to verify that an object is correctly identified and free from (intentional or accidental) corruption (i.e., capable of delivering its original message). Authenticity encompasses identity and integrity (as well as Provenance and Reference). Identity comprises all those attributes necessary to determine what a thing is (e.g., the original recording of a Work). Integrity asserts that none of those essential attributes have changed, i.e., there are no significant differences neither in the same resource over time nor between two resources thought to be copies of the same asset. While identical copies are authentic, authenticity does not require complete equivalence. Thus, a digital version of an analog original may be an authentic copy of the Work if it can be shown that the differences between the two versions are not significant, e.g., all of the content is present and is structured the same way, and all important elements or attributes, such as title, creator, performer, remain the same [176]
Integrity	**Integrity** represents the state of a Digital Item indicating the fact of being complete and unaltered. It can be proven by verifying the presence of all required parts in an unaltered (i.e., not modified) state [176]
Fixity	**Fixity** encompasses the information ensuring that resources (as described by their properties) are not altered in an undocumented manner. This information is also used to verify the integrity of Digital Items. Thus, if the fixity information for an Item changes over time, the Item has changed [176]

to associate it to a specific child of **Information Object**, the **Repository**. In our PoF Middleware we have to manage **CMIS** repositories, i.e., every repository exporting a CMIS interface [312].

Furthermore, the Middleware Perspective in Fig. 6.12 introduces the so-called *Detachment Elements* [47] that are low- level elements such as **File** and **Bitstream** (children of **Component**, aggregated by **Item**) as well as the detailed metadata information represented by **Descriptors** (that are all children of **Information Object**). These **Detachments** have been designed in order to be compliant to the most widely adopted preservation metadata standards, as described in Sect. 6.7.

Furthermore, the **OAIS:PDI** information package has been added to the Middleware Perspective, which embodies the *Preservation Description Information* according to the OAIS model. They are mostly **Descriptors** needed for expressing digital preservation information. We have identified a **Descriptor** stereotyped as *Metadata* that inherits from the more generic **Information Object**. The latter is inherited by many low level descriptive information elements. Among others we have reported here the **Provenance**, the **Reference**, the **Authenticity**, **Integrity**, and **Fixity**. As described in the Fig. 6.12, in order to assess the Authenticity we need to make use of the other descriptors, expressed by the *uses* dependency dashed arrows: **Fixity** is needed for guaranteeing the **Integrity** which is needed for assuring the **Authenticity** that needs also **Provenance** information [148] and related resources and references. Together with the OAIS Preservation Description Information we have added some other *Elements* coming from other standards and best practices in digital preservation (see Sect. 6.7).

The OAIS Descriptor expressing the *Rights* has been improved: the Descriptor **OAIS Rights** has quite general purposes. The experience matured in professional environments (e.g., broadcasting) where archived digital contents have strict rules for their government has induced us to split the **Rights Descriptor** into two main elements: **Exploitation Rights** and **Usage Rights**. Without this distinction, it may happen that many *preservation actions* can be blocked and/or forbidden: there are many cases where the lack of *usage rights* are practically freezing the DPS, leading to the impossibility to preserve and curate the stored contents. Even if the DPS has a copy of the contents (and is ideally able to preserve it), if it is not sure about the exact rights and permission on their modifications and changes it cannot undertake any preservation action. To this end we need to clearly state as **preservation description information** (PDI) this difference and clear it.

We split exploitation and usage. Separating the Rights about **Exploitation** (eventually described into **Contracts**) from the **Usage** allows the DPS to execute the needed preservation actions without infringing the copyright laws. As good practice in digital preservation, during the submission and ingestion of digital contents into preservation storage systems, it must be explicitly granted the usage rights, especially if the digital archive has not the ownership of the contents and cannot commercially exploit them. We have expressed the *rights* to perform these actions with the *hasRights* association between **Actor** and the generic **Rights**. As already discussed above, an **Actor** can be a **Person** as well as a **System Instance**.

A **Descriptor** not planned in the OAIS but vitally important especially for media contents, is the **Quality** (represented as child of **Descriptor** as well) and implementing all the digital properties related to the quality of a digital item. An image can have, for instance, a quality property expressing the blurriness level and a video can have a property for the *lossy* or *lossless* compression adopted (e.g., YUV 4:2:2).

The complete list of **Elements** introduced in the Information Model is provided in Table 6.3. It is worth noticing that due to the close correspondence of some elements to the MP-AF standard those elements are also described according to [176].

6.5 Mapping to PoF Architecture

In the following, we describe the architecture of an integrated framework, which we refer to in the following as the PoF Framework, based on the core concepts of the model described above. We describe how the model can be mapped to the architecture of the framework and propose a reference implementation.

6.5.1 PoF Framework Architecture

The architecture of the PoF Framework is made up of three layers: Active System, PoF Middleware, and DPS, as depicted in Fig. 6.13.

The Active System represents user applications, while the PoF Middleware is intended to enable seamless transition from Active System to the DPS (and vice versa) for the synergetic preservation, and to provide the necessary functionality for supporting managed forgetting and contextualized remembering. The PoF Middleware provides also the integration framework for all components implementing the functional entities of the model.

The DPS is composed by two sub-systems: the Digital Repository and the Preservation-aware Storage, which includes also a Cloud Storage Service. The Digital Repository is an OAIS-compliant system which implements the core OAIS functionalities such as Ingest, Access, Administration and Data Management and supports Information Packages. As already mentioned before, in the PoF Reference Model a few OAIS functionalities have been extended, so the Digital Preservation System and the Information Packages must also implement additional features such as those related to contextualization. The Digital Repository is complemented by a dedicated storage system, the Preservation-aware Storage, which implements the OAIS Archival Storage functionality but is also used to extend some OAIS functionalities such as Preservation Planning and therefore the storage system also includes such preservation-aware functionalities. In the designed architecture, taking into account recent developments in the most popular open-source digital preservation systems, we also included a cloud-based storage to support long-term preservation. The DPS, therefore, provides both content management and typical archive functionalities required for the synergetic preservation.

The representation of the PoF architecture in Fig. 6.13 contains a synthetic description and additional details for each component, which cannot be discussed here in detail. It is important to stress again the role of the OAIS Reference Model [67] in the overall architecture: since OAIS nowadays is the most recognizable conceptualization of a DPS, it was considered as one of the building blocks of PoF approach. However, the model described in Sects. 6.3 and 6.4 complements and supersedes this initial approach towards the OAIS model.

6.5.2 Relationship with PoF Architecture

The mapping between each functional entity in the PoF Functional Model and the architectural components of the PoF Middleware is reported in Table 6.4. A detailed description of the purpose of each component can be found in Fig. 6.13. It is worth noting that for some components the mapping with model entities is not one-to-one, because more than one component can participate in the implementation of a given functional entity of the model.

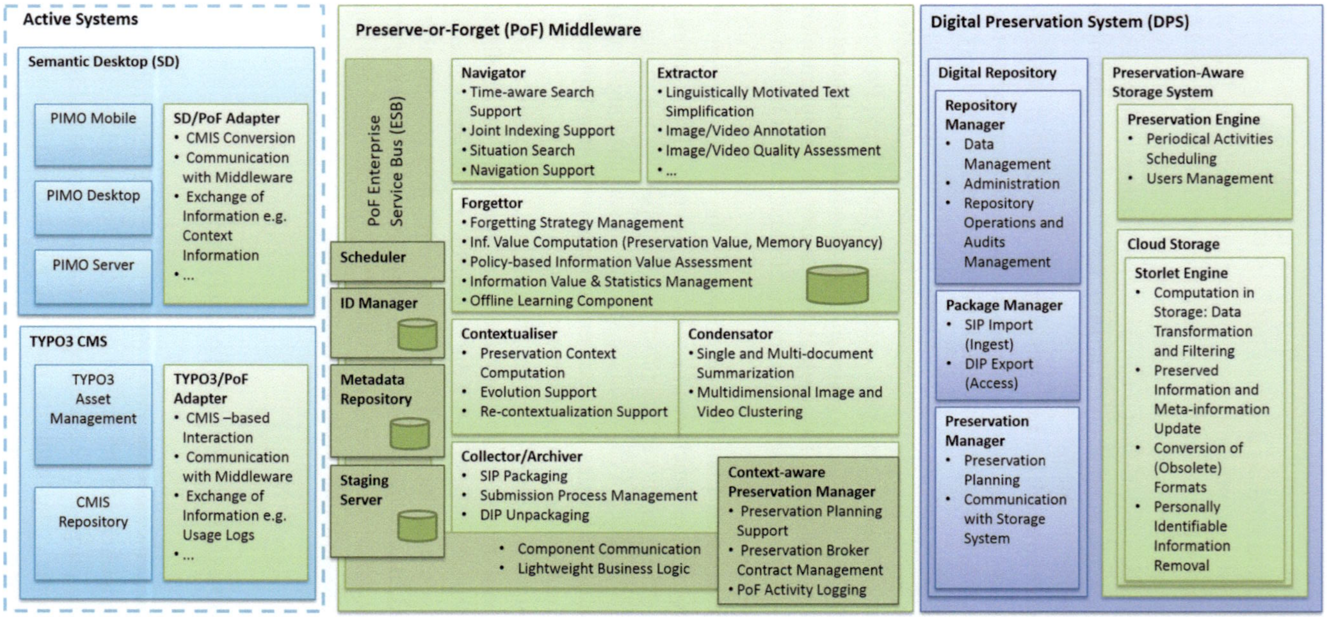

Fig. 6.13 Architecture diagram of the PoF Framework

Table 6.4 Mapping between PoF Reference Model functional entities and the PoF Middleware components

Functional entity	Model layers	PoF middleware components
ID Management	*Core, remember and forget*	`ID Manager`
Exchange support	*Core, remember and forget*	`Collector`, `Archiver`, `Metadata Repository`
Content value assessment	*Remember and forget*	`Forgettor`
Managed forgetting and appraisal	*Remember and forget*	`Forgettor`
De-contextualization	*Remember and forget*	`Contextualizer`
Contextualization	*Remember and forget*	`Contextualizer`, `Extractor`, `Condensator`
Preservation contract management	*Remember and forget*	`Context-aware Preservation Manager`
Re-contextualization	*Remember and forget*	`Contextualizer`, `Archiver`
Search and navigation	*Remember and forget*	`Navigator`
Metadata management	*Remember and forget*	`Forgettor`, `Extractor`, `Condensator`, `Contextualizer`, `Metadata Repository`, `Collector`, `Archiver`
Content value re-assessment	*Remember and forget*	`Forgettor`, `Contextualizer`
Context-aware preservation management	*Evolution*	`Context-aware Preservation Manager`
Evolution monitoring	*Evolution*	`Context-aware Preservation Manager`
Context evolution management	*Evolution*	`Context-aware Preservation Manager`, `Contextualizer`

The PoF Functional Model described in Sect. 6.3 includes several workflows spanning across the three model layers. The different steps of such workflows involve different PoF Framework components, mainly for what concerns the PoF Middleware. The activation of the different components in each workflow can be obtained from Table 6.4.

Compared to Fig. 6.13, the `Scheduler` component is not explicitly mentioned in Table 6.4, because it mainly provides process management functionalities supporting the different workflows across the three layers described before. As already mentioned in the description of the PoF Functional Model layers, other preservation-related functionalities, which are typically supported by a DPS, also benefit from PoF Middleware components. For example, in terms of OAIS entities, two functionalities which are relevant for the Evolution Layer, such as Preservation Planning and Administration, are partially supported by the Context-aware Preservation Manager. Another typical DPS-related functionality, such as the Pre-ingest, is supported by the Archiver (and a dedicated workflow for Preservation Preparation).

It is worth noting that some components are involved only in one of the layers, e.g., the Remember and Forget Layer or the Evolution Layer (see Table 6.4) and that Fig. 6.8 about the Setting Change workflow includes also the Active System and DPS components, while the others involve only the components within the PoF Middleware.

6.5.3 PoF Reference Implementation

An implementation perspective of the Information Model described in Sect. 6.4 has been provided by the ForgetIT project.

The main challenges in implementing the PoF Reference Model are associated to (a) the integration of the components within the PoF Middleware, (b) the integration of the Active Systems and of the DPS with the PoF Middleware, and (c) the implementation of some specific components which are crucial for the new PoF approach to digital preservation described in this model. Examples of such components are the `Forgettor`, the `Contextualizer`, and the `Context-aware Preservation Manager`, just to name a few.

In the following, we describe the reference implementation of the PoF Framework, providing high-level details about the technologies used for such implementation within the ForgetIT project.

The communication among the components and the business logic for the different workflows have been implemented in the PoF Middleware using a Message-Oriented Middleware (MOM) approach [73], powered by a rule-based engine which activates the different components according to specific Enterprise Integration Patterns (EIP) [170], based on best practices in the field of Enterprise Application Integration (EAI). The choice of the most suitable solution was performed according to ForgetIT requirements and also taking into account the possible future adoption of the PoF Framework.

One suitable solution adopted in ForgetIT for implementing the PoF Middleware was the Apache ServiceMix[1] suite, which provides both the message broker and rule-engine components, is released under an open source license and is supported by an active community of developers and contributors, being included also in other products. Anyway, the adoption of any middleware technology requires some effort by software architects and engineers before it can be used in a effective way. The integration of the Active System and the DPS should be based on standard technologies and robust APIs, to enable the integration with different preservation solutions and user

[1] Apache ServiceMix - http://servicemix.apache.org.

applications. The PoF Middleware implemented in ForgetIT exposes REST APIs for integrating with the Active System and the DPS, the communication protocols were JSON and CMIS [312]. CMIS was used to access content in the Active Systems and also to fetch it after re-activation. By employing CMIS, a standard representation of the user content (including relationships, hierarchies and metadata) is established, which eases later re-use, transformation and migration. For the implementation of the two DPS components we used DSpace[2] for the Digital Repository and OpenStack Swift[3] for the implementation of the Preservation-aware Cloud Storage.

In the previous section, we described how the different components of the PoF Framework are related to the PoF Reference Model functional entities. The final release of the PoF Framework developed by ForgetIT was fully compliant to the model described here. The PoF Framework prototype first focused on two priority workflows for basic synergetic preservation and managed forgetting support, then it was further improved according to the model and provided an implementation of the Preservation Preparation and Re-activation workflow, integrating all components and finally implemented the PoF Information Model with an improved support for the functional model workflows. This approach could be considered a viable implementation schedule for building a PoF reference implementation from scratch.

The main challenge in implementing the PoF Framework components is related to the novelty of the approach and to the lack of similar technologies or applications. Examples of such components are the `Context-aware Preservation Manager` (synergetic preservation), the `Forgettor` (managed forgetting), and the `Contextualizer` (contextualized remembering), just to name a few which are closely related to the core PoF principles. The design and development of such components should be based on a iterative approach, for example as one of those provided by Agile software development methodologies such as SCRUM.[4] Based on one or more digital preservation use cases (for example, personal preservation or organizational preservation), when new requirements are captured they can be converted into specific digital preservation scenarios associated to one or more use cases. Such scenarios, describing the relevant interactions among the users (human or software components) and the PoF Framework, can drive the identification of the main processes and the design of the components.

6.6 Information Management Systems Extensions

The goal of the PoF approach is to keep the impact of introducing preservation into the information management workflow as small as possible. Besides the long-term preservation of selected content—which is the aim—the approach also has

[2]DSpace - http://dspace.org.

[3]OpenStack Swift - http://swift.openstack.org.

[4]SCRUM Alliance - https://www.scrumalliance.org.

the potential to introduce other more immediate benefits into active information management. Both for the basic functionality of supporting preservation as well as for leveraging the benefit enabled by the approach, some extensions are required in the Active System.

These extensions are discussed in more detail in Sect. 6.6.1, while Sect. 6.6.2 elaborates on the benefit that can be created in the Active System. Finally, Sect. 6.6.3 focuses on preservation strategies, discussing different interactions of Active System and DPS.

6.6.1 *Extensions of the Active System*

Extensions to the Active System are required, where it has to interact with a DPS (possibly via a middleware as in the case of PoF architecture) and where information has to be provided for the targeted intelligent preservation processes. This includes the collection of evidence for information value assessment and the collection of information in support of contextualization.

6.6.1.1 Supporting Information Exchanges

A core functionality, which needs to be enabled for synergetic preservation is *information exchange* between the Active System and the DPS.

Information to be exchanged includes the content to be preserved as well as metadata and context information describing this content. Furthermore, it has to be possible to bring content from the DPS back into the Active System (see Re-activation in Sect. 6.3.2). Thus, bidirectional information exchange has to be enabled.

Bidirectional exchange can be enabled for example by a repository used by both sides for making content available to the respective other system (plus possibly a notification channel). We mention here two different approaches adopted in ForgetIT to exchange information with the PoF Middleware in order to show that different strategies are possible with the actual implementation of the PoF architecture. As a first example, we consider TYPO3 CMS, the Active System chosen in the project to implement the organizational preservation use case, empowered with a standard-based repository supporting the content exchange standard CMIS [312], which enabled the exchange between TYPO3 CMS and the PoF Middleware using a CMIS repository as intermediate. Besides these asynchronous channels, more synchronized forms of information exchange are also possible, such as direct service calls. This was done in the second approach, where we considered as a second example the PIMO Server (see Chap. 7), the Active System chosen in the project to implement the personal preservation use case, where we made use of direct service calls between PoF Middleware and the Active System. There, CMIS was used as an exchange format for content objects which enabled the PoF Middleware to retrieve content directly from the PIMO Server. Nevertheless, both approaches use the PoF interfaces for communicating with the PoF Middleware such as registering content, PV updates, restore requests, and so on.

6.6.1.2 Information Value Evidence

The Managed Forgetting and Appraisal function described in Sect. 6.3.3 heavily depends on the idea of Content Value Assessment discussed before. This is true for assessing short-term importance as it is done for computing MB as well as for assessing the long-term value, namely PV.

For substantial Content Value Assessment, evidence have to be collected from the Active System. For the short-term importance, these are for example information about the usage pattern of a resource as well as information about the relationship between resources. In order to provide such evidence, specific interfaces as well as protocols are required defining which evidence are provided, in which format and in which frequency. Furthermore, methods for collecting such evidence have to be implemented in the Active System. In the opposite direction, the Active System might also profit from the computed content value information and use it for advanced functionalities and generate short-term benefits (see Sect. 6.6.2). The Active System can perform such assessments on its own; in such case the exchange is reduced to the calculated values such as the PV categories.

6.6.1.3 Supporting Contextualization

Context information added to the preserved content is meant to ease the interpretation of such content in case of re-activation. Information contextualization has been discussed in Chap. 5.

Context information can also be gained in different ways, since (a) it can be provided by the Active System at the time content is sent to the DPS, (b) the PoF Middleware can automatically extract information from the provided content and other sources such as e.g. a domain-specific ontology or external knowledge sources (e.g., Wikipedia), and (c) it can be a mix of the previous ones.

If this is possible in the considered Active System, harvesting context information which is already explicated in the Active System (option (a) above) looks more promising. In this way, a richer and more quality-controlled form of context can be provided, with respect to what can be automatically extracted in the preservation process.

For example, the approach discussed in Chap. 7 is based on content already annotated using an ontology, i.e., the PIMO. This annotation, obviously, is a good source of context information for preservation. The Semantic Editor described in Chap. 7 allows annotation of textual content during writing which supports early contextualization by a user. The annotation vocabulary consists of above-mentioned personal as well as external knowledge.

However, option (a) also puts higher requirements on the Active System: (1) explicated context has to be available (or it has to be explicated for this purpose) and (2) the Active System has to be extended with a functionality that is able to attach context information to the content information sent for preservation.

6.6.2 Creating Benefit in the Active System

Investment in preservation is typically paying back in the long term only. In order to foster the adoption of preservation technology, it is one of the goals of the PoF approach to also create short-term benefit in the Active Systems—as a kind of positive side-effect of introducing preservation technology. This section summarizes some ideas on how such side-effects can be created in the Active System based on the PoF approach.

6.6.2.1 Forgetful Information Presentation

The functionality for Managed Forgetting and Appraisal and the related Content Value Assessment (see Sect. 6.3.3) can be used to distinguish between content which is of current importance from other content (see discussion about MB in Chap. 4). The values of MB can be used in the Active System to bring the content currently important *closer to the user*, e.g., by showing it on a PC desktop or in special lists, having it on mobile devices, or by preferring search results with high MB, the so-called *forgetful search*. The core idea is to ease access to the things that are currently important: this is related to one of the five characteristics of the PoF Reference Model (*brain-inspired*), as discussed in Sect. 6.2.3 where we described the Digital Working Memory. This would be very similar to the Human Working Memory, thus helping the user to focus on current activities. Examples for implementations of such forgetful information presentation can be found in Chap. 7.

6.6.2.2 Forgetful and Archive-Aware Search

Search is one of the core content access methods. Search and Navigation functionality (see Sect. 6.3.3) in the Active System can be affected in two ways by the introduction of preservation technology, as described in the following. The most obvious way is to smoothly integrate the archived content into the Active System search functionality, i.e., *archive-aware search*. This idea has already been discussed in more detail in Sect. 6.3.3, within the Active System appropriate extensions in support of archive-aware search have to be implemented. As a second way of modifying search in order to benefit from the PoF approach, forgetful search (see above) can be introduced. The idea here is to take MB into account in the ranking function, thus preferring resources of relevance for the current task in the search result list.

6.6.2.3 Creating Awareness for Content Value

On a more conceptual level, the idea of Content Value Assessment as it is used for computing MB and PV in Managed Forgetting can also be used to raise the awareness for the value of content assets. An improved understanding of the value of content, which is based on a variety of factors such as investment, usage, popularity, etc. can become an important building block for next-generation CMS applications. This idea is closely related to organizational preservation and was investigated in ForgetIT, while in the context of personal preservation using the Content Value Assessment also for evolutionary knowledge management can be considered.

6.6.2.4 Content Value Assessment in the Active System

The functional entity Content Value Assessment is responsible for the assessment of resources in the PoF Framework as pointed out in Sect. 6.3.3. Considering its role in the PoF Framework, the Semantic Desktop described in Chap. 7 is an example of Active System which is capable of computing the PV for the preservation decision as well as the MB for Managed Forgetting within the Active System itself. In the light of the benefits discussed above, the Semantic Desktop embeds the Content Value Assessment functional entity into the Active System. In contrast to that, another Active System implementation could not calculate the values by itself but rather deliver the evidence to the PoF Framework where the computation will take place.

Choosing either of the two approaches is also a design decision, which could be made because of the beneficial usage of both MB and PV in the Active System infrastructure, as in the case of Semantic Desktop. The rich semantic model of the PIMO (see Chap. 7) and the usage statistics of the Semantic Desktop allow for a comprehensive view on the resources with respect to MB and PV. Furthermore, the nature of the PIM application scenario implies a lot of access, usage, and changes to resources and the PIMO resulting in a lot of traffic as well as content assessment in the PIMO as a knowledge base. Therefore, both values are computed in the Semantic Desktop and stored directly in the PIMO to be easily accessed by its components and thus, making them an integral part of the PIMO. To enable the PoF Middleware to make decisions based on the PV, the values are reported and updated in certain time intervals to the PoF Middleware.

6.6.3 Preservation Strategies

When preservation is introduced into the content management life-cycle of an Active System, a variety of decisions have to be taken when defining the preservation strategy to be used. This includes decisions about when to preserve and about the granularity of preservation. Furthermore, the interaction between resource versioning and the preservation of a resource has to be defined.

Preservation actions can be triggered in different ways. They can for example be activated by the content management life-cycle: resources might be considered for preservation, when they go out of active use (low MB) or already upon creation or import into the system (e.g., for very valuable resources). Furthermore, preservation can be scheduled, for example, by queuing all resources above a predefined PV threshold for preservation on a regular basis. Finally, it is of course also possible to manually trigger preservation actions for individual resources or resource collections.

The choice of strategy is also dependent on the type of resources considered as well as on the level of control the user wants (or needs) over the preservation process. This could include enabling identification and removal of duplicate objects, or removal of objects with poor quality, as well as if there should be (or has to be) any transformation of objects already at ingest. Decision has to be made on which of the options are best suited for an Active System under consideration. The chosen options influence the way the preservation process is integrated into the Active System beyond enabling the transfer of content to be archived.

Besides deciding *when* to preserve, it is also necessary to decide *what* to preserve. This can be considered along two related dimensions. First, it is possible to either preserve individual resources or entire collections of resources (or other types of complex objects such as sets of related resources) as one unit of archival. Second, resources can be preserved in isolation or together with context, which describes them. This second point is closely related to the work on contextualization discussed in Chap. 5 and the results affect the definition of the archival objects, the basic units of the PoF Information Model (see Sect. 6.4).

The choices with respect to granularity of preservation have consequences for the transfer protocols between Active System and DPS. In addition, it might require methods for selecting (extracting/collecting) relevant context information for a resource to be preserved.

One further aspect of granularity is the possibility to use different service providers for different types of objects. Image objects could for example go to a specialized image preservation provider, while regular documents go to a general preservation service, and moving pictures (and sound) to a media archive. This is supported by the Preservation Contract, Exchange Support, and ID Management entities running in the PoF Middleware, which gives the Active System one single point of contact for interacting with several DPS.

An interesting further aspect of the preservation strategy is to think about the model of co-existence between the copy of the resource in the archive and the resource in the Active System (if the strategy allows for such a co-existence). This has some implications, when the resource is changed in the Active System, after a copy has been archived. Typically, newer versions will not overwrite the archived version. Rather, the changed version will be archived as a new version. There are, however, decisions to be made about, if and when the updated version is put (automatically) into the archive. In any event, there should be a possibility to define how to handle copies in the DPS and if/when the version in the archive should be overwritten/updated, or versioned.

Last but not least, the preservation strategy is also to be considered for a service provider when defining the business model for a preservation service. The strategy will influence service costs including traffic and storage as well as quality of service offered to the customer.

6.7 Digital Preservation Standards

Several digital preservation standards have been developed so far. In the previous sections, we already mentioned the relationships with a few standards, such as OAIS and PAIMAS. In order to better position the model in the context of digital preservation, we mention here a few examples among the most popular digital preservation models, starting from OAIS Reference Model, but also discussing other standard metadata schema conceived for digital preservation applications:

- **Open Archival Information System (OAIS)** [67], according to the definition, is a model for describing an archive, consisting of an organization of people and systems, that has accepted the responsibility to preserve information and make it available for a Designated Community. The reference model introduced by the Consultative Committee for Space Data Systems (CCSDS) is now an ISO standard (ISO 14721:2012). Due to the relevance of OAIS in the digital preservation community, including the available platforms claiming compliance to this model, it has been considered as one of the building blocks of PoF approach. The structure of the PoF Reference Model is similar to the one adopted in OAIS, with functional and information models. The PoF Reference Model has a broader scope, since it considers active information use and preservation as part of such a joint ecosystem, which stresses the smooth transitions and the synergetic interactions rather than the system borders. This is a core distinction from the OAIS model, which is mainly related the DPS. Hence the PoF approach has a different focus and can be integrated with any OAIS-compliant approach because it extends the preservation outside the archive, bridging the gap with the information system.
- **Metadata Encoding and Transmission Standard (METS)** [233] is a standard for encoding descriptive, administrative, and structural metadata regarding objects within a digital library and is maintained by the Library of Congress. Its modular structure allows the integration with virtually any other metadata schema to represent specific information. The METS document acts as a wrapper of several sections, each with a specific set of metadata for the different purposes of digital preservation. Each section can embed any metadata schema, including custom ones. For example METS can embed Dublin Core elements [413] or PREMIS elements (see below) for descriptive metadata. The most popular digital preservation platforms and also solutions for digital repositories typically use METS for internal and external metadata representation and also as an exchange format. Concerning the relationship with the PoF model, due to its flexibility, METS can

be used to represent archived information in the DPS but also as an exchange format when ingesting or accessing content from the PoF Middleware.

- **Preservation Metadata Implementation Strategies (PREMIS)** [235] refers to a popular metadata standard from Library of Congress, supported by several digital preservation standards. The PREMIS Data Dictionary and its supporting documentation is a comprehensive, practical resource for implementing preservation metadata in digital archiving systems. The Data Dictionary is built on a data model that defines five entities: Intellectual Entities, Objects, Events, Rights, and Agents. The Data Dictionary defines preservation metadata supporting viability, renderability, understandability, authenticity, and identity of digital objects in a preservation context. It represents the information necessary to preserve digital materials over the long term and makes no assumptions made about preservation technologies, strategies, metadata storage, and management. PREMIS can be used standalone or to represent preservation metadata within the Administrative section of a METS container. The relationship between PREMIS and the PoF Model lies in the representation of core elements of the Information Model, such as Collections and Items even at the level of Files and Bitstreams, but also to represent some features of the Preservation Contract.
- **Provenance Ontology (PROV-O)** [407] is a standard from World Wide Web Consortium (W3C). PROV-O is a lightweight ontology that can be adopted in a wide range of applications. The PROV Ontology classes and properties can be used to represent provenance information (for example, according to OAIS guidelines), and can also be specialized for modeling application-specific provenance details in a variety of domains or used to create domain-specific provenance ontologies. PROV-O Agents can be used to represent actors in Preservation Contracts and to enrich Collections and Items in the DPS with provenance metadata, as part of the preservation tasks.
- **Multimedia Application Preservation Format (MP-AF)** [176] is a standard defined by ISO IEC SC29 WG11 Moving Picture Expert Group (MPEG). The MP-AF (standard ISO/IEC 23000-15) defines the Multimedia Preservation Description Information (MPDI), extending the concept of OAIS Preservation Description Information (PDI), providing metadata addressing the specific requirements for preserving multimedia content. MP-AF defines a metadata format that enables users to effectively exchange information (metadata) related to multimedia preservation operations and their outcomes. Typical examples include the description of integrity checking and related results, content migration from one system to another, replication of sub-parts or entire contents, content quality evaluation and related quality report, relationships between the source and output of any transformation process, etc. The model has been harmonized with MPEG-21 Digital Item Declaration and the schema reuses considerable parts of existing MPEG technologies, most notably MPEG-21 and MPEG-7. The relationship with the PoF model is mainly related to the representation of Collections and Items, but also for archiving information in the DPS concerning the digital rights associated to the preserved resources and the quality information generated automatically by

tools for quality assessment, which is an essential part of the digital preservation life-cycle.

- **Conceptual Data Model (CCDM)** [123] is a standard maintained by the European Broadcasting Union (EBU). The EBU Class CCDM is an ontology defining a basic set of classes and properties as a common vocabulary to describe business objects, e.g. programmes, articles and other types of content, and their relations in the business processes of media enterprises. Examples are programmes in their different phases of creation from commissioning to delivery, their associated rights or publication events, etc. Properties for describing each of the objects can be found in another EBU standard, EBUCore, or can be customized. The CCDM has been purposefully designed as a minimum and flexible set of classes for a wide range of broadcasting applications, including archives, exchange and media service-oriented production, semantic web, and linked data. The CCDM specification combines several aspects from existing models and specifications into a common framework. It has been built over several EBU attempts to represents broadcasting as a simple logical model. It has benefited from EBU work in metadata modeling (P-META and EBUCore) and semantic web developments. The connection with the PoF model mainly lies in a alternative way of representing Collections and Items in scenarios typical of video broadcasting.

The list provided above is not intended to be exhaustive and is mainly based on the direct experience of the authors in digital preservation research.

Based on the ideas discussed in the previous sections, a detailed model could be derived to represent core information model entities and the representation of such entities should be either based on existing metadata standards such as those mentioned above or based on custom elements in such a way that guarantees interoperability with the adopted technologies, platforms and tools.

6.8 Conclusions

In this chapter, we discussed a model for digital preservation based on the PoF approach. Five main characteristics concerning the foundations of the model were discussed. The resulting model is composed by a functional and a information part. The main entities and workflows of the functional model were described, including three different layers (Core, Remember and Forget, Evolution) which represent the different levels of compliance to the model which can be adopted within an organization or in a preservation process. The information model introduced three main preservation entities (Content, Context, and Situation) and their relationships, also compared to existing digital preservation standards. A reference implementation of the PoF model with an emerging architecture integrating information and preservation systems was described. In this chapter we also discussed the impact of the PoF approach on the information management systems and how to take advantages from the adoption of synergetic preservation.

Part III
Multimedia Preservation in Practice

Chapter 7
Remembering and Forgetting for Personal Preservation

Heiko Maus, Christian Jilek and Sven Schwarz

Abstract Chapter 1 detailed the need for preservation especially for our personal life. Even so, it is not part of most users' regular practice. Preservation challenges users with a manual effort and a somewhat stern discipline to continuously perform the required steps. Being aware of these challenges, the chapter will present the novel approach realized in ForgetIT to embed support for personal preservation in users' daily activities of Personal Information Management (PIM), reducing the effort and users' cognitive burden for preservation. In this approach, the previously introduced concepts of remembering and forgetting play a major role for a successful realization and for providing benefits to users. It is a method rooted in artificial intelligence research that allows us to derive and represent a user's mental model and making data machine understandable. This "semantification" of the user's resources paves the way for more effective functionalities for automated preservation, forgetting, and remembering embedded in the user's daily activities and applications. The chapter will detail a pilot based on this ForgetIT approach realizing remembering and forgetting for preservation. We further investigate how activities from PIM provide context to these. Regarding remembering, we present applications allowing a semantic photo organization and providing a self-generating diary to remember past events. Considering forgetting, we investigate how forgetting functionalities can be embedded in applications and present how different variants for forgetting are used in the pilot. Finally, a comprehensive approach for personal preservation is presented utilizing the PoF Framework introduced in Chap. 6 and overcoming the obstacles for personal preservation. The chapter concludes with a discussion of experience of using the pilot in daily work of our research group.

H. Maus (✉) · C. Jilek · S. Schwarz
German Research Center for AI (DFKI), Kaiserslautern, Germany
e-mail: Heiko.Maus@dfki.de

C. Jilek
e-mail: Christian.Jilek@dfki.de

S. Schwarz
e-mail: Sven.Schwarz@dfki.de

V. Mezaris et al. (eds.), *Personal Multimedia Preservation*, Springer Series on Cultural Computing, https://doi.org/10.1007/978-3-319-73465-1_7

7.1 Motivation for Personal Preservation

When considering preservation for personal, non-professional, or home usage, we have to contend with a vast increase in ways to create digital artifacts (computers, smartphones, tablets, digital cameras, etc.) as well as an ever-increasing amount of storage for this digital material. These days, users' personal information space consists of a substantial number of information objects connected to the person's life such as wedding videos, travel photos, or graduation keepsakes. It requires serious dedication and cognitive effort to organize all this data and keep it accessible as time passes. Moreover, these digital artifacts often represent past moments but are not associated with a physical memento. Therefore, they form a valuable resource for the user and future generations. If the material is lost or corrupted due to improper conservation, it will be useless.

As already discussed in Sect. 1.2, most users still use backups as their main form of preservation (see [186]). Existing recommendations for personal preservation such as the ones of the Library of Congress [232, 234] as well as preliminary technologies such as first cloud storage services (see [331] for an overview) leave most steps for personal preservation to the user, i.e., what to save, how to organize, where to store (hard disk or online storage), and when to migrate. All this is a lot of effort for users, various decisions need to be made and it requires discipline in, e.g., maintaining and updating the archive.

Creating a structure for preservation in particular is one of the major problems. Every person who adds material has to follow this structure every time further material is added, and people who want to search for files need to be aware of this structure. After a long period of time, someone else such as descendants need to be able to interpret the structure.

Considering this current state of personal preservation, the main obstacles we see so far are:

- Users are **not aware of personal preservation** of digital content. There is a huge gap between current practices, such as backup by copying material to a different hard disk, and a proper Preservation Strategy.
- When starting with personal preservation, the user faces **high up-front costs** in terms of time, effort, and resources, and there are **very few tools** to help users prepare material for preservation and interact with an archiving service. The best-practice recommended by Marshall (see Sect. 1.2) is not supported comprehensively.
- There is no **personal preservation service** for the majority of end users which supports the whole preservation process. Cloud storage alone is not preservation.
- The **vast increase in digital content with relevance to a person's life** poses challenges to PIM as well as preservation.
- Designing and organizing an archive so that its **structure can be understood in several decades from now** is cognitively challenging for users.

While some users are concerned about preservation, it is not part of most users' regular practice. Preservation requires manual effort and to actually do it, the users need to think about it which poses a cognitive burden on them. Therefore, the approach for Personal Preservation presented in this chapter is to embed it into the user's activities in the personal information space. This comprises collecting material to be preserved and evidence for preservation values, as well as triggers for preservation while keeping user involvement minimal.

But how can this be achieved? User's Personal Information Management (PIM; see [188])—i.e., all activities to organize one's life and information space—is a major reason to use computers in daily life (apart from recreation with gaming, for example). That means, the interaction with computers and information objects leaves electronic footprints of resources which could be leveraged for supporting preservation activities of users.

Therefore, by concentrating on the users' PIM, we can cover various life events together with associated digital material, usage of the digital material, and derive evidences for preservation values. For example, we can detect whether a file is only relevant for a certain time frame (such as time tables for a trip) or has emotional relevance (e.g., a photo showing the user's children).

Furthermore, it is a chance to derive the user's mental model when dealing with the content, and thus, get a means to describe the preserved material from a user's point of view with less effort. Therefore, providing an ecosystem for PIM will allow to collect resources including relevant context information from their usage to identify candidates to preserve and automate preservation. Ideally, activities for PIM and applications in that area such as photo organization, should be enabled to provide input for preservation as resources as well as context provider.

As part of Artificial Intelligence, research in the Semantic Desktop (see, e.g., [40, 156, 349]) field addresses how to use semantic technologies and knowledge representation to make user's data and activities machine understandable and how to embed this in user applications as well as their devices. Section 7.2.1 will give insights on the Semantic Desktop approach.

Although some of the required ingredients can be seen in some operating systems such as Microsoft's office suite or Apple's iCloud ecosystem with documents, contacts, calendars, or even tags, a knowledge representation as envisioned in the Semantic Desktop approach with its knowledge representation is not available. Therefore, the presented work for personal preservation also presents potentials for future operating systems and application ecosystems to apply semantic technologies and knowledge representation.

By using the Semantic Desktop approach we can:

- use the **Personal Information Model (PIMO)** as knowledge representation to represent a user's mental model over time. The PIMO [351] provides a basic ontology of concepts that a person uses for their desktop and PIM. The PIMO is modeled as a semantic graph of interconnected concepts and information objects. Extensions adapt the ontology to specific domains or tasks.
- provide an **ecosystem of applications and plug-ins** which access the PIMO for vocabulary and knowledge representation. The ecosystem outlined in [273] serves as an implementation of the Semantic Desktop approach and can be extended to

support the goals of Managed Forgetting, Contextual Remembering, and Synergetic Preservation.
- provide means to **continuously update a user's PIMO** and adapt to new situations. The PIMO is capable of long-term use [348, 352] and the oldest PIMO still in use as knowledge base at the DFKI has been evolving steadily for more than 10 years.
- provide **context for information objects** such as files, webpages, or emails by using the PIMO. The PIMO provides the knowledge representation layer both for users and for semantic services [350].
- provide a means to understand—together with observing user actions, access, creation, and deletion of information objects—the **context of the user** [357] and provide services such as context-aware task management [274].

Up until now, research focused on users in a professional setting, e.g., in PIM for research [352] or business administration [217]. This work indicates that people can build up and use rich PIMOs from and in their everyday work in the office. Concepts range from professional topics such as projects, contacts, and meetings to personal concepts such as interests and friends.

7.2 Semantic Desktop Approach to Personal Preservation

In the following, the Semantic Desktop approach is introduced together with the concept behind the PIMO. We will detail how this contributes to the PIM of users and present several PIMO-enabled services and how they contribute to Personal Preservation.

7.2.1 Semantic Desktop in a Nutshell

The Semantic Desktop approach was motivated by the observation that users, especially knowledge workers, would benefit from a support of their personal knowledge management (for details on history—here, most notably the EU Integrated Project Nepomuk (The Social Semantic Desktop; Grant No FP6-027705) was a predecessor for the Semantic Desktop work in ForgetIT—and motivation see [40, 114, 349]) as the modern working environment places high requirements on knowledge workers: they are confronted with various applications, are involved in several projects and processes, work in changing teams, are on the road with a mobile office, and finally, face an ever-increasing flow of information. The result is a knowledge space —a metaphor for the distribution of information and knowledge known by the user, contained in different documents, applications, and in the structuring of folders on the file system, as well as their interconnections which need to be handled by the user.

These knowledge spaces are complex, dynamic, distributed over several applications, and use different vocabulary (i.e., set of names for folders or tags, for example). In this situation, it is hard to handle the complexity of the resulting personal knowledge space.

Therefore, the approach of the Semantic Desktop addresses this challenge. It follows the strategy to embed the mental model—the representation of the world in the user's cognitive system as the user understands it—of the knowledge worker in their daily work by means of a "Personal Information Model" ("PIMO", [351]). The representation of the user's mental model in the PIMO consists of concepts (called "things"; We keep this naming convention from the Semantic Desktop area as it is one step closer to an end user when explaining that all their things are represented in the PIMO instead of talking about concepts.) such as specific topics, projects, persons, tasks, etc.), associations between them (persons are member of projects, a task has topic "Semantic Desktop", etc.), and finally, associated resources (documents, emails, web pages, photos, etc.). Such resources are semantically represented in the PIMO (the Semantic Desktop community denotes this as "rebirth": the resource is introduced with its semantic representation into the PIMO).

The PIMO serves as an easy to understand conceptualization of the knowledge worker's mental model, which can be used as a common vocabulary across different applications. Therefore, the PIMO provides the means required for a multi-criterial document classification considering the user's subjective view. Figure 7.1 shows an example of a representation of resources in the real world within the PIMO. The person Peter Stainer, his holiday trip as an event in a calendar, and the photo on his computer are resources in the real world.

These resources are represented in the PIMO as things having different types (in knowledge representation, these are instances of classes such as "Peter Stainer" is an instance of the class "Person"). The relations between the things can also be

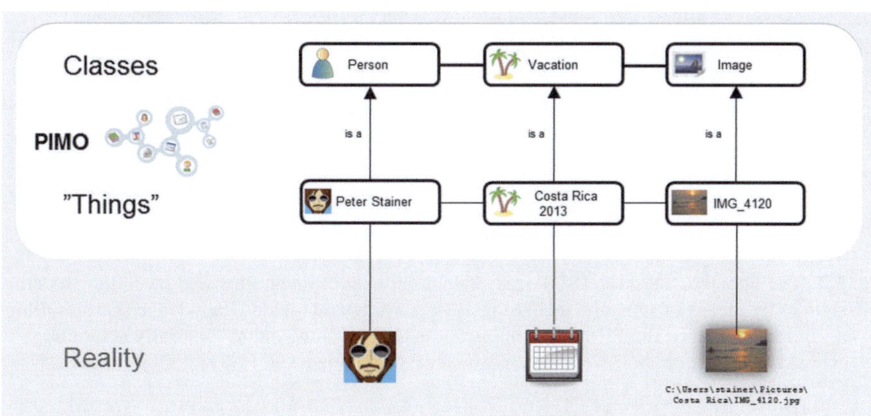

Fig. 7.1 The layers of the PIMO and their connection to the real world

expressed, for instance, that Peter attended the event and a photo has been taken on the trip. The classes and relations that are available for usage are defined in the PIMO ontology: a model of classes, their hierarchy, and allowed relations between them (as shown in the upper layer of Fig. 7.1).

The resulting graph connects various resources, e.g., from the file system with items of a calendar application, with notes written by the user, with web pages about the holiday. The resources can further be associated with topics, locations, tasks, etc. In various applications, this graph then allows to find and access resources or things, to annotate, and to relate them.

The PIMO uses the semantic power of the formal representation of the PIMO as an ontology [351], thus, introducing a knowledge representation layer on the user's computer and beyond. Besides enabling to annotate and interconnect resources over application borders, further semantic services are available which make use of the semantic representation of the user's mental model in the PIMO. Figure 7.2 depicts the Semantic Desktop ecosystem and components.

Therefore, the Semantic Desktop supports a user's PIM (and even Personal Knowledge Management) across various applications, embracing various resources, and connecting them in the PIMO, providing contextual information for value-added services. This support for a user's PIM is detailed in the next section.

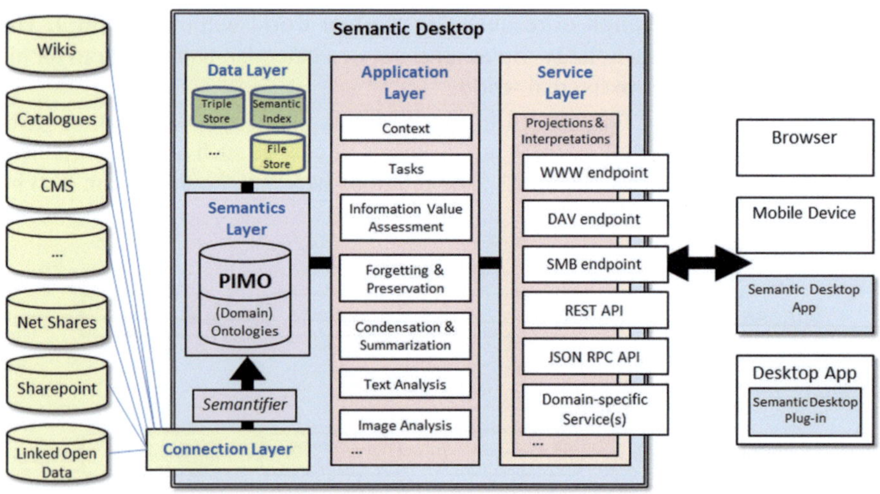

Fig. 7.2 The Semantic Desktop (SD) ecosystem architecture: integrating and leveraging external data sources by means of semantic technologies to provide value-added knowledge services. Plug-ins and endpoints embed the PIMO into applications and reaching out to user daily activities

7.2.2 *Supporting Personal Information Management*

This section provides an overview of selected features of the Semantic Desktop ecosystem for PIM and their contribution to the goals of personal preservation. The Semantic Desktop ecosystem consists of various applications and plug-ins for standard programs that provide support for the users in every day life, and thus, in various scenarios identified for personal preservation. Furthermore, the resources, concepts, and the interaction with them provide evidences for services in the Preserve-or-Forget (PoF) Framework in order to calculate Memory Buoyancy (MB) and Preservation Value (PV). Furthermore, the ability of the PoF Framework to get insights on the user's relation to resources helps in the reduction of effort for actually preserving resources whenever this is embedded and supported by PIM applications.

Therefore, the infrastructure consists of components which support users' PIM. The support addresses the following areas and functionalities:

- **Annotation support**: With its contained concepts (such as topics, persons, events, projects, etc.), PIMO provides a vocabulary to users for annotating (or tagging respectively) resources of different types. By providing access to this vocabulary as a set of tags for third-party applications, tagging with one vocabulary across different applications is enabled. This surpasses what is common today, where each application or service has its own set of tags. The following applications for PIM activities are covered: web browser and email client (with the add-on FireTag for Mozilla Firefox and Thunderbird, also MS Internet Explorer), file system (Semantic File Explorer for Windows), and annotation embedded in special-purpose applications such as photo organization or a text editor.
- **File organization**: With the SemanticFileExplorer (SFE)—a PIMO-enabled sidebar embedded in the Microsoft Windows File Explorer (see Fig. 7.10) —it is possible to annotate, access, filter, and find files using the PIMO embedded in a user's normal desktop environment. The PIMOCloud—a service similar to DropBox or Google Drive, but embedded in the PIMO, semantically representing each file as a resource in the PIMO—extends this to cloud storage with file synchronization across different devices, versioning, and sharing. Embedded in the SFE are various convenience methods such as browsing a file in the PIMO or creating a photo collection from a folder.
- **Task management**: The Semantic Desktop ecosystem supports task management by introducing tasks as dedicated concepts with special-purpose applications such as the Task Management application in PIMO5 (PIMO5 is a web-based user interface for the Semantic Desktop ecosystem using HTML5; see Fig. 7.5). This app supports reminders, due dates, notes, annotations of concepts and resources (across all connected applications and plug-ins such as tagging an email with a task), etc. Besides, it is also possible to connect and synchronize with third-party task management tools.
- **Calendar**: Like tasks, events are also specific concepts in the Semantic Desktop. This allows to manage events and reminders within the PIMO as well as to organize and associate them with everything else represented there, such as topics,

persons, resources, or notes. By offering a CalDAV (a standard internet protocol for accessing scheduling information on a server including events, alarms, and tasks) endpoint, events can be synced and managed in all third-party calendar tools and devices that support CalDAV such as Mozilla Thunderbird (with Lightning calendar) or on iOS (e.g., iPhone) without losing the power of the richer representation of events in the PIMO.
- **Contacts**: In analogy to the "calendar", the Semantic Desktop also offers a CardDAV (a standard internet protocol for accessing address book information on a server) endpoint, thus allowing to access and exchange contacts in the PIMO, i.e., persons in the PIMO will be available via CardDAV and the Semantic Desktop can extract contact information from CardDAV-supporting address books, respectively.
- **Writing**: Taking notes, writing descriptive texts or whole documents is supported by a semantic text editor (see Sect. 7.2.3) which is embedded throughout the infrastructure. This supports all situations in the Semantic Desktop ecosystem where text has to be written such as notes, descriptions of photos (see Fig. 7.4), or task notes.
- **Mobile**: The infrastructure of the PIMO allows to have mobile access to the PIMO—to the concepts as well as to resources via PIMOCloud—either by an HTML client on a mobile device or by the endpoints mentioned above such as calendar or contacts.
- **Collaboration**: Users have their own PIMO with private concepts and resources which can be shared with other users (on the same PIMO server). This supports teams in an organization as well as a family setting. The infrastructure allows to share and reuse concepts as well as any kind of resources from photos to notes, calendar events to tasks. As a default, things created by users are initially private, only visible to the creator. Even annotations of such a private resource to public ones stay private. Thus, users are in control of what to share with others. Furthermore, users can subscribe to interesting things in a PIMO such as topics and get informed about activities of other users. A chat infrastructure allows to chat with users about resources such as appointments or webpages which are then also available in the PIMO. First step toward talking to the PIMO via a chatbot are undertaken such as searching the PIMO for things or let the chatbot explain a thing contained in the PIMO such as a person or an organization. This social aspect of the PIMO fosters its usage and the benefits of actually introducing material. Likewise, sharing of resources and interaction with shared resources of other users provide further evidences for PV.

The open nature of the Semantic Desktop ecosystem—i.e., providing access and semantic services on the user's PIMO but leaving the actual usage in plug-ins or special-purpose apps open to developers —allows a multitude of special-purpose applications or plug-ins to be developed. For instance, tagging in the email client as shown in Fig. 7.3.

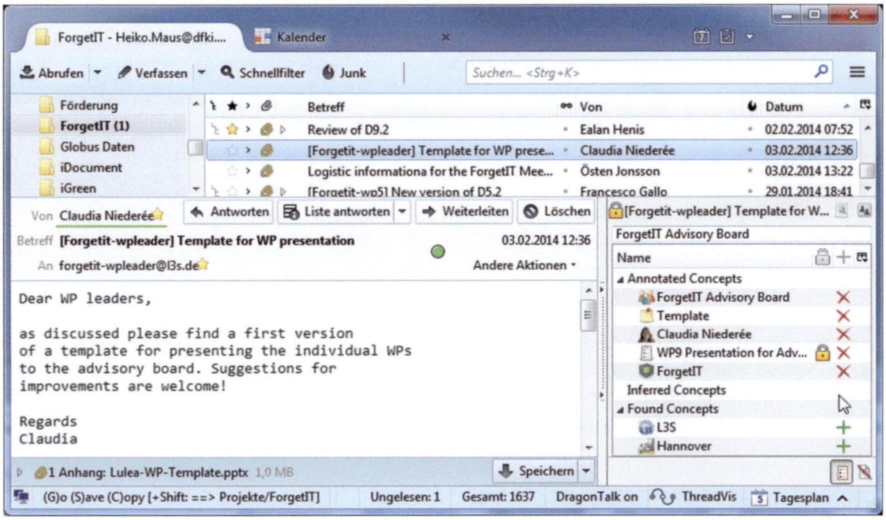

Fig. 7.3 PIM with PIMO: FireTag, an add-on for Mozilla Thunderbird, embedding the PIMO into the email client: by using semantic text analysis, relevant concepts from the PIMO are proposed. Furthermore, anything from the PIMO can be annotated such as tasks or events. Such annotated emails are then available in the PIMO

7.2.3 PIMO-Enabled Services

As previously explained, at the heart of the Semantic Desktop is the PIMO, which models the personal knowledge of the user. Having access to the PIMO and the mental model of the user represented there, various services can be provided. Since it is very useful for personal preservation, we present the semantic text editor "Seed" (short for "Semantic editor").

Seed provides an interface for texts in the PIMO such as notes and is an extensible knowledge-supported natural language text composition tool. It builds upon state-of-the-art technology in the fields of NLP (Natural Language Processing), Linked Open Data, and Semantic Web technologies to provide a user-friendly way of interacting with complex knowledge systems (see [127–129]).

Semantic annotation of texts plays an important role in enabling early contextualization of written texts. These annotations embedded in the text allow to find texts more easily via semantic associations. Moreover, they provide context for preservation in terms of the user's mental model in the PIMO at the time of creation without requiring much additional effort.

Seed is integrated in multiple GUIs of the PIMO where texts appear such as in notes, tasks, or events. It helps in exploring, modifying, and creating semantically annotated textual content. It reduces prerequisite domain knowledge and the accompanying cognitive load on users. Figure 7.4 shows a sample text being composed in Seed. Seed's main features are:

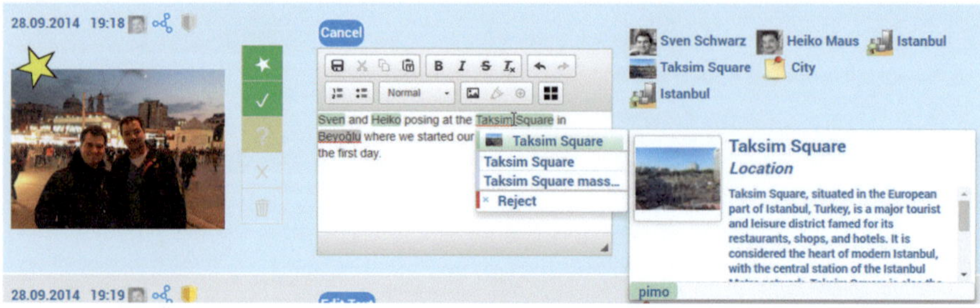

Fig. 7.4 Text being composed using seed (highlights in green: annotated entities from the PIMO). Users are able to view information on entities including information from external sources (here, Taksim Square entry from DBpedia—originating from Wikipedia—as well as the gray highlight for the Beyolu district which gives details on that entity from Wikipedia); such information can also be imported into the PIMO as was the case here

- **Annotate as you type**: Users can naturally compose text in a WYSIWYG (What you see is what you get: The final appearance of the text is directly shown to the user, e.g., headlines are shown in bold) fashion, while Seed analyzes the content in real-time and annotates mentions of PIMO entities in a non-obtrusive way. Furthermore, wrong or unwanted annotations can be rejected.
- **Proactive information delivery**: Seed not only annotates text, it also presents information about the entities annotated in an interactive way allowing the user to discover further knowledge about things mentioned in the text.
- **Access to public knowledge**: Seed also discovers entities mentioned in texts which are not yet represented in the PIMO. It links them to publicly available Linked Open Data sources like DBpedia (which is a semantic representation of Wikipedia) and proposes them to the user (gray highlights in Fig. 7.4). Then, users are able to import them into the PIMO along with their metadata, facilitating the growth of the user's personal knowledge model.
- **Collaboration**: Texts created and annotated in Seed can immediately be reused by others. This allows for many collaborative editing scenarios that make use of the semantic annotations. For example, one user can create and annotate a text, which is later accessed by another user who revises it and modifies shared annotations as well as the content of the text.
- **Immediate contextualization**: By annotating the text with entities from the user's PIMO, Seed saves the context with the text allowing it to be better retrieved, recalled, preserved in context, and ultimately understood. This immediate contextualization reduces the effort during preservation time as well as providing the subjective view of the user.

Seed is an example for the openness of the PIMO infrastructure and available as a service in the application layer shown in Fig. 7.2.

7.2.4 *Contribution of the Semantic Desktop Approach to Personal Preservation*

In this chapter, we will extend PIM with preservation and forgetting and use with the PIMO a personal vocabulary close to the users subjective view. Applying preservation support as part of PIM will ease the burden for users to do this manually. Moreover, using the PoF Framework introduced in Chap. 6 allows for seamlessly embedding preservation in the Semantic Desktop ecosystem.

Second, introducing Managed Forgetting to PIM will provide a whole new way for users in this area. The forgetting will also reduce the user's cognitive burden for past activities and information in PIM but still allow access if needed. Similar to our brain will retrieve details of our past when remembering and getting associations (see Chap. 2), the Semantic Desktop provides such means.

Therefore, the contribution of the Semantic Desktop approach for preservation, forgetting, and remembering is as follows.

7.2.4.1 Preservation

The Semantic Desktop ecosystem (applications, plug-ins, mobile apps) allows us to connect the PIMO to the user's information objects through annotating photos and web pages, organizing documents and emails, and managing tasks as well as reminders. Information objects are connected by reusing concepts such as contacts, which are part of the PIMO, for annotating images and writing emails. The resulting personal information space tightly links resources and concepts. Evidence for PVs and context for preserving an information object can be derived from this information and formalized using the PIMO knowledge representation.

Importantly, the continuously evolving PIMO not only covers information objects in current use but also objects which have already been stored in the archive for later use and are therefore no longer directly accessible for the user.

7.2.4.2 Forgetting

Metadata about and observations on information objects in the Semantic Desktop ecosystem that is held together by the PIMO provide evidences also for assessing topical and long-term relevance. Therefore, investigating activities and changes a user does in the semantic network of the PIMO gives insights on relevance of information objects. For instance, while topics of previous projects might still be relevant to the user, most of the associated resources, such as meetings, notes, and presentations, might no longer be of interest. Here, the PIMO and the Semantic Desktop ecosystem provide insights to identify concepts and resources to be forgotten.

7.2.4.3 Remembering

Like the human brain, the PIMO is still capable to retrieve things which seem to be forgotten. Similar to humans, who can remember things or situations by starting with a cue and then follow associations, PIMO can provide paths through the semantic graph that start from a particular node. For example, starting from a project (ForgetIT) we can follow a path to an associated event (the kick-off meeting in Hannover), then to a photo (the group in front of the town hall), and to a person (the professor from Edinburgh). At each node along the path, the links from the node to other concepts provide the context required to remember. Thus, the PIMO contributes to contextualized remembering.

7.2.4.4 Proof-of-Concept

As a result of the ForgetIT project, the presented approach built on top of the Semantic Desktop shows the potential for personal preservation if provided as part of the user's activities for PIM. Furthermore, it shows how the concepts of Managed Forgetting, Contextual Remembering, and Synergetic Preservation presented in this book can be used for an end user and how they could be part of applications and future operating systems. Therefore, the presented approach realizes the personal preservation application scenario by connecting to the PoF Framework as well as using components presented in this book so far to realize some of its functionality. Most notably, these are multimedia processing as explained in Chap. 3, Memory Buoyancy calculations and initial preservation policy (Chap. 4), contextualization and condensation (Chap. 5), interfacing with preservation workflows, functionality, communication, and the PoF Middleware (Chap. 6).

The goal of the pilot is also to provide applications and services which support needs or desires of users. In the PoF Framework, they are part of the Active System (see Fig. 6.2) to provide benefits for the users and rely on PoF components and features. In turn, they again contribute to the goals for personal preservation, e.g., by allowing to collect and organize photos which enable preservation possibilities.

Two such applications will be presented in the following sections: PIMO Photo Organization and the PIMO Diary.

7.2.5 Organizing Photos with the PIMO

The user survey in Sect. 2.5 and [419] showed that users would appreciate support in organizing their photos. This motivated us to introduce a dedicated application allowing users to organize their photo collections as part of the personal preservation scenario. The resulting PIMO Photo Organization app is an example of how the PIMO and technologies presented in this book can be embedded in user's daily life and be combined to provide semantically enriched resources for preservation.

The idea for the photo organization in the Semantic Desktop, is to provide users with an application that could be part of their usual PIM for the family. Because the application is part of the PoF Framework, evidences can be derived contributing to personal preservation goals without additional effort required by the user. Such evidences can be photos marked as favorites, the event a photo belongs to, further annotations and descriptions of a photo, as well as further material connected to the collection which could provide even more contextual information on the event or on the photo itself.

The challenge such an application faces is how to motivate people to use and contribute information when organizing photos. The approach taken is first to provide a better experience than organizing photos simply by naming folders on the computer (or even keeping them on the camera).

Photo organization software for home users such as Apple's Photos already provides easy organization by events (here, an event is simply a set of photos with a label, with no connection to or interpretation as a calendar event), geo-location, and persons (via face detection). We extend this by allowing to annotate with PIMO concepts and resources, (semantically interpreted) texts, condensation of events, etc. The PIMO introduces the concept of a life situation which can contain photo collections and allows to differ in its view depending on the specific type of life situation such as birth, wedding, or trip.

The application (see Fig. 7.5) allows users to organize their photos by providing the user's mental model (as represented in the PIMO) as well as details of activities and events (such as a trip) from other sources in the Semantic Desktop (events, documents, notes, etc.). Moreover, by using the mental model represented in the PIMO, we reduce effort for the user for organizing photos. And vice versa, that part of the mental model which was explicated in the photo collection, can be reused later in other parts of the Semantic Desktop ecosystem.

Furthermore, annotations added to one photo are aggregated for the photo collection. Combined they comprise an aggregated description of the collection (as shown in Fig. 7.6). And vice versa, annotations to the photo collection are propagated to the contained photos. This helps in finding photos by using annotations of the collection which were not separately added to a photo by the user. Again, this reduces effort for contextualizing each and every photo.

The resulting life situation with its photos is embedded in the PIMO, thus enabling services like preserving, forgetting, reminiscence, cloud storage in the PIMO, and mobile access, contextualizing and condensation, or associative retrieval of photos via PIMO's faceted search.

Please note: By using just this application for photo organization purposes, without all the other Semantic Desktop applications, we are already able to get hold of photo collections, can enrich these with contextual information, and enable the selection for preservation by the PoF Middleware. This is in contrast to the Photo Preservation Application presented in the following Chap. 8 which focuses on supporting users during the selection process for preservation.

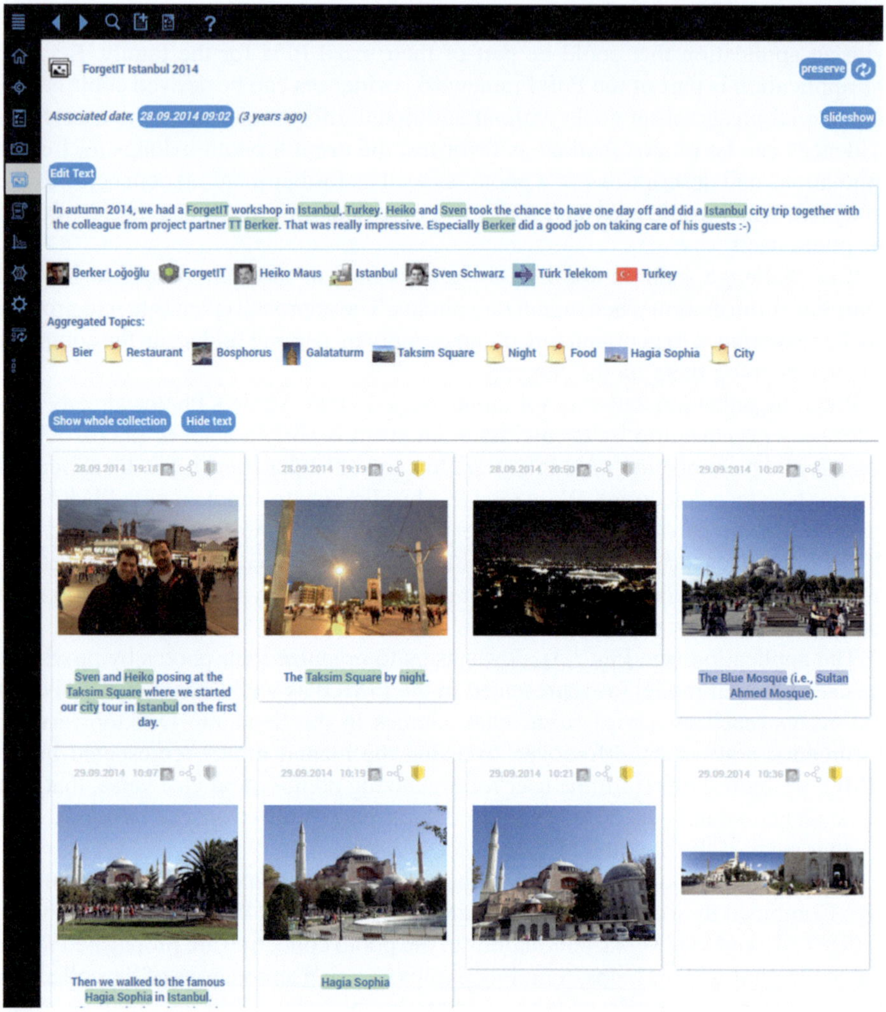

Fig. 7.5 Photo collection in the PIMO: collection from an Istanbul trip with entities such as persons, topics, locations

By integrating part of the image services as presented in Chap. 3, the Semantic Desktop ecosystem and especially the use case of photo organization benefits from three functionalities: image quality assessment, near duplicate detection, and visual concept detection (see Fig. 7.7).

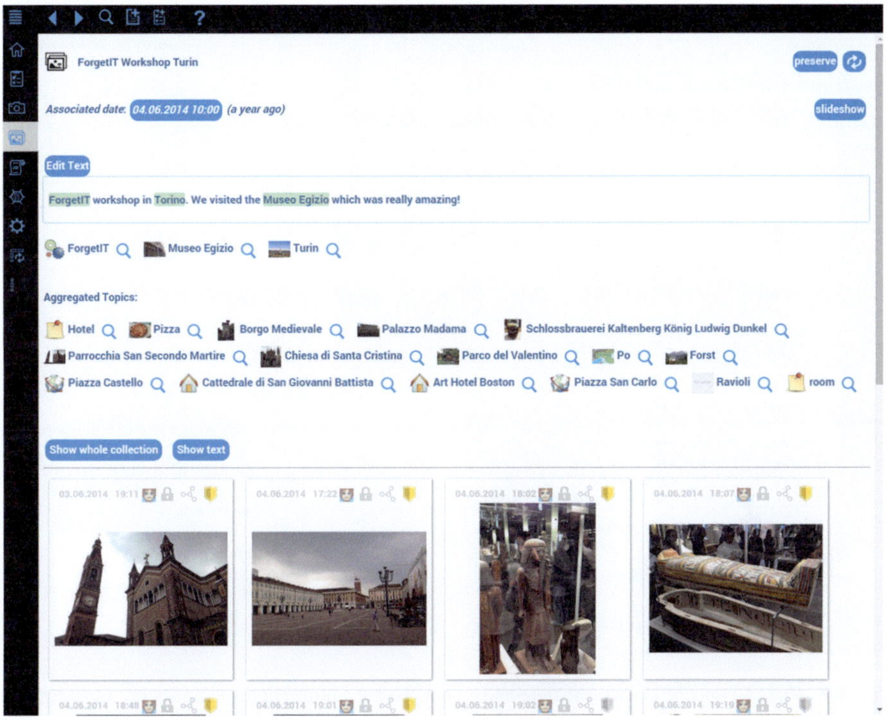

Fig. 7.6 Photo collections in PIMO: the entry page shows the favorite images in a thumbnail gallery, all annotations of this collection, and a descriptive text. This overview serves as a condensed view (favorite photos and PIMO concepts) of the whole photo collection, thus giving an impression on the collection w/o requiring to browse through all photos

7.2.6 Contextual Remembering with PIMO Diary

Using the Semantic Desktop regularly leads to a PIMO enriched with plenty of semantically annotated information, e.g., documents, web pages, emails, calendar events, etc. Sorting, mentally connecting and abstracting from parts of these things in order to remember what actually happened in a given period of time is typically a difficult and time-consuming task.

The PIMO Diary realizes Contextual Remembering by enabling a user to generate a personal (or group) diary based on these information items from the PIMO. To support contextual remembering and at the same time to prevent the diary from being a confusing, large, sequential collection of material, we need to identify semantic relationships among possibly several thousands of individual information items and create suitable abstractions from them. If a user, for example, looks back on the last decade, they should not be overwhelmed with a view showing plenty of individual events, but compact statements like project names, stages of life, life situations, etc. Examples for those are terms like “school years”, “studies”, “wedding”, or the name

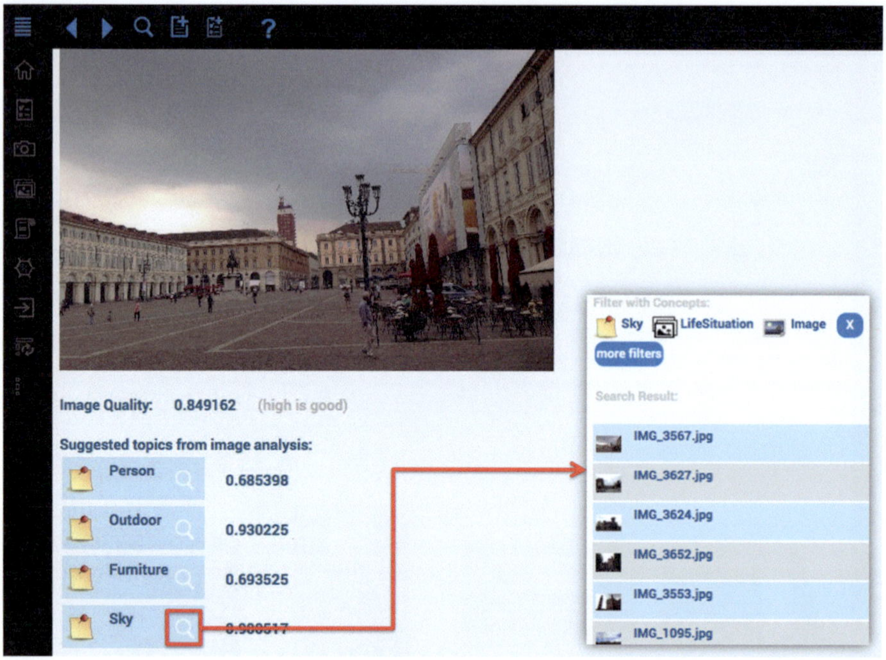

Fig. 7.7 Visual concept detection: detected concepts are automatically annotated as suggested topics. The detail view also shows the confidence of each concept. Clicking the magnifying glass next to a concept starts a semantic search for images and photo collections that were also annotated with it

of a place where a vacation or longer stay abroad has been spent. The user literally *zooms out* of an overwhelming mass of details. If desired, these abstractions can easily be resolved by selecting a subperiod of time for concretization (*zooming in*), e.g., a year of a decade or a month of a year. Concretizations (half-years, quarters, months, weeks, days) can be performed until the user reaches the actual basic material, which are the concrete information items like notes, photos, documents, etc. Clicking any of these items directly opens them in the appropriate app, e.g., notes are opened in the note app.

The system applies a combination of merging and filtering by clustering related or very similar things to diary entries and evaluating their importance for the user. The former aspect fosters a high diversity within the diary, making it interesting and fun to read, whereas the latter aspect is a necessity induced by the fact that the number of diary entries to be generated is usually limited. It is also compliant to ForgetIT's basic idea of forgetting less important, situational short-term information in favor of more important items selected for long-term preservation. In the example screenshot (Fig. 7.8), we see that there are 1420 information items available for the selected month. By using 502 of these items, ten diary entries were generated and displayed. The other 918 items were disregarded in the current diary view, which

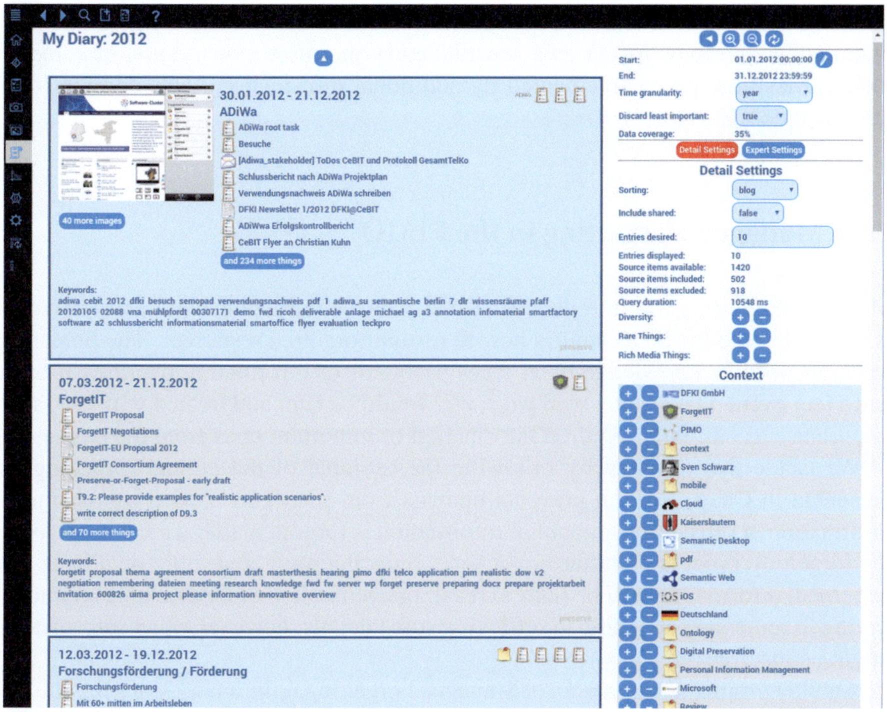

Fig. 7.8 PIMO Diary showing the year 2012 of a ForgetIT member using DFKI's PIMO: most relevant clusters: a project finished in 2012 (ADiWa) and the proposal preparation of the ForgetIT project both containing tasks and documents from the user activities at that time

leads to a data coverage of 35%. Nevertheless, diaries covering 100% of the available data can be generated if desired (in these cases, the feature of sorting out items by their importance is turned off).

As depicted in Fig. 7.8, a typical diary entry consists of a date (or time interval), a headline, and the most prominent things and keywords gathered from all information items that were clustered to form this entry. On an entry's right-hand side there are its most prominent annotations revealing more of its contextual background. Additionally, if a photo is associated with the entry (or more precisely: with one or more of its items), it is displayed on its left-hand side.

In the lower right of Fig. 7.8, another feature called the "concept context" (or "context" for short) is illustrated. It is intended to provide a quick overview of those things of a user's life (reflected by their PIMO) that concerned them the most in a given time period. For example, "DFKI GmbH", the "ForgetIT" project, "PIMO" and the topic of "context" are among the most prominent things in the depicted sample year.

Users also have the possibility to incorporate shared data of their family, friends, or colleagues—represented by a *group information model (GIMO)*—into their own personal diary turning it into a *group diary*. As a consequence, a friend's shared photo collection may appear as a separate entry in a user's own diary, or some of their entries may be complemented by additional information items coming from other people's PIMOs.

7.3 Managed Forgetting in the PIMO

Managed Forgetting was introduced in Chap. 4. In the following, we address how this is realized in the PIMO as well as how to restore forgotten resources. The Semantic Desktop, with its knowledge base, faces problems of information overflow if each and every event, tasks, note, web page, etc. would be kept and treated with the same importance as currently required information or important ones from the past.

We tackle this problem by following the example of the human forgetting as presented in Chap. 2 which prevents humans from problems caused by too much information: a substantial amount of information is forgotten after a mere short time; the forgetting process continues over time, reducing more and more details. If not relearned, information will be hard to recall or eventually not be available anymore. Trying to remember will help in retrieving some details, however, other information might be lost forever.

Another promising approach for Managed Forgetting is the analogy of a lighthouse which identifies an area from far away without actually seeing the patch of land. Getting closer, more and more details get visible. Transferred to our semantic network in the PIMO, we introduce "lighthouse concepts" which will aggregate a complex, detailed network of concepts, content, and relations under a single node in the PIMO. The lighthouse concept represents a cluster of information that could be forgotten as long as the lighthouse is still there. If getting older, even the lighthouse concepts will fade away from the user's direct view.

These views on forgetting are applied in the concept and calculation of the MB. The Semantic Desktop provides two types of evidences for the calculation: First, user interaction events with resources such as "create", "view", or "modify" are analyzed. That means, the Semantic Desktop delivers a user action event containing the type of user action, a timestamp, the active user, and the URI of the respective thing. This information serves as evidence that the user actually did something with the resource and is therefore used in the calculation.) Second, the semantic representation of a resource in the PIMO and its connections to other resources are taken into account. The latter is used, e.g., for the spreading algorithm in the MB calculation enabling it to decide where to spread and which weights to apply to other relevant resources which are connected. This enables the MB to be available for every resource in the PIMO and also ensures that values are always updated if the user interacts with resources or as time elapses (such as decay). Figure 7.9 shows an internal view of a MB graph of several resources.

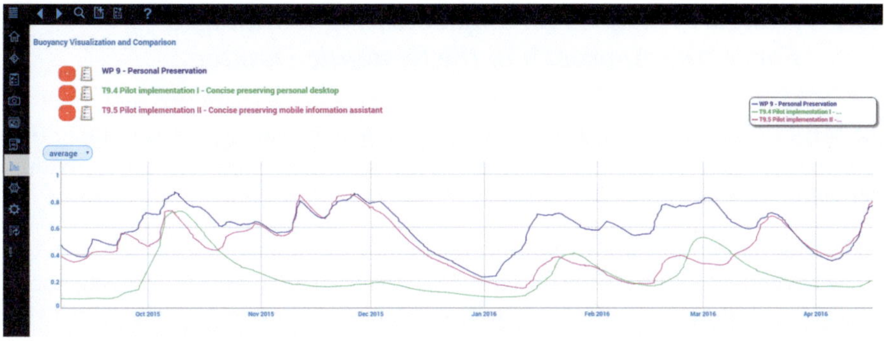

Fig. 7.9 A real-life example of a Memory Buoyancy graph from the DFKI PIMO: a ForgetIT work package task and two subtasks. We see final phase of the project, where the task T9.5 was active and T9.4 was revisited due to deliverables (in December) and final review in April

Currently realized forgetting strategies in the PIMO are:

- **Hiding**: Hiding resources to be forgotten in the user interface (in PIMO5, an HTML-based user interface for the PIMO): Depending on a threshold (which is higher on a mobile device than on a desktop computer), resources below the threshold are not shown immediately to the user but can be retrieved after explicit requests (e.g., via button "show forgotten"). See Fig. 7.11 for an example.
- **Moving**: Moving files from the desktop to the cloud and to the archive: desktop files to be forgotten can be removed from the file system and moved to the cloud (if not already there). The files are still accessible on demand from the cloud. This is done via the PIMOCloud Service (available as desktop and server version). A further escalation strategy is then to move cloud files to the archive and leaving only a condensed version (which could simply be the PIMO representation only containing a reference to the archive) (see Sect. 7.3.2).
- **Condensing**: Condensing several information items to one information object representing original non-relevant/too detailed/to-be-forgotten items: the PIMO Diary (see Sect. 7.2.6, [183]) uses condensation to generate on demand condensed representations for activities in the PIMO within a specific period of time. This condensed representation is presented to the user. First steps toward identifying lighthouse concepts representing a whole cluster is introduced by context elements. Links to the contained material are kept. If this material is then forgotten (e.g., moved to the archive), only the condensation is kept in the PIMO.
- **Synchronizing**: Synchronizing material to a device based on a relevancy assessment: the PIMOCloud Service on a device is capable of syncing files to a device if their relevancy (i.e., MB) is above a certain threshold (which again can be different depending on the device type and available space). It is also capable of removing files from the device again, if the MB drops below a threshold—meaning it should be forgotten (on the device).

7.3.1 Design Principles for Implementing a Managed Forgetting Approach in the Semantic Desktop

The MB calculation in the PIMO follows these design principles: Every thing (i.e., the semantic representation of a resource or concept) in the PIMO has an **individual MB value** for a user.

- The MB value is updated every time the thing is stimulated.
- The strength of a stimulation depends on the user interaction (e.g., viewing, modifying, annotating, etc.), the thing itself, and its connections in the semantic network of the PIMO.
- MB calculation has to cope with activity bursts as well as erratic accesses.
  - MB values are normalized (between 0.0 and 1.0).
  - Single access of an item should not directly lead to a MB of 1.0.
  - Multiple accesses in quick succession (every minute) are treated reluctantly.
  - Over day, multiple accesses will saturate against 1.0.

Realize forgetting by orienting on insights **human brain activity on the mental model** as described in Chap. 2.

- MB drops for things that are not stimulated (first steep decline then a long-tail of slow decline).
- MB increases for things that are stimulated.
- MB decreases slower for things that are repeatedly stimulated over time (learning effect).
- Associations to accessed things are stimulated as well.
  - Especially "lighthouse concepts" allow an orientation for users in a set of resources; allow such lighthouse concepts, let their MB inherit stimulations of connected things.
  - We took an iterative approach: use the expected ones from the PIMO and further domain ontologies (such as projects or life situations).
  - Start to identify such concepts in the PIMO from user evidences (see, e.g., the PIMO Diary).

Apply forgetting **reasonably** and remember important stuff in context to keep the user's **trust**—ensure MB actually helps rather than merely imitates human behavior (mimicking "human forgetting as failure" as well as "remembering it all" is no help).

- Apply rules and heuristics to deal with requirements of various domains. Utilize heuristics derived from PIM to predict individual MB such as
  - upcoming events should stimulate connected things (such as locations, persons, material, topics),
  - finished items shall decrease faster (tasks, events) unless other indicators speak against this, or

  - times with low user interaction (thus sparse or no stimulations such as weekends or holidays) should not lead to massive decay in MB.

- Applications shall use MB including various thresholds to the requirements of the individual use case.

  - For instance, a 3rd-Party calendar which is not capable of dealing with MB should have access to all the events otherwise users might lose trust in interacting with the PIMO. This requires that each thing has its own MB and PIMO Server APIs allowing to set individual MB thresholds.

Utilize the information from the PIMO's **semantic network**. First, we make use of the type of a concept as short- and long-term importance of information items also can be derived from their type. For instance, emails are faster forgotten than persons. Therefore, individual decay curves are used for classes in the PIMO and domain ontologies. Furthermore, as with humans, mentioning things also stimulate associations in their semantic neighborhood:

- As a basis, spreading activation on the semantic network of the PIMO is used for MB calculation.
- Heuristics for the type and number of relations connecting things influence the spreading algorithm.

We considered also **technical requirements** as forgetting is just one among many dimensions in the PIMO. Over time, the PIMO can amount to a huge data collection but still needs a quick response time for MB values. As it is used in daily work, a mere research approach is not feasible. Therefore, the following design decisions to embed MB calculation in the current PIMO Server version were used:

- MB is time-dependent which poses a challenge for calculation as MB values change permanently just as time passes by (i.e., decay).

  - Conceptually splitting MB value into two parts: a static (time-independent) and a dynamic (time-dependent) part.
  - Database stores most recently calculated MB value and calculation timestamp.
  - Decay happens at retrieval time: value stored in database is "decayed" according to time difference between retrieval time and last calculation time.

- MB values must always be up-to-date.

  - Use an online calculation (instead of offline-like overnight calculation).
  - Accessing PIMO things must trigger recalculation of MB involving their semantic neighborhood to also identify hot regions.

- Keep high performance despite additional MB calculation.

  - Requesting MB values is done very often, therefore, retrieval must be fast (processing high-volume access event streams is not feasible at runtime).

- Minimize database updates: updating MB values for all things in the PIMO is not feasible.
- Incremental updates: only recalculate the most minimal set of PIMO things.

These principles are applied in the MB calculation in the Semantic Desktop. In the following sections, two exemplary forgetting services implemented in the Semantic Desktop are presented.

7.3.2 Managed Forgetting in the File System

With the help of the Semantic Desktop ecosystem being embedded in a computer's file system, the forgetting functionality is available on the user's desktop file system. It is now possible that files are removed from the computer if the PoF Framework decides to do so (based on low MB). Depending on the user's chosen policy, these files are either suggested as candidates to be forgotten (awaiting confirmation, see Fig. 7.10) or they are removed automatically in the background.

The Semantic Desktop checks at regular time intervals if there exist local files whose MB dropped under a certain threshold which would indicate that these should be forgotten. This interval can be individually configured. Reasonable time frames

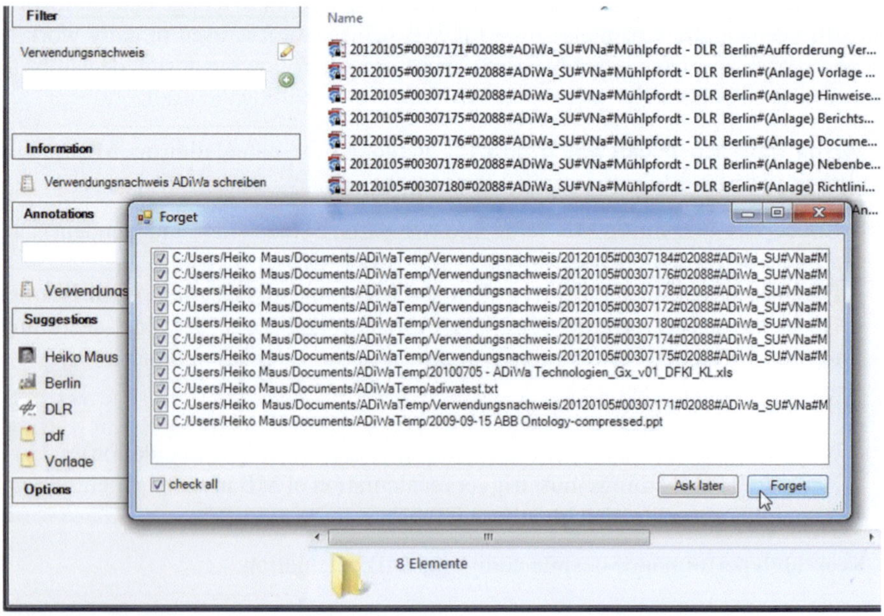

Fig. 7.10 Forgetting of files: the PoF Framework has decided to forget several files on the user's computer. They are presented in a dialog window that also allows modifications to the list before the forgetting is finally executed

range from a daily basis—although no quick changes are to be expected—to a week. Identified files are proposed to the user to be forgotten, i.e., removed from the computer.

The current implementation uses a preservation policy which removes the file from the computer (after user confirmation, see Fig. 7.10), but leaves the file in the PIMOCloud untouched. The preservation decision is left to the PoF Middleware. That means that details pertaining to what happens in the case of removal from the computer w.r.t. preservation will be clarified in a preservation policy. For instance, the file in the PIMOCloud may first be preserved and then deleted in the PIMOCloud, or the file will be preserved and kept in the PIMOCloud until the MB drops below an even lower threshold. As long as the cloud file is available, it can be restored on any computer or accessed on a mobile device. If the cloud file is also removed, only restoring it from the archive will be possible (if actually preserved there).

This strategy keeps high- and medium-buoyant resources on the desktop and gradually removes resources with low MB from the desktop.

Although the files are forgotten, their semantic representation (i.e., the thing) in the PIMO is still there. However, due to the low MB it will not show up in normal browsing (i.e., the user will not stumble upon it easily; see also Sect. 7.3.3). At what time such things shall be removed from the PIMO is subject to the user's policy of trashing things as well as condensing things into a landmark.

Therefore, users are also able to find, inspect, and restore once forgotten files. By using PIMO's associative search, forgotten things can be retrieved. Users may then inspect them and finally decide to restore them on their local computer.

7.3.3 Managed Forgetting in the User Interface

A further benefit of having MB calculations is the possibility to actively hide things from the user when browsing the PIMO if the MB is low. Not showing each and every resource in the PIMO, but only those of current and medium-term relevancy (as expressed by a high MB) prevents the users from an information overload.

The PIMO5 user interface applies hiding of information if the MB of a thing is below a certain threshold (during browsing and during search). This threshold is set differently whether users browse on a desktop computer or a smartphone and can also be adjusted by them.

Figure 7.11 shows an example of a thing's buoyancy over a period of time: whereas in the beginning all connected things are listed directly, after time progresses, things with lower MB are hidden from immediate view. Forgotten things are shown only if the user issues an explicit request ("show forgotten").

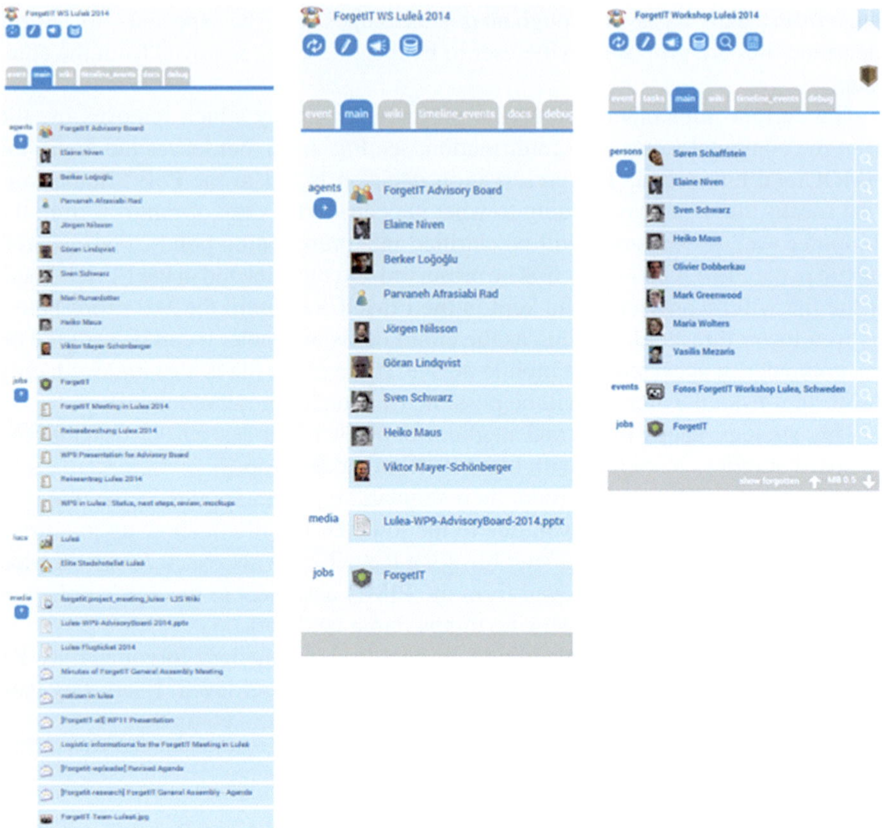

Fig. 7.11 Hiding forgotten things: an example of viewing a workshop in the PIMO at different times: during the workshop (left), after eight months (middle) and after two years (right). Things are hidden when falling below the MB threshold (which is at 0.5 as we see on the right image). Here, documents, emails, and tasks are hidden, while still active things such as project members and the project itself are kept, which results in a condensed view for the user

7.4 Supporting Preservation with the Semantic Desktop

The following sections detail how preservation is supported in the Semantic Desktop. First, Sect. 7.4.1 details how the realization of the Preservation Value (PV) Assessment in the Semantic Desktop allows to embed a detailed and personalized Preservation Strategy into the Semantic Desktop. This Preservation Strategy is based on indicators from the Semantic Desktop and the PIMO specified as policies and rules. These policies and rules are classified along the dimensions for assessment identified by in Sect. 4.3.2. Users can use predefined Preservation Strategies as well as customize their own. This is embedded in a user interface to define the Preservation Service Contract with a service provider including Preservation Levels which is presented in Sect. 7.4.2. The components and examples shown here are taken from the Personal Preservation pilot implemented in the ForgetIT project using the Semantic Desktop ecosystem and the DFKI's PIMO.

7.4.1 Preservation Value Assessment in the Semantic Desktop

Assessing a PV was introduced in Sect. 4.3. In the following, we detail how the Semantic Desktop realizes such a PV Assessment of resources. This will allow for Synergetic Preservation by the PoF Middleware connected to the Semantic Desktop. In the PoF Framework this is done in the functional entity called "Content Value Assessment" (see also the Preservation Preparation Workflow (see Fig. 6.5) in the PoF Reference Model). This entity assesses resources w.r.t. MB and PV. In this Section, we focus on the PV which reflects the long-term importance or relevance of a resource as defined in Sect. 4.3. This PV is then used by the PoF Middleware as a basis for making preservation decisions, e.g., if a resource should be preserved or how much should be invested in its preservation, i.e., which "Preservation Level" should be used (see Sect. 7.4.2.1).

To allow an assessment of resources, first, it must be clarified what aspects in the assessment could possibly contribute to the long-term importance and then consider individual preferences of the user in a so-called "Preservation Strategy" of the PoF Reference Model as introduced in Sect. 6.6.3.

The following sections explain how a personal Preservation Strategy is supported. To ease the usability for the user, such a Preservation Strategy can be defined along specific dimensions for assessment which will be detailed in Sect. 7.4.1.1.

The approach for personal preservation allows to define Preservation Strategies in two ways: presets based on dedicated user profiles (Sect. 7.4.1.2) or a combination of presets and a more detailed customization using policies and rules (Sect. 7.4.1.3).

7.4.1.1 Preservation Strategy

The Preservation Strategy will be based on a set of policies and rules which support an assessment of the PV. For this assessment six dimensions where identified, which are—from the point of view of the Semantic Desktop—relevant for the Personal Preservation Scenario. As identified in Sect. 4.3.2 these are investment, gravity, social graph, popularity, coverage, and quality.

These are the dimensions identified for collecting evidences for the assessment and finally the calculation of the PV. Which evidences are used and how they contribute (weighting) to the calculation of the PV is defined by a Preservation Strategy.

The following sections detail the two realized approaches.

7.4.1.2 Personal Preservation Strategy Based on Personas

To help users who are new to a personal preservation service, it would be useful to have a predefined set of policies and rules defined for the six dimensions mentioned above, so that they do not need to care about defining a rather complex Preservation Strategy.

The survey conducted on personal preservation of photos (see Sect. 2.5) identified four personas representing attitudes toward personal Preservation Strategies (reported in [419]). The personas are defined along two key preservation dimensions of "Loss"—the user is worried about losing important photos—and "Generations"—importance to the user of preserving important photos for future generations.

For each dimension, two habits could be clustered. Regarding "Loss", a group took less precautions against losing their photos (therefore named "Forget") than the "Safety in Redundancy" group which tended to have redundant copies of their photos on different storage units. Regarding "Generations", one group put much effort in organizing their photos (therefore named "Curators"), e.g., by assigning keywords. In contrast, the "Filing First" group almost exclusively relies on files and folders. Using these dimensions, the four personas identified are "Safe Curator", "Safe Filer", "File and Forget", and "File and Forget Curator".

To achieve the aforementioned ease of use, we defined one Preservation Strategy for each persona. We assigned different weights to policies and rules to match the persona's preferences and assumed behavior. The different personas tend to score differently on the six dimensions of PV Assessment presented in Sect. 4.3.2:

- **Investment**: The Curator's investment is on purpose, thus evidences for investment in this group should be ranked higher, whereas in the File and Forget group, the investment might be sporadic.
- **Gravity**: This is assumed to be more helpful to Safe Filers as Curators are supposed to decide on importance on their own.
- **Social Graph**: The relevance of content to social relations is important for all personas. Social aspects are important for every persona.
- **Popularity**: Filers are purposeful in accessing resources valuable to them and ratings might be rare. In contrast, Curators are expected to access more resources especially for curation purposes which does not directly indicate popularity of the resource, thus this evidence should be weighted less.
- **Coverage**: For both Curators and Safe Filers coverage is important; to the Curator more than to the Safe Filer.
- **Quality**: For Filers the quality (expressed by image quality) is more important whereas for Curators the automatically calculated quality assessment is not that important as they will rely on their manual assessment.

To reflect these persona perspectives in the PV Assessment, corresponding profiles were created for the PV calculation (which can be set in the Semantic Desktop as shown in Fig. 7.12). The profiles mirror the basic distinction between "Curators" and "Filers" by mainly basing the preservation suggestions on the investment spent by the former, and an emphasis on popularity and material quality by the latter. For the

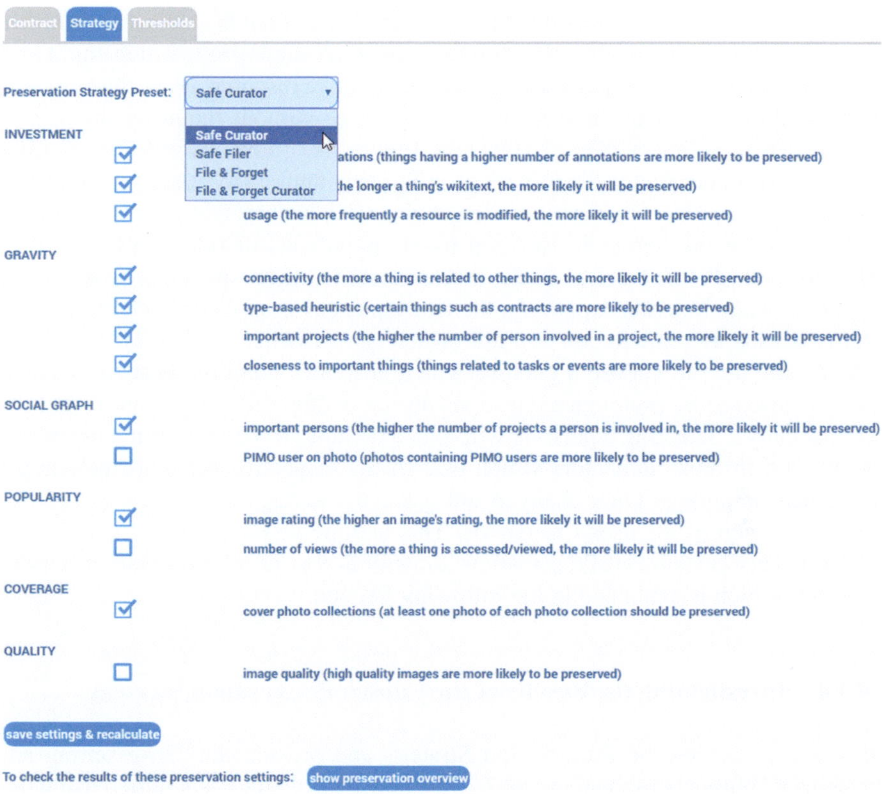
Contract
Strategy
Thresholds
Preservation Strategy Preset:
Safe Curator
Safe Curator
Safe Filer
File & Forget
File & Forget Curator
INVESTMENT
ations (things having a higher number of annotations are more likely to be preserved)
he longer a thing's wikitext, the more likely it will be preserved)
usage (the more frequently a resource is modified, the more likely it will be preserved)
GRAVITY
connectivity (the more a thing is related to other things, the more likely it will be preserved)
type-based heuristic (certain things such as contracts are more likely to be preserved)
important projects (the higher the number of person involved in a project, the more likely it will be preserved)
closeness to important things (things related to tasks or events are more likely to be preserved)
SOCIAL GRAPH
important persons (the higher the number of projects a person is involved in, the more likely it will be preserved)
PIMO user on photo (photos containing PIMO users are more likely to be preserved)
POPULARITY
image rating (the higher an image's rating, the more likely it will be preserved)
number of views (the more a thing is accessed/viewed, the more likely it will be preserved)
COVERAGE
cover photo collections (at least one photo of each photo collection should be preserved)
QUALITY
image quality (high quality images are more likely to be preserved)
save settings & recalculate
To check the results of these preservation settings:
show preservation overview

Fig. 7.12 Setting a more detailed Preservation Strategy in PIMO5: allowing to easily select/deselect those policies and rules which matter the most to the user. Selecting a persona loads a predefined set of choices. Changes are possible and saved as a personal Preservation Strategy

safety-conscious persona profiles, the algorithm tries to ensure a certain coverage of the different subsets (e.g., photo collections) of the material to be preserved.

The next section will describe more comprehensive strategies for including more resources as well as more complex rules.

7.4.1.3 Customization for Preservation Strategies

In the previous section, the Preservation Strategy has been based on personas defining strategies in which the user is not able to influence details but can only change the persona itself. To allow a more fine-grained Preservation Strategy setting for the Semantic Desktop along the preservation policy and rules, the following more detailed strategy setting has been realized as an extension of the aforementioned persona-only approach.

For the application scenario of PIM, several evidences or indicators were identified in the Semantic Desktop along the aforementioned six dimensions which could help in the assessment of the expected long-term benefit of a resource. Now, the Semantic Desktop allows to adapt these to one's preferences without requiring the user to be an expert in policy or rule management. Figure 7.12 shows the PIMO5 interface allowing to set and change the Preservation Strategy applied to a user's resources as introduced above. Here, a more detailed choice of indicators (e.g., allowing further evidences from the Semantic Desktop usage as policies or rules) to be used for calculating the PV of the user's resources are shown. Each indicator is described in human readable terms explaining the consequences if applied. Each indicator is internally used in a calculation or a rule which can be switched on or off.

Users are able to choose a persona which describes them the best (or it rather could be inferred by preference questions during configuration time and is then set automatically). Selecting a persona will load a default profile and set the respective check mark to those indicators which best fit the respective persona (including a predefined weighting). Once changed and saved, the settings are used for calculating the PV for each of the user's resources. This is done periodically in the Semantic Desktop. This customized Preservation Strategy is part of a "Preservation Service Contract" which is explained in the following Section.

7.4.1.4 Investigating the Results of the Chosen Preservation Strategy

Once a user has set the Preservation Strategy and pressed the "Save setting and recalculate" button (as shown in Fig. 7.12), a new PV calculation is started using this new strategy. The "Show preservation overview" button provides the user with an overview of the current material from the PIMO which would be preserved (if the PoF Framework decides to start preserving) according to the selected Preservation Strategy. This view shows all material from the PIMO such as documents, concepts, projects, or persons.

For easier inspection, the view lists those images which would be preserved under their respective photo collection (in the PIMO the class Life Situation). Currently, the list starts with an overview of the resources with the highest PVs first and allowing the user to request more items as shown in Fig. 7.13. Each thing has a so-called badge indicating the PV Category. Clicking on a thing's badge shows an explanation for the PV decision as shown in Figs. 7.14 and 7.15.

7.4.1.5 Preservation Embedded in the File System

The previous sections have shown how the Semantic Desktop is connected to the PoF Framework and can start preservation activity automatically after certain time frames. To bring preservation even closer to users, the Semantic Desktop ecosystem allows to preserve single items at any time by triggering PoF Framework's preservation workflow on manual request.

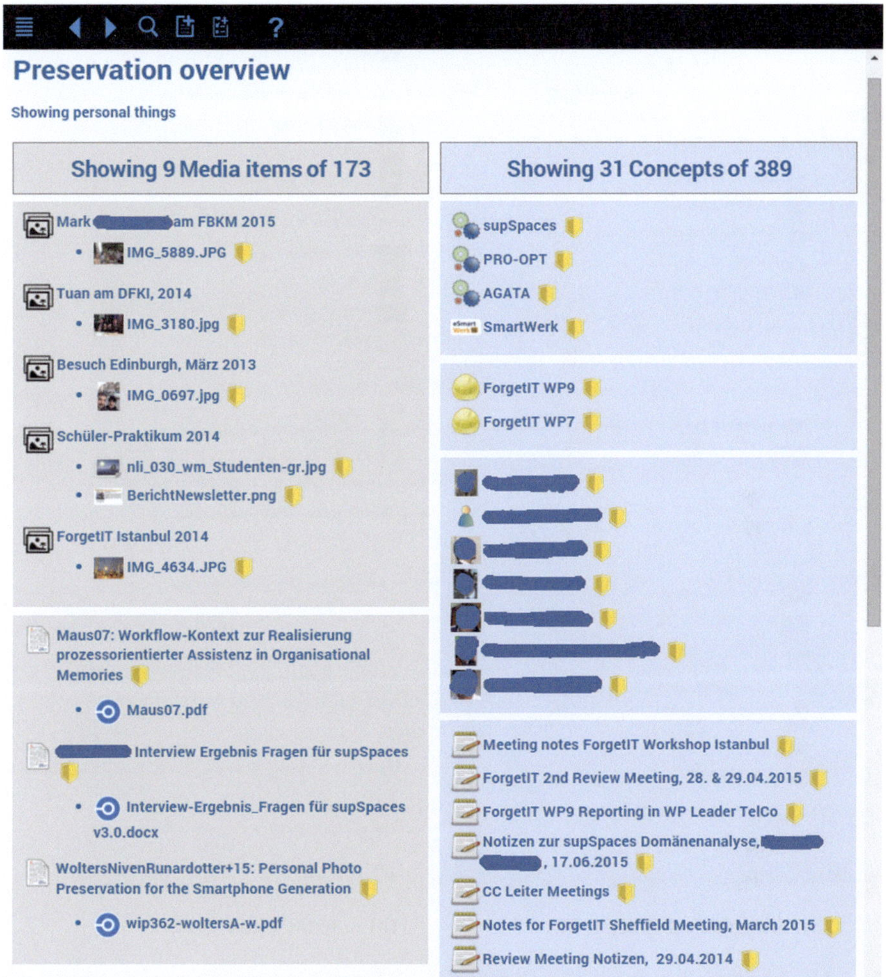

Fig. 7.13 Preservation overview: a dedicated preservation view has been integrated in PIMO5 to check the Preservation Strategy setting. It allows to browse through all resources and concepts to be preserved. The screenshot shows an individual (and partly anonymized) view on the DFKI PIMO with a safe curator profile

As a use case, the Semantic Desktop's plug-in for the Microsoft Windows File Explorer has been extended to enable users to manually preserve resources. To do this, the user could choose a file through the file explorer, as shown in Fig. 7.16, and select "Preserve" in the file's context menu. Preservation of the file is issued without requiring any further interaction by the user with the PoF Middleware. Technically, the manual triggering of "Preserve" on one file sets its PV to maximum. Depending on the preservation policy, the PoF will then decide on the schedule to preserve.

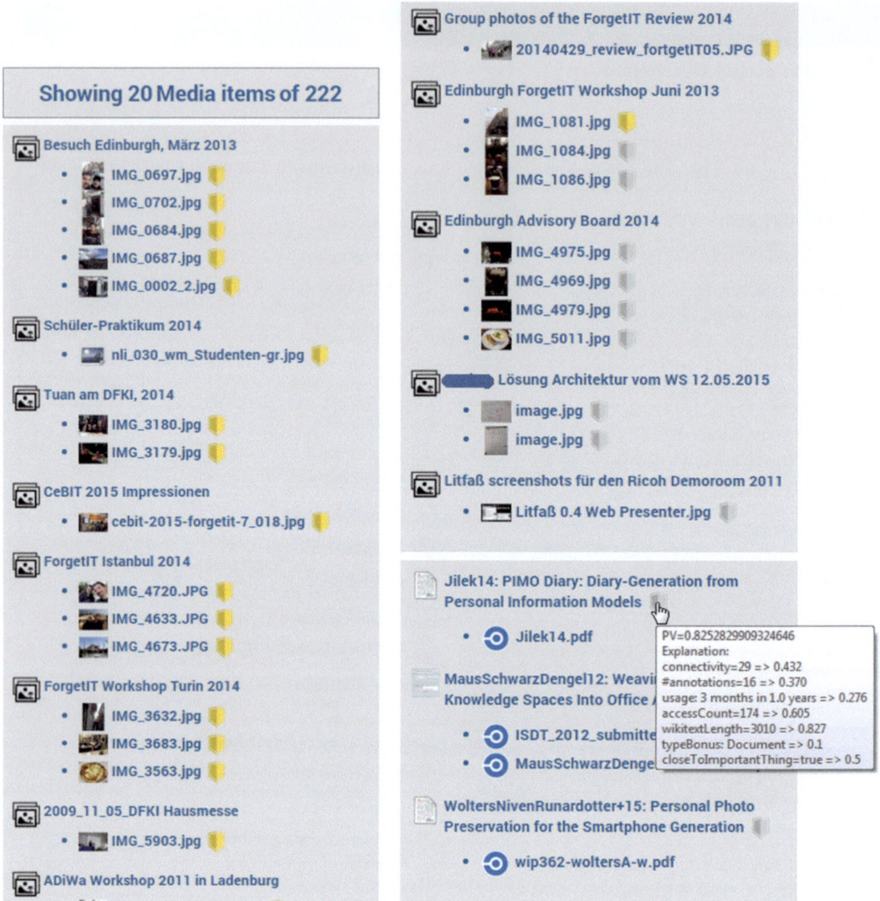

(a) Scrolling down all the photos ... (b) ... to the media items.

Fig. 7.14 Preservation overview: choosing the File and Forget Preservation Strategy generates this list which contains mainly photos as media items

7.4.2 Preservation Service Contract

In addition to the Preservation Strategy, another detail to be considered for personal preservation is which service infrastructure is used for preservation. In other words, who provides the actual service for preservation to the user and what are the conditions? Preservation could be offered as a service by a provider using an instance of the PoF Framework (for the services) and a subset of the Semantic Desktop ecosystem—most prominently the PIMO Photo Organization—as applications for customers. Assuming such a service is established, a contract between the user and the company would state the conditions of the service and its costs. Moreover,

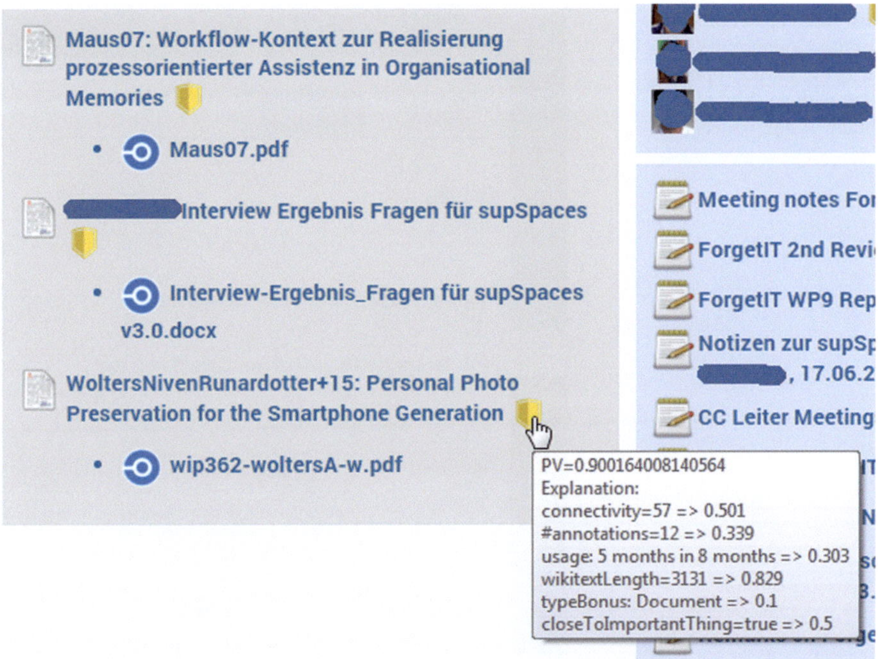

Fig. 7.15 A short explanation of the decision for PV using the Preservation Strategy settings

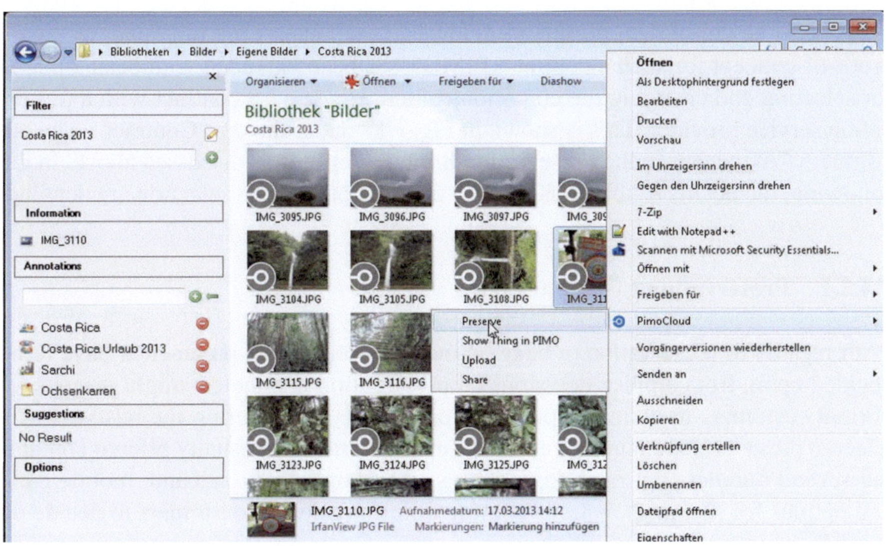

Fig. 7.16 Preserving embedded in the MS windows Explorer context menu of a file: issuing manual preservation

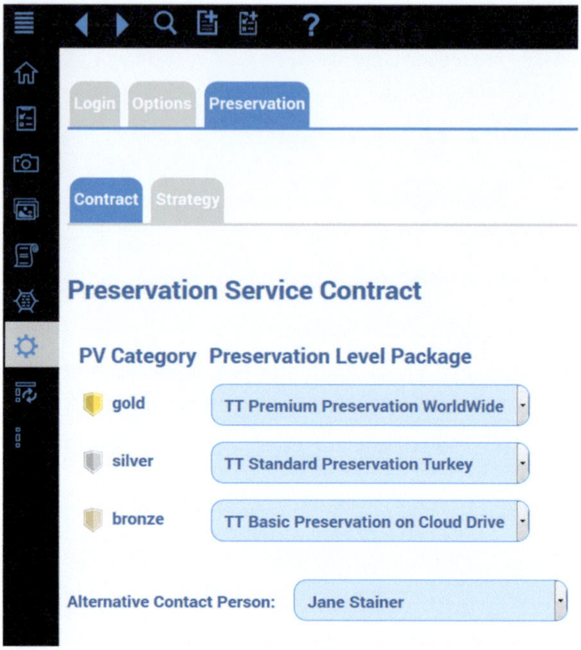

Fig. 7.17 Preservation Service Contract: it can be set in the PIMO5 options. Here with an exemplary choice of a provider

such a contract would also detail how the service would be used, e.g., the amount of space to be consumed, preservation levels, how formats are migrated, etc. As a proof-of-concept for such a contract, PIMO5 has been extended with basic options for selecting and changing the conditions of a user's service contract with a preservation service provider. This is shown in Fig. 7.17 under the tab "Contract". The tab "Strategy" then leads to the Preservation Strategy settings as discussed above. In the following, the details of this basic service contract preference selection are detailed.

7.4.2.1 Preservation Level Package

With regards to preservation, a huge amount of options and parameters have to be decided upon. But complex decisions on preservation parameters might discourage normal customers to choose a preservation service. Considering the business of a telecom provider, for example, pre-configured contracts are usually offered containing several bundles (flat rates for text messages, landline, broadband, mobile data, and options for roaming) making it (more or less) easier for customers to decide on suitable contracts.

As the goal is to reduce the effort for Personal Preservation, offering such bundles for preservation options as in telecom contracts makes sense for the average customer. By additionally providing more detailed options, this still allows advanced users to adapt their contract to their personal preferences. Finally, the bundling of preservation

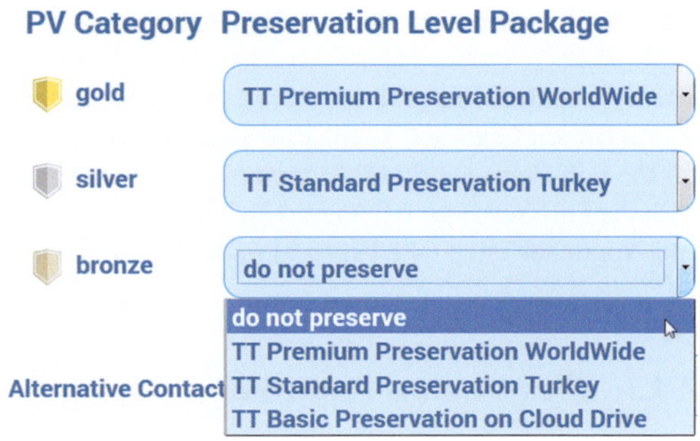

Fig. 7.18 Preservation Level Packages: in PIMO5 the user is able to select Preservation Level Packages for each Preservation Value Category

services with normal telecom contracts holds the potential of bringing preservation to a larger audience.

Offering a preservation service with bundles of preservation functionalities and options as packages would allow customers to choose for the respective Preservation Value Category (gold, silver, bronze), between several preservation levels (offered as "Preservation Level Package") as well as a "do not preserve" for a category as shown in Fig. 7.18. Such a package contains a reasonable default set of preservation functionalities and options for a certain price. These packages could range from a basic package—which could be free with a mobile contract—up to packages with extended functionalities or security with additional costs. Furthermore, some options might be offered to the customer such as allowing storage worldwide (as in the package "Premium Preservation WorldWide") or limit storage to certain countries. Furthermore, we also assume that for a contract bundle, the PV Categories come with a preset for the Preservation Levels as well as for the Preservation Strategy to accomplish an uncomplicated contract activation.

7.4.2.2 Alternative Contact Person

To cope with the case that a user is deceased, a contract has to provide possibilities to identify alternative contacts which are then able to take over the archive. Therefore, the preservation contract tab allows to enter a contact from the PIMO which shall be contacted in the case a user passed away. Figure 7.17 shows the section where a contact can be selected via a dropdown box listing all persons in the PIMO. This contact is actually a `pimo:Person` which can either be imported from an address book together with address details or simply created in the Semantic Desktop. This is realized as a proof-of-concept. It could be extended with more persons, with priorities, situations (death, unable to act, etc.) in which to contact, with a commitment of the selected user, e.g., by exchanging emails, etc.

7.4.2.3 Preservation Broker Contract

The terms of this Preservation Service Contract are transferred in a so-called "Preservation Broker Contract" to the PoF Middleware. This is done via the SD/PoF Adapter (in the PoF Framework, this adapter is part of the Active System and communicates with the PoF; see Figs. 6.2 and 6.13). The contract is used in the "Managed Forgetting and Appraisal" step (see Fig. 6.5) to decide on the preservation actions.

7.4.3 Preservation Preparation Workflow

This section details the connection of the Semantic Desktop as an Active System with the PoF Middleware to enable preservation by relying upon the user's Preservation Strategy and Preservation Value explained in the previous sections. This section describes the preservation steps along the PoF Framework workflow "Preservation Preparation Workflow" as defined in the PoF Functional Model in Sect. 6.3.

The workflow is depicted in Fig. 7.19 with its steps and functional entities involved in these steps (which are explained in the Functional Model; see Fig. 6.2). The additional numbers in the Figure are aligned with the following subsection numbers to explain the steps with involved functional entities.

7.4.3.1 Content Value Assessment

Before the workflow starts, the functional entity "Content Value Assessment" (CVA) is responsible for the assessment of resources in the PoF Framework. As already pointed out in Sect. 7.4.1.1 this step provides the Preservation Value of a resource.

Considering the role of the functional entity CVA in the PoF Framework, the Semantic Desktop as Active System is an example of the situation where the Active System is capable of providing the PV for the preservation decision (as well as the

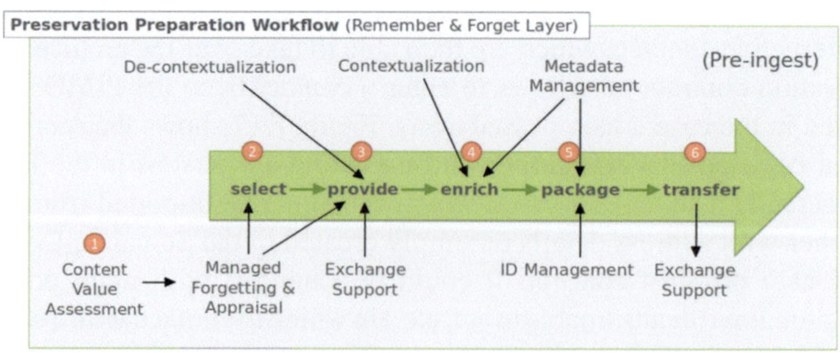

Fig. 7.19 The Preservation Preparation Workflow (adapted from Fig. 6.5)

MB for Managed Forgetting in the Active System) and thus, the functional entity CVA is part of the Active System.

In contrast to that, the implementation chosen for the application scenario using Typo3 in Sect. 6.6.1 is an example of the situation where the Active System does not calculate the values by itself but rather delivers the evidences to the PoF Framework where the computation will take place.

This design decision was made because of the beneficial usage of both MB and PV in the Semantic Desktop ecosystem. The rich semantic model of the PIMO and the usage statistics of the Semantic Desktop allow for a comprehensive view on the resources wrt. MB and PV. Furthermore, the nature of the PIM application scenario implies a lot of access, usage, and changes to resources and the PIMO resulting in a lot of traffic as well as content assessment in the PIMO as a knowledge base. Therefore, both values are computed in the Semantic Desktop and stored directly in the PIMO to be easily accessed by its components and thus, making them an integral part of the PIMO.

Therefore, to enable the PoF Middleware to make decisions based on the PV in the "Select" step, the values are reported and updated in certain time intervals to the PoF Middleware by the SD/PoF Adapter (see Fig. 6.13). The update contains the resource's URI, its Preservation Value, and last modification date of the resource. Adding the last modification date allows the PoF Middleware to decide if the resource might need to be sent to the archive again if the resource changed since the last preservation.

7.4.3.2 Select

The "Select" step uses the functional entity "Managed Forgetting and Appraisal" to make conscious decisions about preservation of resources of the Active System. To accomplish this, the results of the "Content Value Assessment" are used for deciding about preservation actions.

The "Forgettor" component (see Fig. 6.13) selects the set of resources to be preserved based on the selected Preservation Value Categories set in the user's Preservation Strategy. This information is part of the "Preservation Broker Contract" introduced in previous Sect. 7.4.2, set in the Preservation Service Contract, communicated to the PoF Middleware and managed there for each user.

7.4.3.3 Provide

The step "Provide" uses the functional entity "De-Contextualization" to extract a resource from its Active System context in preparation of packaging it for archiving. The PoF Middleware retrieves resources via the "Collector" using the CMIS [312] (see also Sect. 6.6.1) interface embedded in the SD/PoF Adapter. For the PIMO, this means that a thing and its grounding occurrence (i.e., the semantic representation and the actual physical file) is separated: the CMIS interface hands over the resource to be preserved as a `cmis:Item` and the PIMO's model information about its thing will be part of the context information handed over in the `forgetit:context` attribute of the `cmis:Item`. This attribute is then available for the modules in the PoF Middleware, especially the "Contextualizer" in the next step.

Technically, the context information export is an excerpt from the PIMO semantic graph describing the resource in the PIMO and its connection to other things such as topics for a document or persons attending an event. The format used for the exported excerpt is RDF/S using the PIMO Ontology RDF Schema and Turtle[1] (the "Terse RDF Triple Language" is a compact textual syntax for representing RDF) as exchange format.

Furthermore, this interface was enhanced by handling collections of resources and using the additional context delivered by the SD/PoF Adapter. Now every concept in the PIMO can be preserved separately, i.e., the handling was extended to all PIMO classes not only those representing (file) resources such as `pimo:Media` and `pimo:LifeSituation`. Now, it is also possible to preserve a, e.g., `pimo:Project` such as "ForgetIT" in the DFKI PIMO, although it might not have a physical file attached.

7.4.3.4 Enrich

In the "Enrich" step the functional entity "Contextualization" shall provide additional information for the content to be preserved in order to allow archived items to be fully and correctly interpreted at some future date (see Sect. 6.4.2). All resources in the submitted collection are handed over to the "Contextualizer" which runs three different components:

First, the **world knowledge contextualization**—as proposed in Chap. 5—processes each textual resource in the submitted collection. This component creates a "World Context" by applying an entity recognition to the text of a resource (e.g., a document or email) using DBPedia[2] as source to disambiguate entities. Each entity found in the text is added as semantic annotation (i.e., as URI) to the World Context. This World Context is then stored as additional context information to the metadata of the respective resource.

Second, the **visual concept detection**—as proposed in Sect. 5.2.2 for contextualizing images—adds visual concepts detected in images as additional context. Third, the **personal knowledge contextualization** takes the context information provided in the previous step by the Semantic Desktop in the `forgetit:context` attribute as separate context. In terms of the PoF Reference Model, this context information generated from personal knowledge represented in the PIMO is stored in the so-called "Local Context". The context information delivered by the Semantic Desktop satisfies the following context dimensions:

---

[1] http://www.w3.org/TR/turtle/.

[2] https://dbpedia.org.

- **Time**: The excerpt contains the thing's creation time, last modification, and in addition any time information associated with certain things such as events (either a point in time or a time period).
- **Location**: If locations are associated with a resource, e.g., usually for events or also for the subclass `pimo:LifeSituation`.
- **Topic**: Any kind of topics identified for the resource. For the PIMO, this includes manually annotated topics (e.g., with the property `pimo:hasTopic`), suggested ones with `pimo:hasSuggestedTopic` (e.g., suggested by the entity recognition using GATE in FireTag or SemanticFileExplorer, or using the ForgetIT image services), or inferred concepts with `pimo:hasInferredTopic` (e.g., because the photo collection as a whole has this topic, or the super task was annotated with it).
- **Entity Space**: This is comprised by the remaining relations a resource has in the PIMO not already covered above. These are various properties such as `rdfs:partOf` or `pimo:isFundedBy`.
- **Document Space**: This consists of other documents or subclasses such as web pages or emails related to the resource.

7.4.3.5 Package

In this step the functional entity "Archiver" creates from the resource(s) collected from the Semantic Desktop the content and metadata to create a "Submission Information Package" (SIP). This is then handed over to the "Transfer" step.

7.4.3.6 Transfer

The "Transfer" step then submits the SIP to the "Digital Preservation System" (DPS)(see Fig. 6.13) which stores it as an "Archival Information Package" (AIP). In the case of the pilot implementation on the ForgetIT testbed, the DPS is composed of DSpace and Openstack Swift. For the DFKI PIMO pilot it is DSpace only (see Fig. 7.20).

7.4.3.7 Preservation Finished

Once the preservation is finished, the PoF Middleware notifies the Active System of the outcome. Notifying the user of the outcome is twofold: first, the user gets a notification once a collection has been preserved in the PIMO5 home screen as shown in Fig. 7.21. Second, several places in the Semantic Desktop show if a thing is preserved such as in the thing view in Fig. 7.22 or 7.23.

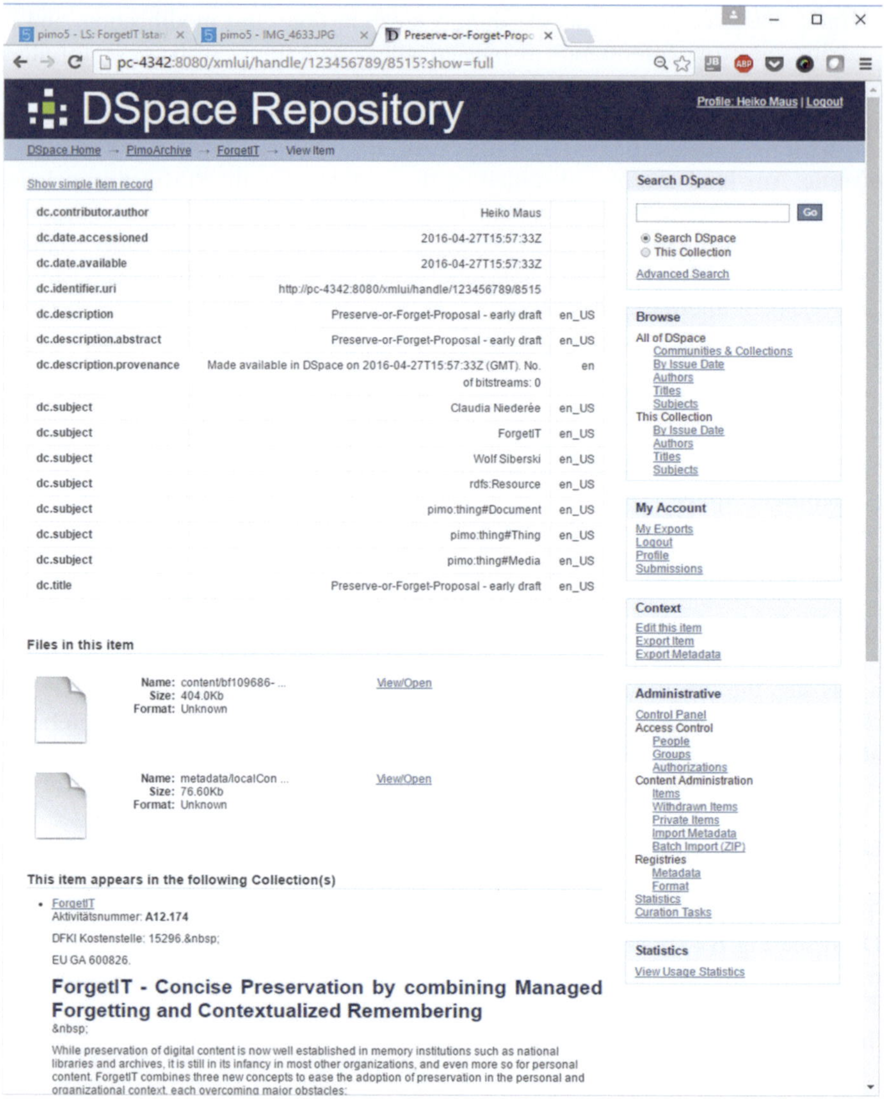
pimo5 - LS: ForgetIT Ista
pimo5 - IMG_4633.JPG
Preserve-or-Forget-Propo
pc-4342:8080/xmlui/handle/123456789/8515?show=full
DSpace Repository
Profile: Heiko Maus | Logout
DSpace Home → PimoArchive → ForgetIT → View Item
Show simple item record
dc.contributor.author Heiko Maus
dc.date.accessioned 2016-04-27T15:57:33Z
dc.date.available 2016-04-27T15:57:33Z
dc.identifier.uri http://pc-4342:8080/xmlui/handle/123456789/8515
dc.description Preserve-or-Forget-Proposal - early draft en_US
dc.description.abstract Preserve-or-Forget-Proposal - early draft en_US
dc.description.provenance Made available in DSpace on 2016-04-27T15:57:33Z (GMT). No. of bitstreams: 0 en
dc.subject Claudia Niederée en_US
dc.subject ForgetIT en_US
dc.subject Wolf Siberski en_US
dc.subject rdfs:Resource en_US
dc.subject pimo:thing#Document en_US
dc.subject pimo:thing#Thing en_US
dc.subject pimo:thing#Media en_US
dc.title Preserve-or-Forget-Proposal - early draft en_US
Files in this item
Name: content/bf109686- ... Size: 404.0Kb Format: Unknown View/Open
Name: metadata/localCon ... Size: 76.60Kb Format: Unknown View/Open
This item appears in the following Collection(s)
ForgetIT
Aktivitätsnummer: A12.174
DFKI Kostenstelle: 15296.
EU GA 600826.
ForgetIT - Concise Preservation by combining Managed Forgetting and Contextualized Remembering

While preservation of digital content is now well established in memory institutions such as national libraries and archives, it is still in its infancy in most other organizations, and even more so for personal content. ForgetIT combines three new concepts to ease the adoption of preservation in the personal and organizational context, each overcoming major obstacles:
Search DSpace
Go
Search DSpace
This Collection
Advanced Search
Browse
All of DSpace
Communities & Collections
By Issue Date
Authors
Titles
Subjects
This Collection
By Issue Date
Authors
Titles
Subjects
My Account
My Exports
Logout
Profile
Submissions
Context
Edit this item
Export Item
Export Metadata
Administrative
Control Panel
Access Control
People
Groups
Authorizations
Content Administration
Items
Withdrawn Items
Private Items
Import Metadata
Batch Import (ZIP)
Registries
Metadata
Format
Statistics
Curation Tasks
Statistics
View Usage Statistics

Fig. 7.20 Preserved document in DSpace: the ForgetIT proposal preserved from the DFKI PIMO

7.5 Toward Using Personal Information Management to Support Personal Preservation

The presented approach for Personal Preservation has three phases:

- In the **Preparation** phase the tasks are connecting to a service provider, choosing a preservation contract, and installing the Semantic Desktop ecosystem.

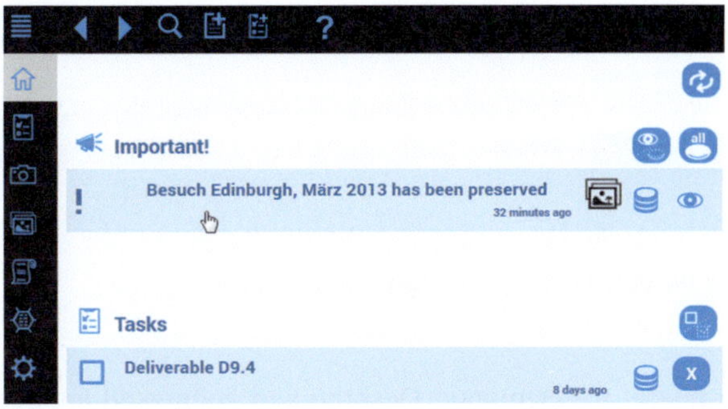

Fig. 7.21 Notification of the successful preservation on the PIMO5 home screen

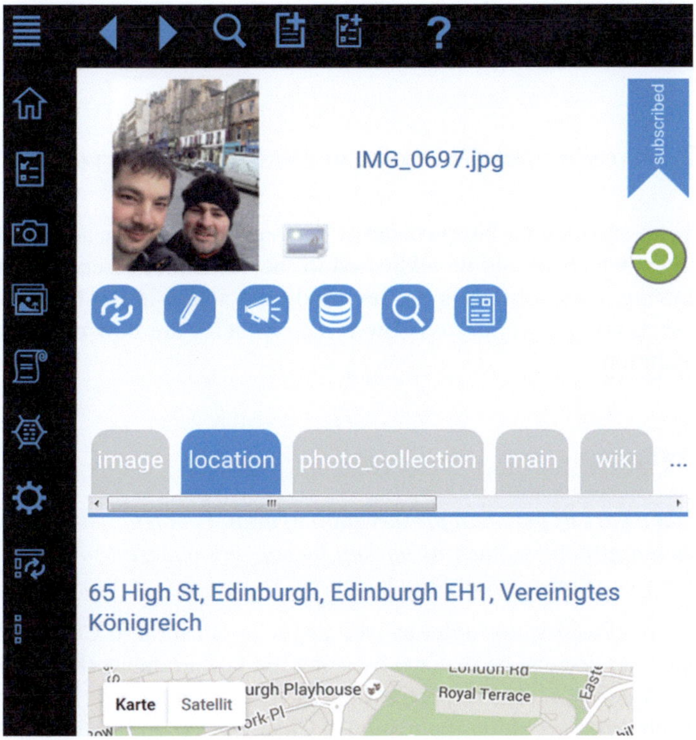

Fig. 7.22 Showing the preservation state of a photo in the PIMO5 image detail view

Besuch Edinburgh, März 2013
Associated date: 13.03.2013 12:00 (3 years ago)
This photo collection has been preserved.
slideshow

Fig. 7.23 Showing the preservation state of a photo collection

- In the **Usage** phase, the Semantic Desktop and connected applications are used for PIM activities. In this phase, resources are continuously preserved (usually without user intervention, but manual preservation is also possible).
- Finally, if the need arises, **Access to Preserved Material** is granted either directly via the Semantic Desktop ecosystem or by the preservation service provider alone.

7.5.1 Overcoming the Obstacles of Personal Preservation

In Sect. 7.1, we assessed the current state of Personal Preservation and identified five main obstacles which should be addressed in the Personal Preservation approach. In the following, those obstacles are revisited (and stated in the beginning of the respective section) and we discuss how these obstacles are now overcome by the presented solution.

7.5.1.1 Awareness

*Users are **not aware of personal preservation** of digital content. There is a huge gap between current practices, such as backup by copying material to a different hard disk, and a proper Preservation Strategy.*

The Personal Preservation Pilot as well as the application in Chap. 8 show how a preservation service can be realized by using the PoF Framework. Although both use the PoF Middleware, the respective approach is different.

First, the photo preservation application of Chap. 8 is a single application extended with preservation abilities by connecting to the PoF Middleware. Thus, it shows how "normal" applications can be extended with a preservation functionality and benefit from services provided by the PoF Middleware.

Second, the Personal Preservation Pilot approach shows how a complete infrastructure such as the Semantic Desktop as well as various applications can be extended with preservation functionality and by their usage, provide valuable resources and context for preservation. Moreover, they show how an application ecosystem can contribute to realize Synergetic Preservation allows to asses the benefits of embedding preservation in users' PIM.

After choosing a Preservation Strategy, the Synergetic Preservation is started with no additional effort for the user apart from occasional checks if the resource selection is sufficient (which would be optimized for product-like services). Furthermore, although setting up a preservation service is easy, the prerequisite of using a Semantic Desktop-like infrastructure still holds. Semantic Desktop applications such as the SemanticFileExplorer or the PIMO Photo Organization app, show that user resources can be covered to some extent with less effort and could be realized as stand-alone applications.

Nevertheless, the Semantic Desktop ecosystem is also a step toward embedding Synergetic Preservation into an operating system. Helpful capabilities such as PIM, photo collections, or tagging, are already prominently introduced, e.g., in Apple's macOS operating system.

7.5.1.2 High Up-Front Costs

*When starting with personal preservation, the user faces **high up-front costs** in terms of time, effort, and resources, and there are* **very few tools** *to help users prepare material for preservation and interact with an archiving service. The best-practice recommended by Marshall is not supported comprehensively.*

The high up-front costs in making personal resources suitable for preservation are reduced by embedding the required functionality for preservation into user's daily PIM activities or at least providing applications supporting selection and connection to a preservation service as shown in Chap. 8. The evaluation with the PIMO Photo Organization app showed that early contextualization is well accepted by users if the benefits are immediate (such as the textual explanation of the context of a photo or automated search capabilities). Furthermore, offering a personal preservation service is a potential business model for, e.g., a telecom provider as additional service for their customers. If that would be accomplished, the high up-front costs would be reduced for finding and connecting to a preservation service for end users.

Concerning the availability of tools, the two application scenarios show that extending an Active System with preservation capabilities is possible and the connection to the PoF Framework by implementing the interfaces is manageable. Thus, both possibilities—embedding preservation services in an infrastructure (such as the Semantic Desktop) or extending a single application with preservation capabilities—are now open to enhance tools with preservation functionality which could foster the availability in future.

7.5.1.3 No Personal Preservation Services

*There is no **personal preservation service** for the majority of end users which supports the whole preservation process. Cloud storage alone is not preservation.*

As mentioned before, services for personal preservation could be offered by a service provider. The business domain of a telecom provider nowadays covers lots of activities (e.g., mobile internet and access at home) and resources of users (e.g., photos, emails, or files on a cloud storage) with potential to extend it even further (calendar, services for friends and family). In this light, extending their services with preservation capability fits well in the existing business models.

The digitalisation of various daily activities (e.g., calendar, chat, photos) including resources held in internet platforms such as social media, lead to challenges of how to access, inherit, and preserve the material after a user's death. Recent lawsuits concerning access to material in internet platforms (such as material in Facebook or resources connected to the Apple account) shed a light on the increasing need for services embracing these sources. However, this will include legal issues to be covered when extending the preservation service. Furthermore, we can predict that the public awareness will increase for such services also including all digital resources. This would be a good market entry for a personal preservation service.

Finally, apart from telecom providers, with the PoF Framework various flavors of Digital Preservation Systems can be supported. Therefore, we see the possibility also for a take-up by specialized service providers offering PoF Middleware as a service.

7.5.1.4 Increasing Amount of Digital Content

The ***vast increase in digital content with relevance to a person's life*** *poses challenges to PIM as well as preservation.*

The variety of applications in the Semantic Desktop ecosystem and its openness to integrate further applications, plug-ins, and information sources allows to include various digital content in the user's PIM. The solution presented in this chapter has shown that applications could support users in handling large amounts of digital data. This is done with the help of the technologies for analyzing digital media presented in the first part of the book. For instance, visual concept detection allows to search large photo collections without any effort for manual annotation. The research presented in Chaps. 3 and 5 show further technologies to manage large media content such as photo and video analysis.

7.5.1.5 Understanding for Future Generations

Designing and organizing an archive so that its **structure can be understood in several decades from now** *is cognitively challenging for users.*

The PIMO—as a semantic representation of the mental model of a user—allows to structure existing digital content of the user's PIM activities. Further extensions such as the life situations ("LifeSituation", an advanced photo collection) can cover more specialized situations and involved material.

Applications in the Semantic Desktop ecosystem take care of structuring this information for the user (using the PIMO) without requiring them to model this by themselves. The PIMO Photo Organization app is an example for this approach. Users organize their photo collections, add texts and maybe also annotations. The app stores this in a machine understandable semantic structure which covers the photo collections. It includes information from the user as well as extracted (e.g., EXIF data) and enriched metadata from components such as visual concept detection.

These structures allow a machine understandable access to the digital content as well as a human understandable presentation. They are used in the Semantic Desktop for providing added value such as semantic search or reusing content for other services such as the PIMO Diary. Moreover, the combination of personal knowledge in the PIMO, early contextualization with PIMO services as well as world knowledge (e.g., entity recognition and annotation in texts using PIMO as well as external knowledge sources such as DBpedia in the semantic text editor) provides an even richer context for the digital content.

This rich semantic structure as well as the enriched digital content builds the basis for an understanding of the structure for future generations. The structure is transferred to the PoF Middleware in the "Local Context" for each and every resource covering semantic information of the resource itself as well as relations to other resources and concepts. Technically, the PIMO is represented using RDF (Resource Description Framework), standardized by the W3C. The "Local Context" handed over to the PoF Middleware is a formalized textual representation. This ensures readability and accessibility for long-term preservation.

Finally, the PoF Framework retrieves the content and adds its own contextualization for interpretation by future generations.

To summarize, the Semantic Desktop approach and the PIMO are the means to reduce the effort for users to generate structures. The combination of the "Local Context"—generated from the semantic information in the PIMO—and the additional contextualization in the PoF Middleware provides the means for the understanding of the content for future generations.

7.6 Conclusions

This chapter presented how PIM activities can be used to derive context to realize Personal Preservation and thus reduce the manual effort for users. This context is enriched with information derived from the user's mental model during usage of the resources by using semantic technologies and the PIMO. A pilot for Personal Preservation built on top of the Semantic Desktop ecosystem showed the potential of embedding semantic technologies in the operating system as well as realizing user applications for preservation, forgetting, and remembering in context.

The work presented here allowed us to deploy and use the functionalities described in DFKI's own installation of the PIMO (which is in use since 2012). This allowed us to gain insights on the applicability of the pilot which will be discussed the following.

7.6.1 Managed Forgetting

By extending the DFKI PIMO Server with a Memory Buoyancy calculation based on the work presented in [390] and Chap. 3 as well as the forgetting extensions in the PIMO5 user interface, we already use part of the Managed Forgetting functionality in daily work (as of now, over 3 years).

We can see benefits for coping with the information overload originating from daily usage of the PIMO as lots of things are created with decreasing relevance on the long run such as tasks, events, web pages, or notes. Such once relevant things are now forgotten over time and are hidden from direct view during browsing and search. Furthermore, due to the PIMO's semantic network, although not accessed directly, things do not drop that much in MB due to their relation to high buoyant concepts preventing them from being forgotten.

While we still need more fine tuning of the algorithm and experience with the MB for the DFKI PIMO, we see that Managed Forgetting already provides benefits for the knowledge work and still offers more potential. On the other hand, we also see further research required considering user behavior and their expectations. For instance, how to predict and cope with the circumstances in the user interface that sometimes users want to access exactly those things long forgotten.

We see lots of potential in the Managed Forgetting approach to tackle challenges of information overload in information systems especially when dealing with an evolutionary approach as supported by the Semantic Desktop.

7.6.2 Contextual Remembering

The PIMO already allowed to see resources in their past context by inspecting explicit relations to other things. With the introduction of the PIMO Diary, we could show the potential for Contextual Remembering by using the rich material in the PIMO including semantic representation as well as content (textual or visual). Personal insights from the diary give an interesting timeline. We found that the PIMO Diary is also enjoyable due to its capabilities to identify and present clustered activities of the user's "electronic footprints" in the PIMO. Although focused on the personal application scenario, by "playing around" with it in the DFKI PIMO we see lots of potential for usage in Knowledge Management applications. For instance, it can serve as a kind of reporting tool giving an overview of one's own activities in a period of time or it can be used as a starting point for explorative search, especially for new colleagues to get an overview of a group's activities.

7.6.3 Synergetic Preservation

In the pilot, a Preservation Strategy has been introduced initially as a predefined set of rules and policies. Taking the advantage of actually having a live PIMO running at the DFKI as a real data set for an organizational application scenario, we introduced a more fine-grained Preservation Strategy with several heuristics and rules which could be applied to the DFKI scenario.

Especially the possibility of changing the strategy, recalculating, and inspecting the results provides interesting insight into the data set. Lots of material is accumulated over the years in this group PIMO. Besides the photo collections, particularly interesting from organizational point of view are other items proposed for preservation such as documents, presentations, notes, or topics. Nevertheless, there are still resources assumed not to be worthwhile to be preserved.

Enhancing the pilot with group functionality (in the personal use case these are family and friends) also provides a group or a team at work with a means for organizational preservation on a group level. Considering the sharing activity in the DFKI PIMO, we see that nearly 47% of the things are public for the group. Thus, the PIMO contains private material as well as material considered relevant for the group. Thus, at least the shared resources would be subject to a preservation for the group.

With lots of professional businesses based on knowledge work such as product development, research, or consulting, companies get the opportunity to acquire and preserve valuable knowledge items from team interaction without requiring effort to document and preserve manually. This is also a contribution from the Semantic Desktop approach to an organizational application scenario.

In this PV Assessment we also see a first step toward Information Value Assessment for Knowledge Management purposes using new evidences for calculating content value provided by the Semantic Desktop ecosystem and the PIMO.

To conclude, the Semantic Desktop approach provides lots of potential to embed personal preservation in personal life. Some of the activities of PIM supported by dedicated applications or recent operating systems could already now realize personal preservation if connected to a preservation service as introduced with the PoF Framework. Further research in the Semantic Desktop area will contribute to the personal preservation scenario as well as to organizational preservation as the experience with the pilot at the DFKI shows.

Chapter 8
Personal Photo Management and Preservation

Andrea Ceroni

Abstract Thanks to the spread of digital photography and available devices, taking photographs has become effortless and tolerated nearly everywhere. This makes people easily ending up with hundreds or thousands of photos, for example, when returning from a holiday trip or taking part in ceremonies, concerts, and other events. Furthermore, photos are also taken of more mundane motives, such as food and aspects of everyday life, further increasing the number of photos to be dealt with. The decreased prices of storage devices make dumping the whole set of photos common and affordable. However, this practice frequently makes the stored collections a kind of dark archives, which are rarely accessed and enjoyed again in the future. The big size of the collections makes revisiting them time demanding. This suggests to identify, with the support of automated methods, the sets of most important photos within the whole collections and to invest some preservation effort for keeping them accessible over time. Evaluating the importance of photos to their owners is a complex process, which is often driven by personal attachment, memories behind the content, and personal tastes that are difficult to capture automatically. Therefore, to better understand the selection process for photo preservation and future revisiting, the first part of this chapter presents a user study on a photo selection task where participants selected subsets of most important pictures from their own collections. In the second part of this chapter, we present methods to automatically select important photos from personal collections, in light of the insights emerged from the user study. We model a notion of photo importance driven by user expectations, which represents what photos users perceive as important and would have selected. We present an expectation-oriented method for photo selection, where information at both photo and collection levels is considered to predict the importance of photos.

A. Ceroni (✉)
L3S Research Center, Leibniz Universität Hannover, Hanover, Germany
e-mail: ceroni@L3S.de

V. Mezaris et al. (eds.), *Personal Multimedia Preservation*, Springer Series on Cultural Computing, https://doi.org/10.1007/978-3-319-73465-1_8

8.1 Introduction

Photos are excellent means for keeping and refreshing memories; they can illustrate situations we have gone through and serve as memory cues [284, 285] to bring back reminiscences of experiences, events, and people from our past. In the recent years, we have been witnessing a huge increase in the production of photographs, mostly due to the wide spread of digital devices such as cameras, smartphones, and tablets. People easily take hundreds or even thousands of photos during relatively short and memorable events, e.g., vacations, ceremonies, concerts, or depicting more mundane aspects of everyday life [301], like shopping, eating, working, and free time. These numbers can amount to Terabytes of data over years. Even, considering only those uploaded in social media like Flickr, Facebook, Instagram, and Snapchat, a study conducted few years ago [290] estimates that 500 million photos (most of them from personal collections) are uploaded to the Internet every day. In addition, this number is expected to double every year.

This scenario points out the significance of properly dealing with such increasing volumes of pictures. Due to decreasing storage prices and offers of cloud storage services, e.g., by Microsoft or Google, it is not a problem to store personal photos somewhere. As a matter of fact, directly dumping photo collections spending little or even no time in activities like pruning, editing, sorting, or naming has turned out to be a popular procedure [206]. This comes at a price: storage devices tend to become a kind of "dark archives" [222] of photo collections, which means that the stored pictures, although still available, are rarely accessed and revisited again in the future. The big size of the stored collections makes going through them such a tedious activity to prevent the viewers from accessing them at all. As an additional challenge, already discussed in Chap. 1, there is the risk of losing photos by a random form of "digital forgetting" [191]: over decades storage devices break down, and formats and storage media become obsolete, making random parts of photo collections inaccessible (Digital Obsolescence [367]). One example is how difficult it would be today to access photos stored years ago in .mos format in a floppy disk.

Both the threats of personal dark archives and digital forgetting raise the following question: how can photos be kept enjoyable and serve their original purpose as memory cues, where large photo collections tend to get dumped on hard disks and other types of storage? We propose a transition from dumped contents to more selective personal digital memories, supported by automatic methods for information value assessment, to support long-term personal data management. Regarding photo collections, this means identifying the most important photos from an entire collection and investing some effort to keep them accessible and enjoyable on the long run. Having a reduced subset of important photos would make the revisiting easier and more pleasant for the user. However, understanding the importance of pictures to their owner for preservation and revisiting purposes is a complex process due to the presence of hidden factors, which are hard to model and capture automatically. These can be, for instance, memories, context, relationships to whom is in the picture, or simply personal tastes.

Therefore, the first part of this chapter summarizes a user study for a photo selection task where participants were asked to provide their personal photo collections and to select the subsets of photos that they would want to preserve and revisit again in the future. The study involved 35 participants, each one contributing at least one personal collection containing some hundreds of photos. The goal of this part is to better understand the human selection process for photo preservation and revisiting, identifying insights, patterns, and challenges that can shape the development of automatic selection approaches. Moreover, the gathered data will be employed for the development and evaluation of automatic selection methods. The user study was complemented by a survey, which we asked the participants to fill after completing the photo selection task.

In the second part of this chapter, we present and compare methods to automatically select important photos from personal collections for the sake of preservation and revisiting, inspired by the insights emerged from the user study. Many approaches to photo selection for summarization are centered around the concept of coverage, aiming at creating summaries that resemble the original collection as much as possible (see Sect. 8.2.2 for an overview). However, we believe that the complex decision-making behind the selection of photos from personal collections, characterized by personal attachment due to memories, might reduce the importance of coverage. Therefore, we model a notion of photo importance driven by user expectations, which represents what photos users perceive as important and would have selected. We present an expectation-oriented selection method, where information at both photo and collection levels (incorporating a relaxed notion of coverage) is considered to predict the importance of photos. We also investigate the role of coverage further by combining the expectation-oriented selection with an explicit modeling of coverage in different ways, showing that coverage plays only a secondary role in this task.

Our approach is an attempt to estimate Preservation Value (PV), previously introduced in Chap. 4, considering personal photos as specific information items. In fact, the notion of importance assigned to each photo by our model reflects what should be kept for future preservation, because the selection decisions collected during our user study and exploited for the development of our model have been taken exactly for that purpose. Furthermore, the input information extracted from photo collections covers different PV dimensions, compatibly with the characteristics of our scenario (e.g., the popularity dimension is not addressed as it refers to sharing and liking behaviors that are not very prominent in a personal scenario, where the data is rather kept private). The PV dimensions that we take into account are discussed in Sect. 8.4.2.1 and their roles within the selection process are summarized in Sect. 8.4.5.6.

The rest of the chapter is structured as follows. In Sect. 8.2, we outline related works and current approaches to photo selection. Section 8.3 describes the user study while the selection methods are presented and compared in Sect. 8.4. Finally, in Sect. 8.5 we summarize and conclude the chapter.

8.2 Related Work

The discussion of previous works relevant to the topic of personal photo selection and preservation is organized into two parts. The first one mentions previous empirical and rather qualitative user studies, while the second one reviews automatic approaches to the photo selection and summarization tasks.

8.2.1 User Studies and Surveys

A considerable research effort has been dedicated to investigate issues related to photo management and preservation from a human–computer interaction perspective [95, 206, 408, 418, 419]. Kirk et al. [206] introduced the notion of "photowork" as the set of activities performed with digital photos after capturing them and before any end usage like sharing or revisiting. One of their findings was that people spend little time in activities like reviewing, pruning, editing, and sorting, because these are cumbersome and time-consuming procedures. This fact clearly supports the topic and objective of this chapter. In the context of preservation of public photos, a qualitative study assessing their value for representing social history is reported in [95]. This study is mostly limited in (a) not considering personal photos and (b) the small number of photos considered. The evaluators were asked to rate five images, selected from Flickr, considering their worthiness for long-term preservation. Interestingly, the participants expressed a clear inclination to preserve all the pictures irrespective of their actual value. The authors hypothesized two possible reasons for this, namely the difficulty of anticipating a future information need and the effort required for organizing and pruning increasing amounts of data. In any case, they recognized this as a problem and pointed to the need of methodologies for information appraisal and selection.

Wolters et al. [418] investigated which photos from an event people tend to delete over time. In this study, described in Chap. 2, the participants took photos during a common event and then they were asked for deletion decisions at different points in time. While this work is certainly related to our study, which drew inspiration from it especially regarding the formulation of the survey, there are nevertheless some differences. Despite preservation ("keep") and "delete" decisions are related, we explicitly asked our evaluators to make selection decisions for the purposes of preservation and revisiting of images, rather than for deletion. Moreover, in our study, the users were asked to make joint selection decisions (i.e., select a subcollection) instead of making decisions for each individual picture in isolation. This is potentially a key difference, since selecting one photo might affect the decisions for other similar photos. Finally, instead of taking pictures of a common event explicitly for the study, we work with personal real-world collections belonging to diversified events. A subsequent work by Wolters et al. [419] presented a large-scale survey of 72 young people and students, with the goal of supporting the design of personal and mobile preservation systems. The main message of the study is coherent with what emerged from our survey: a large part of the participants acknowledge the importance of preserving photos for future generations. Interestingly, however, only a small fraction of them carries out practices to support photo management and preservation. Another user study has been presented in [408], where participants wearing eye-tracking devices were asked to select subsets of photos from two collections depicting two social events. This work focuses more on the selection process than on preservation matters. The survey on the aspects driving the selection process shares with our experiment both similarities (e.g., most of the highly rated aspects were subjective) and differences (e.g., quality was highly rated there).

8.2.2 Photo Selection and Summarization

Automated photo selection has already been studied in various other contexts, such as photo summarization [229, 358, 365, 389, 412], identification of appealing photos based on quality and aesthetics [228, 425], selection of representative photos [78, 408], and the creation of photo books from social media content [333]. We consider the task of selecting important photos from personal collections (e.g., for revisiting or preservation), which meet user expectations.

The work of Wang et al. [412] is probably the most related to ours, as their model of image importance does not explicitly include coverage and diversity aspects. They introduce the notion of "event-specific image importance", meaning that the importance of photos for selection purposes depends on the category of the event they belong to. The main assumption is that, within a photo collection depicting a certain type of event, the set of images commonly perceived as important by most people can be identified based on the event type. There are, however, substantial differences regarding the task definition and the way the ground truth was built. First, the ground truth was not gathered considering photo selection, since ratings were assigned by the evaluators to each image in isolation without explicitly deciding what subset of the collection should be kept. Second, individuals different than the collection owner rated the importance of images, potentially ignoring any personal attachment due to memories or hidden context. Image importance has been also considered in [228, 425]; nevertheless, it was based on quality and aesthetic criteria. Instead, we explicitly consider selections preferences and expectations of users for both training our model and an evaluation criterion. Walber et al. [408] also consider human judgments to evaluate selections, but the users have to wear eye trackers when using the system to make automatic selections because gaze information is used as features in the model.

Different photo selection and summarization works consider coverage by identifying clusters of images based on time and visual content [78, 229, 333]. Differently, our approach does not impose such a strict notion of coverage but rather considers clusters and other global information together with image-level information, learning their different impacts on a single model. The works in [299, 358, 365, 389] are closer to ours, as they consider coverage in a relaxed way as part of a multi-goal optimization, but they still consider coverage as a key component. Moreover, [358, 365] do not consider user assessments in their evaluation and make partial use of manually created text to associate semantic descriptors to images, while our method does not require any manual input, once the models for both feature extraction and importance estimation have been learned. Image collection summarization is performed in [299, 389] by applying structured prediction methods for learning weighted mixtures of submodular functions. The attention is drawn to two aspects that good summaries should exhibit, namely fidelity (coverage) and diversity, which are represented as a set of nonnegative submodular functions and combined together in a single weighted submodular scoring function. There are two main differences with respect to the work presented in this chapter. First, their goal is purely summarization, aiming at optimizing coverage and diversity of output summaries, without considering whether they contain the most valuable pictures. This is strengthened by the utilization of the recall-based V-ROUGE metric (a criterion for summary evaluation inspired by the ROUGE metric [239], used for document summarization) within the loss function. Second, the way the ground truth has been collected is heavily oriented toward coverage: the evaluators, not the owners of the collections, were explicitly told to produce reference summaries that summarize the original collections in the best possible way, and those exhibiting low coverage were discarded. Conversely, we asked the collection's owners to select the most important photos according to their memories and perceptions, without any mention to coverage or diversity.

Besides [358, 365], other works in the literature rely on external knowledge to accomplish the task of image summarization [59, 346, 429]. Camargo et al. [59] combine textual and visual contents of a collection in the same latent semantic space, using convex nonnegative matrix factorization, to generate multimodal image collection summaries. Domain-specific ontologies are required as further input in [346]. They provide the knowledge about the concepts in a domain and are used to derive a set of ontology-based features for measuring the semantic similarity between images. Finally, [429] jointly leverages image content and associated tags and encodes the selection of images in two vectors, for the visual and textual domains, respectively, whose nonzero elements represent the images to be included in the summary. The optimization process makes use of a similarity-inducing regularizer imposed on the two vectors to encourage the summary images to be representative in both visual and textual domains.

Summarizing, our approach is different from all the previous works under at least one of the following aspects: (a) our notion of photo importance is based on selection decisions made by people on their own photo collections; (b) we do not estimate photo importance using single indicators (e.g., quality, presence of faces, and representativeness of the cluster a photo belongs to), but we rather learn the impact of such aspects through a single prediction model; (c) we use selection decision made by the collection owners themselves as ground truth for evaluation; and (d) we do not rely on any kind of photo tagging or descriptive annotation provided manually.

8.3 User Study

As a preliminary step toward the development of automatic methods, we describe a user study conducted on a photo selection task, whose objective is the gathering of insights, challenges, and behaviors exhibited by humans when selecting personal photos for preservation and revisiting purposes [69]. Using their own photo collections depicting personal events, participants were asked to select a subset of photos that they would like to stay accessible and enjoyable in the future. Such data, i.e., the whole collections along with the selections done by the users, will be used for the training and evaluation of the selection methods described in Sect. 8.4. Upon completion of the task, the participants were also asked to fill a survey about it, which is described and analyzed in Sect. 8.3.2. This study is closely related to the one described in Chap. 2 and has been partially inspired by it. However, as already elaborated during the survey of the literature in Sect. 8.2.1, there are some important differences. First, we asked the participants to jointly select a subcollection for the sake of preservation and revisiting instead of making "keep" or "delete" decisions for each image in isolation. Second, our study involves personal collections spontaneously taken and belonging to diversified events rather than photos of a common event taken explicitly for the study. This section is mainly organized into three parts: Sect. 8.3.1 elaborates on the setup of the study, Sect. 8.3.2 reports the insights learned from the study and the survey, and in Sect. 8.3.3 we show a comparison between event-based clustering and human selections.

8.3.1 Task Setup

The setup of the performed photo selection task involves the gathering of both participants and their photo collections, instructions on how the task should be accomplished, and, of course, the development of a software application to perform the selection in a comfortable way.

The experiment involved 35 users (28.6% females and 71.4% males) with 15 nationalities: 25.7% of the participants came from Greece, 17.1% from Germany, 11.4% from Italy, 11.4% from China, 5.7% from Vietnam, and the rest from Ethiopia, Turkey, Kosovo, Iran, UK, Thailand, Sweden, Brazil, Albania, and Georgia. Regarding their ages, 60.0% of the participants are between 20 and 30 years, 25.7% between 30 and 40, 11.4% between 40 and 50, and 2.9% between 50 and 60.

Previous works mostly consider either public photo collections, for instance, available on social media like Facebook and Flickr [59, 333, 346, 412], or pictures from a shared event in which all the evaluators took part [408]. One difficulty we see with using public collections of photos from different people, even if they attended the same event, is that according to the different experiences of the individuals in the event they might also have a different level of appreciation for the same photo, thus influencing their decisions. In contrast, we use personal photo collections. For instance, these can be photos from business trips, vacations, ceremonies, or other personal events the evaluator participated in. This means that each collection is not just a bunch of pictures, which might exhibit different degrees of quality and aesthetics, but there are experiences, sub-events, and memories that might influence the selection behavior. We decided to focus on such personal collections because we wanted to observe the personal photo selection decisions in a setting that is as realistic as possible. In total, 39 collections were used in the experiment (four users evaluated two collections), resulting in 8,528 photos. The size of the collections ranges between 100 and 625 pictures, with an average size of 219 and a standard deviation of 128.7. These collection sizes also emphasize the need for automated selection support, since manually browsing for photo selection becomes time-consuming. We asked users for further information about their collections, such as the main topic of the collection, whether they were previously pruned (e.g., by discarding low-quality photos) and when they were taken. Overall, 51% of the collections represent vacations, 30% business trips, and 19% other events like music festivals and graduation ceremonies. In addition, 23% of the collections were already pruned before the evaluation. The time when the collections were taken spans from 2007 to 2014 (64% in 2013–2014, 17% in 2011–2012, the rest in 2007–2010).

Since our task of selecting photos for preservation is not an everyday task for the users, it was important to find a good metaphor for supporting the task. After discussing a number of options with cognitive experts, we decided to use the metaphor of a "magic digital vault", which incorporates the ideas of protection, durability, and a sort of advanced technologies to keep things accessible in the long term. Therefore, the task consisted in selecting a subset of valuable photos to be put in the magic digital vault, which would protect them against loss and would ensure that they remain readable and accessible over the next decades.

To perform the photo selection task, we developed a desktop application, which enabled the participants to import their own collections and to select photos in a comfortable way. It is depicted in Fig. 8.1, where the photos contained in the imported collection are displayed in the bottom panel, while the ones selected are shown in the top panel. Note that faces appearing in Fig. 8.1 have been blurred for the sake of privacy (only for inclusion in this book). The photos are selected and deselected by double-clicking on them, and they can be enlarged to inspect them better and appreciate their quality, although no explicit reference to the quality aspect was made in our instructions to the users. The photos in the collection were shown in the same order in which they were taken, since this makes the browsing, remembering, and selection easier and more realistic for the users. Nevertheless, we also made a preliminary evaluation where the photos were shuffled before being presented. This resulted in higher evaluation time and a higher mental effort for the selection process, because it made picking from a set of related photos very difficult. We verified that keeping the original order did not introduce any significant bias in the selection toward the early photos in the collection. This could have been a risk, since users might lose attention or even complete the selection without going through the entire collection.

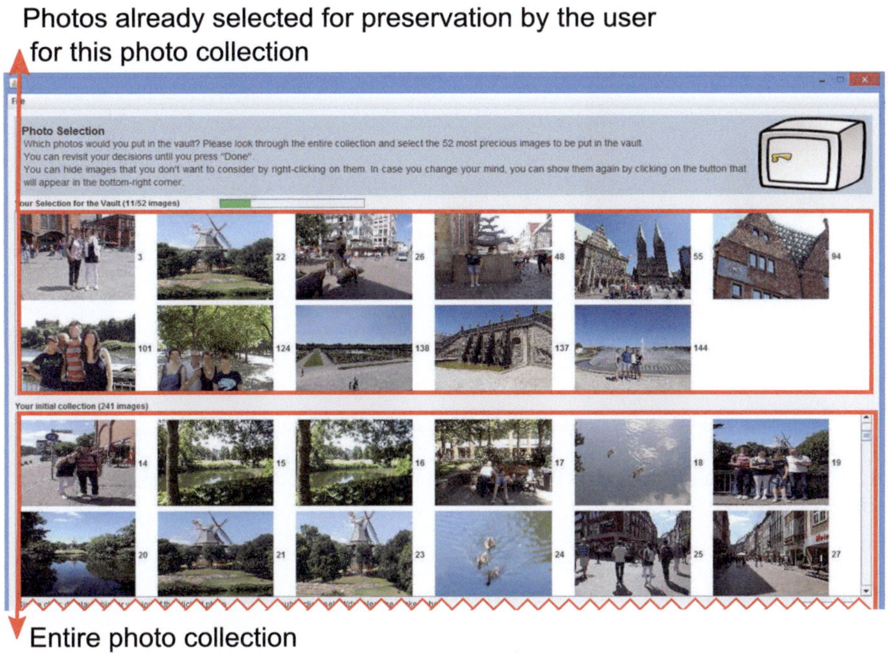

Fig. 8.1 GUI used by participants to browse the collections and select the photos to preserve

Before starting the evaluation, the users were personally introduced to the photo selection task as well as to the application that they were asked to use. Further remarks and clarifications about both the task and the usage of the application were given, where needed. However, no guidelines were given about the criteria to use for selection, in order not to influence the selection process. After the users imported their collections, the application asked them to select 20% of photos from them for preservation and revisiting purposes. This selection percentage (20%) has been empirically identified as a reasonable amount of representative photos, after a discussion with a subset of users before the study. We also checked the adequacy of this chosen amount with the users in the survey by asking them whether they would have selected more photos if they could: 45% of them answered yes, the rest no. This balance means that 20% was a meaningful threshold, neither being too low (the majority of the users would have answered "yes" in this case) or too high.

8.3.2 *Survey and Discussion*

After the photo selection step, the users were asked to fill a survey that can be conceptually split into two parts. The first group of questions refers to the scenario

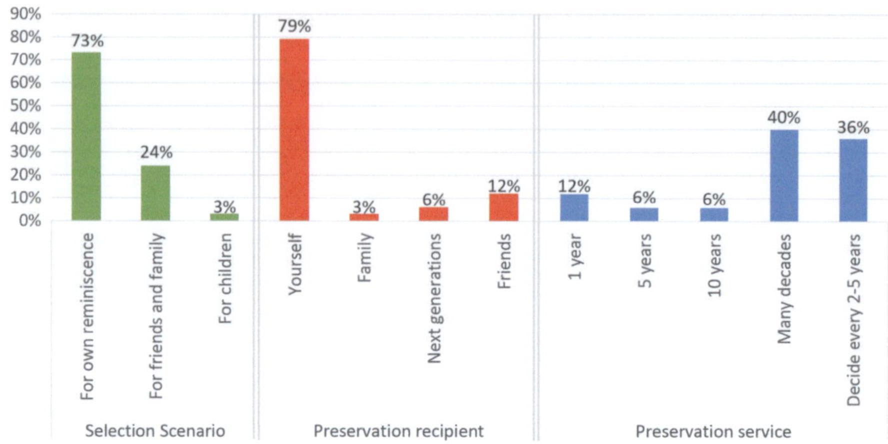

Fig. 8.2 Survey results with respect to preservation scenario, preservation target group, and preservation as a service

of photo selection process for personal preservation, while the second one looks into the criteria that were considered during the selection.

Regarding the first group of questions, the users were asked to provide information about (a) which scenario they had in mind when selecting the photos; (b) for whom they are preserving the photos; and (c) whether they would be ready to pay, and for how many years, if preservation was a paid service. The answers to each question were posed as multiple choices and are reported in Fig. 8.2. The answers to questions (a) and (b) reveal that the long-term preservation process is centered around the owner of the photos: more than 70% of the evaluators said that they thought about own future reminiscence when they selected the photos, and almost 80% indicated themselves as a main consumer of the preservation outcome. Looking at the preservation as a valuable service to be paid (question (c)), the evaluators were mostly split into two groups: either being ready to pay for many decades (39%) or needing flexibility to make new preservation decisions every 2–5 years (36%). In both cases, these answers highlight a clear need for preservation of personal photo collections.

In the second group of questions, we suggested different photo selection criteria and asked the users to rate how much each criterion was considered during the selection. The suggested criteria, which are in line with the insights on "keep" and "delete" decisions in [418], were rated via star ratings on a scale between 1 and 5 (5 stars mean very important, 1 means not important at all). The criteria along with statistics about their ratings are reported as box plots in Fig. 8.3. Note that medians are represented as horizontal bold bars, while sample mean is indicated with a bold cross. For the sake of clarity, we grouped the criteria into three classes: "content-based criteria" refer to objective and subjective measures for individual photos such as quality, typicality (i.e., how suitable it is for serving as an iconic summary of the event), the presence of important people in them, whether photos are generally important, and the evocation

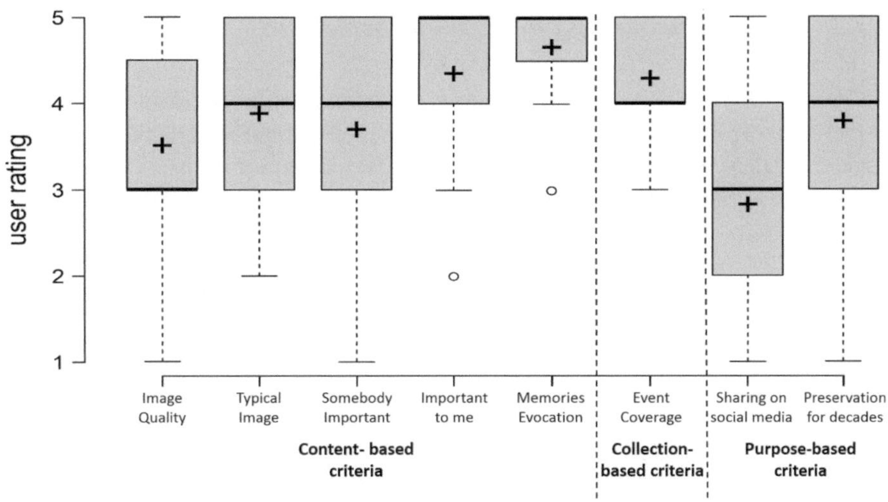

Fig. 8.3 Boxplots of the different selection criteria

of memories; "collection-based criteria"—here represented by coverage of events—consider a photo in the context of its collection; "purpose-based criteria", indicating the importance of different selection goals (in our case, sharing and preservation).

An important finding of this evaluation is that the objective quality of photos is rated as the second least important selection criterion, after the sharing intent. This shows that quality and aesthetics, although being important and used for general-purpose photo selection [228], are not considered very important in case of selecting photos for preservation. In contrast, criteria more related to reminiscence, such as event coverage, typical image, and "the picture evokes (positive) memories" are all rated high, with highest ratings for memory evocation. The remaining two criteria "picture is important to me" and picture "shows somebody important" refer to the personal relationship to the picture and are also both rated high. These results anticipate that the task of predicting photos to be selected for long-term preservation is likely to be difficult, since many of the criteria that are rated high, e.g., memory evocation, personal importance and "typical image", are difficult to assess for a machine, because they contain a high level of subjectivity. Another complicating fact is that there is no single dominant selection criterion, but a combination of highly rated criteria. In these ratings, we can observe differences with respect to the ones given to the partially overlapping set of criteria reported in [408], where photos on shared events were used and the selection was not directly related to preservation and reminiscence. In that work, much higher ratings are given to criteria such as quality, whereas event coverage and importance of depicted persons are rated relatively low (although with high variance). Interestingly, photos that capture a memory are also rated high in this case.

8.3.3 Image Clustering and Human Selections

We analyze the applicability of current selection and summarization approaches to the scenario of personal photo selection for preservation, highlighting possible issues that they might face in this situation. The main uncertainties in applying state-of-the-art methods to our task are (a) that they are developed with other photo selection scenarios in mind and (b) that they often do not compare the performances of their output with selections done by users. They, for example, identify subsets of photos that provide comprehensive summaries of the initial collections [333, 365, 389], without checking if the summary meets the user expectations, or they consider judgments based on more objective criteria such as aesthetics [228, 425]. Since a wide part of the state-of-the-art methods for photo selection and summarization considers clustering and/or coverage for generating selections and summaries (as discussed in Sect. 8.2.2), we clustered photos by applying the event-based clustering technique described in Chap. 3 (Sect. 3.5) and compared the clustering results with the human selections. This analysis is corroborated by the fact that the event coverage criterion, representable through clustering, has been identified as important during our study (Sect. 8.3.2).

In our opinion, one of the main risks of applying clustering to emulate human selections for long-term preservation is that not all the clusters might be important for the users. There might be photos from a sub-event that the user either simply does not like or considers less important than others. We supported this hypothesis by counting the number of human-selected photos in each cluster identified in our collections. As to be expected, only for a few clusters (7.3%) all the photos within the same cluster were selected. However, for a considerable part of the clusters (43%), no photos were selected at all. Given these statistics, the selection done by any pure coverage-based method that picks an equal number of photos from each cluster will contain at least 43% of them that would not have been selected by the user. Another statistics worth to be mentioned refers to the possibility for cluster-based selections of picking centroids as representative photos. From our collections, it resulted that only the 26% of the centroids was actually selected by the users. This reveals that information about how much a photo is representative of a wider group is only one of the aspects considered by the users when selecting photos.

Finally, making the assumption that bigger clusters might be more important for the users (as indicated by the users' choice to take more photos that capture that part of the event), we consider the size of the clusters with respect to the number of user-selected photos that they contain. Figure 8.4 shows the correlation between relative size of clusters (x-axis) and the percentage of selected photos in them (y-axis). It is possible to observe that the selections done by the users result in many clusters with few selected photos in each, which is coherent with the notion of coverage. However, what is more interesting is that the size of the cluster seems to be only marginally correlated with the importance of the cluster (i.e., the number of selected photos it contains). This is potentially another limitation for all those methods that select an amount of photos from each cluster proportionally to its size.

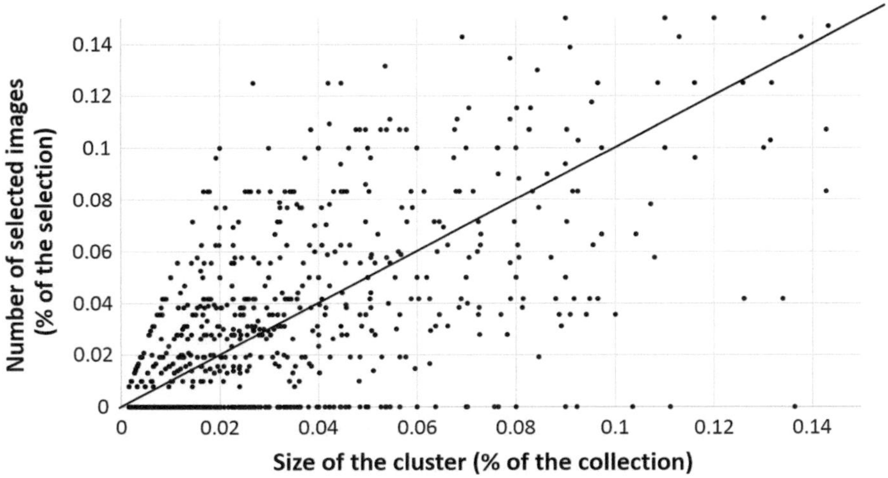

Fig. 8.4 Amount of selected photos in clusters (with respect to the size of selection) versus relative size of clusters

8.4 Photo Selection

We present in this section an automatic method [70] to identify, within big personal collections, those photos that are most important to the user, in order to invest more effort for keeping them accessible and enjoyable in the future. The availability of such a method alleviates the problems of "digital forgetting" and "dark archives", discussed in Sect. 8.1, which affect the archival of images and their access, respectively. From one side, preservation effort could be invested only on those photos that are worth to be preserved for the owner. From the other side, having a reduced subset of important photos would make the revisiting and enjoying easier and pleasant for the user. Moreover, to foster adoption, such automated selection method has to keep the level of user investment low. We do not rely on any additional user investment such as photo annotation with text [333, 358, 365] or eye-tracking information [408], because we believe it is exactly the reluctance of further investment that lets large photo collections unattended on our hard disks. To alleviate errors in automatically generated selections as well as accommodate user preferences, our approach can be regarded as a semi-automatized procedure, where the user can interact with it and modify the suggested selections.

When developing methods for semi-automatic photo selection, it is important to consider human expectations and practices. Photo selection is a complex and partially subjective process, where the selection decision taken for a given image both affects the decisions for other photos and depends on the ones already selected. For this reason, many state-of-the-art methods for photo selection and summarization are driven by the aspect of coverage, which means attempting to create summaries that resemble the content of the original collection as much as possible. Some of them perform a two-step process of first clustering the photo collection (for reflecting sub-events in the collection) and subsequently picking the most representative photos from the clusters [229, 333]. Others [358, 365, 389] consider coverage as part of a multi-goal optimization, along with the concepts of quality and diversity within the summary. While coverage surely plays an important role for many photo selection tasks (see e.g., [408]), we believe that the complex decision-making behind the selection of photos from personal collections, characterized by subjectivity and personal attachment possibly due to memories, might reduce the importance of coverage. For instance, considering photos taken during a trip, the user might want to discard the ones depicting boring or joyless moments.

Therefore, we model a multifaceted notion of photo importance driven by user expectations, which represents what photos users perceive as important and would have selected. User expectations have been acquired during the study described in Sect. 8.3, where participants have been asked to provide their own photo collections and to select those most important to them for preservation and revisiting. We present an expectation-oriented method for photo selection, where information at both photo and collection levels is considered to predict the importance of photos (Sect. 8.4.2). This information consists of (a) concept detection, to capture the semantic content of images beyond aesthetic and quality indicators; (b) face detection, reflecting the importance of the presence of people within photos; (c) near-duplicate detection, to take the redundancy of many pictures of the same scene as a signal of importance, and to eliminate very similar ones; (d) quality assessment, since good quality photos might be preferred in case of comparable photos. This is complemented by (e) temporal event clustering and, more generally, collection-level information, to reflect the role of coverage in photo selection. The impact of the different features is learned through a single model to predict the importance of each photo. Information regarding the selections performed by the users from their own collections is explicitly used to train the selection model, so that the predicted importance of photos represents what the user would have selected. For sake of comparison, in Sect. 8.4.3, we investigate how the expectation-oriented selection can be combined with more explicit ways of modeling coverage, showing that coverage plays only a secondary role in this task.

Before delving into the details of the selection method, a general consideration on the comparison between the features considered in the model and the user study presented in Sect. 8.3 has to be done. The aspects that resulted to be important from the user study, e.g., evocation of positive memories, image typicality, and personal importance of photos, are highly subjective and not directly recognizable by a machine, especially when only relying on the visual content without any other contextual information. Given these challenges and constraints imposed by the task, our attempt to address the insights emerged from the study is threefold: (a) we model event coverage, which resulted to be an important aspect in the user study, through clustering and the hybrid selection methods described in Sect. 8.4.3; (b) we employ concept detection to model more semantic and abstract aspects; and (c) we also include image quality, although perceived as not very important within the user study, for the sake of comparison with the other features.

8.4.1 Overview

The problem that we tackle in this chapter can be formalized as follows.

Definition 1 Let a photo collection P be a set of N photos, where $P = \{p_1, p_2, \ldots, p_N\}$. The photo selection problem is to select a subset S of size θ ($S \subset P$ and $|S| = \theta$), which is as close as possible to the subset S* that the user would select as the photos most important to her, i.e., S meets user expectations.

We represent each photo collection as a set $C = \{P, CL, ND\}$, where P is the set of original photos, and CL and ND are sets of clusters and near-duplicate photos identified in the collection, respectively. A cluster $cl \in CL$ contains a set of photos P_{cl} grouped together with respect to a defined notion of similarity, whereas a near-duplicate set $nd \in ND$ is a set of highly similar photos P_{nd}. Each photo $p \in P$ is modeled as a set of features $p = \{\mathbf{q}, \mathbf{c}, F, t\}$, where $\mathbf{q} \in \mathbb{R}^{n_q}$ is the quality vector of the photo, $\mathbf{c} \in \mathbb{R}^{n_c}$ is the concept vector of the photo, F is the set of faces f appearing in the photo, and t is its timestamp. Each face $f = \{f_l, f_s\}$ is described by its location f_l and relative size f_s in the photo. For each photo p, we will estimate the importance value I using the extracted features.

Figure 8.5 depicts the overview of our approach to photo selection. Given a photo collection, we extract information from the photos it contains by applying different image processing techniques described in Chap. 3 and in [70], such as concept detection, image quality assessment, face detection, event clustering, and near-duplicate detection. Our main approach is named expectation-oriented selection (Sect. 8.4.2), which learns to generate selections by taking into account user selections from personal collections as training data. Furthermore, we present three different hybrid selection methods (coverage-driven, filtered expectation-oriented, and optimization-driven), with the goal of investigating whether our method can be improved by combining it with state-of-the-art methods that explicitly consider coverage. The hybrid selection methods will be discussed in detail in Sect. 8.4.3.

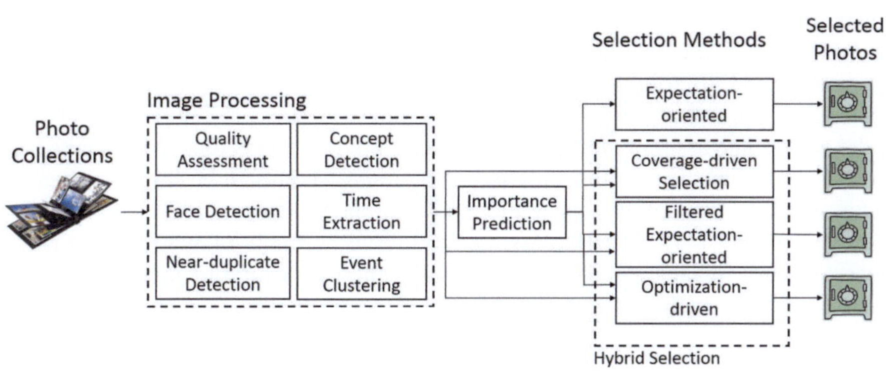

Fig. 8.5 Approach overview of automatic photo selection

8.4.2 Expectation-Oriented Selection

The photo selection model presented in this section aims at meeting human expectations when selecting photos that are most important to the user from a collection, for revisiting or preservation purposes. We believe that selecting photos that are important to a user from personal collections is a different task than generating comprehensive summaries: the set of images important to the user might not be a proportioned subsample of the original collection. For this reason, we do not impose a strict notion of coverage but rather consider clusters and other global information as a set of features, along with photo-level features, learning their different impacts on a single selection model by mean of supervised machine learning.

While we do not employ deep learning techniques, they can be used for either computing new features or replacing the computation of the current ones, still leaving the rest of the approach intact. For instance, image representations learned by convolutional neural networks (e.g., GoogLeNet [377]) can be used for concept detection as shown in Sect. 3.2. This is indeed one of our goals for the next future.

A key characteristic of our features is that they do not require any manual annotation (e.g., tags, textual descriptions, and file names) or external knowledge, differently from other works [333, 346, 358, 365] that make partial use of manually created text associated to photos. This means that the user does not have to invest time and effort in preparing the photos before feeding them into our system.

8.4.2.1 Features

Four groups of features have been designed to be used in the photo selection task, based on the information extracted from photos as presented in Chap. 3 and [70]. The correspondence between these features and the PV dimensions defined in Chap. 4 is made explicit in their descriptions.

Quality-Based Features

They consist of the five quality measures, namely, blur, contrast, darkness, noise, and their fused value (weighted pooling using Minkowski metric), which have been extracted as in [70], following the procedure presented in [275]. They are all numeric features whose values are between 0 and 1, where 0 represents the best quality and 1 the worst. The assumption behind using this information is that users might tend to select good quality photos, although their impact seems to be less important in subjective selections of humans as emerged from previous work [408] and from our user study (Sect. 8.3). Nevertheless, quality might probably play a role in case of near-duplicate images with different qualities: the user would pick the best one in these cases. This family of features corresponds to the quality PV dimension defined in Chap. 4.

Face-Based Features

The presence and position of faces in a picture might be an indicator of importance and might influence the selection. Some people might prefer photos depicting persons instead of landscapes, others might like group photos more than single portraits. We capture this by considering, for each photo, the number of faces within it as well as their positions and relative sizes. Faces have been detected through the approach presented in [70], which combines several face detectors (all incorporating the Haar-like-feature-based detector by Viola and Jones [405]) to maximize the number of detected faces. Then, each photo is divided into nine quadrants and the number of faces and their size in each quadrant are computed, resulting in 19 features: two for number and size of faces in each quadrant, plus an aggregated one representing the total number of faces in the photo. These features, to some extent, can be associated to the social graph PV dimension defined in Chap. 4, because the presence of people in a picture could indicate relationships between the appearing people and the owner of the photo. The notion of who is in a picture, for instance, obtainable via face clustering and tagging, would provide more precise and complex relationships among the owners and the people appearing in their collections. However, this would also introduce additional effort for the user, who would have to manually make the system aware of the kind of relationship with respect to any unknown person found in a new collection.

Concept-Based Features

High-level and semantic information has been thoroughly investigated in the past years within the scope of digital summarization (e.g., [358, 365]). The semantic content of photos, which we model in terms of concepts appearing in them, is expected to be a better indicator than low-level visual features, because it is closer to what a picture encapsulates. We consider the 346 concepts defined as part of the TRECVID 2013 benchmarking activity [6] and previously mentioned in Chap. 3, Sect. 3.2.3.1. The concept set includes both abstract concepts, such as "joy", "entertainment", "greeting", and more concrete concepts, such as "animal", "building", and "mountain". We trained a Support Vector Machine (SVM) as concept detector for each of them, using the TRECVID 2013 dataset (described in Chap. 3, Sect. 3.2.3.1) as training corpus. We used SIFT, SURF, and ORB local descriptors and their color variants [5] for visual feature extraction. Then, PCA was applied on each descriptor for reducing their dimensionality to 80, and VLAD encoding [19] was applied to calculate the final image representation. The applied methodology is described in [5] in more detail. Having such detectors available, we associate to each photo a vector of 346 elements, one for each concept, where the ith value represents the probability for the ith concept to appear in the photo. The correspondence between this class of features and the PV dimensions is not strict and depends on which concepts are included in the concept space. Concepts might be related to the gravity dimension, in case they represent aspects related to the events in the collection, or to the social graph dimension, in case they represent appearance of people, groups, or crowds.

Collection-Based Features

All the previously mentioned features are extracted from photos in isolation. However, when users have to identify a subset of important photos, instead of just making decisions for each photo separately, the characteristics of the collection a photo belongs to might influence the overall selection of the subset. For the same reasons, but moving to a finer granularity, it might be worth considering information about the cluster a photo belongs to. This family of features is a representative of the coverage PV dimension. For each photo, we consider collection-based features to describe the collection and, if any, the cluster and near-duplicate set the photo belongs to. Regarding the whole collection, we consider its size, the number of clusters and near-duplicate sets in the collection, the number of not near-duplicate photos, the size of the clusters (avg, std, min, and max) in the collection, the size of near-duplicate sets (avg, std, min, and max) in the collection, the quality of the collection (avg and std), and the number of faces in the collection (avg, std, max, and min). Regarding clusters, we first perform event-based clustering by applying the method described in Chap. 3, Sect. 3.5. Then, given the cluster a given photo belongs to, we compute its size, its quality (avg, std, max, and min), and the number of faces within it (avg). Finally, since the redundancy introduced by shooting many pictures of the same scene can be evidence of its importance for the user, we also extract features regarding whether the given photo has near-duplicates or not, as well as how many they are. Near-duplicates are detected by mean of the methodology described in Sect. 3.4. Shooting many similar photos of the same scene can be regarded as a form of "investment", because the user puts effort in replicating a scene to ensure its availability and quality.

8.4.2.2 Importance Prediction and Ranking

Given a set of photos p_i, their vectors $\mathbf{f}_{p_i}$ containing the features presented above, and their selection labels l_{p_i} (i.e., "selected" or "not selected") available for training, a prediction model represented by an SVM is trained to predict the selection probabilities of new unseen photos, i.e., their importance (see Sect. 8.4.4 for details regarding the training process). Figure 8.6 shows how the importance prediction and ranking of photos is performed for new unseen collections. First, feature vectors $\mathbf{f}_p$ are constructed based on the information extracted from the collections as described before and the importance of each unseen photo p is computed as

$$I_p = M\left(\mathbf{f}_p\right), \tag{8.1}$$

which is the probability of the photo to be selected by the user. Second, once the importance of each photo in the collection has been predicted, they are ranked based on these values and the top-k are finally selected. The parameter k represents the requested size of the selection and has to be specified in advance. The choice of k will be discussed during our evaluation (Sect. 8.4.4).

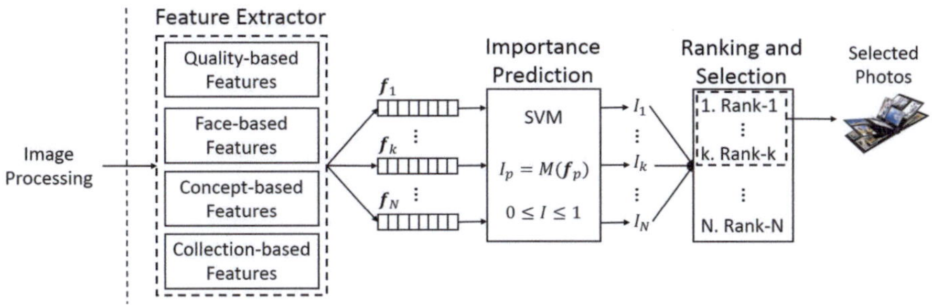

Fig. 8.6 Workflow of the importance prediction and photo selection

8.4.3 *Hybrid Selection*

In Sect. 8.4.2, we have presented an expectation-oriented photo selection model to explicitly meet selection decisions of humans via Machine Learning. As the evaluation will show (Sect. 8.4.5), our expectation-oriented selection clearly outperforms state-of-the-art methods for photo selection based on explicit modeling of coverage. However, given the wide exploitation of the concept of coverage in many state-of-the-art methods, we want to better understand its role in photo selection, in order to see if and in which way our method can be improved by combining it with explicit consideration of coverage. The notion of coverage resulted to be highly important from our user study (Sect. 8.3) as well, which is another motivation for further investigating its potential contributions and limitations. It is interesting to note that, despite the participants declared coverage as highly important, the selections that they made in the study exhibited a poor degree of coverage.

We propose and investigate three ways of combining our importance prediction model with coverage-oriented photo selection methods, denoted as "hybrid selection" methods and described hereafter. The coverage PV dimension, although kept into account within the expectation-oriented selection via the collection-based features (Sect. 8.4.2.1), becomes more dominant in this new family of selection methods. While our discussion is centered around the role of coverage, it is worth mentioning that also the diversity PV dimension is considered within one of the hybrid methods (described in Sect. 8.4.3.3).

8.4.3.1 Coverage-Driven Selection

The coverage-driven selection is based on the widely used two-step process of first clustering and subsequently picking photos from the clusters. First, for a given collection C, a set of clusters CL_C is computed as described in Chap. 3 (Sect. 3.5) and the importance $I(p)$ of each photo $p \in P_C$ is computed according to our importance prediction model (Eq. (8.1)). Given the clusters CL_C, we use the importance $I(p)$ for each photo $p \in P_C$ to pick an equal number of top-ranked photos from each cluster in order to produce the selection S of required size k.

Cluster Visiting

When picking photos from each cluster, there are different possible ways of iterating over them until the requested size of the selection is reached. After experimenting a number of alternatives, we identified a round-robin strategy with a greedy selection at each round as the best performing one. The pseudocode is listed in Algorithm 1. Given an initial set of candidate clusters CL_{cand}, the greedy strategy in each step selects the cluster cl^* containing the photo p^* with the highest importance, according to the prediction model M. The photo p^* is added to the selection S and removed from its cluster cl^*. The cluster cl^* is then removed from the set of candidate clusters for this iteration, and the greedy strategy is repeated until the candidate set is empty. Once it is, all the not empty clusters are considered available again and a new iteration of the cluster visiting starts. This procedure continues until the requested selection size k is reached. We also experimented with a regression model to predict the number of photos to select from each cluster, but it did not lead to satisfactory results.

Cluster Filtering

The intuition behind cluster filtering is that not all the clusters identified in a collection are equally important to the user. For instance, considering photos taken during a trip, there might be some of them depicting exciting moments along with other more boring situations, which the user might want to discard. We tackle this issue by proposing a cluster filtering method to automatically predict the clusters that are not important for the user, in order to ignore them when picking photos from each cluster. We train a classifier (SVM) to detect and filter out clusters which are not important

Algorithm 1 Coverage-driven Selection (Greedy)

Input: clusters CL, size k, prediction model M
Output: selection S

```
Set S = ∅
while |S| < k do
   Set CL_cand = CL
   while |CL_cand| > 0 do
      {cl*, p*} = get_most_important_cluster (CL_cand, M)
      S = S ∪ {p*}
      P_cl* = P_cl* − {p*}
      CL_cand = CL_cand − {cl*}
      if |cl*| = 0 then
         CL = CL − {cl*}
      end if
   end while
end while

return S
```

to the user. First, each cluster is described with the following features: size, quality vector (avg and std), average concept vector, number of faces (avg, std, min, and max), number of near-duplicate sets and near-duplicate photos in it, near-duplicate sets size (avg, std, min, and max), photo time (avg, std, min, and max), and photo importance (avg, std, min, and max). The label associated to a cluster is "good" if it contains at least one selected photo, "bad" otherwise. Given a training set made of clusters c_i, their corresponding feature vectors $\mathbf{f}_{c_i}$, and their classes l_{c_i}, an SVM is trained and the learned model N is used to predict the class $L = N\left(\mathbf{f}_{c_{new}}\right)$ of new unseen clusters c_{new}. Details regarding the training process are reported in Sect. 8.4.4.

Given the clusters CL_C in a collection and a classifier trained on a different portion of the dataset, applying cluster filtering removes from CL_C all those clusters that are classified as *bad* by the classifier. The iteration and picking phase are then performed only with the remaining "good" clusters.

8.4.3.2 Filtered Expectation-Oriented Selection

The coverage-driven selection is characterized by two steps: first clusters are identified and handled by possibly filtering and sorting them, and then photos in each cluster are ranked based on their predicted importance. Differently, within the filtered expectation-oriented selection, we give priority to importance prediction. The photos in a collection are first ranked based on the predicted importance and then cluster filtering is applied. The result is a ranked list of photos, where those belonging to clusters classified as "bad" have been removed. Note that the second phase of this paradigm, which contains cluster filtering in our case, can incorporate any other computation that exploits cluster information. The way photos are selected after applying cluster filtering is the same as the one described in Sect. 8.4.2.2: the selection S of size k is created by choosing the top-k photos in the list.

8.4.3.3 Optimization-Driven Selection

Besides applying clustering, another way of explicitly incorporating coverage into a photo selection process is to consider it as part of a multi-goal optimization problem. This has been done in [365] to generate representative summaries from personal photo collections, with the objective of having concise subcollections that resemble the original one as much as possible. In more detail, in this work quality, coverage, and diversity are jointly optimized and the optimal summary S^* of a requested size k is defined as

$$S^* = \underset{S \subset P_C}{\arg\max}\, F\left(Qual\left(S\right), Div\left(S\right), Cov\left(S, P_C\right)\right), \tag{8.2}$$

where $Qual\left(S\right)$ determines the interestingness of the summary S and it aggregates the "interest" values of the individual photos within S, $Div\left(S\right)$ is an aggregated measure of the diversity of the summary measured as $Div\,(S) = \min_{p_i, p_j \in S, i \neq j} Dist\,(p_i, p_j)$, and $Cov\,(S, P_C)$ denotes the number of photos in the original collection C that are represented by the photos in the summary S with respect to a concept space.

We incorporate our expectation-oriented selection within this framework, creating the optimization-driven selection, by computing the $Qual\,(\cdot)$ function in Eq. (8.2) based on the importance prediction model (Eq. (8.1)), that is,

$$Qual\,(S) = \sum_{p \in S} M\,(p) \tag{8.3}$$

Since parts of the concepts in [365] are discrete categorical attributes, associated to photos using textual information and external knowledge bases not available in our task, we binarized the elements of our automatically detected concept vector (which includes the probability that a given concept appears in the photo) by using a threshold τ such that $c_i = 1\ if\ c_i > \tau$, and $c_i = 0$ otherwise. The threshold has been empirically identified as $\tau = 0.4$ as the value that led to the most meaningful binary results. The rest of the calculation of the $Div\,(\cdot)$ and $Cov\,(\cdot)$ functions in Eq. (8.2) is performed as in the original work. In more detail, the distance between two photos, used to measure the diversity within a summary, is computed based on Exif features, time, and concept vectors (as in the original work, however we use the automatically extracted concepts), while the coverage of a summary is calculated based on the number of photos in the original collection that are represented by the ones within the summary in a concept space (considering binarized concepts vectors when needed).

Regarding the resolution of Eq. (8.2), which is an NP-Hard problem, we experimented with the different approaches presented in [365] and the best performing one consisted in combining quality, diversity, and coverage in a linear way:

$$S^* = \arg\max_{S \subset P_C} \left[\alpha \cdot Qual\,(S) + \beta \cdot Div\,(S) + \gamma \cdot Cov\,(S, P_C)\right] \tag{8.4}$$

and performing a greedy optimization, which has proved performance guarantees (please refer to [365] for further details). We will discuss the values used for the α, β, γ parameters in the experimental analysis.

8.4.4 Experimental Setup

8.4.4.1 Dataset

For our experiments, we use personal photo collections with importance judgments given by the owners of the collections as dataset. These can be photos from business trips, vacations, ceremonies, or other personal events a person participated in. We decided to focus on personal collections because we wanted to observe the personal photo selection decisions in a setting that is as realistic as possible. This gives us a ground truth for assessing user expectations.

Given the unavailability of such a dataset of real-world personal collections, with selections done by the owners based on their perceived importance, we considered the data collected during the user study previously described in Sect. 8.3. As a short reminder, participants were asked to provide their personal photo collections and to select the 20% that they perceive as the most important for revisiting or preservation purposes. The selection percentage (20%) was empirically identified as a reasonable amount of representative photos, after discussing this matter with a subset of participants before the study. In order to make the evaluation results more statistically significant, we expanded the originally collected dataset (Sect. 8.3.1) by repeating the same evaluation procedure with other participants and photo collections. Such extended dataset consists in 18,147 photos organized in 91 collections and belonging to 42 users. The collection sizes range between 100 and 625 photos, with an average of 199.4 (SD = 101.03).

Near-duplicates have been detected and filtered by considering the centroid of each set as representative photo, as done in [78]. For sets containing two photos, the one with better quality is chosen as representative. Similarly to [353], each representative is marked as selected if at least one photo in its set has been marked as selected, and marked as not selected otherwise.

8.4.4.2 Evaluation Metrics

Since the overall goal of our work is emulating the human behaviors in selecting the subsets of photos from a personal collection, we compare the automatic selections generated by our methods with the ones done by the users.

The selection methods presented in this chapter can generate a selection S of size k from the original collection, where k can assume different values. We evaluate the different methods considering the precision P@k of the selection S of size k that they produce, computed as the ratio between number of photos in S that were originally selected by the user and the size of S. Since the collections in our dataset have high size variability (from 100 to 625 photos), absolute values of k, although traditionally used in information retrieval tasks, would result in selecting very different relative portions of the collections depending on their sizes. This makes the impact of the selection different among collections. We, therefore, decided to express k as a percentage of the collection size, instead of an absolute value. In particular, we compute the precision for $k = 5, 10, 15, 20\%$, which are indicated as P@5, P@10, P@15, and P@20%, respectively. We concentrate the discussion on P@20%, because our ground truth was gathered by asking users to select the 20% of their collections. We will also give comments about the recall of the selections generated by the different methods.

The 91 collections in our dataset have been split by 10-fold cross validation (used for training and evaluating the classifiers) and all the values reported in the rest of this section are averaged over the test sets of each split. Statistical significance tests were performed using a two-tailed paired t test, and significant improvements are marked as ▲ and △ (with $p < 0.01$ and $p < 0.05$, respectively). If not stated otherwise, the significance outcome reported in the tables always refers to the comparisons with both the baselines described in Sect. 8.4.4.4.

8.4.4.3 Parameter Settings

The classifiers employed in this chapter for importance prediction and cluster filtering, built using the SVM implementation of LibSVM,[1] have radial basis functions as Kernels and their hyper-parameters are the following. The ones of the SVM used within the expectation-oriented method for importance prediction are $C = 1.0$, $\gamma = 1.0$, while the SVM used for cluster filtering has parameters $C = 3.0$, $\gamma = 1.5$. All of them were tuned by grid search and 10-fold cross validation.

8.4.4.4 Baselines

We compare our method with two baselines, one based on clustering and one representing the optimization framework presented in [365].

Clustering

Similarly to what was described at the beginning of Sect. 8.4.3.1, for a given collection C, a set of clusters CL_C is computed. The selection is built by iterating the clusters, temporally sorted, in a round-robin fashion and picking at each round the most important photo from the current cluster (until the requested selection size is reached). Instead of using our expectation-based model, the importance of each photo $p \in P_C$ is modeled as

$$I(p) = \alpha \cdot \left\| \mathbf{q}_p \right\| + (1 - \alpha) \cdot \dim \left(F_p \right) \tag{8.5}$$

which is a weighted sum of the quality vector of the photo and the number of faces in it. This notion of image importance covers different works in the literature, for instance [229, 333]. We experimented with different values of the parameter α, identifying the best value as $\alpha = 0.3$, which gives more importance to the number of faces in the photos. We report the performances obtained with this parameter value in our evaluation.

Summary Optimization

We implemented the approach presented in [365] as another baseline, where summaries are generated by optimizing quality, coverage, and diversity as in Eq. (8.2). It differs from the hybrid method described in Sect. 8.4.3.3 in how photo importance is modeled, as here the expectation-oriented model is not considered. Instead, the quality of summaries is computed by summing the "interest" of photos in it, defined as a measure dependent on photo quality and presence of portraits, groups,

[1] http://www.csie.ntu.edu.tw/~cjlin/libsvm/.

and panoramas. We computed the interest of photos as in the original work, using the concepts “face”, “3 or more people”, and “landscape” available in our concept set to represent portraits, groups, and panoramas, respectively. Also, the diversity and coverage of summaries are computed coherently with their original computation, as already described in Sect. 8.4.3.3. Assigning equal weights to the α, β, γ parameters gave us the best results, and thus we will report the performances for only this setup in the following evaluation, denoting it *SummOpt*.

8.4.5 Results

The discussion of the results is organized as follows. First, we show the performances of our expectation-oriented selection with respect to the baselines, discussing the impact of different features subsets in the selection (Sect. 8.4.5.1). We also analyze the correlation between single features and selections in Sect. 8.4.5.2. Second, we present the results of the hybrid selection methods and we compare them both with the baselines (Sect. 8.4.5.3) and with the expectation-oriented selection (Sect. 8.4.5.4). Third, we make a general comparison of the methods based on recall performances (Sect. 8.4.5.5).

Besides providing the numeric performances, we discuss and compare the dominant criteria behind each method, and we map such analysis to the PV dimensions introduced in Chap. 4. These considerations are summarized in Sect. 8.4.5.6.

8.4.5.1 Expectation-Oriented Selection

This section presents the evaluation of our expectation-oriented selection with respect to the two baselines defined in Sect. 8.4.4.4. Different importance prediction models have been trained by using the subsets of the features described in Sect. 8.4.2.1, so that the impact of different groups of features on the precision can be analyzed. Since each group is linked to part of the PV dimensions (Chap. 4), our analysis provides insights about the importance of the dimensions in the context of personal photo selection for preservation.

To reduce the dimensionality of the *concepts* features, consisting of 346 numerical values, we performed feature selection based on Information Gain [141] and we kept the top-160 features for training. The amount of 160 features has been empirically identified as a compromise between simplicity and expressiveness of the model. We did not apply any feature selection on *quality* and *faces* features because their dimensionality is small.

The results for different selection sizes (k) are listed in Table 8.1. The two baselines exhibit comparable performances, with *SummOpt* performing slightly better for all considered values of k (5, 10, 15, and 20%). Regarding our model, *quality* features are the ones that perform weakest individually, which has already been observed for other photo selection tasks [408]. This corroborates the idea that low-quality

Table 8.1 Precision of the expectation-oriented selection, distinguishing different sets of features

	P@5%	P@10%	P@15%	P@20%
Baselines				
Clustering	0.3741	0.3600	0.3436	0.3358
SummOpt	0.3858	0.3843	0.3687	0.3478
Expectation-oriented selection				
Quality	0.3431	0.3261	0.3204	0.3168
Faces	0.4506▲	0.3968▲	0.3836△	0.3747△
Concepts	0.5464▲	0.4599▲	0.4257▲	0.4117▲
Photo-level	0.5482▲	0.4760▲	0.4434▲	0.4266▲
All (Expo)	**0.7124**▲	**0.5500**▲	**0.4895**▲	**0.4652**▲

photos might be kept anyway because they contain and recall memories and events important to the user. *Faces* features alone already show better performances than the baselines: the presence, number, and position of people in photos, largely used as one selection criterion in other works, is indeed a meaningful indicator of importance. The performance achieved when only using *concepts* features is better than the ones of *quality* and *faces*: they are able to capture the semantic content of the photos, going beyond their superficial aesthetic and quality. Examples of concepts with a high importance in the model are "person", "joy", "entertainment", and "crowd". The model trained with the combination of all the aforementioned features, denoted by *photo-level* because the features are extracted from each picture in isolation, slightly improves the performance of using concept features alone. This indicates that leveraging quality and faces features in addition to semantic measures, such as concepts, can ameliorate the overall performance.

If we include global features for each photo representing information about the collection, the cluster, and the near-duplicate set the photo belongs to, we get a comprehensive set of features, which we call *all*. Similarly to the case of *concepts* features, we performed feature selection based on Information Gain on the whole set of *all* features and we retained the top-200 features for training. Again, the set size has been empirically identified as a compromise between simplicity and expressiveness of the model. The precision of the selection for this global model further increases for every selection size: this suggests that decisions for single photos are not taken in isolation but they are also driven by considering general characteristics of the collection the photo belongs to, e.g., number of photos, clusters, average quality of photos in the collection and in the same cluster, and how many duplicates for the photo there are. This is a point of distinction with respect to state-of-the-art methods (represented by the two baselines), because our selection approach does not strictly handle collection-level information by imposing clustering (*Clustering*) or optimizing measures like coverage and diversity along with photo importance only based on quality and presence of people (*SummOpt*). It rather takes this global information in consideration in a flexible way through a set of features, whose impact on the selection is learned from user selections and expectations. The expectation-oriented model using all the available features (named *Expo* in the rest of the evaluation) leads to a relative improvement of 38.5 and 33.75% over *Clustering* and *SummOpt*, respectively, considering P@20%, and even higher improvements when considering smaller values of k (90.4 and 84.6% for P@5%).

The P@20% metric is of primary importance because we asked users to select exactly 20% of their collections during the data acquisition. However, another point of discussion is the trend of precision performances over different values of k: all the models reach higher precision values for smaller selection sizes. This can be due to the presence of a limited number of selected photos that are relatively easy to identify for the methods, which give them highest selection probability.

Summarizing, modeling different promising aspects in terms of features and flexibly combining them through Machine Learning leads (except when using quality information alone) to consistent and statistically significant improvements over state-of-the-art summarization and selection methods.

8.4.5.2 Feature Analysis

For sake of completeness, in Table 8.2 we report the top-30 features ranked based on the Information Gain with respect to the class (i.e., user selections). Despite the presence of similar and redundant features, the table still provides an overview of the features that are correlated to the class the most. The symbol † for features related to

Table 8.2 Top-30 features ranked by information gain with respect to the class

Info gain	Feature name	Info gain	Feature name
0.10836	ND of photos	0.01561	Avg aggr. quality in collection
0.02569	Images without ND in collection	0.01538	Std ND set size
0.02258	Min darkness in cluster†	0.01523	Min ND set size
0.02251	Std aggr. quality in collection	0.01469	Std faces in collection
0.02240	Norm of concepts in collection	0.01440	Concept "person"
0.02189	Count of faces in photo	0.01414	Count of faces in cluster†
0.02177	Avg size of ND sets in collection	0.01321	Std aggr. quality in cluster†
0.02144	Avg contrast in cluster†	0.01306	Concept "dresses"
0.02009	Max cluster size in collection	0.01291	Concept "joy"
0.01863	Avg contrast in collection	0.01273	Avg blur in cluster†
0.01760	Count of central faces in photo	0.01147	Avg blur in collection
0.01732	Avg count of faces in collection	0.00952	Concept "two people"
0.01610	Min clusters size	0.00889	Concept "entertainment"
0.01609	ND sets in collection	0.00873	Contrast of photo
0.01565	Size of central faces in photo	0.00826	Concept "girl"

clusters means that the cluster containing the input photo is considered. For instance, given an input photo, the feature "Min darkness in cluster" represents the minimum darkness over all the images within the cluster the input photo belongs to. The first-ranked feature, whose Information Gain value is significantly higher than the ones of the other features, represents the number of near-duplicates that the input photo has. This reveals that the redundancy introduced by taking many shoots of the same scene is a strong signal of importance for that scene. Besides this feature, the other ones in the table have much smaller and similar Information Gain values. Many other high-ranked features are computed considering global information from clusters and collections, which confirms what already discussed: the decisions taken for single photos implicitly take into account general characteristics of the collection the photo belongs to. Features computed based on faces are also important, namely the total number of faces in the picture and the number and size of faces in the center of the photo. Quality is mostly considered in relation to collections and clusters (i.e., quality statistics with respect to the whole collection or a given cluster). A relatively low number of features represent concepts, which is somewhat counterintuitive if compared with the selection results of the *concepts* features reported in Table 8.1. Nevertheless, the high-performance values, if compared to those of *quality* and *faces* features, might be due to the combination of many concept features, although they are not all top ranked.

8.4.5.3 Hybrid Selection

This section discusses the precision of the hybrid selection methods presented in Sect. 8.4.3 with respect to the baselines, along with a comparative analysis between the different hybrid selection methods. The results are listed in Table 8.3, where they have been split based on the three different classes of hybrid selection described in Sect. 8.4.3. For coverage-driven selection, we report results of different combinations: *basic* refers to the coverage-driven selection which only uses our importance prediction model defined in Sect. 8.4.2.2 as photo importance measure, picking photos in a round-robin fashion from clusters temporally ordered; the term *filtered* means the use of cluster filtering, while the presence of the term *greedy* indicates the use of the greedy visiting strategy. The filtered expectation-oriented selection is denoted as *F-Expo*.

For the optimization-driven method, we experimented with the different optimization methods described in [365] after introducing our importance prediction model in place of the original importance measure used in that work ($Qual(\cdot)$). We found out that the best performing method was still the greedy optimization of a linear cost functional combining importance, diversity, and coverage (Eq. (8.4)) but with a parameter combination that gives more importance to the quality of the photos (0.6 *Qual*, 0.3 *Cov*, 0.1 *Div*). We consider the results of this setup in the following evaluation. This difference in weights with respect to the *SummOpt* baseline already anticipates that our expectation-based measure of importance has a bigger impact on

Table 8.3 Precision of the hybrid selection methods

	P@5%	P@10%	P@15%	P@20%
Baselines				
Clustering	0.3741	0.3600	0.3436	0.3358
SummOpt	0.3858	0.3843	0.3687	0.3478
Coverage-driven selection				
Basic	0.4732▲	0.4113▲	0.3902△	0.3809△
Filtered	0.5351▲	0.4617▲	0.4325▲	0.4170▲
Filtered+greedy	0.6271▲	0.4835▲	0.4391▲	0.4262▲
F-Expo	0.7065▲	0.5502▲	0.4863▲	0.4600▲
SummOpt++	0.7115▲	**0.5533▲**	**0.4937▲**	**0.4708▲**
Expo	**0.7124▲**	0.5500▲	0.4895▲	0.4652▲
Filtering with oracle				
Greedy+oracle	0.6499▲	0.5107▲	0.4665▲	0.4484▲
F-Expo+oracle	0.7150▲	0.5606▲	0.4982▲	0.4753▲

the performances than the native quality measure defined in [365]. The method will be referred as *SummOpt++*.

The results in Table 8.3 show that all hybrid methods outperform the baselines, with statistical significance, showing that the inclusion of the importance prediction model to assess photo importance has a strong impact compared to the baselines methods, which model photo importance with simple functions of quality and people occurrence. Similarly to the performances of the expectation-oriented models, both the absolute precision values and the improvements with respect to the baselines increase for decreasing *k*.

Focusing on the *coverage-driven selection*, the results in Table 8.3 also show that cluster filtering increments the precision of the *basic* approach of an amount between 9.48% (P@20%) and 13.1% (P@10%). The greedy visiting strategy leads to improvements as well. Statistical significance tests revealed that the improvements introduced by *filtered* and *filtered+greedy* are statistically significant.

Comparing the results of the different hybrid selection methods, *F-Expo* and *SummOpt++* achieve better precision performances than the coverage-driven methods, and a t test confirms that these improvements are statistically significant. This shows that the measure of photo importance modeled by our importance prediction has a bigger impact on the precision of the selection than coverage, and those methods that strictly model it through clustering (*coverage-driven selection*) get a smaller benefit when incorporating the expectation-oriented model. On the other side, methods that either give priority to expectations (*F-Expo*) or consider expectations, coverage, and global information in a flexible way via optimization (*SummOpt++*) can better exploit the expectation-oriented model.

8.4.5.4 Expectation Versus Hybrid Analysis

In this section, we make a comparative analysis between the expectation-oriented selection model exploiting all the available features (*Expo*) and the hybrid selection models. Considering Table 8.3, we can observe that the performances of *Expo* are better or comparable with the ones of the hybrid selection models. In particular, the improvements of *Expo* with respect to the *coverage-driven* methods are statistically significant. The only improvements over *Expo* (which anyway are not statistically significant) are obtained when considering methods that prioritize expectations (*F-Expo*) or possess a relaxed consideration of coverage and global information in general (*SummOpt++*). These results further support our assumption that, for the photo selection task involving personal data, a strong consideration of coverage overstresses this aspect as a selection criterion. Instead, the users might not follow a strict idea of coverage when making selections, generating selections that are not as proportioned samples of the original collections as purely coverage-based methods would suggest. Only for the methods with a more flexible consideration of coverage, the performances are similar to the pure expectation-oriented method.

Cluster filtering is an attempt to eliminate clusters uninteresting to the user, and in order to further alleviate this aspect we conducted experiments considering only important clusters, i.e., those ones containing at least one selected photo. This is done by assuming to have a perfect classifier, i.e., an "oracle", to filter out not important clusters and to focus the hybrid selection strategies only on the important ones. Although getting improvements compared to *filtered+greedy* and *F-Expo*, the performances when using such Oracle, reported in the bottom part of Table 8.3, did not lead to consistent and statistically significant improvements with respect to *Expo*. *Greedy+oracle* does not beat *Expo*, while *F-Expo+oracle* only introduces a limited and not statistically significant improvement. These results show that the aspect that mostly drives user selections and expectations is the personal perception of importance, although this can produce unbalanced selections which are not representative of the original collection. Another problem related to clustering, even considering the important ones, might be the decision of how many photos to pick from each of them.

8.4.5.5 Recall-Based Analysis

We make a comparative analysis of the different methods based on recall. The motivation of considering recall is that a user might accept to increase the size of the automatically created selection in order to include more important photos than the ones included when remaining strict to the ideal size of 20% (considered during the user study). In Table 8.4, we show the recalls of the best performing methods from each selection class, computed for different selection sizes. Note that R@20% always coincides with P@20%, since users were asked to select 20% of their collections. The results are coherent with the analysis already done for the precision: both the expectation-based model and the hybrid selection methods outperform the

Table 8.4 Recall of different selection methods

	R@20%	R@30%	R@50%	R@75%
Clustering	0.3358	0.4555	0.7000	0.9231
SummOpt	0.3478	0.4354	0.6884	0.9253
Expo	0.4652▲	0.5310▲	0.7356△	0.9310
Filtered+greedy	0.4262▲	0.5129△	0.7232	0.9231
Filtered Expo	0.4600▲	0.5361▲	0.7433△	0.9275
SummOpt++	**0.4708▲**	**0.5408▲**	**0.7405△**	**0.9315**

baselines, and the former is overall better than or comparable to the latter class. Only methods that prioritize user selections (*filtered expectation-based*) or consider expectations, coverage, and global information in a flexible way via optimization (*optimization-driven selection*) can reach slightly higher recall values than one of the expectation-based models. In the future, this consideration could be the starting point for a photo selection method that maximizes recall, or at least considers it in the learning model along with precision-based criteria.

8.4.5.6 Features and Preservation Value Dimensions

We now summarize the main insights obtained from this work, linking the results of the photo selection methods to the high-level dimensions of the PV introduced in Chap. 4.

From the results reported in Sect. 8.4.5.1, *quality* features are the ones that perform worst, revealing that the quality PV dimension is not of primary importance for preservation in personal scenarios. As an example, one might want to keep a photo because it evokes memories of the time when we took the photo, despite its low quality. The *faces* class of features alone, although performing better than *quality* features, was not as a good indicator as expected from its common usage in photo summarization and selection. The introduction of face clustering and tagging, to know who is actually appearing in the photos and what the relationship with the collection owner is, might probably help make the social graph dimension more important. However, this would also require a certain investment of the user in tagging and annotating, as well as the awareness of social relationships, which are both not assumed to be available in the considered scenario.

Since a wide part of the state-of-the-art methods for photo selection and summarization [78, 333, 358, 365] considers clustering and, more generally, coverage as primary criterion for generating selections and summaries, we applied selection methods based on temporal clustering and on summary optimization to our scenario. These high expectations on the coverage dimension were not confirmed by the experimental results. We observed that emphasizing coverage, either strictly by selecting photos fairly from each cluster or more flexibly via summary optimization, did not yield significant improvements over the pure expectation-oriented selection, which incorporates global information in a more relaxed way through a set of features. The only positive result related to coverage is the high correlation between the presence of near-duplicates and selection decisions (Table 8.2), which shows that people tend to shoot many similar photos of what they like the most and is most important to them. However, this fact is more related to the concepts of redundancy and investment than coverage. In our opinion, one of the main pitfalls of stressing coverage to emulate human selections from personal collections for preservation is that not all the clusters are usually equally important for the users. There might be photos from a sub-event that the user either simply does not like or considers less important than others. The optimal parameter values identified for the optimization-driven selection (Sect. 8.4.3.3), jointly considering importance, coverage, and diversity, showed that also the diversity dimension had a low impact on the selection. While being widely considered for photo summarization, diversity resulted to have only a marginal role in emulating user selections for preservation.

8.4.6 Personalization

Although the expectation-oriented method presented in Sect. 8.4.2 has been proved to be more effective in meeting user expectations than state-of-the-art approaches based on coverage, it applies the learned selection model for any user and collection. Nevertheless, the photo selection process (especially for personal data) can be highly subjective and the factors that drive the selection can vary from individual to individual [314, 353, 425]. General selection models, although capable of representing common selection patterns (e.g., photos depicting people might be usually appreciated), might be improved by considering the preferences of each single user separately and derive personalized models for them. Some users might be particularly interested in photos depicting many people, while others might prefer pictures with landscapes or buildings. Besides variations in the set of appreciated concepts, also selection aspects that are ignored by some people might become more important for others. It is therefore worth spending some thoughts on how personalized selection models that adapt to the preferences of different users could be developed. To this aim, we have performed a preliminary study in [143] to investigate how personalized models can be derived from the photo selection approach described in Sect. 8.4.2, denoted by "general model" hereafter. We highlight the applied methodology and its findings in the rest of this section.

8.4.6.1 Methodology

A recurrent matter in Machine Learning is continuously managing new data, so that the existing model can be updated to accommodate new information and to adapt to it. Two common approaches for updating the model to new incoming data are

Online Learning [46], where the model is updated only considering the new data, and Incremental Learning [65], where the model update considers the old training data along with the incoming data. We considered the latter strategy and retrain the model each time new data (i.e., selection decisions) was provided by the user because, in our scenario, the updated model has to be aware of the entire data available, not just of the most recent one. Although efficient and effective incremental versions of off-line learning algorithms exist (e.g., [65]), we performed the model update by including the new data in the training set and retrain the model from scratch. We implemented such more straightforward but functionally equivalent approach because our scenario does not impose strict temporal constraints for the model update, thus making the efficiency benefit of incremental versions of secondary importance. The time taken by a user to produce a new collection (e.g., after a trip or vacation) can be considered sufficient to retrain the model with the whole available data. Should the temporal constraints of the envisioned scenario become stricter, the incremental version of the employed algorithm could be plugged in without changing the functionalities of the whole application.

The personalization workflow is summarized in Fig. 8.7, which emulates the application of the personalized model in real-world settings. The personalized photo selection models, one for each given user, are built by re-training the model every time that a new collection is imported and the automatic selection done by the current selection model is revised by the user. The annotated photo collections available to train the general model are first preprocessed through image processing techniques and features are extracted from them, in the same way as described before in this chapter.

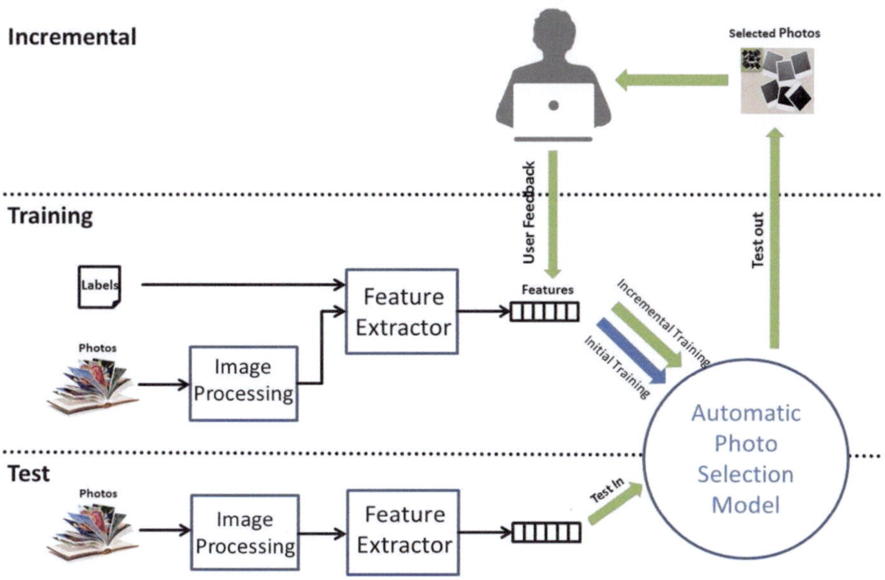

Fig. 8.7 Overview of the personalization of the general photo selection model

For each new collection provided by the user, a first selection is made by the trained general model as described in Sect. 8.4.2.2 and the selected photos are displayed to the user, who gives feedback revising the automatically generated selection. The training dataset is then expanded by adding the feedback data and the general model is retrained with the updated training dataset. Iterating this process, it is expected that the gap between user expectations and model's selections gets lower, due to the adaptation of the model toward the selection preferences of the user. This workflow represents the envisioned behavior once the whole system has been finalized and released to the end user. However, in order to easily repeat evaluations when designing and implementing the model, we collected the data from each user once for all, i.e., users evaluated all the collections from scratch without revising any automatically generated selection. Although we are aware that the selections done by the user starting from an automatically generated selection might differ from those done when selecting photos from scratch, repeating the evaluation multiple times when designing the system would have been unfeasible for the users. Moreover, acquiring evaluations done from scratch is unbiased from the initial selection proposed automatically.

Usually, the adaptation of a system within the initial rounds of user interactions is affected by the so-called "cold-start problem": there is not enough (or even not at all) training data to let the model adapt to the user. This holds in our scenario as well, where the selection model might not make proper predictions due to the lack of annotated collections in the initial training set. We considered two ways of building the initial training set. One consists in using one annotated collection of the given user as initial training set. The other is based on using annotated collections from other users to train the initial selection model, hopefully boosting the adaptation of the model to a given user when a limited amount of personal training data is available. The latter approach is based on the assumption that, despite the subjectivity of the task, common selection patterns exist and could be captured through a sample of selections done by other users.

8.4.6.2 Findings

We used the dataset already described in Sect. 8.4.4 as basis of our experiments. In order to assess personalization performances, we consider users who contributed at least five collections as test users. Among the overall 91 photo collections, there are 11 users who provided at least 5 collections (10 users contributed 5 collections, 1 user contributed 6 collections) which result in 56 collections totally. Afterward, the original dataset is split into two parts: one part contains 35 collections from 31 users, whereby each user provided at most 2 collections, which is named *general dataset*; another part contains 56 collections from 11 users, whereby each user provided at least 5 collections, which is called *personalized dataset*.

Given the aforementioned general distinction between *general* and *personalized* dataset, we evaluate the performances of the model update over different rounds of adaptation. The *personalized dataset* is split based on users where each one owns 5 collections (one user owns 6). At each iteration k, for each user with N collections, k collections are added to the initial training set to learn the personalized model of the user, and $N - k$ collections are used for testing. We considered three ways of building training sets. In the *stand-alone* procedure, the initial model is trained with one random collection of the user, and the model update is incrementally done considering the remaining collections of the same user. In this case, we are considering each test user in isolation, ignoring any data from others. The *collaborative* strategy fills the initial training set with all the collections within the *general dataset*. This case represents the situation where, in the absence of large amount of annotated personal data for training, annotated collections of other users are used to alleviate the cold-start problem. The *user-agnostic* method, similarly to the *collaborative* case, uses the *general dataset* as initial training set. However, at each iteration, instead of including collections of the user under consideration, we add randomly selected collections from the other test users. This case is motivated by the assumption that if one collection, which is not from the user that we are considering, is included in the training set at each iteration, then the adaptation performances should be smaller than including collections that are from the user that we are considering. This would highlight the importance of incorporating selection information of the user in the training set when making selections for new collections of the same user.

We observed from the experiments that the precision of both *stand-alone* and *collaborative* increases at each iteration, i.e., with the increase of the number of user's collections considered for training the model. This suggests that having a selection model partially aware of the user preferences (by exploiting a certain amount of the selection behavior in the training phase) can improve the precision of new unseen collections of the same user. The precision of *collaborative* was higher than the one of *stand-alone*, especially at the first iterations, showing that the selection data from other users can alleviate the cold-start problem. We also measured the relative gain obtained by each strategy between any two consecutive iterations. The gain of *stand-alone* at each iteration resulted to be higher than the one of *collaborative*, because the initial model was weaker (due to the limited training set) and the inclusion of new training collections had a higher impact on the learning. Comparing *user-agnostic* and *collaborative*, the former exhibited an almost null or even negative gain over iterations, while the latter led to a bigger and increasing performance gain at every iteration. This demonstrated that the increase of performance at each iteration was due to the inclusion of a new collection of the same user in the training set and not simply caused by expanding the training set at each iteration, since in this case the gain of *user-agnostic* should have been higher as well.

As a conclusion, this evaluation led to promising results, showing that (a) including new annotated collections for the same user when training the model can benefit the selections on new unseen collections of the same user, and (b) exploiting annotated collections from other users as initial training data can boost the system performances in cold-start scenarios. It is important to clarify that the standard deviation observed in these experiments was relatively high. This can be due to a mixture of aspects, such as a limited size of test set (both in terms of users and iterations) and intrinsic changes of difficulty among collections of the same user. For this reason, although a promising user adaptation emerged from this study, the inclusion of an extended amount of users, collections, and iterations would help make the results more evident and statistically significant.

8.5 Conclusions

In this chapter, we considered the problem of keeping personal photo collections enjoyable over time. Given the explosion in the production of digital photos within the recent years and the common practice of merely dumping such data on cheap storage devices or using storage services, the stored photo collections are rarely accessed and revisited afterward. To some extent, their content tends to be forgotten because the big collection size makes their revisiting a fatiguing process.

As a remedy, we proposed a selective approach to long-term data management that aims at identifying what is most important to the user and investing in the longevity and enrichment of this content, in order to make the future revisiting more enjoyable and less tedious. The development of such automated method was preceded by a user study, to lay the foundations of the task and better understand its challenges.

The user study was centered around a photo selection task where 35 participants contributed their own collections, from which they selected the photos most important to them, namely the ones that they would like to preserve for future revisiting. One important outcome was that many hidden and subjective criteria (memory evocation, personal importance, and photo typicality) were rated high, anticipating the difficulty of automatizing the selection task. Moreover, the more objective criterion of photo quality was rated as less important. Another aspect emerged as important was coverage, which means that the set of selected pictures should fairly represent the content of the original collection. Although this was stated by the participants, their selections exhibited a poor degree of coverage.

Afterward, we presented an expectation-oriented method for photo selection exploiting an extensive set of photo- and collection-level features, to estimate the long-term photo importance based on user expectations. The evidence of user expectations has been derived from the personal data provided during the user study and has been used to train the selection model. The goal of this method is supporting users in selecting the most important photos for creating an enjoyable subcollection of a personal collection for preservation and revisiting purposes. Since a wide part of state-of-the-art methods is driven by the concept of coverage, which resulted to be highly rated in our user study as well, we also investigated how to combine the expectation-oriented selection with more explicit modelings of coverage. Experiments with real-world photo collections showed that (a) our method outperforms such state-of-the-art works when considering human selections as evaluation criterion and (b) comparable results to our method can be achieved only when coverage is not considered as a primary selection aspect.

References

1. Foundations of forgetting and remembering final report. Deliverable 2.4 for eu fp7: Project forgetit - concise preservation by combining managed forgetting and contextualization remembering. https://www.forgetit-project.eu/fileadmin/fm-dam/deliverables/ForgetIT_WP2_D2.4.new.pdf. Accessed 10 July 2017
2. Foundations of forgetting and remembering intermediate report. Deliverable 2.3 for eu fp:7 project forgetit - concise preservation by combining managed forgetting and contextualization remembering. https://www.forgetit-project.eu/fileadmin/fm-dam/deliverables/ForgetIT_WP2_D2.3.pdf. Accessed 10 July 2017
3. Afrasiabi Rad, P., Nilsson, J., Päivärinta, T.: Administration of digital preservation services in the cloud over time: design issues and challenges for organizations. In: Endicott-Popovsky B. (ed.) The Proceedings of the 2nd International Conference on Cloud Security Management, Proceedings of the International Conference on Cloud Security Management. Academic Conferences and Publishing International Ltd (2014)
4. Agrawal, R., Gollapudi, S., Halverson, A., Ieong, S.: Diversifying search results. In: Proceedings of the Second ACM International Conference on Web Search and Data Mining, WSDM '09, pp. 5–14. ACM, New York, NY, USA (2009). http://doi.acm.org/10.1145/1498759.1498766
5. Markatopoulou et al., F.: A study on the use of a binary local descriptor and color extensions of local descriptors for video concept detection. In: MultiMedia Modeling Conference. LNCS, vol. 8935, pp. 282–293. Springer, Berlin (2015)
6. Over et al., P.: Trecvid 2013 – an overview of the goals, tasks, data, evaluation mechanisms and metrics. In: Proceedings of TRECVID 2013. NIST, USA (2013)
7. Alberdi, E.: Accommodating surprise in taxonomic tasks: a psychological and computational investigation. Ph.D. thesis, University of Aberdeen (1996)
8. Alberdi, E., Sleeman, D.H.: Retax: a step in the automation of taxonomic revision. Artif. Intell. **91**(2), 257–279 (1997)
9. Alexe, B., Deselaers, T., Ferrari, V.: Measuring the objectness of image windows. IEEE Trans. Pattern Anal. Mach. Intell. **34**(11), 2189–2202 (2012)
10. Ames, M., Eckles, D., Naaman, M., Spasojevic, M., Van House, N.: Requirements for mobile photoware. Pers. Ubiquitous Comput. **14**(2), 95–109 (2010)
11. Anastasiu, D.C., Karypis, G.: L2ap: fast cosine similarity search with prefix l-2 norm bounds. In: 30th International Conference on Data Engineering (ICDE), pp. 784–795. IEEE (2014)
12. Anderson, J.R., Schooler, L.J.: Reflections of the environment in memory. Psychol. Sci. **6**(2), 396–408 (1991)

V. Mezaris et al. (eds.), *Personal Multimedia Preservation*, Springer Series on Cultural Computing, https://doi.org/10.1007/978-3-319-73465-1

13. Anderson, M.C., Baddeley, A., Eysenck, M., Anderson, M.: Retrieval. Memory pp. 163–189 (2009)
14. Andersson, I., Lindqvist, G., Randers, F.: Preservation services planning: a decision support framework. In: The Proceedings of the 2nd International Conference on Cloud Security Management (2014)
15. Andoni, A.: Locality-sensitive hashing scheme based on p-stable distributions. Nearest neighbor methods in learning and vision: Theory and practice (2006)
16. Apostolidis, E., Mezaris, V.: Fast shot segmentation combining global and local visual descriptors. In: Proceedings of International Conference on Acoustics, Speech and Signal Processing (ICASSP), pp. 6583–6587. IEEE (2014)
17. Apostolidis, K., Papagiannopoulou, C., Mezaris, V.: CERTH at MediaEval 2014 synchronization of multi-user event media task. In: Proceedings of the MediaEval Workshop (2014)
18. Apostolidis, K., Solachidis, V., Papadopoulou, O., Mezaris, V.: Photo collection contextualization. In: 2015 IEEE International Conference on Multimedia Expo Workshops (ICMEW), pp. 1–6 (2015). https://doi.org/10.1109/ICMEW.2015.7169761
19. Arandjelovic, R., Zisserman, A.: All about VLAD. In: Proceedings of the Conference on Computer Vision and Pattern Recognition, pp. 1578–1585. IEEE (2013)
20. Argyriou, A., Evgeniou, T., Pontil, M.: Multi-task feature learning. In: Advances in Neural Information Processing Systems (NIPS 2007). MIT Press, Cambridge (2007)
21. Argyriou, A., Evgeniou, T., Pontil, M.: Convex multi-task feature learning. Mach. Learn. **73**(3), 243–272 (2008)
22. Awad, M., Khan, L., Thuraisingham, B.: Predicting www surfing using multiple evidence combination. VLDB J. **17**(3), 401–417 (2008). https://doi.org/10.1007/s00778-006-0014-1
23. Babenko, A., Lempitsky, V.: Aggregating local deep features for image retrieval. In: Proceedings of the International Conference on Computer Vision (ICCV), pp. 1269–1277. IEEE (2015)
24. Backstrom, L., Leskovec, J.: Supervised random walks: predicting and recommending links in social networks. In: Proceedings of the Fourth ACM International Conference on Web Search and Data Mining, WSDM '11, pp. 635–644. ACM, New York, NY, USA (2011). https://doi.org/10.1145/1935826.1935914
25. Baddeley, A.: Essentials of Human Memory, pp. 139–144. Psychology Press, Abingdon (1999)
26. Baddeley, A., Eysenck, M., Anderson, M.: Memory. Psychology Press, Abingdon (2009)
27. Baddeley, A., Eysenck, M., Anderson, M.: Memory. Taylor & Francis, New York (2015). https://books.google.gr/books?id=nxNWBQAAQBAJ
28. Baddeley, A., Logie, R.: Working memory: the multiple-component model. In: Miyake, A., Shah, P. (eds.) Models of Working Memory: Mechanisms of Active Maintenance and Executive Control, pp. 28–61 (1999)
29. Baddeley, A.D., Hitch, G.: Working memory. Psychol. Learn. Motiv. **8**, 47–89 (1974)
30. Baeza-Yates, R., Gionis, A., Junqueira, F., Murdock, V., Plachouras, V., Silvestri, F.: The impact of caching on search engines. In: Proceedings of the 30th Annual International ACM SIGIR Conference on Research and Development in Information Retrieval, SIGIR '07, pp. 183–190. ACM, New York, NY, USA (2007). https://doi.org/10.1145/1277741.1277775
31. Bahrick, H.P.: Semantic memory content in permastore: fifty years of memory for spanish learned in school. J. Exp. Psychol. Gen. **113**(1), 1 (1984)
32. Banks, R., Kirk, D., Sellen, A.: A design perspective on three technology heirlooms. Human-Comput. Interact. **27**(1–2), 63–91 (2012)
33. Barthel, R., Mackley, K.L., Hudson-Smith, A., Karpovich, A., de Jode, M., Speed, C.: An internet of old things as an augmented memory system. Pers. Ubiquitous Comput. **17**(2), 321–333 (2013)
34. Bartlett, F.C., Burt, C.: Remembering: a study in experimental and social psychology. B. J. Educ. Psychol. **3**(2), 187–192 (1933)
35. Barua, D., Kay, J., Kummerfeld, B., Paris, C.: Theoretical foundations for user-controlled forgetting in scrutable long term user models. In: Proceedings of the 23rd Australian Computer-Human Interaction Conference, pp. 40–49. ACM (2011)

36. Basave, A.E.C., Rizzo, G., Varga, A., Rowe, M., Stankovic, M., Dadzie, A.: Making sense of microposts (#microposts2014) named entity extraction and linking challenge. In: 4th Workshop on Making Sense of Microposts (2014)
37. Bendersky, M., Croft, W.B.: Discovering key concepts in verbose queries. In: Proceedings of the 31st Annual International ACM SIGIR Conference on Research and Development in Information Retrieval, SIGIR '08, pp. 491–498 (2008)
38. Berberich, K., Bedathur, S., Alonso, O., Weikum, G.: A language modeling approach for temporal information needs. In: Proceedings of the 32 European Conference on Advances in Information Retrieval, ECIR'2010, pp. 13–25 (2010)
39. Berdan, R.: Composition and the elements of visual design. Photo composition articles (2004)
40. Bernardi, A., Grimnes, G.A., Groza, T., Scerri, S.: The NEPOMUK semantic desktop. In: Warren, P., Davies, J., Simperl, E. (eds.) Context and Semantics for Knowledge Management - Technologies for Personal Productivity. The NEPOMUK Semantic Desktop, pp. 255–274. Springer, Berlin (2011)
41. Berntsen, D., Rubin, D.C.: Cultural life scripts structure recall from autobiographical memory. Mem. Cognit. **32**(3), 427–442 (2004)
42. Bhattacharya, S., Nojavanasghari, B., Chen, T., Liu, D., Chang, S.F., Shah, M.: Towards a comprehensive computational model foraesthetic assessment of videos. In: Proceedings of the 21st International Conference on Multimedia, pp. 361–364. ACM (2013)
43. Blanken, H.M., de Vries, A.P., Blok, H.E., Feng, L.: Multimedia Retrieval. Springer, Berlin (2005)
44. Blei, D.M., Ng, A.Y., Jordan, M.I.: Latent dirichlet allocation. J. Mach. Learn. Res. (2003)
45. Bontcheva, K., Derczynski, L., Funk, A., Greenwood, M.A., Maynard, D., Aswani, N.: TwitIE: an open-source information extraction pipeline for microblog text. In: Proceedings of the International Conference on Recent Advances in Natural Language Processing. Association for Computational Linguistics (2013)
46. Bordes, A., Ertekin, S., Weston, J., Bottou, L.: Fast kernel classifiers with online and active learning. J. Mach. Learn. Res. **6**(Sep), 1579–1619 (2005)
47. Borghoff, U., Rdig, P., Scheffczyk, J.: Long-term preservation of digital documents. In: Uwe, M.B., Rodig, P., Schmitz, L., Jan S. Principles and Practices, Online-Ausg. edn. Springer, Berlin (2006). https://doi.org/10.1007/978-3-540-33640-2
48. Bos, E.: We can make forgetting impossible, but should we? Interactions **2**(3), 11–14 (1995)
49. Bote, J., Fernandez-Feijoo, B., Ruiz, S.: The cost of digital preservation: a methodological analysis. Proc. Technol. **5**, 103–111 (2012)
50. Bottou, L.: Large-scale machine learning with stochastic gradient descent. In: Proceedings of COMPSTAT, pp. 177–186. Springer (2010)
51. Brand, S.: Escaping the digital dark age. Libr. J. **124**(2), 4669 (1999)
52. Bransford, J.: Human Cognition: Learning, Understanding, and Remembering. Thomson Brooks/Cole (1979)
53. Brewer, W.F.: Qualitative Analysis of the Recalls of Randomly Sampled Autobiographical Events. Cambridge University Press, Cambridge (1988)
54. Brighton, H., Mellish, C.: Advances in instance selection for instance-based learning algorithms. Data Min. Knowl. Discov. **6**(2), 153–172 (2002)
55. Brown, R., Kulik, J.: Flashbulb memories. Cognition **5**(1), 73–99 (1977)
56. Broyden, C.G.: The convergence of a class of double rank minimization algorithms 1. general considerations. J. Appl. Math. **6**(1), 76–90 (1970)
57. Brubaker, J.R., Callison-Burch, V.: Legacy contact: Designing and implementing post-mortem stewardship at facebook. In: Proceedings of the 2016 CHI Conference on Human Factors in Computing Systems, CHI '16, pp. 2908–2919. ACM, New York, NY, USA (2016). https://doi.org/10.1145/2858036.2858254
58. Cabeza, R., St Jacques, P.: Functional neuroimaging of autobiographical memory. Trends Cognit. Sci. **11**(5), 219–227 (2007)
59. Camargo, J.E., González, F.A.: Multimodal latent topic analysis for image collection summarization. Inf. Sci. **328**, 270–287 (2016)

60. Campos, V., Salvador, A.: Giro-i Nieto, X., Jou, B.: Diving deep into sentiment: Understanding fine-tuned CNNs for visual sentiment prediction. In: Proceedings of the 1st International Workshop on Affect and Sentiment in Multimedia. ASM '15, pp. 57–62. ACM, New York, NY, USA (2015)
61. Carmel, D., Cohen, D., Fagin, R., Farchi, E., Herscovici, M., Maarek, Y.S., Soffer, A.: Static index pruning for information retrieval systems. In: Proceedings of the 24th Annual International ACM SIGIR Conference on Research and Development in Information Retrieval, SIGIR '01, pp. 43–50. ACM, New York, NY, USA (2001). https://doi.org/10.1145/383952.383958
62. Carmel, D., Kurland, O.: Query performance prediction for ir. In: Proceedings of the 35th International ACM SIGIR Conference on Research and Development in Information Retrieval, SIGIR '12, pp. 1196–1197 (2012)
63. Carmel, D., Yom-Tov, E.: Estimating the query difficulty for information retrieval. In: Proceedings of the 33rd International ACM SIGIR Conference on Research and Development in Information Retrieval, SIGIR '10, pp. 911–911 (2010)
64. Carpenter, G.A., Grossberg, S.: Adaptive Resonance Theory. Springer, Berlin (2017)
65. Cauwenberghs, G., Poggio, T.: Incremental and decremental support vector machine learning. In: Proceedings of the 13th International Conference on Neural Information Processing Systems, NIPS'00, pp. 388–394 (2000)
66. CCSDS: Producer-Archive Interface Methodology Abstract Standard (PAIMAS) - Recommended Practice, CCSDS 651.0-M-1 (Magenta Book) Issue 1. Equivalent to ISO 20652:2006 (2004). http://public.ccsds.org/publications/archive/651x0m1.pdf. Accessed Sep 2017
67. CCSDS: Reference Model for an Open Archival Information System (OAIS) - Recommended Practice, CCSDS 650.0-M-2 (Magenta Book) Issue 2. Equivalent to ISO 14721:2012 (2012). http://public.ccsds.org/publications/archive/650x0m2.pdf. Accessed Sep. 2017
68. CCSDS Secretariat, S.C., Office, N.: Reference Model for an Open Archival Information System (OAIS). Space Operations Mission Directorate (2009)
69. Ceroni, A., Solachidis, V., Fu, M., Kanhabua, N., Papadopoulou, O., Niederée, C., Mezaris, V.: Investigating human behaviors in selecting personal photos to preserve memories. In: Proceedings of the 2015 IEEE International Conference on Multimedia and Expo (ICME) Workshop on Human Memory-Inspired Multimedia Organization and Preservation (HMMP'15) (2015)
70. Ceroni, A., Solachidis, V., Niederée, C., Papadopoulou, O., Kanhabua, N., Mezaris, V.: To keep or not to keep: an expectation–oriented photo selection method for personal photo collections. In: Proceedings of the ACM International Conference on Multimedia Retrieval (ICMR'2015) (2015)
71. Ceroni, A., Tran, N.K., Kanhabua, N., Niederée, C.: Bridging temporal context gaps using time-aware re-contextualization. In: Proceedings of the 37th International ACM SIGIR Conference on Research and Development in Information Retrieval, SIGIR '14, pp. 1127–1130 (2014)
72. Chang, Y.W., Lin, C.J.: Feature ranking using linear SVM. In: Proceedings of WCCI Causation and Prediction Challenge, pp. 53–64 (2008)
73. Chappell, D.: Enterprise Service Bus. O'Reilly Media, Inc., California (2004)
74. Chatfield, K., Simonyan, K., Vedaldi, A., Zisserman, A.: Return of the devil in the details: delving deep into convolutional nets. In: British Machine Vision Conference (2014)
75. Chen, J., Hibino, S.: Reminiscing view: Event-based browsing of consumer's photo and video-clip collections. In: Tenth IEEE International Symposium on Multimedia, pp. 23–30 (2008). https://doi.org/10.1109/ISM.2008.104
76. Chen, R.C., Lee, C.J., Croft, W.B.: On divergence measures and static index pruning. In: Proceedings of the 2015 International Conference on The Theory of Information Retrieval, ICTIR '15, pp. 151–160. ACM, New York, NY, USA (2015). https://doi.org/10.1145/2808194.2809472
77. Chen, Y.: Information valuation for information lifecycle management. In: Proceedings of International Conference on Autonomic Computing (2005)

78. Chu, W.T., Lin, C.H.: Automatic selection of representative photo and smart thumbnailing using near-duplicate detection. In: Proceedings of the 16th ACM International Conference on Multimedia, MM '08, pp. 829–832. ACM (2008)
79. Ciglan, M., Nørvåg, K.: Wikipop: personalized event detection system based on Wikipedia page view statistics. In: Proceedings of the 19th ACM International Conference on Information and Knowledge Management, CIKM '10, pp. 1931–1932 (2010)
80. Cocchini, G., Logie, R.H., Della Sala, S., MacPherson, S.E., Baddeley, A.D.: Concurrent performance of two memory tasks: evidence for domain-specific working memory systems. Mem. Cognit. **30**(7), 1086–1095 (2002)
81. Cohen, J., Mihailidis, P.: Storify and news curation: teaching and learning about digital storytelling. Second Ann. Soc. Media Technol. Conf. Workshop **1**, 27–31 (2012)
82. Conci, N., De Natale, F.G., Mezaris, V., Matton, M.: Synchronization of multi-user event media (SEM) at mediaeval 2014: task description, datasets, and evaluation. In: MediaEval (2014)
83. Conci, N., Natale, F.D., Mezaris, V.: Synchronization of multi-user event media (SEM) at mediaeval 2014: task description, datasets, and evaluation. In: MediaEval 2014 Workshop, Barcelona, Spain (2014)
84. Connor, M., Spitzer, S.: The places freqency algorithm. https://developer.mozilla.org/en-US/docs/Mozilla/Tech/Places/Frecency_algorithm (2015). Accessed 31 Aug 2015
85. Conway, M.A.: Memory and the self. J. Mem. Lang. **53**(4), 594–628 (2005)
86. Conway, M.A.: Episodic memories. Neuropsychologia **47**(11), 2305–2313 (2009)
87. Conway, M.A., Anderson, S.J., Larsen, S.F., Donnelly, C.M., McDaniel, M.A., McClelland, A.G., Rawles, R.E., Logie, R.H.: The formation of flashbulb memories. Mem. Cognit. **22**(3), 326–343 (1994)
88. Conway, M.A., Cohen, G., Stanhope, N.: Very long-term memory for knowledge acquired at school and university. Appl. Cognit. Psychol. **6**(6), 467–482 (1992)
89. Conway, M.A., Loveday, C.: Accessing autobiographical memories. Act of Remembering: Toward an Understanding of How We Recall the Past, pp. 56–70 (2010)
90. Conway, M.A., Loveday, C.: Accessing Autobiographical Memories, the Act of Remembering: Toward an Understanding of How We Recall the Past, pp. 56–70. Wiley Blackwell, New Jersey (2010)
91. Conway, M.A., Pleydell-Pearce, C.W.: The construction of autobiographical memories in the self-memory system. Psychol. Rev. **107**(2), 261 (2000)
92. Conway, P.: Overview: Rationale for Digitization and Preservation, Chap. 2, pp. 5–20. NEDCC (2000)
93. Cook, T.: Macroappraisal in theory and practice: origins, characteristics, and implementation in Canada, 19502000. Arch. Sci. **5**(2–4), 101–161 (2005). http://dx.doi.org/10.1007/s10502-005-9010-2
94. Cooper, M., Foote, J., Girgensohn, A., Wilcox, L.: Temporal event clustering for digital photo collections. ACM Trans. Multimed. Comput. Commun. Appl. (TOMM) **1**(3), 269–288 (2005)
95. Copeland, A.: The use of personal value estimations to select images for preservation in public library digital community collections. Future Internet **6**(2) (2014)
96. Cosley, D., Sosik, V.S., Schultz, J., Peesapati, S.T., Lee, S.: Experiences with designing tools for everyday reminiscing. Hum. Comput. Interact. **27**(1–2), 175–198 (2012)
97. da Costa Pinto, A.a.n., Baddeley, A.D.: Where did you park your car? Analysis of a naturalistic long-term recency effect. Eur. J. Cognit. Psychol. **3**(3), 297–313 (1991)
98. Cowan, N.: Working Memory Capacity. Psychology Press (2012)
99. Crestani, F., Lee, P.L.: Searching the web by constrained spreading activation. Inf. Process. Manag. **36**(4), 585–605 (2000). https://doi.org/10.1016/S0306-4573(99)00073-4. http://www.sciencedirect.com/science/article/pii/S0306457399000734
100. Crovitz, H.F., Schiffman, H.: Frequency of episodic memories as a function of their age. Bull. Psychon. Soc. **4**(5), 517–518 (1974)
101. Csurka, G., Dance, C., Fan, L., Willamowski, J., Bray, C.: Visual categorization with bags of keypoints. In: ECCV Workshop on Statistical Learning in Computer Vision, 1–22, pp. 1–2. Prague (2004)

102. Cubelli, R., Della Sala, S.: Flashbulb memories: special but not iconic. Cortex **44**(7), 908–909 (2008)
103. Cubelli, R., Della Sala, S.: Flashbulb memories: sorry, no flash!. Cortex **1**(49), 356–357 (2013)
104. Cunningham, H., Tablan, V., Roberts, I., Greenwood, M.A., Aswani, N.: Information extraction and semantic annotation for multi-paradigm information management. In: Lupu, M., Mayer, K., Tait, J., Trippe, A.J. (eds.) Current Challenges in Patent Information Retrieval. The Information Retrieval Series, vol. 29, pp. 307–327. Springer, Berlin (2011). https://doi.org/10.1007/978-3-642-19231-9_15
105. Curci, A., Conway, M.A.: Playing the flashbulb memory game: a comment on cubelli and della sala. Cortex **49**(1), 352–355 (2013)
106. Cutrell, E., Dumais, S.T., Teevan, J.: Searching to eliminate personal information management. Commun. ACM **49**(1), 58–64 (2006)
107. Daelemans, W., Van Den Bosch, A., Zavrel, J.: Forgetting exceptions is harmful in language learning. Mach. Learn. **34**(1–3), 11–41 (1999)
108. Dang, V., Croft, W.B.: Feature selection for document ranking using best first search and coordinate ascent. In: Proceedings of SIGIR'10 Workshop on Feature Generation and Selection for Information Retrieval (2010)
109. Das, M., Loui, A.: Detecting significant events in personal image collections. In: IEEE International Conference on Semantic Computing, 2009. ICSC '09, pp. 116–123 (2009)
110. Datta, R., Li, J., Wang, J.Z.: Studying aesthetics in photographic images using a computational approach. US Patent App. 13/542,326, 2012
111. Datta, R., Wang, J.Z.: ACQUINE: aesthetic quality inference engine-real-time automatic rating of photo aesthetics. In: Proceedings of the International Conference on Multimedia information retrieval, pp. 421–424. ACM (2010)
112. Daumé III, H.: Bayesian multitask learning with latent hierarchies. In: Proceedings of the 25th Conference on Uncertainty in Artificial Intelligence (UAI '09), pp. 135–142. AUAI Press, Arlington, Virginia, US (2009)
113. De Groot, A.D.: Thought and Choice in Chess, vol. 4. Walter de Gruyter GmbH & Co KG (1978)
114. Dengel, A. (ed.): Semantische Technologien. Spektrum (2012)
115. Dhar, S., Ordonez, V., Berg, T.L.: High level describable attributes for predicting aesthetics and interestingness. In: IEEE Conference on Computer Vision and Pattern Recognition (CVPR), pp. 1657–1664 (2011)
116. Djafari Naini, K., Altingovde, I.S.: Exploiting result diversification methods for feature selection in learning to rank. In: de Rijke, M., Kenter, T., de Vries, A.P., Zhai, C., de Jong, F., Radinsky, K. Hofmann, K. (eds.) Advances in Information Retrieval: 36th European Conference on IR Research, ECIR 2014, Amsterdam, The Netherlands, April 13–16, 2014. Proceedings, pp. 455–461. Springer International Publishing, Cham (2014). https://doi.org/10.1007/978-3-319-06028-6_41
117. Djafari Naini, K., Kawase, R., Kanhabua, N., Niederee, C.: Characterizing high-impact features for content retention in social web applications. In: Proceedings of the 23rd International Conference on World Wide Web, WWW '14 Companion, pp. 559–560. ACM, New York, NY, USA (2014). https://doi.org/10.1145/2567948.2576954
118. Douze, M., Jégou, H., Sandhawalia, H., Amsaleg, L., Schmid, C.: Evaluation of gist descriptors for web-scale image search. In: Proceedings of the International Conference on Image and Video Retrieval, p. 19. ACM (2009)
119. Drucker, H., Burges, C.J.C., Kaufman, L., Smola, A.J., Vapnik, V.: Support vector regression machines. In: Mozer, M.C., Jordan, M.I., Petsche T. (eds.) Advances in Neural Information Processing Systems, vol. 9, pp. 155–161 (1997)
120. Duan, L.Y., Lin, J., Wang, Z., Huang, T., Gao, W.: Weighted component hashing of binary aggregated descriptors for fast visual search. IEEE Trans. Multimed. **17**(6), 828–842 (2015)
121. Eaton, E., Ruvolo, P.L.: Ella: An efficient lifelong learning algorithm. In: Dasgupta, S., Mcallester D. (eds.) Proceedings of the 30th International Conference on Machine Learning (ICML-13), vol. 28, pp. 507–515. JMLR Workshop (2013)

122. Ebbinghaus, H.: Memory: A Contribution to Experimental Psychology (1964)
123. EBU: Class Conceptual Data Model (CCDM) - TECH 3351. https://tech.ebu.ch/metadata (2016). Accessed Sep 2017
124. Eder, J., Koncilia, C.: Modelling changes in ontologies. In: Proceedings of the On The Move - Federated Conferences (OTM 2004) (2004)
125. Edworthy, J., Hellier, E.: Fewer but better auditory alarms will improve patient safety. In: BMJ Quality and Safety **14**(3), 212–215 (2005). https://doi.org/10.1136/qshc.2004.013052. http://qualitysafety.bmj.com/content/14/3/212
126. Eiter, T., Wang, K.: Semantic forgetting in answer set programming. Artif. Intell. **172**(14), 1644–1672 (2008)
127. Eldesouky, B., Bakry, M., Maus, H., Dengel, A.: Supporting early contextualization of textual content in digital documents on the web. In: Proceedings of the 13th International Conference on Document Analysis and Recognition. Nancy, France (2015)
128. Eldesouky, B., Bakry, M., Maus, H., Dengel, A.: Seed, an end-user text composition tool for the semantic web. In: The Semantic Web - ISWC 2016, 15th International Semantic Web Conference, Proceedings. International Semantic Web Conference (ISWC-2016), 15th, October 17–21, Kobe, Japan. Springer (2016)
129. Eldesouky, B., Maus, H., Schwarz, S., Dengel, A.: Seed, a natural language interface to knowledge bases. In: Yamamoto, S. (ed.) Human Interface and the Management of Information. Information and Knowledge Design, *LNCS*, vol. 9172, pp. 280–290. Springer (2015)
130. Ericcson, K.A., Chase, W.G., Faloon, S.: Acquisition of a memory skill. Science **208**(4448), 1181–1182 (1980)
131. Everingham, M., Van Gool, L., Williams, C.K.I., Winn, J., Zisserman, A.: The PASCAL Visual Object Classes Challenge 2012 (VOC2012) Results
132. Evgeniou, T., Pontil, M.: Regularized multi–task learning. In: Proceedings of the 10th ACM SIGKDD International Conference on Knowledge Discovery and Data Mining (KDD '04), pp. 109–117. ACM, NY, USA (2004)
133. Fagni, T., Perego, R., Silvestri, F., Orlando, S.: Boosting the performance of web search engines: caching and prefetching query results by exploiting historical usage data. ACM Trans. Inf. Syst. **24**(1), 51–78 (2006). https://doi.org/10.1145/1125857.1125859
134. Faidi, T., Chaieb, F., Ghorbel, F.: A new multi-resolution affine invariant planar contour descriptor. In: International Conference on Image Analysis and Processing, pp. 494–505. Springer (2015)
135. Fang, Y., Chang, M.W.: Entity linking on microblogs with spatial and temporal signals. Trans. Assoc. Comput. Linguist. **2**, 259–272 (2014)
136. Ferragina, P., Scaiella, U.: Fast and accurate annotation of short texts with wikipedia pages. IEEE Softw. 70–75 (2012)
137. Firth, J.R.: A Synopsis of Linguistic Theory, 1930–1955. Special Volume of The Philological Society (1957)
138. Fischer, P., Dosovitskiy, A., Brox, T.: Descriptor Matching with Convolutional Neural Networks: a Comparison to Sift (2014). arXiv:1405.5769
139. Fitchett, S., Cockburn, A.: Accessrank: Predicting what users will do next. In: Proceedings of the SIGCHI Conference on Human Factors in Computing Systems, CHI '12, pp. 2239–2242. ACM, New York, NY, USA (2012). https://doi.org/10.1145/2207676.2208380
140. Fitzgerald, J.M., Lawrence, R.: Autobiographical memory across the life-span. J. Gerontol. **39**(6), 692–698 (1984)
141. Forman, G.: An extensive empirical study of feature selection metrics for text classification. J. Mach. Learn. Res. **3**, 1289–1305 (2003)
142. Frohlich, D., Fennell, J.: Sound, paper and memorabilia: resources for a simpler digital photography. Personal Ubiquitous Comput. **11**(2), 107–116 (2007)
143. Fu, M., Ceroni, A., Solachidis, V., Niederée, C., Papadopoulou, O., Kanhabua, N., Mezaris, V.: Learning personalized expectation-oriented photo selection models for personal photo collections. In: IEEE International Conference on Multimedia and Expo Workshops, ICME Workshops, pp. 1–6 (2015)

144. Galton, F.: Psychometric experiments. Brain **2**(2), 149–162 (1879)
145. Gargi, U.: Consumer media capture: Time-based analysis and event clustering. HP-Labs Tech Report (2003)
146. Geng, X., Liu, T.Y., Qin, T., Li, H.: Feature selection for ranking. In: Proceedings of SIGIR'07, pp. 407–414 (2007)
147. Girshick, R., Donahue, J., Darrell, T., Malik, J.: Rich feature hierarchies for accurate object detection and semantic segmentation. In: Proceedings of the IEEE Conference on Computer Vision and Pattern Recognition (CVPR) (2014)
148. Gladney, H.M.: Preserving Digital Information. Springer, Berlin (2007). https://doi.org/10.1007/978-3-540-37887-7
149. Glück, J., Bluck, S.: Looking back across the life span: a life story account of the reminiscence bump. Mem. Cognit. **35**(8), 1928–1939 (2007)
150. Goetz, T.: Harnessing the Power of Feedback Loops. WIRED Magazine (2011). http://www.wired.com/magazine/2011/06/ff_feedbackloop/
151. Goldberg, D., Nichols, D., Oki, B.M., Terry, D.: Using collaborative filtering to weave an information tapestry. Commun. ACM **35**(12), 61–70 (1992). https://doi.org/10.1145/138859.138867
152. Gorrell, G., Petrak, J., Bontcheva, K.: Using @Twitter conventions to improve #lod-based named entity disambiguation. In: The Semantic Web. Latest Advances and New Domains, pp. 171–186. Springer, Berlin (2015)
153. Gowans, G., Campbell, J., Alm, N., Dye, R., Astell, A., Ellis, M.: Designing a multimedia conversation aid for reminiscence therapy in dementia care environments. In: CHI'04 Extended Abstracts on Human Factors in Computing Systems, pp. 825–836. ACM (2004)
154. Grand Challenge at ACM Multimedia Conference (MM'13): NHK Where is beauty (2013). http://acmmm13.org/subm-issions/call-for-multimedia-grand-challenge-solutions/task-where-is-beauty/
155. Greenberg, D.L.: President bush's false [flashbulb] memory of 9/11/01. Appl. Cognit. Psychol. **18**(3), 363–370 (2004)
156. Grimnes, G.A., Adrian, B., Schwarz, S., Maus, H., Schumacher, K., Sauermann, L.: Semantic desktop for the end-user. i-com **8**(3), 25–32 (2009)
157. Guo, S., Chang, M.W., Kıcıman, E.: To link or not to link? a study on end-to-end tweet entity linking. NAACL-HLT **2013**, 1020–1030 (2013)
158. Hanley, J.A., McNeil, B.J.: The meaning and use of the area under a receiver operating characteristic (roc) curve. Radiology **143**(1), 29–36 (1982)
159. Harada, S., Naaman, M., Song, Y.J., Wang, Q., Paepcke, A.: Lost in memories: interacting with photo collections on PDAS. In: Proceedings of the 4th ACM/IEEE-CS Joint Conference on Digital Libraries, pp. 325–333. ACM (2004)
160. Harvey, R.: Appraisal and Selection, Chapter 1, pp. 6–39. Digital Curation Center (2007)
161. Harvey, R., Thompson, D.: Automating the appraisal of digital materials. Libr. Hi Tech **28**(2), 313–322 (2010). https://doi.org/10.1108/07378831011047703
162. He, B., Ounis, I.: Inferring query performance using pre-retrieval predictors. In: Proceedings of the Symposium on String Processing and Information Retrieval (2004)
163. Henkel, L.A.: Point-and-shoot memories: the influence of taking photos on memory for a museum tour. Psychol. Sci. **25**(2), 396–402 (2014)
164. Heutelbeck, D., Brunsmann, J., Wilkes, W., Hundsdörfer, A.: Motivations and challenges for digital preservation in design and engineering InDP 2009. In: Proceedings of the First International Workshop on Innovation in Digital Preservation in Conjunction with JCDL 2009. Austin TX, USA (2009)
165. Ho, W.C., Dautenhahn, K., Lim, M.Y., Vargas, P.A., Aylett, R., Enz, S.: An initial memory model for virtual and robot companions supporting migration and long-term interaction. In: The 18th IEEE International Symposium on Robot and Human Interactive Communication, 2009. RO-MAN 2009, pp. 277–284. IEEE (2009)
166. Ho, W.C., Dautenhahn, K., Nehaniv, C.L.: Computational memory architectures for autobiographic agents interacting in a complex virtual environment: a working model. Connect. Sci. **20**(1), 21–65 (2008)

167. Hodges, S., Berry, E., Wood, K.: Sensecam: a wearable camera that stimulates and rehabilitates autobiographical memory. Memory **19**(7), 685–696 (2011)
168. Hoffart, J., Yosef, M.A., Bordino, I., Fürstenau, H., Pinkal, M., Spaniol, M., Taneva, B., Thater, S., Weikum, G.: Robust disambiguation of named entities in text. In: Proceedings of the Conference on Empirical Methods in Natural Language Processing, EMNLP '11, pp. 782–792 (2011)
169. Hohman, T.J., Peynircioğlu, Z.F., Beason-Held, L.L.: Flexibility of event boundaries in autobiographical memory. Memory **21**(2), 249–260 (2013)
170. Hohpe, G., Woolf, B.: Enterprise Integration Patterns: Designing, Building, and Deploying Messaging Solutions. Addison-Wesley Longman Publishing Co., Inc., Boston, MA, USA (2003)
171. Hook, E.: Where to Position that Horizon? (Published in Digital Photography School, May, 2013). http://goo.gl/vU1g46
172. van den Hoven, E., Eggen, B.: Informing augmented memory system design through autobiographical memory theory. Personal Ubiquitous Comput. **12**(6), 433–443 (2008)
173. Hutař, J.: Archives New Zealand Migration from Fedora Commons to the Rosetta Digital Preservation System. iPRES2013 Proceedings (2013)
174. Hyun, J., Kim, H.K., Oh, W.G.: Study on performance of mpeg-7 visual descriptors for deformable object retrieval. In: 21st Korea-Japan Joint Workshop on Frontiers of Computer Vision (FCV), pp. 1–5. IEEE (2015)
175. Ingwersen, P., Järvelin, K.: The Turn: Integration of Information Seeking and Retrieval in Context (The Information Retrieval Series). Springer, New York Inc., Secaucus, NJ, USA (2005)
176. ISO/IEC: FDIS 23000-15 - Information technology – Multimedia application format (MPEG-A) – Part 15: Multimedia preservation application. http://www.iso.org/iso/catalogue_detail.htm?csnumber=66430 (2016). Accessed Sep 2017
177. Isurin, L., Mcdonald, J.L.: Retroactive interference from translation equivalents: implications for first language forgetting. Mem. Cognit. **29**(2), 312–319 (2001)
178. Jégou, H., Chum, O.: Negative evidences and co-occurences in image retrieval: the benefit of pca and whitening. Comput. Vis. ECCV **2012**, 774–787 (2012)
179. Jegou, H., Douze, M., Schmid, C.: Hamming embedding and weak geometric consistency for large scale image search. Comput. Vis. ECCV 304–317 (2008)
180. Jégou, H., Douze, M., Schmid, C., Pérez, P.: Aggregating local descriptors into a compact image representation. In: Conference on Computer Vision and Pattern Recognition (CVPR), pp. 3304–3311. IEEE (2010)
181. Jia, Y., Shelhamer, E., Donahue, J., Karayev, S., Long, J., Girshick, R., Guadarrama, S., Darrell, T.: Caffe: Convolutional architecture for fast feature embedding. In: Proceedings of the 22nd ACM International Conference on Multimedia, pp. 675–678. ACM (2014)
182. Jiang, Y.G., Ngo, C.W., Yang, J.: Towards optimal bag-of-features for object categorization and semantic video retrieval. In: Proceedings of the 6th ACM International Conference on Image and Video Retrieval, CIVR '07, pp. 494–501. ACM, NY, USA (2007)
183. Jilek, C., Maus, H., Schwarz, S., Dengel, A.: Diary generation from personal information models to support contextual remembering and reminiscence. In: IEEE International Conference on Multimedia and Expo Workshops, ICME Workshops 2015, Turin, Italy, pp. 1–6 (2015)
184. Jinda-Apiraksa, A., Vonikakis, V., Winkler, S.: California-ND: an annotated dataset for near-duplicate detection in personal photo collections. In: 5th International Workshop on Quality of Multimedia Experience (QoMEX), pp. 142–147. IEEE (2013)
185. Joachims, T.: Optimizing search engines using clickthrough data. In: Proceedings of KDD'02, pp. 133–142 (2002)
186. John, J.L., Rowlands, I., Williams, P., Dean, K.: Digital lives: Personal digital archives for the 21st century – an initial synthesis. Research paper Beta Version 0.2, British Library (2010). http://britishlibrary.typepad.co.uk/files/digital-lives-synthesis02-1.pdf. Accessed 16 Oct 2016

187. John Walker, S.: Big Data: A Revolution that Will Transform How We Live, Work, and Think (2014)
188. Jones, W.: Keeping Found Things Found: The Study and Practice of Personal Information Management. Morgan Kaufmann (2007)
189. Julius, M.: Themen in Sozialen Netzwerken (topics in social networks). blog (2013). http://multimedia-memories.tumblr.com/post/45185122672/. Accessed 16 Oct 2017
190. Kalnikaitė, V., Whittaker, S.: A saunter down memory lane: digital reflection on personal mementos. Int. J. Hum. Comput. Stud. **69**(5), 298–310 (2011)
191. Kanhabua, N., Niederée, C., Siberski, W.: Towards concise preservation by managed forgetting: Research issues and case study. In: Proceedings of the 10th International Conference on Preservation of Digital Objects (iPres) (2013)
192. Kanhabua, N., Nørvåg, K.: Determining time of queries for re-ranking search results. In: Proceedings of the 14th European Conference on Research and Advanced Technology for Digital Libraries, ECDL'10, pp. 261–272 (2010)
193. Kao, S.H., Day, W.Y., Cheng, P.J.: An aesthetic-based approach to re-ranking web images. In: Information Retrieval Technology, pp. 610–623. Springer, Berlin (2010)
194. Kärkkäinen, T., Kaakinen, A., Vainio, T., Väänänen-Vainio-Mattila, K.: Design guidelines for managing metadata for personal content on mobile devices. In: Proceedings of the 7th International Conference on Mobile and Ubiquitous Multimedia, pp. 162–167. ACM (2008)
195. Karpicke, J.D., Roediger, H.L.: Repeated retrieval during learning is the key to long-term retention. J. Mem. Lang. **57**(2), 151–162 (2007)
196. Katifori, A., Vassilakis, C., Dix, A.: Ontologies and the brain: Using spreading activation through ontologies to support personal interaction. Cognit. Syst. Res. **11**(1), 25 – 41 (2010). https://doi.org/10.1016/j.cogsys.2009.02.001. http://www.sciencedirect.com/science/article/pii/S1389041709000138. Brain Informatics
197. Kawase, R., Papadakis, G., Herder, E., Nejdl, W.: Beyond the usual suspects: context-aware revisitation support. In: ACM Hypertext, pp. 27–36 (2011). https://doi.org/10.1145/1995966.1995974
198. Kaya Kızılöz, B., Tekcan, A.I.: Canonical categories in flashbulb memories. Appl. Cognit. Psychol. **27**(3), 352–359 (2013)
199. Kaye, J.J., Vertesi, J., Avery, S., Dafoe, A., David, S., Onaga, L., Rosero, I., Pinch, T.: To have and to hold: exploring the personal archive. In: Proceedings of the SIGCHI Conference on Human Factors in Computing Systems, CHI '06, pp. 275–284. ACM, New York, NY, USA (2006). https://doi.org/10.1145/1124772.1124814
200. Ke, Y., Tang, X., Jing, F.: The design of high-level features for photo quality assessment. In: IEEE Computer Society Conference on Computer Vision and Pattern Recognition, vol. 1, pp. 419–426 (2006)
201. Kejser, U.B., Nielsen, A.B., Thirifays, A.: Cost model for digital preservation: cost of digital migration. IJDC **6**(1), 255–267 (2011)
202. Kelly, P., Marshall, S.J., Badland, H., Kerr, J., Oliver, M., Doherty, A.R., Foster, C.: An ethical framework for automated, wearable cameras in health behavior research. Am. J. Prev. Med. **44**(3), 314–319 (2013)
203. Kesireddi, R.C., Raj, G.: Embedding, extracting and matching of fingerprint images using digital watermarking. In: Proceedings of the International Conference on Advanced Research in Computer Science Engineering and Technology (ICARCSET), ICARCSET '15. ACM, New York, NY, USA (2015)
204. Kimeldorf, G., Wahba, G.: Some results on Tchebycheffian spline functions. J. Math. Anal. Appl. **33**(1), 82–95 (1971)
205. Kindberg, T., Spasojevic, M., Fleck, R., Sellen, A.: How and why people use camera phones. HP Laboratories Technical Report HPL-2004–216 (2004)
206. Kirk, D., Sellen, A., Rother, C., Wood, K.: Understanding photowork. In: Proceedings of the SIGCHI Conference on Human Factors in Computing Systems, pp. 761–770. ACM (2006)
207. Koppel, J., Brown, A.D., Stone, C.B., Coman, A., Hirst, W.: Remembering president barack obama's inauguration and the landing of us airways flight 1549: a comparison of the predictors of autobiographical and event memory. Memory **21**(7), 798–806 (2013)

208. Koutstaal, W., Schacter, D.L., Johnson, M.K., Angell, K.E., Gross, M.S.: Post-event review in older and younger adults: improving memory accessibility of complex everyday events. Psychol. Aging **13**(2), 277 (1998)
209. Koutstaal, W., Schacter, D.L., Johnson, M.K., Galluccio, L.: Facilitation and impairment of event memory produced by photograph review. Mem. Cognit. **27**(3), 478–493 (1999)
210. Krizhevsky, A., Ilya, S., Hinton, G.: ImageNet classification with deep convolutional neural networks. In: Advances in Neural Information Processing Systems (NIPS 2012), pp. 1097–1105. Curran Associates, Inc., New York (2012)
211. Kumar, A., Daume, H.: Learning task grouping and overlap in multi-task learning. In: Langford, J., Pineau, J. (eds.) Proceedings of the 29th International Conference on Machine Learning (ICML-12), pp. 1383–1390. ACM, NY, USA (2012)
212. Kuny, T.: A digital dark ages? Challenges in the preservation of electronic information. In: 63RD IFLA Council and General Conference, Workshop on Audiovisual and Multimedia joint with Preservation and Conservation, Information Technology, Library Buildings and Equipment, and the PAC Core Programme (1997)
213. Kurby, C.A., Zacks, J.M.: Segmentation in the perception and memory of events. Trends Cognit. Sci. **12**(2), 72–79 (2008)
214. Kuwahara, N., Abe, S., Yasuda, K., Kuwabara, K.: Networked reminiscence therapy for individuals with dementia by using photo and video sharing. In: Proceedings of the 8th international ACM SIGACCESS Conference on Computers and Accessibility, pp. 125–132. ACM (2006)
215. Kvavilashvili, L., Mirani, J., Schlagman, S., Kornbrot, D.E.: Comparing flashbulb memories of september 11 and the death of princess diana: effects of time delays and nationality. Appl. Cognit. Psychol. **17**(9), 1017–1031 (2003)
216. Lakatos, I.: Proofs and refutations (i). Br. J. Philos. Sci. **14**(53), 1–25 (1963)
217. Lampasona, C., Rostanin, O., Maus, H.: Seamless integration of order processing in ms outlook using smartoffice: an empirical evaluation. In: ESEM '12 Proceedings of the ACM-IEEE International Symposium on Empirical Software Engineering and Measurement. ACM Press (2012). https://doi.org/10.1145/2372251.2372281
218. Landauer, T.K., Bjork, R.A.: Optimum rehearsal patterns and name learning. Pract. Asp. Mem. **1**, 625–632 (1978)
219. Lang, J., Marquis, P.: Reasoning under inconsistency: a forgetting-based approach. Artif. Intell. **174**(12–13), 799–823 (2010)
220. Lantz, B.: Photography Composition Tips and Techniques (Published in Macro Photography, 2013). http://goo.gl/fsx20y
221. Lappas, T., Arai, B., Platakis, M., Kotsakos, D., Gunopulos, D.: On burstiness-aware search for document sequences. In: Proceedings of the 15th ACM SIGKDD International Conference on Knowledge Discovery and Data Mining, KDD '09, pp. 477–486 (2009)
222. Lavoie, B., Dempsey, L.: Thirteen ways of looking at...digital preservation. D-Lib Mag. **10**(7/8) (2004). http://dblp.uni-trier.de/db/journals/dlib/dlib10.html
223. LeCun, Y., Bengio, Y., Hinton, G.: Deep learning. Nature **521**(7553), 436–444 (2015)
224. Lee, C.J., Chen, R.C., Kao, S.H., Cheng, P.J.: A term dependency-based approach for query terms ranking. In: Proceedings of the 18th ACM Conference on Information and Knowledge Management, CIKM '09, pp. 1267–1276 (2009)
225. Lehmann, J., Gonçalves, B., Ramasco, J.J., Cattuto, C.: Dynamical classes of collective attention in twitter. In: Proceedings of the 21st International Conference on World Wide Web, WWW '12, pp. 251–260 (2012)
226. Lei, Y., Zheng, L., Huang, J.: Geometric invariant features in the radon transform domain for near-duplicate image detection. Pattern Recognit. Lett. **47**(11), 3630–3640 (2014)
227. Levine, B., Svoboda, E., Hay, J.F., Winocur, G., Moscovitch, M.: Aging and autobiographical memory: dissociating episodic from semantic retrieval. Psychol. Aging **17**(4), 677 (2002)
228. Li, C., Loui, A.C., Chen, T.: Towards aesthetics: a photo quality assessment and photo selection system. In: Proceedings of the International Conference on Multimedia, pp. 827–830. ACM (2010)

229. Li, J., Lim, J.H., Tian, Q.: Automatic summarization for personal digital photos. In: Fourth International Conference on Information, Communications and Signal Processing, 2003 and the Fourth Pacific Rim Conference on Multimedia. Proceedings of the 2003 Joint, vol. 3, pp. 1536–1540 vol.3 (2003)
230. Li, X., Larson, M., Hanjalic, A.: Pairwise geometric matching for large-scale object retrieval. In: Proceedings of the Conference on Computer Vision and Pattern Recognition, pp. 5153–5161. IEEE (2015)
231. Li, Y., Sheopuri, A.: Applying image analysis to assess food aesthetics and uniqueness. In: Proceedings of International Conference on Image Processing (ICIP), pp. 311–314. IEEE (2015)
232. Library of Congress: Personal archiving: preserving your digital memories. http://www.digitalpreservation.gov/personalarchiving. Accessed 16 Oct 2017
233. Library of Congress, M.E.B.: Metadata encoding and transmission standard, Version 1.11. http://www.loc.gov/standards/mets (2015). Accessed Sep 2017
234. Library of Congress: Preserving digital memories. In: 7th International Conference on Preservation of Digital Objects (iPRES 2010) (2010). http://www.digitalpreservation.gov/personalarchiving/documents/NDIIP_PA_poster.pdf Accessed 16 Oct 2017
235. Library of Congress, P.E.C.: PREMIS data dictionary for preservation metadata, Version 3.0. http://www.loc.gov/standards/premis/v3/index.html (2015). Accessed Sep 2017
236. Lim, M.Y.: Memory Models for Intelligent Social Companions (2012)
237. Lim, M.Y., Aylett, R., Ho, W.C., Enz, S., Vargas, P.: A socially-aware memory for companion agents. In: International Workshop on Intelligent Virtual Agents, pp. 20–26. Springer (2009)
238. Lim, M.Y., Aylett, R., Vargas, P.A., Ho, W.C., Dias, J.: Human-like memory retrieval mechanisms for social companions. In: The 10th International Conference on Autonomous Agents and Multiagent Systems, vol. 3, pp. 1117–1118. International Foundation for Autonomous Agents and Multiagent Systems (2011)
239. Lin, C.Y.: Rouge: a package for automatic evaluation of summaries. In: Text Summarization Branches Out: Proceedings of the ACL-04 Workshop, vol. 8 (2004)
240. Lindley, S.E.: Before i forget: from personal memory to family history. Hum. Comput. Interact. **27**(1–2), 13–36 (2012)
241. Lindsay, R.C.: Handbook Of Eyewitness Psychology 2 Volume Set. Psychology Press (2014)
242. Linton, M.: Memory for Real-world Events. Explorations in Cognition, pp. 376–404 (1975)
243. Liu, D.C., Nocedal, J.: On the limited memory BFGS method for large scale optimization. Math. Progr. **45**(1–3), 503–528 (1989)
244. Liu, J., Huang, Z., Cai, H., Shen, H.T., Ngo, C.W., Wang, W.: Near-duplicate video retrieval: current research and future trends. Comput. Surv. (CSUR) **45**(4), 44 (2013)
245. Liu, T.Y.: Learning to rank for information retrieval. Found. Trends Inf. Retr. **3**(3), 225–331 (2009)
246. Lo, K.Y., Liu, K.H., Chen, C.S.: Assessment of photo aesthetics with efficiency. In: 21st International Conference on Pattern Recognition (ICPR), pp. 2186–2189. IEEE (2012)
247. Lo, K.Y., Liu, K.H., Chen, C.S.: Intelligent photographing interface with on-device aesthetic quality assessment. In: Computer Vision-ACCV 2012 Workshops, pp. 533–544. Springer (2013)
248. Loftus, E.F., Palmer, J.C.: Reconstruction of automobile destruction: an example of the interaction between language and memory. J. Verb. Learn. Verb. Behav. **13**(5), 585–589 (1974)
249. Logie, R., Hunter, J., McIntosh, N., Gilhooly, K., Alberdi, E., Reiss, J.: Medical cognition and computer support in the intensive care unit: a cognitive engineering approach. In: Engineering Psychology and Cognitive Ergonomics: Integration of Theory and Application, pp. 167–174 (1997)
250. Logie, R., Wright, R., Decker, S.: Recognition memory performance and residential burglary. Appl. Cognit. Psychol. **6**(2), 109–123 (1992)
251. Logie, R.H.: Spatial and visual working memory: a mental workspace. Psychol. Learn. Mot. **42**, 37–78 (2003)

252. Logie, R.H.: The functional organization and capacity limits of working memory. Current Directions Psychol. Sci. **20**(4), 240–245 (2011). https://doi.org/10.1177/0963721411415340
253. Logie, R.H.: Visuo-spatial Working Memory. Psychology Press (2014)
254. Loui, A.C., Savakis, A.: Automated event clustering and quality screening of consumer pictures for digital albuming. IEEE Trans. Multimed. **5**(3), 390–402 (2003)
255. Lowe, D.G.: Distinctive image features from scale-invariant keypoints. Int. J. Comput. Vis. **60**(2), 91–110 (2004)
256. Lu, Y., Wan, Y.: PHA: a fast potential-based hierarchical agglomerative clustering method. Pattern Recognit. Lett. **46**(5), 1227–1239 (2013)
257. Lucero, A., Boberg, M., Uusitalo, S.: Image space: capturing, sharing and contextualizing personal pictures in a simple and playful way. In: Proceedings of the International Conference on Advances in Computer Entertainment Technology, ACE '09, pp. 215–222. ACM, New York, NY, USA (2009). https://doi.org/10.1145/1690388.1690424
258. Luminet, O., Curci, A.: Flashbulb Memories: New Issues and New Perspectives. Psychology Press (2008)
259. Luo, Y., Tang, X.: Photo and video quality evaluation: focusing on the subject. In: Computer Vision–ECCV, pp. 386–399. Springer, Berlin (2008)
260. Maguire, E.A.: Neuroimaging studies of autobiographical event memory. Philos. Trans. R. Soc. Lond. B Biol. Sci. **356**(1413), 1441–1451 (2001)
261. Maji, S., Berg, A., Malik, J.: Classification using intersection kernel support vector machines is efficient. In: IEEE Conference on Computer Vision and Pattern Recognition, 2008. CVPR 2008, pp. 1–8 (2008)
262. Manning, C.D., Raghavan, P., Schütze, H.: Introduction to Information Retrieval. Cambridge University Press, New York, NY, USA (2008)
263. Manning, C.D., Surdeanu, M., Bauer, J., Finkel, J., Bethard, S.J., McClosky, D.: The Stanford CoreNLP natural language processing toolkit. In: ACL '14 (2014)
264. Marchesotti, L., Perronnin, F., Larlus, D., Csurka, G.: Assessing the aesthetic quality of photographs using generic image descriptors. In: IEEE International Conference on Computer Vision (ICCV), pp. 1784–1791 (2011)
265. Marée, R., Geurts, P., Wehenkel, L.: Content-based image retrieval by indexing random subwindows with randomized trees. In: Asian Conference on Computer Vision, pp. 611–620. Springer (2007)
266. Markatopoulou, F., Mezaris, V., Patras, I.: Cascade of classifiers based on binary, non-binary and deep convolutional network descriptors for video concept detection. In: Proceedings of the IEEE International Conference on Image Processing (ICIP 2015), pp. 1786–1790 (2015)
267. Markatopoulou, F., Mezaris, V., Patras, I.: Online multi-task learning for semantic concept detection in video. In: IEEE International Conference on Image Processing (ICIP), pp. 186–190 (2016)
268. Markatopoulou, F., Mezaris, V., Pittaras, N., Patras, I.: Local features and a two-layer stacking architecture for semantic concept detection in video. IEEE Trans. Emerg. Top. Comput. **3**(2), 193–204 (2015)
269. Markatopoulou, F., Pittaras, N., Papadopoulou, O., Mezaris, V., Patras, I.: A Study on the Use of a Binary Local Descriptor and Color Extensions of Local Descriptors for Video Concept Detection, pp. 282–293. Springer International Publishing, Cham (2015)
270. Marshall, C.C.: Challenges and Opportunities for Personal Digital Archiving. Digital: Personal Collections in the Digital Era, pp. 90–114 (2011)
271. Marshall, C.C.: I, Digital: Personal Collections in the Digital Era. Society of American Archivists (2011)
272. Mather, M., Carstensen, L.L.: Aging and motivated cognition: the positivity effect in attention and memory. Trends Cognit. Sci. **9**(10), 496–502 (2005)
273. Maus, H., Schwarz, S., Dengel, A.: Weaving personal knowledge spaces into office applications. In: Integration of Practice-Oriented Knowledge Technology: Trends and Prospectives, pp. 71–82. Springer, Berlin (2013)

274. Maus, H., Schwarz, S., Haas, J., Dengel, A.: CONTASK: context-sensitive task assistance in the semantic desktop. In: Filipe, J., Cordeiro, J. (eds.) Enterprise Information Systems. 12th International Conference, ICEIS 2010, Funchal-Madeira, Portugal, June 8–12, 2010, Revised Selected Papers. Lecture Notes in Business Information Processing, vol. 73, pp. 177–192. Springer (2011). https://doi.org/10.1007/978-3-642-19802-1_13
275. Mavridaki, E., Mezaris, V.: No-reference blur assessment in natural images using fourier transform and spatial pyramids. In: Proceedings of International Conference on Image Processing (ICIP). IEEE (2014)
276. Mavridaki, E., Mezaris, V.: A comprehensive aesthetic quality assessment method for natural images using basic rules of photography. In: 2015 IEEE International Conference on Image Processing (ICIP), pp. 887–891. IEEE (2015)
277. Maxwell, K.T., Croft, W.B.: Compact query term selection using topically related text. In: Proceedings of the 36th International ACM SIGIR Conference on Research and Development in Information Retrieval, SIGIR '13, pp. 583–592 (2013)
278. Mayer-Schönberger, V.: Delete - The Virtue of Forgetting in the Digital Age. Morgan Kaufmann Publishers, Massachusetts (2009)
279. Mayer-Schönberger, V.: Delete: The Virtue of Forgetting in the Digital Age. Princeton University Press, Princeton (2011)
280. Maynard, D., Greenwood, M.A.: Who cares about sarcastic tweets? Investigating the impact of sarcasm on sentiment analysis. In: Proceedings of LREC 2014. Reykjavik, Iceland (2014)
281. Maynard, D., Roberts, I., Greenwood, M.A., Rout, D., Bontcheva, K.: A Framework for Real-time Semantic Social Media Analysis. Web Semantics: Science, Services and Agents on the World Wide Web (2017). https://doi.org/10.1016/j.websem.2017.05.002. http://www.sciencedirect.com/science/article/pii/S1570826817300240
282. McCamy, C.S.: Correlated color temperature as an explicit function of chromaticity coordinates. Color Res. Appl. **17**(2), 142–144 (1992)
283. McDaniel, M.A., Einstein, G.O.: Strategic and automatic processes in prospective memory retrieval: a multiprocess framework. Appl. Cognit. Psychol. **14**(7) (2000)
284. McDaniel, M.A., Einstein, G.O.: Strategic and automatic processes in prospective memory retrieval: a multiprocess framework. Appl. Cognit. Psychol. **14**, 127–144 (2000)
285. McDaniel, M.A., Einstein, G.O.: Prospective Memory: An Overview and Synthesis of an Emerging Field. SAGE Publications, Inc., California (2007)
286. McGee-Lennon, M.R., Wolters, M.K., Brewster, S.: User-centred multimodal reminders for assistive living. In: Proceedings of the SIGCHI Conference on Human Factors in Computing Systems, pp. 2105–2114. ACM (2011)
287. McGeoch, J.A., McDonald, W.T.: Meaningful relation and retroactive inhibition. Am. J. Psychol. **43**(4), 579–588 (1931)
288. McKENNA, S.P., Glendon, A.: Occupational first aid training: decay in cardiopulmonary resuscitation (CPR) skills. J. Occup. Organ. Psychol. **58**(2), 109–117 (1985)
289. McLaren, K.: Xiiithe development of the cie 1976 (l* a* b*) uniform colour space and colour-difference formula. J. Soc. Dyers Colour. **92**(9), 338–341 (1976)
290. Meeker, M., Wu, L.: Internet trends. Technical report, Kleiner Perkins Caufield and Byers (2013)
291. Mei, T., Wang, B., Hua, X.S., Zhou, H.Q., Li, S.: Probabilistic multimodality fusion for event based home photo clustering. In: 2006 IEEE International Conference on Multimedia and Expo, pp. 1757–1760. IEEE (2006)
292. Meij, E., Weerkamp, W., de Rijke, M.: Adding semantics to microblog posts. In: Proceedings of the Fifth ACM International Conference on Web Search and Data Mining, pp. 563–572 (2012)
293. Meyer, J.: Emotional Images: How to add Feeling with Muted Tones and Harmonious Color (Published in Digital Camera World, March 28, 2013). https://goo.gl/7uV9iz
294. Mezaris, V., Sidiropoulos, P., Dimou, A., Kompatsiaris, I.: On the use of visual soft semantics for video temporal decomposition to scenes. In: 2010 IEEE Fourth International Conference on Semantic Computing (ICSC), pp. 141–148 (2010). https://doi.org/10.1109/ICSC.2010.23

295. Mihalcea, R., Csomai, A.: Wikify!: Linking documents to encyclopedic knowledge. In: Proceedings of the Sixteenth ACM Conference on Conference on Information and Knowledge Management, CIKM '07, pp. 233–242 (2007)
296. Mikolajczyk, K., Tuytelaars, T., Schmid, C., Zisserman, A., Matas, J., Schaffalitzky, F., Kadir, T., Van Gool, L.: A comparison of affine region detectors. Int. J. Comput. Vis. **65**(1–2), 43–72 (2005)
297. Miller, G.A.: The magical number seven, plus or minus two: some limits on our capacity for processing information. Psychol. Rev. **63**(2), 81 (1956)
298. Milne, D., Witten, I.H.: Learning to link with wikipedia. In: Proceedings of the 17th ACM Conference on Information and Knowledge Management, CIKM '08, pp. 509–518 (2008)
299. Mirzasoleiman, B., Badanidiyuru, A., Karbasi, A.: Fast constrained submodular maximization: Personalized data summarization. In: Proceedings of the 33nd International Conference on Machine Learning, ICML, pp. 1358–1367 (2016)
300. Mitra, S., Winslett, M., Hsu, W.W.: Query-based partitioning of documents and indexes for information lifecycle management. In: Proceedings of the 2008 ACM SIGMOD international conference on Management of data, SIGMOD '08, pp. 623–636 (2008). https://doi.org/10.1145/1376616.1376680
301. Mols, I., Hoven, E.v.d., Eggen, B.: Making memories: a cultural probe study into the remembering of everyday life. In: Proceedings of the 8th Nordic Conference on Human-Computer Interaction: Fun, Fast, Foundational, NordiCHI '14, pp. 256–265. ACM (2014)
302. Moorthy, A.K., Obrador, P., Oliver, N.: Towards computational models of the visual aesthetic appeal of consumer videos. In: Proceedings of the 11th European Conference on Computer Vision (ECCV), Heraklion, Crete, Greece, 2010, pp. 1–14. Springer (2010)
303. Morris, P.E., Tweedy, M., Gruneberg, M.M.: Interest, knowledge and the memorizing of soccer scores. Br. J. Psychol. **76**(4), 415–425 (1985)
304. Mothe, J., Tanguy, L.: Linguistic features to predict query difficulty. In: ACM SIGIR 2005 Workshop on Predicting Query Difficulty - Methods and Applications (2005)
305. Mousavi, H., Srinivas, U., Monga, V., Suo, Y., Dao, M., Tran, T.: Multi-task image classification via collaborative, hierarchical spike-and-slab priors. In: Proceedings of the IEEE International Conference on Image Processing (ICIP 2014), pp. 4236–4240 (2014)
306. Murray, N., Marchesotti, L., Perronnin, F.: AVA: a large-scale database for aesthetic visual analysis. In: IEEE Conference on Computer Vision and Pattern Recognition (CVPR), pp. 2408–2415 (2012)
307. Murray, N., Marchesotti, L., Perronnin, F., Meylan, F.: Learning to rank images using semantic and aesthetic labels. In: BMVC, pp. 1–10 (2012)
308. Nathan, L., Shaffer, E.: Preserving social media: opening a multi-disciplinary dialogue. In: Proceedings of the The Memory of the World in the Digital Age: Digitization and Preservation. Vancouver, BC, 26–28 September 2012. UNESCO (2013)
309. Ng, J., Yang, F., Davis, L.: Exploiting local features from deep networks for image retrieval. In: Proceedings of the Conference on Computer Vision and Pattern Recognition Workshops, pp. 53–61. IEEE (2015)
310. Niederee, C., Kanhabua, N., Gallo, F., Logie, R.H.: Forgetful digital memory: towards brain-inspired long-term data and information management. SIGMOD Rec. **44**(2), 41–46 (2015). https://doi.org/10.1145/2814710.2814718
311. Niu, Y., Liu, F.: What makes a professional video? a computational aesthetics approach. IEEE Trans. Circuits Syst. Video Technol. **22**(7), 1037–1049 (2012)
312. OASIS: Content Management Interoperability Services (CMIS) Version 1.1. OASIS Standard. https://docs.oasis-open.org/cmis/CMIS/v1.1/CMIS-v1.1.html (2013). Accessed Sep 2017
313. Obozinski, G., Taskar, B.: Multi-task feature selection. In: Proceedings of the 23rd International Conference on Machine Learning (ICML 2006). Workshop of Structural Knowledge Transfer for Machine Learning. Pittsburgh, Pennsylvania (2006)
314. Obrador, P., De Oliveira, R., Oliver, N.: Supporting personal photo storytelling for social albums. In: Proceedings of the 18th ACM International Conference on Multimedia, pp. 561–570. ACM (2010)

315. Oliva, A., Torralba, A.: Modeling the shape of the scene: a holistic representation of the spatial envelope. Int. J. Comput. Vis. **42**(3), 145–175 (2001)
316. Oquab, M., Bottou, L., Laptev, I., Sivic, J.: Learning and transferring mid-level image representations using convolutional neural networks. In: CVPR (2014)
317. Owoputi, O., O'Connor, B., Dyer, C., Gimpel, K., Schneider, N., Smith, N.A.: Improved part-of-speech tagging for online conversational text with word clusters. NAACL-HLT **2013**, 380–390 (2013)
318. Page, L., Brin, S., Motwani, R., Winograd, T.: The pagerank citation ranking: Bringing order to the web. In: Proceedings of the 7th International World Wide Web Conference, pp. 161–172. Brisbane, Australia (1998). https://citeseer.nj.nec.com/page98pagerank.html
319. Päivärinta, T., Westerlund, P., Nilsson, J.: Integrating Contemporary Content Management and Long-term Digital Preservation: a Design Problem. Springer Verlag, Luleå University of Technology, Information Systems (2015)
320. Papadakis, G., Kawase, R., Herder, E., Niederée, C.: A layered approach to revisitation prediction. In: Proceedings of the 11th International Conference on Web Engineering, ICWE'11, pp. 258–273. Springer, Berlin (2011). http://dl.acm.org/citation.cfm?id=2027776.2027796
321. Papagiannopoulou, C., Mezaris, V.: Concept-based image clustering and summarization of event-related image collections. In: Proceedings of the 1st ACM International Workshop on Human Centered Event Understanding from Multimedia, pp. 23–28. ACM (2014)
322. Peetz, M.H., de Rijke, M.: Cognitive temporal document priors. In: Proceedings of the 35th European Conference on Advances in Information Retrieval, ECIR'13, pp. 318–330. Springer, Berlin (2013). https://doi.org/10.1007/978-3-642-36973-5_27
323. Perronnin, F., Sánchez, J., Mensink, T.: Improving the fisher kernel for large-scale image classification. In: Computer Vision ECCV, pp. 143–156 (2010)
324. Petrelli, D., van den Hoven, E., Whittaker, S.: Making history: intentional capture of future memories. In: Proceedings of the SIGCHI Conference on Human Factors in Computing Systems, CHI '09, pp. 1723–1732. ACM, New York, NY, USA (2009). https://doi.org/10.1145/1518701.1518966
325. Petrelli, D., Whittaker, S.: Family memories in the home: contrasting physical and digital mementos. Personal Ubiquitous Comput. **14**(2), 153–169 (2010)
326. Pezdek, K.: Event memory and autobiographical memory for the events of September 11, 2001. Appl. Cognit. Psychol. **17**(9), 1033–1045 (2003)
327. Philbin, J., Chum, O., Isard, M., Sivic, J., Zisserman, A.: Object retrieval with large vocabularies and fast spatial matching. In: Conference on Computer Vision and Pattern Recognition (CVPR), pp. 1–8. IEEE (2007)
328. Piolino, P., Desgranges, B., Eustache, F.: Episodic autobiographical memories over the course of time: cognitive, neuropsychological and neuroimaging findings. Neuropsychologia **47**(11), 2314–2329 (2009)
329. Pittaras, N., Markatopoulou, F., Mezaris, V., et al.: Comparison of Fine-Tuning and Extension Strategies for Deep Convolutional Neural Networks, pp. 102–114. Springer, Cham (2017)
330. Ponte, J.M., Croft, W.B.: A language modeling approach to information retrieval. In: Proceedings of the 21st Annual International ACM SIGIR Conference on Research and Development in Information Retrieval, SIGIR '98, pp. 275–281 (1998)
331. POWRR: Tool-grid (2013). http://digitalpowrr.niu.edu/tool-grid/. Accessed 16 Oct 2017
332. Pritchett, A.R.: Aviation automation: General perspectives and specific guidance for the design of modes and alerts. Rev. Hum. Factors Ergon. **5**(1), 82–113 (2009). https://doi.org/10.1518/155723409X448026
333. Rabbath, M., Sandhaus, P., Boll, S.: Automatic creation of photo books from stories in social media. In: Proceedings of Second ACM SIGMM Workshop on Social Media, WSM '10, pp. 15–20. ACM (2010)
334. Raiber, F., Kurland, O.: Query-performance prediction: setting the expectations straight. In: Proceedings of the 37th International ACM SIGIR Conference on Research and Development in Information Retrieval, SIGIR '14, pp. 13–22 (2014)

335. Rauch, J., Braud, M., Edelstein, O., Rabinovici-Cohen, S., Nagin, K., Marberg, J., Voets, D., Sanya, I., Badawy, M., Shebab, E., Randers, F., Droppert, J., Klecha, M.: Ensure: long term digital preservation of health care, clinical trial and financial data. In: Borbinha, J., Nelson, M., Knight, S. (eds.) iPRES 2013: Proceedings of the 10th International Conference on Preservation of Digital Objects (2013)
336. Reason, J.: Human Error. Cambridge University Press, Cambridge (1990)
337. Renoult, L., Davidson, P.S., Palombo, D.J., Moscovitch, M., Levine, B.: Personal semantics: at the crossroads of semantic and episodic memory. Trends Cognit. Sci. **16**(11), 550–558 (2012)
338. Richards, D., Bransky, K.: Forgetmenot: what and how users expect intelligent virtual agents to recall and forget personal conversational content. Int. J. Hum. Comput. Stud. **72**(5), 460–476 (2014)
339. Ritter, A., Clark, S., Mausam, Etzioni, O.: Named entity recognition in tweets: an experimental study. In: Proceedings of the Conference on Empirical Methods in Natural Language Processing, pp. 1524–1534 (2011)
340. Robertson, S.: A new interpretation of average precision. In: Proceedings of the 31st Annual International ACM SIGIR Conference on Research and Development in Information Retrieval, pp. 689–690. ACM (2008)
341. Robusto, C.C.: The cosine-haversine formula. Am. Math. Mon. **64**(1), 38–40 (1957)
342. Rocha, C., Schwabe, D., Aragao, M.P.: A hybrid approach for searching in the semantic web. In: Proceedings of the 13th International Conference on World Wide Web, WWW '04, pp. 374–383. ACM, New York, NY, USA (2004). https://doi.org/10.1145/988672.988723
343. Roediger, H.L., Marsh, E.J.: Episodic and Autobiographical Memory. Handbook of Psychology (2003)
344. Russ, A.L., Zillich, A.J., McManus, M.S., Doebbeling, B.N., Saleem, J.J.: Prescribers interactions with medication alerts at the point of prescribing: a multi-method, in situ investigation of the human-computer interaction. Int. J. Med. Inf. **81**(4), 232–243 (2012)
345. Russakovsky, O., Deng, J., et al., H.S.: ImageNet large scale visual recognition challenge. Int. J. Comput. Vis. (IJCV) **115**(3), 211–252 (2015). https://doi.org/10.1007/s11263-015-0816-y
346. Samani, Z.R., Moghaddam, M.E.: A knowledge-based semantic approach for image collection summarization. Multimed. Tools Appl. 1–23 (2016)
347. Sansone, E., Apostoldis, K., Conci, N., Boato, G., Mezaris, V., Natale, F.G.B.D.: Automatic synchronization of multi-user photo galleries. IEEE Trans. Multimed. (2017). https://doi.org/10.1109/TMM.2017.2655446
348. Sauermann, L.: The Gnowsis Semantic Desktop Approach to Personal Information Management. Ph.D. thesis, Fachbereich Informatik der Universitt Kaiserslautern (2009). http://www.dfki.uni-kl.de/~sauermann/papers/Sauermann2009phd.pdf
349. Sauermann, L., Bernardi, A., Dengel, A.: Overview and outlook on the semantic desktop. In: Decker, S., Park, J., Quan, D., Sauermann, L. (eds.) Proceedings of the First Semantic Desktop Workshop at the ISWC Conference 2005 (2005). http://www.dfki.uni-kl.de/~sauermann/papers/Sauermann+2005d.pdf
350. Sauermann, L., Dengel, A., van Elst, L., Lauer, A., Maus, H., Schwarz, S.: Personalization in the EPOS project. In: Proceedings of the Semantic Web Personalization Workshop at the ESWC 2006 (2006)
351. Sauermann, L., van Elst, L., Dengel, A.: PIMO – A Framework for Representing Personal Information Models. In: Pellegrini, T., Schaffert, S. (eds.) I-SEMANTICS Conference 5–7 September 2007, Graz, Austria, J.UCS, pp. 270–277. Know-Center, Austria (2007)
352. Sauermann, L., Heim, D.: Evaluating long-term use of the gnowsis semantic desktop for PIM. In: The Semantic Web. 7th International Semantic Web Conference (ISWC-2008), 7th International Semantic Web Conference, October 26–30, Karlsruhe, Germany. LNCS, vol. 5318, pp. 467–482. Springer (2008). http://www.springerlink.com/content/c7u686mq27751373/
353. Savakis, A.E., Etz, S.P., Loui, A.C.: Evaluation of image appeal in consumer photography. In: Electronic Imaging, pp. 111–120. International Society for Optics and Photonics (2000)

354. Schacter, D.L., Koutstaal, W., Johnson, M.K., Gross, M.S., Angell, K.E.: False recollection induced by photographs: a comparison of older and younger adults. Psychol. Aging **12**(2), 203 (1997)
355. Schellenberg, T.R.: The appraisal of modern records. Bull. Natl. Arch. **8**, 46 (1956)
356. Schölkopf, B., Herbrich, R., Smola, A.J.: A generalized representer theorem. In: Proceeding of 14th Annual Conference on Computational Learning Theory, pp. 416–426 (2001)
357. Schwarz, S.: Context-Awareness and Context-Sensitive Interfaces for Knowledge Work Support. Ph.D thesis, University of Kaiserslautern, Fachbereich Informatik (2010). http://www.dr.hut-verlag.de/978-3-86853-388-0.html
358. Seah, B.S., Bhowmick, S.S., Sun, A.: Prism: concept-preserving social image search results summarization. In: Proceedings of the 37th International ACM SIGIR Conference on Research and Development in Information Retrieval, SIGIR '14, pp. 737–746. ACM (2014)
359. Seamon, J.G., Moskowitz, T.N., Swan, A.E., Zhong, B., Golembeski, A., Liong, C., Narzikul, A.C., Sosan, O.A.: Sensecam reminiscence and action recall in memory-unimpaired people. Memory **22**(7), 861–866 (2014)
360. Sellen, A.J., Fogg, A., Aitken, M., Hodges, S., Rother, C., Wood, K.: Do life-logging technologies support memory for the past?: an experimental study using senseCam. In: Proceedings of the SIGCHI Conference on Human Factors in Computing Systems, pp. 81–90. ACM (2007)
361. Shen, W., Wang, J., Luo, P., Wang, M.: Linking named entities in tweets with knowledge base via user interest modeling. In: Proceedings of the 19th ACM SIGKDD International Conference on Knowledge Discovery and Data Mining, KDD '13, pp. 68–76 (2013)
362. Simond, F., Arvanitopoulos Darginis, N., Süsstrunk, S.: Image aesthetics depends on context. In: Proceedings of International Conference on Image Processing (ICIP). IEEE (2015)
363. Simonyan, K., Zisserman, A.: Very deep convolutional networks for large-scale image recognition. In: CoRR (2014). arXiv:abs/1409.1556
364. Singh, V., Elamvazuthi, I.: Fingerprint matching algorithm for poor quality images. J. Eng. **1**(1) (2015)
365. Sinha, P., Mehrotra, S., Jain, R.: Summarization of personal photologs using multidimensional content and context. In: Proceedings of the 1st ACM International Conference on Multimedia Retrieval, ICMR '11, pp. 4:1–4:8. ACM (2011)
366. Skobeltsyn, G., Junqueira, F., Plachouras, V., Baeza-Yates, R.: Resin: A combination of results caching and index pruning for high-performance web search engines. In: Proceedings of the 31st Annual International ACM SIGIR Conference on Research and Development in Information Retrieval, SIGIR '08, pp. 131–138. ACM, New York, NY, USA (2008). https://doi.org/10.1145/1390334.1390359
367. Smit, E., Van Der Hoeven, J., Giaretta, D.: Avoiding a digital dark age for data: why publishers should care about digital preservation. Learn. Publ. **24**(1), 35–49 (2011)
368. Snoek, C., Fontijne, D., van de Sande, K.E., Stokman, H.e.a.: Qualcomm research and university of Amsterdam at TRECVID 2015: recognizing concepts, objects, and events in video. In: Proceedings of TRECVID 2015. NIST, USA (2015)
369. Snoek, C.G.M., Worring, M.: Concept-based video retrieval. Found. Trends Inf. Retr. **2**(4), 215–322 (2009)
370. Sokal, R.R.: Classification: purposes, principles, progress, prospects. Science **185**(4157), 1115–1123 (1974)
371. Solli, M., Lenz, R.: Color emotions for image classification and retrieval. In: Conference on Colour in Graphics, Imaging, and Vision, vol. 2008, pp. 367–371. Society for Imaging Science and Technology (2008)
372. Spyromitros-Xioufis, E., Papadopoulos, S., Kompatsiaris, I.Y., Tsoumakas, G., Vlahavas, I.: A comprehensive study over vlad and product quantization in large-scale image retrieval. IEEE Trans. Multimed. **16**(6), 1713–1728 (2014)
373. St. Jacques, P.L., Levine, B.: Ageing and autobiographical memory for emotional and neutral events. Memory **15**(2), 129–144 (2007)
374. St. Jacques, P.L., Schacter, D.L.: Modifying memory: selectively enhancing and updating personal memories for a museum tour by reactivating them. Psychol. Sci. **24**(4), 537–543 (2013)

375. Subagdja, B., Wang, W., Tan, A.H., Tan, Y.S., Teow, L.N.: Memory formation, consolidation, and forgetting in learning agents. In: Proceedings of the 11th International Conference on Autonomous Agents and Multiagent Systems, vol. 2, pp. 1007–1014. International Foundation for Autonomous Agents and Multiagent Systems (2012)
376. Sun, G., Chen, Y., Liu, X., Wu, E.: Adaptive multi-task learning for fine-grained categorization. In: Proceedings of the IEEE International Conference on Image Processing (ICIP 2015), pp. 996–1000 (2015)
377. Szegedy, C., Liu, W., Jia, Y., Sermanet, P., Reed, S., Anguelov, D., Erhan, D., Vanhoucke, V., Rabinovich, A.: Going deeper with convolutions. In: Proceedings of the IEEE Conference on Computer Vision and Pattern Recognition, pp. 1–9 (2015)
378. Talarico, J.M., Rubin, D.C.: Confidence, not consistency, characterizes flashbulb memories. Psychol. Sci. **14**(5), 455–461 (2003)
379. Tang, X., Luo, W., Wang, X.: Content-based photo quality assessment. IEEE Trans. Multimed. (TMM) **15**, 1930–1943 (2013)
380. Tarjan, R.: Depth-first search and linear graph algorithms. SIAM J. Comput. **1**(2), 146–160 (1972)
381. Thimbleby, H.: Improving safety in medical devices and systems. In: 2013 IEEE International Conference on Healthcare Informatics (ICHI), pp. 1–13. IEEE (2013)
382. Tong, H., Li, M., Zhang, H.J., He, J., Zhang, C.: Classification of digital photos taken by photographers or home users. In: Advances in Multimedia Information Processing-PCM 2004, pp. 198–205. Springer, Berlin (2005)
383. Trad, M.R., Joly, A., Boujemaa, N.: Large scale visual-based event matching. In: Proceedings of the 1st ACM International Conference on Multimedia Retrieval, ICMR '11, pp. 53:1–53:7. ACM, New York, NY, USA (2011). https://doi.org/10.1145/1991996.1992049
384. Tran, N.K., Ceroni, A., Kanhabua, N., Niederée, C.: Back to the past: supporting interpretations of forgotten stories by time-aware re-contextualization. In: Proceedings of the Eighth ACM International Conference on Web Search and Data Mining, WSDM '15, pp. 339–348 (2015)
385. Tran, N.K., Ceroni, A., Kanhabua, N., Niederée, C.: Time-travel translator: automatically contextualizing news articles. In: Proceedings of the 24th International Conference on World Wide Web, WWW '15 Companion, pp. 247–250 (2015)
386. Tran, T., Nguyen, T.N.: Hedera: Scalable indexing and exploring entities in Wikipedia revision history. In: Proceedings of the 2014 International Conference on Posters and Demonstrations Track, ISWC-PD'14, vol. 1272, pp. 297–300 (2014)
387. Tran, T., Tran, N.K., Teka Hadgu, A., Jschke, R.: Semantic annotation for microblog topics using Wikipedia temporal information. In: Proceedings of the 2015 Conference on Empirical Methods in Natural Language Processing (EMNLP) (2015)
388. Tsagkias, M., de Rijke, M., Weerkamp, W.: Linking online news and social media. In: Proceedings of the Fourth ACM International Conference on Web Search and Data Mining, WSDM '11, pp. 565–574 (2011)
389. Tschiatschek, S., Iyer, R.K., Wei, H., Bilmes, J.A.: Learning mixtures of submodular functions for image collection summarization. In: Advances in Neural Information Processing Systems, pp. 1413–1421 (2014)
390. Tuan, T., Schwarz, S., Niederée, C., Maus, H., Kanhabua, N.: The forgotten needle in my collections: task-aware ranking of documents in semantic information space. In: Proceedings of the 1st ACM SIGIR Conference on Human Information Interaction and Retrieval (CHIIR-16), March 13–17, Chapel Hill, North Carolina, USA. ACM, ACM Press (2016)
391. Tulving, E.: Elements of Episodic Memory (1985)
392. Tulving, E.: Episodic memory: from mind to brain. Ann. Rev. Psychol. **53**(1), 1–25 (2002)
393. Tulving, E., Schacter, D.L., McLachlan, D.R., Moscovitch, M.: Priming of semantic autobiographical knowledge: a case study of retrograde amnesia. Brain Cognit. **8**(1), 3–20 (1988)
394. Tulving, E., et al.: Episodic and semantic memory. Organ. Mem. **1**, 381–403 (1972)
395. Tzelepis, C., Mavridaki, E., Mezaris, V., Patras, I.: Video aesthetic quality assessment using kernel support vector machine with isotropic gaussian sample uncertainty (KSVM-IGSU).

In: 2016 IEEE International Conference on Image Processing (ICIP), pp. 2410–2414. IEEE (2016)
396. Tzelepis, C., Mezaris, V., Patras, I.: Linear Maximum Margin Classifier for Learning from Uncertain Data (2015). arXiv:1504.03892
397. Tzelepis, C., Mezaris, V., Patras, I.: Video event detection using kernel support vector machine with isotropic Gaussian sample uncertainty (KSVM-IGSU). In: International Conference on Multimedia Modeling, pp. 3–15. Springer (2016)
398. Underwood, B.J.: Interference and forgetting. Psychol. Rev. **64**(1), 49 (1957)
399. Vaittinen, T., Kärkkäinen, T., Roimela, K.: Experience explorer: context-based browsing of personal media. In: Symposium on Human Interface, pp. 111–120. Springer (2011)
400. Van Der Meulen, M., Logie, R.H., Freer, Y., Sykes, C., McIntosh, N., Hunter, J.: When a graph is poorer than 100 words: a comparison of computerised natural language generation, human generated descriptions and graphical displays in neonatal intensive care. Appl. Cognit. Psychol. **24**(1), 77–89 (2010)
401. Van Opdenbosch, D., Steinbach, E.: AVLAD: Optimizing the VLAD image signature for specific feature descriptors. In: 2016 IEEE International Symposium on Multimedia (ISM), pp. 545–550. IEEE (2016)
402. Vargas, P.A., Fernaeus, Y., Lim, M.Y., Enz, S., Ho, W.C., Jacobsson, M., Ayllet, R.: Advocating an ethical memory model for artificial companions from a Human-centred perspective. AI Soc. **26**(4), 329–337 (2011)
403. Vargas, P.A., Freitas, A.A., Lim, M., Enz, S., Ho, W.C., Aylett, R.: Forgetting and generalisation in memory modelling for robot companions: a data mining approach. In: Proceedings of the Human Memory for Artificial Agents Symposium (AISB 2010), De Montfort University, Leicester, UK (2010)
404. Vennelakanti, R., Madhvanath, S., Subramanian, A., Sowndararajan, A., David, A., Dey, P.: Pixene: creating memories while sharing photos. In: Proceedings of the 14th ACM International Conference on Multimodal Interaction, pp. 59–60. ACM (2012)
405. Viola, P., Jones, M.J.: Robust real-time face detection. Int. J. Comput. Vis. (IJCV) **57** (2004)
406. Vliegendhart, R., Larson, M., Pouwelse, J.A.: Discovering user perceptions of semantic similarity in near-duplicate multimedia files. In: CrowdSearch, pp. 54–58. Citeseer (2012)
407. W3C: PROV-O: The PROV Ontology - Technical report (2013). http://www.w3.org/TR/prov-o/. Accessed Sep 2017
408. Walber, T., Scherp, A., Staab, S.: Smart photo selection: interpret gaze as personal interest. In: Proceedings of CHI '14 (2014)
409. Wang, J., Allebach, J.: Automatic assessment of online fashion shopping photo aesthetic quality. In: Proceedings of International Conference on Image Processing (ICIP), pp. 2915–2919. IEEE (2015)
410. Wang, L., Wang, H., Zhu, F.: Twin feature and similarity maximal matching for image retrieval. In: Proceedings of the 5th International Conference on Multimedia Retrieval, pp. 59–66. ACM (2015)
411. Wang, Y., Dai, Q., Feng, R., Jiang, Y.G.: Beauty is here: Evaluating aesthetics in videos using multimodal features and free training data. In: Proceedings of the 21st ACM International Conference on Multimedia, pp. 369–372. ACM (2013)
412. Wang, Y., Lin, Z., Shen, X., Mech, R., Miller, G., Cottrell, G.W.: Event-specific image importance. In: Proceedings of the IEEE Conference on Computer Vision and Pattern Recognition, pp. 4810–4819 (2016)
413. Weibel, S.: The dublin core: a simple content description model for electronic resources. Bull. Am. Soc. Inf. Sci. Technol. **24**(1), 9–11 (1997). https://doi.org/10.1002/bult.70.
414. Weiss, Y., Torralba, A., Fergus, R.: Spectral hashing. In: Advances in Neural Information Processing Systems, pp. 1753–1760 (2009)
415. Wheeler, M.A., Stuss, D.T., Tulving, E.: Toward a theory of episodic memory: the frontal lobes and autonoetic consciousness. Psychol. Bull. **121**(3), 331 (1997)
416. White, R.W., Bennett, P.N., Dumais, S.T.: Predicting short-term interests using activity-based search context. In: Proceedings of the 19th ACM International Conference on Information

and Knowledge Management, CIKM '10, pp. 1009–1018 (2010). https://doi.org/10.1145/1871437.1871565
417. Williams, H., Conway, M., Baddeley, A.: The boundaries of Episodic Memories, pp. 589–616. Oxford University Press, Oxford (2008)
418. Wolters, M.K., Niven, E., Logie, R.H.: The art of deleting snapshots. In: CHI'14 Extended Abstracts on Human Factors in Computing Systems, pp. 2521–2526. ACM (2014)
419. Wolters, M.K., Niven, E., Runardotter, M., Gallo, F., Maus, H., Logie, R.H.: Personal photo preservation for the smartphone generation. In: Proceedings of the 33rd Annual ACM Conference Extended Abstracts on Human Factors in Computing Systems, pp. 1549–1554. ACM (2015)
420. Wu, X., Hauptmann, A.G., Ngo, C.W.: Practical elimination of near-duplicates from web video search. In: Proceedings of the 15th International Conference on Multimedia, pp. 218–227. ACM (2007)
421. Xie, L., Hong, R., Zhang, B., Tian, Q.: Image classification and retrieval are one. In: Proceedings of the 5th International Conference on Multimedia Retrieval, pp. 3–10. ACM (2015)
422. Yan, L., Zou, F., Guo, R., Gao, L., Zhou, K., Wang, C.: Feature aggregating hashing for image copy detection. World Wide Web **19**(2), 217–229 (2016)
423. Yang, C.Y., Yeh, H.H., Chen, C.S.: Video aesthetic quality assessment by combining semantically independent and dependent features. In: Proceedings of International Conference on Acoustics, Speech and Signal Processing (ICASSP), pp. 1165–1168. IEEE (2011)
424. Yao, L., Suryanarayan, P., Qiao, M., Wang, J.Z., Li, J.: Oscar: on-site composition and aesthetics feedback through exemplars for photographers. Int. J. Comput. Vis. **96**(3), 353–383 (2012)
425. Yeh, C.H., Ho, Y.C., Barsky, B.A., Ouhyoung, M.: Personalized photograph ranking and selection system. In: Proceedings of the 18th ACM International Conference on Multimedia, MM '10, pp. 211–220. ACM (2010)
426. Yeh, H.H., Yang, C.Y., Lee, M.S., Chen, C.S.: Video aesthetic quality assessment by temporal integration of photo-and motion-based features. IEEE Trans. Multimed. **15**(8), 1944–1957 (2013)
427. Yilmaz, E., Kanoulas, E., Aslam, J.A.: A simple and efficient sampling method for estimating AP and NDCG. In: 31st ACM SIGIR International Conference on Research and Development in Information Retrieval, pp. 603–610. ACM, USA (2008)
428. Yosinski, J., Clune, J., Bengio, Y., Lipson, H.: How transferable are features in deep neural networks? In: CoRR (2014). arXiv:abs/1411.1792
429. Yu, H., Deng, Z.H., Yang, Y., Xiong, T.: A joint optimization model for image summarization based on image content and tags. In: Proceedings of the Twenty-Eighth AAAI Conference on Artificial Intelligence, AAAI'14, pp. 215–221. AAAI Press (2014)
430. Zacks, J.M., Speer, N.K., Swallow, K.M., Braver, T.S., Reynolds, J.R.: Event perception: a mind-brain perspective. Psychol. Bull. **133**(2), 273 (2007)
431. Zacks, J.M., Swallow, K.M.: Event segmentation. Current Direct. Psychol. Sci. **16**(2), 80–84 (2007)
432. Zagoruyko, S., Komodakis, N.: Learning to compare image patches via convolutional neural networks. In: Conference on Computer Vision and Pattern Recognition (CVPR). IEEE (2015)
433. Zhang, J., Marszalek, M., Lazebnik, S., Schmid, C.: Local features and kernels for classification of texture and object categories: a comprehensive study. Int. J. Comput. Vis. **73**(2), 213–238 (2007)
434. Zhang, W., Ji, J., Zhu, J., Li, J., Xu, H., Zhang, B.: BitHash: an efficient bitwise locality sensitive hashing method with applications. Knowl. Based Syst. **97**, 40–47 (2016)
435. Zhang, Y., Callan, J., Minka, T.: Novelty and redundancy detection in adaptive filtering. In: Proceedings of the 25th Annual International ACM SIGIR Conference on Research and Development in Information Retrieval, SIGIR '02, pp. 81–88 (2002)
436. Zhao, W.L., Tan, S., Ngo, C.W.: Large-scale near-duplicate web video search: challenge and opportunity. In: International Conference on Multimedia and Expo (ICME), pp. 1624–1627. IEEE (2009)

437. Zhao, Y., Hong, R., Jiang, J.: Visual summarization of image collections by fast ransac. Neurocomputing **172**, 48–52 (2016)
438. Zhou, J., Chen, J., Ye, J.: Clustered multi-task learning via alternating structure optimization. In: Advances in Neural Information Processing Systems (NIPS 2011) (2011)
439. Zhou, W., Li, H., Lu, Y., Tian, Q.: Sift match verification by geometric coding for large-scale partial-duplicate web image search. Trans. Multimed. Comput. Commun. Appl. (TOMM) **9**(1), 4 (2013)
440. Zhou, W., Li, H., Lu, Y., Tian, Q.: SIFT match verification by geometric coding for large-scale partial-duplicate web image search. Trans. Multimed. Comput. Commun. Appl. (TOMM) **9**(1), 4 (2013)

Index

V. Mezaris et al. (eds.), *Personal Multimedia Preservation*, Springer Series on Cultural Computing, https://doi.org/10.1007/978-3-319-73465-1

MIX
Papier aus verantwortungsvollen Quellen
Paper from responsible sources
FSC® C105338

FSC
www.fsc.org

If you have any concerns about our products,
you can contact us on
ProductSafety@springernature.com

In case Publisher is established outside the EU,
the EU authorized representative is:
Springer Nature Customer Service Center GmbH
Europaplatz 3, 69115 Heidelberg, Germany

Printed by Libri Plureos GmbH
in Hamburg, Germany